WORLD HEALTH ORGANIZATION
INTERNATIONAL AGENCY FOR RESEARCH ON CANCER

IARC Monographs on the Evaluation of Carcinogenic Risks to Humans

VOLUME 88

Formaldehyde, 2-Butoxyethanol and 1-*tert*-Butoxypropan-2-ol

This publication represents the views and expert opinions
of an IARC Working Group on the
Evaluation of Carcinogenic Risks to Humans,
which met in Lyon,

2–9 June 2004

2006

IARC MONOGRAPHS

In 1969, the International Agency for Research on Cancer (IARC) initiated a programme on the evaluation of the carcinogenic risk of chemicals to humans involving the production of critically evaluated monographs on individual chemicals. The programme was subsequently expanded to include evaluations of carcinogenic risks associated with exposures to complex mixtures, life-style factors and biological and physical agents, as well as those in specific occupations.

The objective of the programme is to elaborate and publish in the form of monographs critical reviews of data on carcinogenicity for agents to which humans are known to be exposed and on specific exposure situations; to evaluate these data in terms of human risk with the help of international working groups of experts in chemical carcinogenesis and related fields; and to indicate where additional research efforts are needed.

The lists of IARC evaluations are regularly updated and are available on Internet: http://monographs. iarc.fr/

This programme has been supported by Cooperative Agreement 5 UO1 CA33193 awarded since 1982 by the United States National Cancer Institute, Department of Health and Human Services. Additional support has been provided since 1986 by the European Commission, Directorate-General EMPL (Employment, and Social Affairs), Health, Safety and Hygiene at Work Unit, and since 1992 by the United States National Institute of Environmental Health Sciences.

This publication was made possible, in part, by a Cooperative Agreement between the United States Environmental Protection Agency, Office of Research and Development (USEPA-ORD) and the International Agency for Research on Cancer (IARC) and does not necessarily express the views of USEPA-ORD.

Published by the International Agency for Research on Cancer,
150 cours Albert Thomas, 69372 Lyon Cedex 08, France
©International Agency for Research on Cancer, 2006

Distributed by WHO Press, World Health Organization, 20 Avenue Appia, 1211 Geneva 27, Switzerland
(tel.: +41 22 791 3264; fax: +41 22 791 4857; e-mail: bookorders@who.int).

IARC Library Cataloguing in Publication Data

Formaldehyde, 2-Butoxyethanol and 1-*tert*-Butoxypropan-2-ol/
IARC Working Group on the Evaluation of Carcinogenic Risks to Humans (2004 : Lyon, France)

(IARC monographs on the evaluation of carcinogenic risks to humans ; v. 88)

1. Carcinogens, Environmental – toxicity   2. Ethylene Glycols – toxicity
3. Formaldehyde – toxicity   4. Propylene Glycols – toxicity
I. IARC Working Group on the Evaluation of Carcinogenic Risks to Humans   II. Series

ISBN 92 832 1288 6   (NLM Classification: W1)
ISSN 1017-1606

PRINTED IN FRANCE

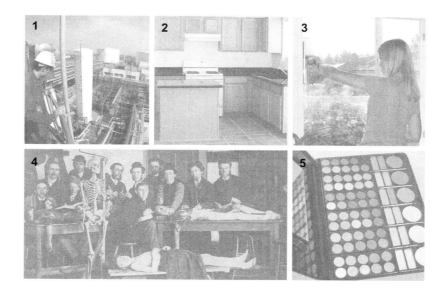

1   Formaldehyde and 2-butoxyethanol are intermediates used in the chemical industry.

2   Formaldehyde-based resins are used in the manufacture of plywood, particleboard, furniture, cabinets and other composite wood products.

3   The general population can be exposed to 2-butoxyethanol and 1-*tert*-butoxypropan-2-ol by inhalation or skin contact with cleaning products containing these glycol ethers.

4   Embalmers, pathologists and anatomists are exposed to formaldehyde, a preservative and embalming agent.

5   Formaldehyde is also present as an antimicrobial agent in many cosmetic products.

Cover design: Georges Mollon, IARC

CONTENTS

NOTE TO THE READER

The term 'carcinogenic risk' in the *IARC Monographs* series is taken to mean that an agent is capable of causing cancer under some circumstances. The *Monographs* evaluate cancer hazards, despite the historical presence of the word 'risks' in the title.

Inclusion of an agent in the *Monographs* does not imply that it is a carcinogen, only that the published data have been examined. Equally, the fact that an agent has not yet been evaluated in a monograph does not mean that it is not carcinogenic.

The evaluations of carcinogenic risk are made by international working groups of independent scientists and are qualitative in nature. No recommendation is given for regulation or legislation.

Anyone who is aware of published data that may alter the evaluation of the carcinogenic risk of an agent to humans is encouraged to make this information available to the Carcinogen Identification and Evaluation Group, International Agency for Research on Cancer, 150 cours Albert Thomas, 69372 Lyon Cedex 08, France, in order that the agent may be considered for re-evaluation by a future Working Group.

Although every effort is made to prepare the monographs as accurately as possible, mistakes may occur. Readers are requested to communicate any errors to the Carcinogen Identification and Evaluation Group, so that corrections can be reported in future volumes.

IARC WORKING GROUP ON THE EVALUATION OF CARCINOGENIC RISKS TO HUMANS: FORMALDEHYDE, 2-BUTOXYETHANOL AND 1-*tert*-BUTOXYPROPAN-2-OL

Lyon, 2–9 June 2004

LIST OF PARTICIPANTS

Members

Ulrich Andrae, GSF-Forschungszentrum für Umwelt und Gesundheit, Institut für Toxikologie, Ingolstädter Landstrasse 1, 85764 Neuherberg, Germany

Sherwood Burge, Occupational Lung Disease Unit, Birmingham Heartlands Hospital, Bordesley Green East, Birmingham B9 5SS, United Kingdom

Rajendra S. Chhabra, National Toxicology Program, National Institute of Environmental Health Sciences, 111 Alexander Drive, PO Box 12233, Research Triangle Park, NC 27709, USA

John Cocker, Head, Biological Monitoring, Health and Safety Laboratory, Broad Lane, Sheffield 3 7HQ, United Kingdom

David Coggon, Medical Research Council, Environmental Epidemiology Unit, University of Southampton, Southampton General Hospital, Southampton SO16 6YD, United Kingdom

Paul A. Demers, School of Occupational and Environmental Hygiene, Centre for Health and Environment Research, University of British Columbia, 2206 E. Mall, Vancouver, BC V6T 1Z3, Canada (*Subgroup Chair; Exposure Data*)

Elaine M. Faustman, Institute for Risk Analysis and Risk Communication, Department of Environmental and Occupational Health Sciences, University of Washington, 4225 Roosevelt Way NE, Suite 100, Seattle, WA 98105-6099, USA

Victor Feron, TNO Nutrition and Food Research, Utrechtseweg 48, 3704 HE Zeist, The Netherlands

Michel Gérin, Département de Santé environnementale et Santé au Travail, Faculté de Médecine, Université de Montréal, Pavillon Marguerite d'Youville, bureau 4095, 2375 chemin de la côte Sainte-Catherine, Montréal, Québec H3T1A8, Canada (*Overall Chair*)

Marcel Goldberg, Director, INSERM Unité 88, Epidemiology, Public Health and Occupational and General Environment, Hôpital National de Saint-Maurice, 14, rue du Val d'Osne, 94415 Saint-Maurice Cédex, France

Bernard D. Goldstein, A625 Crabtree Hall, Graduate School of Public Health, University of Pittsburgh, 130 DeSoto Street, Pittsburgh, PA 15261, USA

Roland Grafström, Experimental Carcinogenesis Group, Institute of Environmental Medicine, Nobelsv 13, Karolinska Institutet, 171 77 Stockholm, Sweden

Johnni Hansen, Danish Cancer Society, Institute of Cancer Epidemiology, Strandboulevarden 49, 2100 Copenhagen O, Denmark

Michael Hauptmann, Division of Cancer Epidemiology and Genetics, National Cancer Institute, Department of Health & Human Sciences, 6120 Executive Boulevard, Bethesda, MD 20892-7244, USA

Kathy Hughes, Health Canada, Room 209, Environmental Health Centre, Tunney's Pasture, Address Locator 0802B1, Ottawa, Ontario K1A 0L2, Canada

Daniel Krewski, McLaughlin Centre for Population Health Risk Assessment, University of Ottawa, Institute of Population Health, Room 320, One Stewart Street, Ottawa, Ontario K1N 6N5, Canada

Martine Reynier, Chemical and Biological Risks Department, Institut National de Recherche et de Sécurité, 30 rue Olivier Noyer, 75680 Paris Cedex 14, France

Judith Shaham, Occupational Cancer Department, National Institute of Occupational and Environmental Health, Loewenstein Hospital, 278 Ahuza Street, POB 3, Raanana 43100, Israel

Morando Soffritti, Cancer Research Centre, Ramazzini Foundation, Via Saliceto 3, 40010 Bentivoglio, Italy (*Subgroup Chair; Cancer in Experimental Animals*)

Leslie Stayner, Director of Epidemiology and Biostatistics, Division of Epidemiology and Biostatistics, UIC School of Public Health (M/C 923), 1603 West Taylor Street, Room 971, Chicago, IL 60612, USA (*Subgroup Chair; Cancer in Humans*)

Douglas Wolf, Environmental Carcinogenesis Division, US Environmental Protection Agency, 109 TW Alexander Drive, Research Triangle Park, NC 27711, USA (*Subgroup Chair; Other Relevant Data*)

Invited Specialists

Rory Conolly, CIIT Centers for Health Research, 6 Davis Drive, Research Triangle Park, NC 27709, USA

David Eastmond, Environmental Toxicology Graduate Program, University of California, 5429 Alfred M. Boyce Hall, Riverside, CA 92521-0314, USA

Ted Junghans, Technical Resources International Inc., 6500 Rock Spring Drive, Suite 650, Bethesda, MD 20817-1197, USA

Steve Olin, ILSI Risk Science Institute, One Thomas Circle, NW, 9th Floor, Washington DC 20005-5802, USA

Patricia Stewart, Division of Cancer Epidemiology and Genetics, National Cancer Institute, National Institutes of Health, Executive Plaza South 8118, 6120 Executive Blvd MSC 7240, Bethesda, MD 20892-7240, USA (*unable to attend*)

Representatives
US National Cancer Institute
David G. Longfellow, Cancer Etiology Branch, Division of Cancer Biology, National Cancer Institute, 6130 Executive Blvd, Suite 5000, MSC7398, Rockville, MD 20892-7398, USA

US Environmental Protection Agency
Jennifer Jinot, National Center for Environmental Assessment (8623-D), US Environmental Protection Agency, 808 17th St. NW, Washington DC 20006, USA
Peter W. Preuss, National Center for Environmental Assessment (8601-D), US Environmental Protection Agency, 808 17th Street NW, Suite 400, Washington DC 20074, USA

Australian National Industrial Chemical and Notification Assessment Scheme (NICNAS)
Paul D. Harvey, National Industrial Chemical and Notification Assessment Scheme, 334-336 Illawarra Road, Marrickville, NSW 2204, GPO Box 58, Sydney, NSW 2001, Australia

Observers
American Chemistry Council and European Chemical Industry Council
James J. Collins, The Dow Chemical Company, Epidemiology, 1803 Building, Midland, MI 48674, USA

European Center for Ecotoxicology and Toxicology of Chemicals
Heinz-Peter Gelbke, Consultant in Toxicology, Dr Kausch Strasse 6a, 67251 Freinsheim, Germany

Formaldehyde Council Inc.
James Swenberg, Center for Environmental Health and Susceptibility, School of Public Health, University of North Carolina at Chapel Hill, 253-C Rosenau Hall, Box 7431, South Columbia Street, Chapel Hill, NC 27599, USA

International Federation of Building and Wood Workers
Lars Vedsmand, BAT-Kartellet, Kampmannsgade 4, 1790 Copenhagen V, Denmark

IARC Secretariat
Robert A. Baan, Carcinogen Identification and Evaluation (*Co-Rapporteur; Subgroup on Other Relevant Data*)

Vincent James Cogliano, Carcinogen Identification and Evaluation (*Head of Programme*)

Fatiha El Ghissassi, Carcinogen Identification and Evaluation (*Co-Rapporteur; Subgroup on Other Relevant Data*)

Tony Fletcher, Environmental Cancer Epidemiology

Marlin Friesen, Nutrition and Cancer

Yann Grosse, Carcinogen Identification and Evaluation (*Responsible Officer; Rapporteur; Subgroup on Cancer in Experimental Animals*)

Jane Mitchell, Carcinogen Identification and Evaluation (*Editor*)

Nikolai Napalkov, Carcinogen Identification and Evaluation

Tomohiro Sawa

Béatrice Secretan, Carcinogen Identification and Evaluation (*Rapporteur; Subgroup on Exposure Data*)

Kurt Straif, Carcinogen Identification and Evaluation (*Rapporteur; Subgroup on Cancer in Humans*)

Administrative assistance

Sandrine Egraz, Carcinogen Identification and Evaluation

Michel Javin, Administrative Services

Martine Lézère, Carcinogen Identification and Evaluation

Georges Mollon, Communications

Elspeth Perez, Carcinogen Identification and Evaluation

PREAMBLE

IARC MONOGRAPHS PROGRAMME ON THE EVALUATION OF CARCINOGENIC RISKS TO HUMANS

PREAMBLE

1. BACKGROUND

In 1969, the International Agency for Research on Cancer (IARC) initiated a programme to evaluate the carcinogenic risk of chemicals to humans and to produce monographs on individual chemicals. The *Monographs* programme has since been expanded to include consideration of exposures to complex mixtures of chemicals (which occur, for example, in some occupations and as a result of human habits) and of exposures to other agents, such as radiation and viruses. With Supplement 6 (IARC, 1987a), the title of the series was modified from *IARC Monographs on the Evaluation of the Carcinogenic Risk of Chemicals to Humans* to *IARC Monographs on the Evaluation of Carcinogenic Risks to Humans*, in order to reflect the widened scope of the programme.

The criteria established in 1971 to evaluate carcinogenic risk to humans were adopted by the working groups whose deliberations resulted in the first 16 volumes of the *IARC Monographs series*. Those criteria were subsequently updated by further ad-hoc working groups (IARC, 1977, 1978, 1979, 1982, 1983, 1987b, 1988, 1991a; Vainio *et al.*, 1992).

2. OBJECTIVE AND SCOPE

The objective of the programme is to prepare, with the help of international working groups of experts, and to publish in the form of monographs, critical reviews and evaluations of evidence on the carcinogenicity of a wide range of human exposures. The *Monographs* may also indicate where additional research efforts are needed.

The *Monographs* represent the first step in carcinogenic risk assessment, which involves examination of all relevant information in order to assess the strength of the available evidence that certain exposures could alter the incidence of cancer in humans. The second step is quantitative risk estimation. Detailed, quantitative evaluations of epidemiological data may be made in the *Monographs*, but without extrapolation beyond the range of the data available. Quantitative extrapolation from experimental data to the human situation is not undertaken.

The term 'carcinogen' is used in these monographs to denote an exposure that is capable of increasing the incidence of malignant neoplasms; the induction of benign neoplasms may in some circumstances (see p. 19) contribute to the judgement that the exposure is carcinogenic. The terms 'neoplasm' and 'tumour' are used interchangeably.

Some epidemiological and experimental studies indicate that different agents may act at different stages in the carcinogenic process, and several mechanisms may be involved. The aim of the *Monographs* has been, from their inception, to evaluate evidence of carcinogenicity at any stage in the carcinogenesis process, independently of the underlying mechanisms. Information on mechanisms may, however, be used in making the overall evaluation (IARC, 1991a; Vainio *et al.*, 1992; see also pp. 25–27).

The *Monographs* may assist national and international authorities in making risk assessments and in formulating decisions concerning any necessary preventive measures. The evaluations of IARC working groups are scientific, qualitative judgements about the evidence for or against carcinogenicity provided by the available data. These evaluations represent only one part of the body of information on which regulatory measures may be based. Other components of regulatory decisions vary from one situation to another and from country to country, responding to different socioeconomic and national priorities. **Therefore, no recommendation is given with regard to regulation or legislation, which are the responsibility of individual governments and/or other international organizations.**

The *IARC Monographs* are recognized as an authoritative source of information on the carcinogenicity of a wide range of human exposures. A survey of users in 1988 indicated that the *Monographs* are consulted by various agencies in 57 countries. About 2500 copies of each volume are printed, for distribution to governments, regulatory bodies and interested scientists. The Monographs are also available from IARC*Press* in Lyon and via the Marketing and Dissemination (MDI) of the World Health Organization in Geneva.

3.   SELECTION OF TOPICS FOR MONOGRAPHS

Topics are selected on the basis of two main criteria: (a) there is evidence of human exposure, and (b) there is some evidence or suspicion of carcinogenicity. The term 'agent' is used to include individual chemical compounds, groups of related chemical compounds, physical agents (such as radiation) and biological factors (such as viruses). Exposures to mixtures of agents may occur in occupational exposures and as a result of personal and cultural habits (like smoking and dietary practices). Chemical analogues and compounds with biological or physical characteristics similar to those of suspected carcinogens may also be considered, even in the absence of data on a possible carcinogenic effect in humans or experimental animals.

The scientific literature is surveyed for published data relevant to an assessment of carcinogenicity. The IARC information bulletins on agents being tested for carcinogenicity (IARC, 1973–1996) and directories of on-going research in cancer epidemiology (IARC, 1976–1996) often indicate exposures that may be scheduled for future meetings. Ad-hoc working groups convened by IARC in 1984, 1989, 1991, 1993 and

1998 gave recommendations as to which agents should be evaluated in the IARC Monographs series (IARC, 1984, 1989, 1991b, 1993, 1998a,b).

As significant new data on subjects on which monographs have already been prepared become available, re-evaluations are made at subsequent meetings, and revised monographs are published.

4. DATA FOR MONOGRAPHS

The *Monographs* do not necessarily cite all the literature concerning the subject of an evaluation. Only those data considered by the Working Group to be relevant to making the evaluation are included.

With regard to biological and epidemiological data, only reports that have been published or accepted for publication in the openly available scientific literature are reviewed by the working groups. In certain instances, government agency reports that have undergone peer review and are widely available are considered. Exceptions may be made on an ad-hoc basis to include unpublished reports that are in their final form and publicly available, if their inclusion is considered pertinent to making a final evaluation (see pp. 25–27). In the sections on chemical and physical properties, on analysis, on production and use and on occurrence, unpublished sources of information may be used.

5. THE WORKING GROUP

Reviews and evaluations are formulated by a working group of experts. The tasks of the group are: (i) to ascertain that all appropriate data have been collected; (ii) to select the data relevant for the evaluation on the basis of scientific merit; (iii) to prepare accurate summaries of the data to enable the reader to follow the reasoning of the Working Group; (iv) to evaluate the results of epidemiological and experimental studies on cancer; (v) to evaluate data relevant to the understanding of mechanism of action; and (vi) to make an overall evaluation of the carcinogenicity of the exposure to humans.

Working Group participants who contributed to the considerations and evaluations within a particular volume are listed, with their addresses, at the beginning of each publication. Each participant who is a member of a working group serves as an individual scientist and not as a representative of any organization, government or industry. In addition, nominees of national and international agencies and industrial associations may be invited as observers.

6. WORKING PROCEDURES

Approximately one year in advance of a meeting of a working group, the topics of the monographs are announced and participants are selected by IARC staff in consultation with other experts. Subsequently, relevant biological and epidemiological data are collected by the Carcinogen Identification and Evaluation Unit of IARC from recognized sources of information on carcinogenesis, including data storage and retrieval systems such as MEDLINE and TOXLINE.

For chemicals and some complex mixtures, the major collection of data and the preparation of first drafts of the sections on chemical and physical properties, on analysis, on production and use and on occurrence are carried out under a separate contract funded by the United States National Cancer Institute. Representatives from industrial associations may assist in the preparation of sections on production and use. Information on production and trade is obtained from governmental and trade publications and, in some cases, by direct contact with industries. Separate production data on some agents may not be available because their publication could disclose confidential information. Information on uses may be obtained from published sources but is often complemented by direct contact with manufacturers. Efforts are made to supplement this information with data from other national and international sources.

Six months before the meeting, the material obtained is sent to meeting participants, or is used by IARC staff, to prepare sections for the first drafts of monographs. The first drafts are compiled by IARC staff and sent before the meeting to all participants of the Working Group for review.

The Working Group meets in Lyon for seven to eight days to discuss and finalize the texts of the monographs and to formulate the evaluations. After the meeting, the master copy of each monograph is verified by consulting the original literature, edited and prepared for publication. The aim is to publish monographs within six months of the Working Group meeting.

The available studies are summarized by the Working Group, with particular regard to the qualitative aspects discussed below. In general, numerical findings are indicated as they appear in the original report; units are converted when necessary for easier comparison. The Working Group may conduct additional analyses of the published data and use them in their assessment of the evidence; the results of such supplementary analyses are given in square brackets. When an important aspect of a study, directly impinging on its interpretation, should be brought to the attention of the reader, a comment is given in square brackets.

7.   EXPOSURE DATA

Sections that indicate the extent of past and present human exposure, the sources of exposure, the people most likely to be exposed and the factors that contribute to the exposure are included at the beginning of each monograph.

Most monographs on individual chemicals, groups of chemicals or complex mixtures include sections on chemical and physical data, on analysis, on production and use and on occurrence. In monographs on, for example, physical agents, occupational exposures and cultural habits, other sections may be included, such as: historical perspectives, description of an industry or habit, chemistry of the complex mixture or taxonomy. Monographs on biological agents have sections on structure and biology, methods of detection, epidemiology of infection and clinical disease other than cancer.

For chemical exposures, the Chemical Abstracts Services Registry Number, the latest Chemical Abstracts primary name and the IUPAC systematic name are recorded; other synonyms are given, but the list is not necessarily comprehensive. For biological agents, taxonomy and structure are described, and the degree of variability is given, when applicable.

Information on chemical and physical properties and, in particular, data relevant to identification, occurrence and biological activity are included. For biological agents, mode of replication, life cycle, target cells, persistence and latency and host response are given. A description of technical products of chemicals includes trade names, relevant specifications and available information on composition and impurities. Some of the trade names given may be those of mixtures in which the agent being evaluated is only one of the ingredients.

The purpose of the section on analysis or detection is to give the reader an overview of current methods, with emphasis on those widely used for regulatory purposes. Methods for monitoring human exposure are also given, when available. No critical evaluation or recommendation of any of the methods is meant or implied. The IARC published a series of volumes, *Environmental Carcinogens: Methods of Analysis and Exposure Measurement* (IARC, 1978–93), that describe validated methods for analysing a wide variety of chemicals and mixtures. For biological agents, methods of detection and exposure assessment are described, including their sensitivity, specificity and reproducibility.

The dates of first synthesis and of first commercial production of a chemical or mixture are provided; for agents which do not occur naturally, this information may allow a reasonable estimate to be made of the date before which no human exposure to the agent could have occurred. The dates of first reported occurrence of an exposure are also provided. In addition, methods of synthesis used in past and present commercial production and different methods of production which may give rise to different impurities are described.

Data on production, international trade and uses are obtained for representative regions, which usually include Europe, Japan and the United States of America. It should not, however, be inferred that those areas or nations are necessarily the sole or major sources or users of the agent. Some identified uses may not be current or major applications, and the coverage is not necessarily comprehensive. In the case of drugs, mention of their therapeutic uses does not necessarily represent current practice, nor does it imply judgement as to their therapeutic efficacy.

Information on the occurrence of an agent or mixture in the environment is obtained from data derived from the monitoring and surveillance of levels in occupational environments, air, water, soil, foods and animal and human tissues. When available, data on the generation, persistence and bioaccumulation of the agent are also included. In the case of mixtures, industries, occupations or processes, information is given about all agents present. For processes, industries and occupations, a historical description is also given, noting variations in chemical composition, physical properties and levels of occupational exposure with time and place. For biological agents, the epidemiology of infection is described.

Statements concerning regulations and guidelines (e.g., pesticide registrations, maximal levels permitted in foods, occupational exposure limits) are included for some countries as indications of potential exposures, but they may not reflect the most recent situation, since such limits are continuously reviewed and modified. The absence of information on regulatory status for a country should not be taken to imply that that country does not have regulations with regard to the exposure. For biological agents, legislation and control, including vaccines and therapy, are described.

8.   STUDIES OF CANCER IN HUMANS

(a)   Types of studies considered

Three types of epidemiological studies of cancer contribute to the assessment of carcinogenicity in humans — cohort studies, case–control studies and correlation (or ecological) studies. Rarely, results from randomized trials may be available. Case series and case reports of cancer in humans may also be reviewed.

Cohort and case–control studies relate the exposures under study to the occurrence of cancer in individuals and provide an estimate of relative risk (ratio of incidence or mortality in those exposed to incidence or mortality in those not exposed) as the main measure of association.

In correlation studies, the units of investigation are usually whole populations (e.g. in particular geographical areas or at particular times), and cancer frequency is related to a summary measure of the exposure of the population to the agent, mixture or exposure circumstance under study. Because individual exposure is not documented, however, a causal relationship is less easy to infer from correlation studies than from cohort and case–control studies. Case reports generally arise from a suspicion, based on clinical experience, that the concurrence of two events — that is, a particular exposure and occurrence of a cancer — has happened rather more frequently than would be expected by chance. Case reports usually lack complete ascertainment of cases in any population, definition or enumeration of the population at risk and estimation of the expected number of cases in the absence of exposure. The uncertainties surrounding interpretation of case reports and correlation studies make them inadequate, except in rare instances, to form the sole basis for inferring a causal relationship. When taken together with case–control and cohort studies, however, relevant case reports or correlation studies may add materially to the judgement that a causal relationship is present.

Epidemiological studies of benign neoplasms, presumed preneoplastic lesions and other end-points thought to be relevant to cancer are also reviewed by working groups. They may, in some instances, strengthen inferences drawn from studies of cancer itself.

(*b*)   *Quality of studies considered*

The Monographs are not intended to summarize all published studies. Those that are judged to be inadequate or irrelevant to the evaluation are generally omitted. They may be mentioned briefly, particularly when the information is considered to be a useful supplement to that in other reports or when they provide the only data available. Their inclusion does not imply acceptance of the adequacy of the study design or of the analysis and interpretation of the results, and limitations are clearly outlined in square brackets at the end of the study description.

It is necessary to take into account the possible roles of bias, confounding and chance in the interpretation of epidemiological studies. By 'bias' is meant the operation of factors in study design or execution that lead erroneously to a stronger or weaker association than in fact exists between disease and an agent, mixture or exposure circumstance. By 'confounding' is meant a situation in which the relationship with disease is made to appear stronger or weaker than it truly is as a result of an association between the apparent causal factor and another factor that is associated with either an increase or decrease in the incidence of the disease. In evaluating the extent to which these factors have been minimized in an individual study, working groups consider a number of aspects of design and analysis as described in the report of the study. Most of these considerations apply equally to case–control, cohort and correlation studies. Lack of clarity of any of these aspects in the reporting of a study can decrease its credibility and the weight given to it in the final evaluation of the exposure.

Firstly, the study population, disease (or diseases) and exposure should have been well defined by the authors. Cases of disease in the study population should have been identified in a way that was independent of the exposure of interest, and exposure should have been assessed in a way that was not related to disease status.

Secondly, the authors should have taken account in the study design and analysis of other variables that can influence the risk of disease and may have been related to the exposure of interest. Potential confounding by such variables should have been dealt with either in the design of the study, such as by matching, or in the analysis, by statistical adjustment. In cohort studies, comparisons with local rates of disease may be more appropriate than those with national rates. Internal comparisons of disease frequency among individuals at different levels of exposure should also have been made in the study.

Thirdly, the authors should have reported the basic data on which the conclusions are founded, even if sophisticated statistical analyses were employed. At the very least, they should have given the numbers of exposed and unexposed cases and controls in a case–control study and the numbers of cases observed and expected in a cohort study. Further tabulations by time since exposure began and other temporal factors are also important. In a cohort study, data on all cancer sites and all causes of death should have been given, to reveal the possibility of reporting bias. In a case–control study, the effects of investigated factors other than the exposure of interest should have been reported.

Finally, the statistical methods used to obtain estimates of relative risk, absolute rates of cancer, confidence intervals and significance tests, and to adjust for confounding should have been clearly stated by the authors. The methods used should preferably have been the generally accepted techniques that have been refined since the mid-1970s. These methods have been reviewed for case–control studies (Breslow & Day, 1980) and for cohort studies (Breslow & Day, 1987).

(c)   Inferences about mechanism of action

Detailed analyses of both relative and absolute risks in relation to temporal variables, such as age at first exposure, time since first exposure, duration of exposure, cumulative exposure and time since exposure ceased, are reviewed and summarized when available. The analysis of temporal relationships can be useful in formulating models of carcino-genesis. In particular, such analyses may suggest whether a carcinogen acts early or late in the process of carcinogenesis, although at best they allow only indirect inferences about the mechanism of action. Special attention is given to measurements of biological markers of carcinogen exposure or action, such as DNA or protein adducts, as well as markers of early steps in the carcinogenic process, such as proto-oncogene mutation, when these are incorporated into epidemiological studies focused on cancer incidence or mortality. Such measurements may allow inferences to be made about putative mecha-nisms of action (IARC, 1991a; Vainio et al., 1992).

(d)   Criteria for causality

After the individual epidemiological studies of cancer have been summarized and the quality assessed, a judgement is made concerning the strength of evidence that the agent, mixture or exposure circumstance in question is carcinogenic for humans. In making its judgement, the Working Group considers several criteria for causality. A strong asso-ciation (a large relative risk) is more likely to indicate causality than a weak association, although it is recognized that relative risks of small magnitude do not imply lack of causality and may be important if the disease is common. Associations that are replicated in several studies of the same design or using different epidemiological approaches or under different circumstances of exposure are more likely to represent a causal relation-ship than isolated observations from single studies. If there are inconsistent results among investigations, possible reasons are sought (such as differences in amount of exposure), and results of studies judged to be of high quality are given more weight than those of studies judged to be methodologically less sound. When suspicion of carcino-genicity arises largely from a single study, these data are not combined with those from later studies in any subsequent reassessment of the strength of the evidence.

If the risk of the disease in question increases with the amount of exposure, this is considered to be a strong indication of causality, although absence of a graded response is not necessarily evidence against a causal relationship. Demonstration of a decline in risk after cessation of or reduction in exposure in individuals or in whole populations also supports a causal interpretation of the findings.

Although a carcinogen may act upon more than one target, the specificity of an association (an increased occurrence of cancer at one anatomical site or of one morphological type) adds plausibility to a causal relationship, particularly when excess cancer occurrence is limited to one morphological type within the same organ.

Although rarely available, results from randomized trials showing different rates among exposed and unexposed individuals provide particularly strong evidence for causality.

When several epidemiological studies show little or no indication of an association between an exposure and cancer, the judgement may be made that, in the aggregate, they show evidence of lack of carcinogenicity. Such a judgement requires first of all that the studies giving rise to it meet, to a sufficient degree, the standards of design and analysis described above. Specifically, the possibility that bias, confounding or misclassification of exposure or outcome could explain the observed results should be considered and excluded with reasonable certainty. In addition, all studies that are judged to be methodologically sound should be consistent with a relative risk of unity for any observed level of exposure and, when considered together, should provide a pooled estimate of relative risk which is at or near unity and has a narrow confidence interval, due to sufficient population size. Moreover, no individual study nor the pooled results of all the studies should show any consistent tendency for the relative risk of cancer to increase with increasing level of exposure. It is important to note that evidence of lack of carcinogenicity obtained in this way from several epidemiological studies can apply only to the type(s) of cancer studied and to dose levels and intervals between first exposure and observation of disease that are the same as or less than those observed in all the studies. Experience with human cancer indicates that, in some cases, the period from first exposure to the development of clinical cancer is seldom less than 20 years; studies with latent periods substantially shorter than 30 years cannot provide evidence for lack of carcinogenicity.

9.   STUDIES OF CANCER IN EXPERIMENTAL ANIMALS

All known human carcinogens that have been studied adequately in experimental animals have produced positive results in one or more animal species (Wilbourn *et al.*, 1986; Tomatis *et al.*, 1989). For several agents (aflatoxins, 4-aminobiphenyl, azathioprine, betel quid with tobacco, bischloromethyl ether and chloromethyl methyl ether (technical grade), chlorambucil, chlornaphazine, ciclosporin, coal-tar pitches, coal-tars, combined oral contraceptives, cyclophosphamide, diethylstilboestrol, melphalan, 8-methoxypsoralen plus ultraviolet A radiation, mustard gas, myleran, 2-naphthylamine, nonsteroidal estrogens, estrogen replacement therapy/steroidal estrogens, solar radiation, thiotepa and vinyl chloride), carcinogenicity in experimental animals was established or highly suspected before epidemiological studies confirmed their carcinogenicity in humans (Vainio *et al.*, 1995). Although this association cannot establish that all agents and mixtures that cause cancer in experimental animals also cause cancer in humans, nevertheless, **in the absence of adequate data on humans, it is biologically plausible and prudent to regard agents and mixtures for which there is *sufficient evidence* (see p. 24) of carcinogenicity in experimental animals as if they presented a carcinogenic risk to humans**. The possibility that a given agent may cause cancer through a species-specific mechanism which does not operate in humans (see p. 27) should also be taken into consideration.

The nature and extent of impurities or contaminants present in the chemical or mixture being evaluated are given when available. Animal strain, sex, numbers per group, age at start of treatment and survival are reported.

Other types of studies summarized include: experiments in which the agent or mixture was administered in conjunction with known carcinogens or factors that modify carcinogenic effects; studies in which the end-point was not cancer but a defined precancerous lesion; and experiments on the carcinogenicity of known metabolites and derivatives.

For experimental studies of mixtures, consideration is given to the possibility of changes in the physicochemical properties of the test substance during collection, storage, extraction, concentration and delivery. Chemical and toxicological interactions of the components of mixtures may result in nonlinear dose–response relationships.

An assessment is made as to the relevance to human exposure of samples tested in experimental animals, which may involve consideration of: (i) physical and chemical characteristics, (ii) constituent substances that indicate the presence of a class of substances, (iii) the results of tests for genetic and related effects, including studies on DNA adduct formation, proto-oncogene mutation and expression and suppressor gene inactivation. The relevance of results obtained, for example, with animal viruses analogous to the virus being evaluated in the monograph must also be considered. They may provide biological and mechanistic information relevant to the understanding of the process of carcinogenesis in humans and may strengthen the plausibility of a conclusion that the biological agent under evaluation is carcinogenic in humans.

(a)   Qualitative aspects

An assessment of carcinogenicity involves several considerations of qualitative importance, including (i) the experimental conditions under which the test was per-formed, including route and schedule of exposure, species, strain, sex, age, duration of follow-up; (ii) the consistency of the results, for example, across species and target organ(s); (iii) the spectrum of neoplastic response, from preneoplastic lesions and benign tumours to malignant neoplasms; and (iv) the possible role of modifying factors.

As mentioned earlier (p. 11), the *Monographs* are not intended to summarize all published studies. Those studies in experimental animals that are inadequate (e.g., too short a duration, too few animals, poor survival; see below) or are judged irrelevant to the evaluation are generally omitted. Guidelines for conducting adequate long-term carcinogenicity experiments have been outlined (e.g. Montesano *et al.*, 1986).

Considerations of importance to the Working Group in the interpretation and evaluation of a particular study include: (i) how clearly the agent was defined and, in the case of mixtures, how adequately the sample characterization was reported; (ii) whether the dose was adequately monitored, particularly in inhalation experiments; (iii) whether the doses and duration of treatment were appropriate and whether the survival of treated animals was similar to that of controls; (iv) whether there were adequate numbers of animals per group; (v) whether animals of each sex were used; (vi) whether animals were allocated randomly to groups; (vii) whether the duration of observation was adequate; and (viii) whether the data were adequately reported. If available, recent data on the incidence of specific tumours in historical controls, as well as in concurrent controls, should be taken into account in the evaluation of tumour response.

When benign tumours occur together with and originate from the same cell type in an organ or tissue as malignant tumours in a particular study and appear to represent a stage in the progression to malignancy, it may be valid to combine them in assessing tumour incidence (Huff *et al.*, 1989). The occurrence of lesions presumed to be preneoplastic may in certain instances aid in assessing the biological plausibility of any neoplastic response observed. If an agent or mixture induces only benign neoplasms that appear to be end-points that do not readily progress to malignancy, it should nevertheless be suspected of being a carcinogen and requires further investigation.

(b)   Quantitative aspects

The probability that tumours will occur may depend on the species, sex, strain and age of the animal, the dose of the carcinogen and the route and length of exposure. Evidence of an increased incidence of neoplasms with increased level of exposure strengthens the inference of a causal association between the exposure and the development of neoplasms.

The form of the dose–response relationship can vary widely, depending on the particular agent under study and the target organ. Both DNA damage and increased cell division are important aspects of carcinogenesis, and cell proliferation is a strong determinant of dose–response relationships for some carcinogens (Cohen & Ellwein, 1990). Since many chemicals require metabolic activation before being converted into their reactive intermediates, both metabolic and pharmacokinetic aspects are important in determining the dose–response pattern. Saturation of steps such as absorption, activation, inactivation and elimination may produce nonlinearity in the dose–response relationship, as could saturation of processes such as DNA repair (Hoel *et al.*, 1983; Gart *et al.*, 1986).

(c)   *Statistical analysis of long-term experiments in animals*

Factors considered by the Working Group include the adequacy of the information given for each treatment group: (i) the number of animals studied and the number examined histologically, (ii) the number of animals with a given tumour type and (iii) length of survival. The statistical methods used should be clearly stated and should be the generally accepted techniques refined for this purpose (Peto *et al.*, 1980; Gart *et al.*, 1986). When there is no difference in survival between control and treatment groups, the Working Group usually compares the proportions of animals developing each tumour type in each of the groups. Otherwise, consideration is given as to whether or not appropriate adjustments have been made for differences in survival. These adjustments can include: comparisons of the proportions of tumour-bearing animals among the effective number of animals (alive at the time the first tumour is discovered), in the case where most differences in survival occur before tumours appear; life-table methods, when tumours are visible or when they may be considered 'fatal' because mortality rapidly follows tumour development; and the Mantel-Haenszel test or logistic regression, when occult tumours do not affect the animals' risk of dying but are 'incidental' findings at autopsy.

In practice, classifying tumours as fatal or incidental may be difficult. Several survival-adjusted methods have been developed that do not require this distinction (Gart *et al.*, 1986), although they have not been fully evaluated.

10.   OTHER DATA RELEVANT TO AN EVALUATION OF CARCINOGENICITY AND ITS MECHANISMS

In coming to an overall evaluation of carcinogenicity in humans (see pp. 25–27), the Working Group also considers related data. The nature of the information selected for the summary depends on the agent being considered.

For chemicals and complex mixtures of chemicals such as those in some occupational situations or involving cultural habits (e.g. tobacco smoking), the other data considered to be relevant are divided into those on absorption, distribution, metabolism and excretion; toxic effects; reproductive and developmental effects; and genetic and related effects.

Concise information is given on absorption, distribution (including placental transfer) and excretion in both humans and experimental animals. Kinetic factors that may affect the dose–response relationship, such as saturation of uptake, protein binding, metabolic activation, detoxification and DNA repair processes, are mentioned. Studies that indicate the metabolic fate of the agent in humans and in experimental animals are summarized briefly, and comparisons of data on humans and on animals are made when possible. Comparative information on the relationship between exposure and the dose that reaches the target site may be of particular importance for extrapolation between species. Data are given on acute and chronic toxic effects (other than cancer), such as organ toxicity, increased cell proliferation, immunotoxicity and endocrine effects. The presence and toxicological significance of cellular receptors is described. Effects on reproduction, teratogenicity, fetotoxicity and embryotoxicity are also summarized briefly.

Tests of genetic and related effects are described in view of the relevance of gene mutation and chromosomal damage to carcinogenesis (Vainio *et al.*, 1992; McGregor *et al.*, 1999). The adequacy of the reporting of sample characterization is considered and, where necessary, commented upon; with regard to complex mixtures, such comments are similar to those described for animal carcinogenicity tests on p. 18. The available data are interpreted critically by phylogenetic group according to the end-points detected, which may include DNA damage, gene mutation, sister chromatid exchange, micro-nucleus formation, chromosomal aberrations, aneuploidy and cell transformation. The concentrations employed are given, and mention is made of whether use of an exogenous metabolic system *in vitro* affected the test result. These data are given as listings of test systems, data and references. The data on genetic and related effects presented in the *Monographs* are also available in the form of genetic activity profiles (GAP) prepared in collaboration with the United States Environmental Protection Agency (EPA) (see also Waters *et al.*, 1987) using software for personal computers that are Microsoft Windows® compatible. The EPA/IARC GAP software and database may be downloaded free of charge from *www.epa.gov/gapdb*.

Positive results in tests using prokaryotes, lower eukaryotes, plants, insects and cultured mammalian cells suggest that genetic and related effects could occur in mammals. Results from such tests may also give information about the types of genetic effect produced and about the involvement of metabolic activation. Some end-points described are clearly genetic in nature (e.g., gene mutations and chromosomal aberra-tions), while others are to a greater or lesser degree associated with genetic effects (e.g. unscheduled DNA synthesis). In-vitro tests for tumour-promoting activity and for cell transformation may be sensitive to changes that are not necessarily the result of genetic alterations but that may have specific relevance to the process of carcinogenesis. A critical appraisal of these tests has been published (Montesano *et al.*, 1986).

Genetic or other activity detected in experimental mammals and humans is regarded as being of greater relevance than that in other organisms. The demonstration that an agent or mixture can induce gene and chromosomal mutations in whole mammals indi-cates that it may have carcinogenic activity, although this activity may not be detectably expressed in any or all species. Relative potency in tests for mutagenicity and related effects is not a reliable indicator of carcinogenic potency. Negative results in tests for mutagenicity in selected tissues from animals treated *in vivo* provide less weight, partly because they do not exclude the possibility of an effect in tissues other than those examined. Moreover, negative results in short-term tests with genetic end-points cannot be considered to provide evidence to rule out carcinogenicity of agents or mixtures that act through other mechanisms (e.g. receptor-mediated effects, cellular toxicity with regenerative proliferation, peroxisome proliferation) (Vainio *et al.*, 1992). Factors that may lead to misleading results in short-term tests have been discussed in detail elsewhere (Montesano *et al.*, 1986).

When available, data relevant to mechanisms of carcinogenesis that do not involve structural changes at the level of the gene are also described.

The adequacy of epidemiological studies of reproductive outcome and genetic and related effects in humans is evaluated by the same criteria as are applied to epidemiological studies of cancer.

Structure–activity relationships that may be relevant to an evaluation of the carcinogenicity of an agent are also described.

For biological agents — viruses, bacteria and parasites — other data relevant to carcinogenicity include descriptions of the pathology of infection, molecular biology (integration and expression of viruses, and any genetic alterations seen in human tumours) and other observations, which might include cellular and tissue responses to infection, immune response and the presence of tumour markers.

11.   SUMMARY OF DATA REPORTED

In this section, the relevant epidemiological and experimental data are summarized. Only reports, other than in abstract form, that meet the criteria outlined on p. 11 are considered for evaluating carcinogenicity. Inadequate studies are generally not summarized: such studies are usually identified by a square-bracketed comment in the preceding text.

(*a*)   *Exposure*

Human exposure to chemicals and complex mixtures is summarized on the basis of elements such as production, use, occurrence in the environment and determinations in human tissues and body fluids. Quantitative data are given when available. Exposure to biological agents is described in terms of transmission and prevalence of infection.

(*b*)   *Carcinogenicity in humans*

Results of epidemiological studies that are considered to be pertinent to an assessment of human carcinogenicity are summarized. When relevant, case reports and correlation studies are also summarized.

(*c*)   *Carcinogenicity in experimental animals*

Data relevant to an evaluation of carcinogenicity in animals are summarized. For each animal species and route of administration, it is stated whether an increased incidence of neoplasms or preneoplastic lesions was observed, and the tumour sites are indicated. If the agent or mixture produced tumours after prenatal exposure or in single-dose experiments, this is also indicated. Negative findings are also summarized. Dose–response and other quantitative data may be given when available.

(*d*) *Other data relevant to an evaluation of carcinogenicity and its mechanisms*

Data on biological effects in humans that are of particular relevance are summarized. These may include toxicological, kinetic and metabolic considerations and evidence of DNA binding, persistence of DNA lesions or genetic damage in exposed humans. Toxicological information, such as that on cytotoxicity and regeneration, receptor binding and hormonal and immunological effects, and data on kinetics and metabolism in experimental animals are given when considered relevant to the possible mechanism of the carcinogenic action of the agent. The results of tests for genetic and related effects are summarized for whole mammals, cultured mammalian cells and nonmammalian systems.

When available, comparisons of such data for humans and for animals, and particularly animals that have developed cancer, are described.

Structure–activity relationships are mentioned when relevant.

For the agent, mixture or exposure circumstance being evaluated, the available data on end-points or other phenomena relevant to mechanisms of carcinogenesis from studies in humans, experimental animals and tissue and cell test systems are summarized within one or more of the following descriptive dimensions:

(i) Evidence of genotoxicity (structural changes at the level of the gene): for example, structure–activity considerations, adduct formation, mutagenicity (effect on specific genes), chromosomal mutation/aneuploidy

(ii) Evidence of effects on the expression of relevant genes (functional changes at the intracellular level): for example, alterations to the structure or quantity of the product of a proto-oncogene or tumour-suppressor gene, alterations to metabolic activation/inactivation/DNA repair

(iii) Evidence of relevant effects on cell behaviour (morphological or behavioural changes at the cellular or tissue level): for example, induction of mitogenesis, compensatory cell proliferation, preneoplasia and hyperplasia, survival of premalignant or malignant cells (immortalization, immunosuppression), effects on metastatic potential

(iv) Evidence from dose and time relationships of carcinogenic effects and interactions between agents: for example, early/late stage, as inferred from epidemiological studies; initiation/promotion/progression/malignant conversion, as defined in animal carcinogenicity experiments; toxicokinetics

These dimensions are not mutually exclusive, and an agent may fall within more than one of them. Thus, for example, the action of an agent on the expression of relevant genes could be summarized under both the first and second dimensions, even if it were known with reasonable certainty that those effects resulted from genotoxicity.

12. EVALUATION

Evaluations of the strength of the evidence for carcinogenicity arising from human and experimental animal data are made, using standard terms.

It is recognized that the criteria for these evaluations, described below, cannot encompass all of the factors that may be relevant to an evaluation of carcinogenicity. In considering all of the relevant scientific data, the Working Group may assign the agent, mixture or exposure circumstance to a higher or lower category than a strict inter-pretation of these criteria would indicate.

> (*a*)   *Degrees of evidence for carcinogenicity in humans and in experimental animals and supporting evidence*

These categories refer only to the strength of the evidence that an exposure is carcino-genic and not to the extent of its carcinogenic activity (potency) nor to the mechanisms involved. A classification may change as new information becomes available.

An evaluation of degree of evidence, whether for a single agent or a mixture, is limited to the materials tested, as defined physically, chemically or biologically. When the agents evaluated are considered by the Working Group to be sufficiently closely related, they may be grouped together for the purpose of a single evaluation of degree of evidence.

> (i)   *Carcinogenicity in humans*

The applicability of an evaluation of the carcinogenicity of a mixture, process, occu-pation or industry on the basis of evidence from epidemiological studies depends on the variability over time and place of the mixtures, processes, occupations and industries. The Working Group seeks to identify the specific exposure, process or activity which is considered most likely to be responsible for any excess risk. The evaluation is focused as narrowly as the available data on exposure and other aspects permit.

The evidence relevant to carcinogenicity from studies in humans is classified into one of the following categories:

Sufficient evidence of carcinogenicity: The Working Group considers that a causal relationship has been established between exposure to the agent, mixture or exposure circumstance and human cancer. That is, a positive relationship has been observed between the exposure and cancer in studies in which chance, bias and confounding could be ruled out with reasonable confidence.

Limited evidence of carcinogenicity: A positive association has been observed between exposure to the agent, mixture or exposure circumstance and cancer for which a causal interpretation is considered by the Working Group to be credible, but chance, bias or confounding could not be ruled out with reasonable confidence.

Inadequate evidence of carcinogenicity: The available studies are of insufficient quality, consistency or statistical power to permit a conclusion regarding the presence or absence of a causal association between exposure and cancer, or no data on cancer in humans are available.

Evidence suggesting lack of carcinogenicity: There are several adequate studies covering the full range of levels of exposure that human beings are known to encounter, which are mutually consistent in not showing a positive association between exposure to the agent, mixture or exposure circumstance and any studied cancer at any observed level of exposure. A conclusion of 'evidence suggesting lack of carcinogenicity' is inevitably limited to the cancer sites, conditions and levels of exposure and length of observation covered by the available studies. In addition, the possibility of a very small risk at the levels of exposure studied can never be excluded.

In some instances, the above categories may be used to classify the degree of evidence related to carcinogenicity in specific organs or tissues.

(ii)   *Carcinogenicity in experimental animals*

The evidence relevant to carcinogenicity in experimental animals is classified into one of the following categories:

Sufficient evidence of carcinogenicity: The Working Group considers that a causal relationship has been established between the agent or mixture and an increased incidence of malignant neoplasms or of an appropriate combination of benign and malignant neoplasms in (a) two or more species of animals or (b) in two or more independent studies in one species carried out at different times or in different laboratories or under different protocols.

Exceptionally, a single study in one species might be considered to provide sufficient evidence of carcinogenicity when malignant neoplasms occur to an unusual degree with regard to incidence, site, type of tumour or age at onset.

Limited evidence of carcinogenicity: The data suggest a carcinogenic effect but are limited for making a definitive evaluation because, e.g. (a) the evidence of carcinogenicity is restricted to a single experiment; or (b) there are unresolved questions regarding the adequacy of the design, conduct or interpretation of the study; or (c) the agent or mixture increases the incidence only of benign neoplasms or lesions of uncertain neoplastic potential, or of certain neoplasms which may occur spontaneously in high incidences in certain strains.

Inadequate evidence of carcinogenicity: The studies cannot be interpreted as showing either the presence or absence of a carcinogenic effect because of major qualitative or quantitative limitations, or no data on cancer in experimental animals are available.

Evidence suggesting lack of carcinogenicity: Adequate studies involving at least two species are available which show that, within the limits of the tests used, the agent or mixture is not carcinogenic. A conclusion of evidence suggesting lack of carcinogenicity is inevitably limited to the species, tumour sites and levels of exposure studied.

(b)   *Other data relevant to the evaluation of carcinogenicity and its mechanisms*

Other evidence judged to be relevant to an evaluation of carcinogenicity and of sufficient importance to affect the overall evaluation is then described. This may include data on preneoplastic lesions, tumour pathology, genetic and related effects, structure–activity relationships, metabolism and pharmacokinetics, physicochemical parameters and analogous biological agents.

Data relevant to mechanisms of the carcinogenic action are also evaluated. The strength of the evidence that any carcinogenic effect observed is due to a particular mechanism is assessed, using terms such as weak, moderate or strong. Then, the Working Group assesses if that particular mechanism is likely to be operative in humans. The strongest indications that a particular mechanism operates in humans come from data on humans or biological specimens obtained from exposed humans. The data may be considered to be especially relevant if they show that the agent in question has caused changes in exposed humans that are on the causal pathway to carcinogenesis. Such data may, however, never become available, because it is at least conceivable that certain compounds may be kept from human use solely on the basis of evidence of their toxicity and/or carcinogenicity in experimental systems.

For complex exposures, including occupational and industrial exposures, the chemical composition and the potential contribution of carcinogens known to be present are considered by the Working Group in its overall evaluation of human carcinogenicity. The Working Group also determines the extent to which the materials tested in experimental systems are related to those to which humans are exposed.

(c)   Overall evaluation

Finally, the body of evidence is considered as a whole, in order to reach an overall evaluation of the carcinogenicity to humans of an agent, mixture or circumstance of exposure.

An evaluation may be made for a group of chemical compounds that have been evaluated by the Working Group. In addition, when supporting data indicate that other, related compounds for which there is no direct evidence of capacity to induce cancer in humans or in animals may also be carcinogenic, a statement describing the rationale for this conclusion is added to the evaluation narrative; an additional evaluation may be made for this broader group of compounds if the strength of the evidence warrants it.

The agent, mixture or exposure circumstance is described according to the wording of one of the following categories, and the designated group is given. The categorization of an agent, mixture or exposure circumstance is a matter of scientific judgement, reflecting the strength of the evidence derived from studies in humans and in experimental animals and from other relevant data.

Group 1 — The agent (mixture) is carcinogenic to humans.
The exposure circumstance entails exposures that are carcinogenic to humans.

This category is used when there is *sufficient evidence* of carcinogenicity in humans. Exceptionally, an agent (mixture) may be placed in this category when evidence of carcinogenicity in humans is less than sufficient but there is *sufficient evidence* of carcinogenicity in experimental animals and strong evidence in exposed humans that the agent (mixture) acts through a relevant mechanism of carcinogenicity.

Group 2

This category includes agents, mixtures and exposure circumstances for which, at one extreme, the degree of evidence of carcinogenicity in humans is almost sufficient, as well as those for which, at the other extreme, there are no human data but for which there is evidence of carcinogenicity in experimental animals. Agents, mixtures and exposure circumstances are assigned to either group 2A (probably carcinogenic to humans) or group 2B (possibly carcinogenic to humans) on the basis of epidemiological and experimental evidence of carcinogenicity and other relevant data.

Group 2A — The agent (mixture) is probably carcinogenic to humans.
The exposure circumstance entails exposures that are probably carcinogenic to humans.

This category is used when there is *limited evidence* of carcinogenicity in humans and *sufficient evidence* of carcinogenicity in experimental animals. In some cases, an agent (mixture) may be classified in this category when there is *inadequate evidence* of carcinogenicity in humans, *sufficient evidence* of carcinogenicity in experimental animals and strong evidence that the carcinogenesis is mediated by a mechanism that also operates in humans. Exceptionally, an agent, mixture or exposure circumstance may be classified in this category solely on the basis of *limited evidence* of carcinogenicity in humans.

Group 2B — The agent (mixture) is possibly carcinogenic to humans.
The exposure circumstance entails exposures that are possibly carcinogenic to humans.

This category is used for agents, mixtures and exposure circumstances for which there is *limited evidence* of carcinogenicity in humans and less than *sufficient evidence* of carcinogenicity in experimental animals. It may also be used when there is *inadequate evidence* of carcinogenicity in humans but there is *sufficient evidence* of carcinogenicity in experimental animals. In some instances, an agent, mixture or exposure circumstance for which there is *inadequate evidence* of carcinogenicity in humans but *limited evidence* of carcinogenicity in experimental animals together with supporting evidence from other relevant data may be placed in this group.

Group 3 — The agent (mixture or exposure circumstance) is not classifiable as to its carcinogenicity to humans.

This category is used most commonly for agents, mixtures and exposure circumstances for which the *evidence of carcinogenicity* is *inadequate* in humans and *inadequate* or *limited* in experimental animals.

Exceptionally, agents (mixtures) for which the *evidence of carcinogenicity* is *inadequate* in humans but *sufficient* in experimental animals may be placed in this category when there is strong evidence that the mechanism of carcinogenicity in experimental animals does not operate in humans.

Agents, mixtures and exposure circumstances that do not fall into any other group are also placed in this category.

Group 4 — The agent (mixture) is probably not carcinogenic to humans.

This category is used for agents or mixtures for which there is *evidence suggesting lack of carcinogenicity* in humans and in experimental animals. In some instances, agents or mixtures for which there is *inadequate evidence* of carcinogenicity in humans but *evidence suggesting lack of carcinogenicity* in experimental animals, consistently and strongly supported by a broad range of other relevant data, may be classified in this group.

13. REFERENCES

Breslow, N.E. & Day, N.E. (1980) *Statistical Methods in Cancer Research*, Vol. 1, *The Analysis of Case–Control Studies* (IARC Scientific Publications No. 32), Lyon, IARC*Press*

Breslow, N.E. & Day, N.E. (1987) *Statistical Methods in Cancer Research*, Vol. 2, *The Design and Analysis of Cohort Studies* (IARC Scientific Publications No. 82), Lyon, IARC*Press*

Cohen, S.M. & Ellwein, L.B. (1990) Cell proliferation in carcinogenesis. *Science*, **249**, 1007–1011

Gart, J.J., Krewski, D., Lee, P.N., Tarone, R.E. & Wahrendorf, J. (1986) *Statistical Methods in Cancer Research*, Vol. 3, *The Design and Analysis of Long-term Animal Experiments* (IARC Scientific Publications No. 79), Lyon, IARC*Press*

Hoel, D.G., Kaplan, N.L. & Anderson, M.W. (1983) Implication of nonlinear kinetics on risk estimation in carcinogenesis. *Science*, **219**, 1032–1037

Huff, J.E., Eustis, S.L. & Haseman, J.K. (1989) Occurrence and relevance of chemically induced benign neoplasms in long-term carcinogenicity studies. *Cancer Metastasis Rev.*, **8**, 1–21

IARC (1973–1996) *Information Bulletin on the Survey of Chemicals Being Tested for Carcinogenicity/Directory of Agents Being Tested for Carcinogenicity*, Numbers 1–17, Lyon, IARC*Press*

IARC (1976–1996), Lyon, IARC*Press*

Directory of On-going Research in Cancer Epidemiology 1976. Edited by C.S. Muir & G. Wagner

Directory of On-going Research in Cancer Epidemiology 1977 (IARC Scientific Publications No. 17). Edited by C.S. Muir & G. Wagner

Directory of On-going Research in Cancer Epidemiology 1978 (IARC Scientific Publications No. 26). Edited by C.S. Muir & G. Wagner

Directory of On-going Research in Cancer Epidemiology 1979 (IARC Scientific Publications No. 28). Edited by C.S. Muir & G. Wagner

Directory of On-going Research in Cancer Epidemiology 1980 (IARC Scientific Publications No. 35). Edited by C.S. Muir & G. Wagner

Directory of On-going Research in Cancer Epidemiology 1981 (IARC Scientific Publications No. 38). Edited by C.S. Muir & G. Wagner

Directory of On-going Research in Cancer Epidemiology 1982 (IARC Scientific Publications
  No. 46). Edited by C.S. Muir & G. Wagner

Directory of On-going Research in Cancer Epidemiology 1983 (IARC Scientific Publications
  No. 50). Edited by C.S. Muir & G. Wagner

Directory of On-going Research in Cancer Epidemiology 1984 (IARC Scientific Publications
  No. 62). Edited by C.S. Muir & G. Wagner

Directory of On-going Research in Cancer Epidemiology 1985 (IARC Scientific Publications
  No. 69). Edited by C.S. Muir & G. Wagner

Directory of On-going Research in Cancer Epidemiology 1986 (IARC Scientific Publications
  No. 80). Edited by C.S. Muir & G. Wagner

Directory of On-going Research in Cancer Epidemiology 1987 (IARC Scientific Publications
  No. 86). Edited by D.M. Parkin & J. Wahrendorf

Directory of On-going Research in Cancer Epidemiology 1988 (IARC Scientific Publications
  No. 93). Edited by M. Coleman & J. Wahrendorf

Directory of On-going Research in Cancer Epidemiology 1989/90 (IARC Scientific Publications No. 101). Edited by M. Coleman & J. Wahrendorf

Directory of On-going Research in Cancer Epidemiology 1991 (IARC Scientific Publications
  No.110). Edited by M. Coleman & J. Wahrendorf

Directory of On-going Research in Cancer Epidemiology 1992 (IARC Scientific Publications
  No. 117). Edited by M. Coleman, J. Wahrendorf & E. Démaret

Directory of On-going Research in Cancer Epidemiology 1994 (IARC Scientific Publications
  No. 130). Edited by R. Sankaranarayanan, J. Wahrendorf & E. Démaret

Directory of On-going Research in Cancer Epidemiology 1996 (IARC Scientific Publications
  No. 137). Edited by R. Sankaranarayanan, J. Wahrendorf & E. Démaret

IARC (1977) *IARC Monographs Programme on the Evaluation of the Carcinogenic Risk of
  Chemicals to Humans.* Preamble (IARC intern. tech. Rep. No. 77/002)

IARC (1978) *Chemicals with* Sufficient Evidence *of Carcinogenicity in Experimental Animals —*
  IARC Monographs *Volumes 1–17* (IARC intern. tech. Rep. No. 78/003)

IARC (1978–1993) *Environmental Carcinogens. Methods of Analysis and Exposure Measurement,* Lyon, IARC*Press*

  Vol. 1. Analysis of Volatile Nitrosamines in Food (IARC Scientific Publications No. 18).
    Edited by R. Preussmann, M. Castegnaro, E.A. Walker & A.E. Wasserman (1978)

  *Vol. 2. Methods for the Measurement of Vinyl Chloride in Poly(vinyl chloride), Air, Water and
    Foodstuffs* (IARC Scientific Publications No. 22). Edited by D.C.M. Squirrell & W.
    Thain (1978)

  Vol. 3. Analysis of Polycyclic Aromatic Hydrocarbons in Environmental Samples (IARC
    Scientific Publications No. 29). Edited by M. Castegnaro, P. Bogovski, H. Kunte & E.A.
    Walker (1979)

  Vol. 4. Some Aromatic Amines and Azo Dyes in the General and Industrial Environment
    (IARC Scientific Publications No. 40). Edited by L. Fishbein, M. Castegnaro, I.K.
    O'Neill & H. Bartsch (1981)

  Vol. 5. Some Mycotoxins (IARC Scientific Publications No. 44). Edited by L. Stoloff,
    M. Castegnaro, P. Scott, I.K. O'Neill & H. Bartsch (1983)

  Vol. 6. N-Nitroso Compounds (IARC Scientific Publications No. 45). Edited by R. Preuss-
    mann, I.K. O'Neill, G. Eisenbrand, B. Spiegelhalder & H. Bartsch (1983)

Vol. 7. Some Volatile Halogenated Hydrocarbons (IARC Scientific Publications No. 68). Edited by L. Fishbein & I.K. O'Neill (1985)

Vol. 8. Some Metals: As, Be, Cd, Cr, Ni, Pb, Se, Zn (IARC Scientific Publications No. 71). Edited by I.K. O'Neill, P. Schuller & L. Fishbein (1986)

Vol. 9. Passive Smoking (IARC Scientific Publications No. 81). Edited by I.K. O'Neill, K.D. Brunnemann, B. Dodet & D. Hoffmann (1987)

*Vol. 10. Benzene and Alkylated Benzenes (*IARC Scientific Publications No. 85). Edited by L. Fishbein & I.K. O'Neill (1988)

Vol. 11. Polychlorinated Dioxins and Dibenzofurans (IARC Scientific Publications No. 108). Edited by C. Rappe, H.R. Buser, B. Dodet & I.K. O'Neill (1991)

Vol. 12. Indoor Air (IARC Scientific Publications No. 109). Edited by B. Seifert, H. van de Wiel, B. Dodet & I.K. O'Neill (1993)

IARC (1979) *Criteria to Select Chemicals for* IARC Monographs (IARC intern. tech. Rep. No. 79/003)

IARC (1982) *IARC Monographs on the Evaluation of the Carcinogenic Risk of Chemicals to Humans*, Supplement 4, *Chemicals, Industrial Processes and Industries Associated with Cancer in Humans* (IARC Monographs, Volumes 1 to 29), Lyon, IARC*Press*

IARC (1983) *Approaches to Classifying Chemical Carcinogens According to Mechanism of Action* (IARC intern. tech. Rep. No. 83/001)

IARC (1984) *Chemicals and Exposures to Complex Mixtures Recommended for Evaluation in IARC Monographs and Chemicals and Complex Mixtures Recommended for Long-term Carcinogenicity Testing* (IARC intern. tech. Rep. No. 84/002)

IARC (1987a) *IARC Monographs on the Evaluation of Carcinogenic Risks to Humans*, Supplement 6, *Genetic and Related Effects: An Updating of Selected* IARC Monographs *from Volumes 1 to 42*, Lyon, IARC*Press*

IARC (1987b) *IARC Monographs on the Evaluation of Carcinogenic Risks to Humans*, Supplement 7, *Overall Evaluations of Carcinogenicity: An Updating of* IARC Monographs *Volumes 1 to 42*, Lyon, IARC*Press*

IARC (1988) *Report of an IARC Working Group to Review the Approaches and Processes Used to Evaluate the Carcinogenicity of Mixtures and Groups of Chemicals* (IARC intern. tech. Rep. No. 88/002)

IARC (1989) *Chemicals, Groups of Chemicals, Mixtures and Exposure Circumstances to be Evaluated in Future IARC Monographs, Report of an ad hoc Working Group* (IARC intern. tech. Rep. No. 89/004)

IARC (1991a) *A Consensus Report of an IARC Monographs Working Group on the Use of Mechanisms of Carcinogenesis in Risk Identification* (IARC intern. tech. Rep. No. 91/002)

IARC (1991b) *Report of an ad-hoc* IARC Monographs *Advisory Group on Viruses and Other Biological Agents Such as Parasites* (IARC intern. tech. Rep. No. 91/001)

IARC (1993) *Chemicals, Groups of Chemicals, Complex Mixtures, Physical and Biological Agents and Exposure Circumstances to be Evaluated in Future* IARC Monographs, *Report of an ad-hoc Working Group* (IARC intern. Rep. No. 93/005)

IARC (1998a) *Report of an ad-hoc* IARC Monographs *Advisory Group on Physical Agents* (IARC Internal Report No. 98/002)

IARC (1998b) *Report of an ad-hoc* IARC Monographs *Advisory Group on Priorities for Future Evaluations* (IARC Internal Report No. 98/004)

McGregor, D.B., Rice, J.M. & Venitt, S., eds (1999) *The Use of Short and Medium-term Tests for Carcinogens and Data on Genetic Effects in Carcinogenic Hazard Evaluation* (IARC Scientific Publications No. 146), Lyon, IARC*Press*

Montesano, R., Bartsch, H., Vainio, H., Wilbourn, J. & Yamasaki, H., eds (1986) *Long-term and Short-term Assays for Carcinogenesis — A Critical Appraisal* (IARC Scientific Publications No. 83), Lyon, IARC*Press*

Peto, R., Pike, M.C., Day, N.E., Gray, R.G., Lee, P.N., Parish, S., Peto, J., Richards, S. & Wahrendorf, J. (1980) Guidelines for simple, sensitive significance tests for carcinogenic effects in long-term animal experiments. In: *IARC Monographs on the Evaluation of the Carcinogenic Risk of Chemicals to Humans*, Supplement 2, *Long-term and Short-term Screening Assays for Carcinogens: A Critical Appraisal*, Lyon, IARC*Press*, pp. 311–426

Tomatis, L., Aitio, A., Wilbourn, J. & Shuker, L. (1989) Human carcinogens so far identified. *Jpn. J. Cancer Res.*, **80**, 795–807

Vainio, H., Magee, P.N., McGregor, D.B. & McMichael, A.J., eds (1992) *Mechanisms of Carcinogenesis in Risk Identification* (IARC Scientific Publications No. 116), Lyon, IARC*Press*

Vainio, H., Wilbourn, J.D., Sasco, A.J., Partensky, C., Gaudin, N., Heseltine, E. & Eragne, I. (1995) Identification of human carcinogenic risk in IARC Monographs. *Bull. Cancer*, **82**, 339–348 (in French)

Waters, M.D., Stack, H.F., Brady, A.L., Lohman, P.H.M., Haroun, L. & Vainio, H. (1987) Appendix 1. Activity profiles for genetic and related tests. In: *IARC Monographs on the Evaluation of Carcinogenic Risks to Humans*, Suppl. 6, *Genetic and Related Effects: An Updating of Selected IARC Monographs from Volumes 1 to 42*, Lyon, IARC*Press*, pp. 687–696

Wilbourn, J., Haroun, L., Heseltine, E., Kaldor, J., Partensky, C. & Vainio, H. (1986) Response of experimental animals to human carcinogens: an analysis based upon the IARC Monographs Programme. *Carcinogenesis*, **7**, 1853–1863

GENERAL REMARKS ON THE SUBSTANCES CONSIDERED

This eighty-eighth volume of *IARC Monographs* evaluates the available evidence on the carcinogenic potential in humans of formaldehyde, 2-butoxyethanol and 1-*tert*-butoxypropan-2-ol. Formaldehyde, a potential carcinogen that is found in the workplace and in the environment, has been studied the most widely and has been evaluated three times previously. In Volume 29 (IARC, 1982), the experimental animal data were evaluated as having *sufficient evidence* and the epidemiological studies as having *inadequate evidence* of carcinogenicity. In Supplement 7 (IARC, 1987), these data were updated and an overall evaluation was made that formaldehyde is *probably carcinogenic to humans* (Group 2A), based on *limited evidence* of carcinogenicity from studies in humans and *sufficient evidence* of carcinogenicity from studies in experimental animals. Formaldehyde was reconsidered again in Volume 62 (IARC, 1995), when the existing classification was reaffirmed. It is being re-evaluated this time following a recommendation from an Advisory Group (IARC, 2003) that identified formaldehyde as a high priority for future re-evaluation, based on the availability of complex mechanistic data and the anticipated publication of new epidemiological studies that became available soon afterwards. The same Advisory Group also identified 2-butoxyethanol and other glycol ethers as high priorities, based on the availability of new carcinogenesis bioassays conducted by the US National Toxicology Program. This is the first evaluation that IARC has made of the two glycol ethers.

A theme common to these three evaluations is the consideration of mechanistic information to develop and evaluate hypotheses on the sequence of steps that lead to the induction of tumours in experimental animals. The hypothesized mechanisms described in this volume provide an interesting set of cases that range from a vast literature on respiratory tract tumours in rats induced by the inhalation of formaldehyde to some more tentative hypotheses on the various tumours observed in animals following exposure to glycol ethers. Both types of mechanistic datasets were of use in the evaluation process.

This evaluation emphasizes the importance of mechanistic information in the classification of carcinogens. For example, the Working Group considered the extensive scientific database on the mechanisms by which formaldehyde can induce cancer in humans. The extensive mechanistic data for formaldehyde-induced respiratory cancer provide strong support for the empirical observation of nasopharyngeal cancer in humans. In contrast, the lack of such information on possible mechanisms by which formaldehyde might increase the risk for leukaemia in humans tempered the interpretation of the epidemiological data on that cancer.

The evaluations in this volume also reveal that the Working Group grappled with questions of interpretation and scientific judgement. A recurring issue was the criteria that characterize a rare tumour or an unusual set of observations that can carry greater weight than a typical bioassay result. Another issue was how to introduce additional information to resolve difficult questions; for example, how to consider the results of historical controls or alternative statistical tests. When the Working Group tried to, but could not reach, consensus on a question of interpretation or scientific judgement, the evaluation presents the differing positions favoured by its members.

Although the *IARC Monographs* focus on a qualitative assessment of the carcinogenic potential of an agent, subsequent predictions of the risks for cancer from formaldehyde could consider pertinent information on mechanisms of carcinogenesis, including dose-dependent cytoxicity and genotoxicity. Information on human biomarkers may facilitate a comparison of the relative susceptibility of animals and humans, as well as describe the variation in the susceptibility of different human populations.

It is important to note that an evaluation of an agent as *not classifiable as to its carcinogenicity to humans* is not a determination of safety, with respect to both cancer and effects other than cancer. Rather, it can indicate the need for further testing and information, particularly when there is widespread human exposure or another reason for public health concern. In these cases, it is important that investigators who represent different scientific disciplines and perspectives conduct further research.

References

IARC (1982) *IARC Monographs on the Evaluation of the Carcinogenic Risk of Chemicals to Humans*, Vol. 29, *Some Industrial Chemicals and Dyestuffs*, Lyon, pp. 345–389

IARC (1987) *IARC Monographs on the Evaluation of Carcinogenic Risks to Humans*, Suppl. 7, *Overall Evaluations of Carcinogenicity: An Updating of* IARC Monographs *Volumes 1–42*, Lyon

IARC (1995) *IARC Monographs on the Evaluation of Carcinogenic Risks to Humans*, Vol. 62, *Wood Dust and Formaldehyde*, Lyon, pp. 217–362

IARC (2003) *Report of an ad-hoc* IARC Monographs *Advisory Group on Priorities for Future Evaluations* (IARC Internal Report No. 03/001), Lyon

THE MONOGRAPHS

FORMALDEHYDE

FORMALDEHYDE

This substance was considered by previous working groups in October 1981 (IARC, 1982), March 1987 (IARC, 1987a) and October 1994 (IARC, 1995). Since that time, new data have become available, and these have been incorporated in the monograph and taken into consideration in the evaluation.

1. Exposure Data

1.1 Chemical and physical data

1.1.1 *Nomenclature*

Chem. Abstr. Serv. Reg. No.: 50-00-0
Deleted CAS Reg. Nos.: 8005-38-7; 8006-07-3; 8013-13-6; 112068-71-0
Chem. Abstr. Name: Formaldehyde
IUPAC Systematic Name: Methanal
Synonyms: Formaldehyde, gas; formic aldehyde; methaldehyde; methyl aldehyde; methylene oxide; oxomethane; oxymethylene

1.1.2 *Structural and molecular formulae and relative molecular mass*

$$\begin{array}{c} H \\ \diagdown \\ \diagup \\ H \end{array} C{=}O$$

CH$_2$O   Relative molecular mass: 30.03

1.1.3 *Chemical and physical properties of the pure substance*

From Lide (2003), unless otherwise specified
(*a*) *Description*: Colourless gas with a pungent odour (Reuss *et al.*, 2003)
(*b*) *Boiling-point*: –19.1 °C
(*c*) *Melting-point*: –92 °C
(*d*) *Density*: 0.815 at –20 °C

(e) *Spectroscopy data*: Infrared [prism, 2538], ultraviolet [3.1] and mass spectral data have been reported (Weast & Astle, 1985; Sadtler Research Laboratories, 1991).

(f) *Solubility*: Soluble in water, ethanol and chloroform; miscible with acetone, benzene and diethyl ether

(g) *Stability*: Commercial formaldehyde–alcohol solutions are stable; the gas is stable in the absence of water; incompatible with oxidizers, alkalis, acids, phenols and urea (IARC, 1995; Reuss *et al.*, 2003; Gerberich & Seaman, 2004).

(h) *Reactivity*: Reacts explosively with peroxide, nitrogen oxide and performic acid; can react with hydrogen chloride or other inorganic chlorides to form bis(chloromethyl) ether (see IARC, 1987b) (IARC, 1995; Reuss *et al.*, 2003; Gerberich & Seaman, 2004).

(i) *Octanol/water partition coefficient (P)*: log P = 0.35 (Hansch *et al.*, 1995)

(j) *Conversion factor*: $mg/m^3 = 1.23 \times ppm$[1]

1.1.4   *Technical products and impurities*

Trade names: BFV; FA; Fannoform; Floguard 1015; FM 282; Formalin; Formalin 40; Formalith; Formol; FYDE; Hoch; Ivalon; Karsan; Lysoform; Morbicid; Paraform; Superlysoform

Formaldehyde is most commonly available commercially as a 30–50% (by weight) aqueous solution, commonly referred to as 'formalin'. In dilute aqueous solution, the predominant form of formaldehyde is its monomeric hydrate, methylene glycol. In more concentrated aqueous solutions, oligomers and polymers that are mainly polyoxymethylene glycols are formed and may predominate. Methanol and other substances (e.g. various amine derivatives) are usually added to the solutions as stabilizers, in order to reduce intrinsic polymerization. The concentration of methanol can be as high as 15%, while that of other stabilizers is of the order of several hundred milligrams per litre. Concentrated liquid formaldehyde–water systems that contain up to 95% formaldehyde are also available, but the temperature necessary to maintain the solution and prevent separation of the polymer increases from room temperature to 120 °C as the concentration in solution increases. Impurities include formic acid, iron and copper (Cosmetic Ingredient Review Expert Panel, 1984).

Formaldehyde is marketed in solid form as its cyclic trimer, trioxane $((CH_2O)_3)$, and its polymer, paraformaldehyde, with 8–100 units of formaldehyde (WHO, 1991; IARC, 1995; Reuss *et al.*, 2003).

---

[1] Calculated from: $mg/m^3 = $ (relative molecular mass/24.45) $\times$ ppm, assuming normal temperature (25 °C) and pressure (103.5 kPa)

1.1.5   *Analysis*

Selected methods for the determination of formaldehyde in various matrices are presented in Table 1.

The most widely used methods for the determination of the concentration of formaldehyde in air are based on spectrophotometry, with which sensitivities of 0.01–0.03 mg/m^3 can be achieved. Other methods include colorimetry, fluorimetry, high-performance liquid chromatography (HPLC), polarography, gas chromatography (GC), infrared detection and gas detector tubes. Most methods require the formation of a derivative for separation and detection.

HPLC is the most sensitive method (limit of detection, 2 μg/m^3 or less). Gas detector tubes (Draeger Safety, undated; Sensidyne, undated; WHO, 1989; MSA, 1998; Matheson Tri-Gas®, 2004; Sensidyne, 2004; SKC®, 2005) that have sensitivities of about 0.05–0.12 mg/m^3 [0.04–0.1 ppm] and infrared analysers (Interscan Corporation, undated; Environmental Protection Agency, 1999a,b; MKS Instruments, 2004a,b; Thermo Electron Corporation, 2005) that have sensitivities of about 1.2–230 μg/m^3 [1–110 ppb] are often used to monitor workplace atmospheres.

Based on these methods, several standards have been established to determine levels of formaldehyde emissions from wood products (European Commission, 1989; ASTM International, 1990; Groah *et al.*, 1991; Jann, 1991; Deutsche Norm, 1992, 1994, 1996; Standardiseringen i Sverige, 1996; Composite Panel Association, 1999; ASTM International, 2000; Japanese Standards Association, 2001; ASTM International, 2002a,b; Composite Panel Association, 2002).

Sandner *et al.* (2001) reported a modification of the existing method 1 of the Deutsche Forschungsgemeinschaft (1993) to monitor formaldehyde in the workplace that uses adsorption to 2,4-dinitrophenylhydrazine-coated sorbents followed by HPLC with ultraviolet (UV)/diode array detection. The detection limit decreased from approximately 15 μg/m^3 for the original method to 0.07 μg/m^3 for the modified method.

In the development of new methods to monitor formaldehyde in air, emphasis has been on direct optical sensors and on increased sensitivity (Friedfeld *et al.*, 2000; Lancaster *et al.*, 2000; Chan *et al.*, 2001; Mathew *et al.*, 2001; Alves Pereira *et al.*, 2002; Werle *et al.*, 2002).

Methods for the analysis of formaldehyde in biological matrices (e.g. blood and urine) have been reviewed (ATSDR, 1999), and new methods continue to be reported (Carraro *et al.*, 1999; Spanel *et al.*, 1999; Luo *et al.*, 2001; Kato *et al.*, 2001). Formaldehyde has been measured in blood by gas chromatography–mass spectrometry (GC–MS) after derivatization to pentafluorophenylhydrazone (Heck *et al.*, 1982, 1985). Formic acid or formate is produced from formaldehyde and can be measured in blood and urine (Baumann & Angerer, 1979). However, biological monitoring of exposure to formaldehyde is not common practice.

Table 1. Methods for the analysis of formaldehyde in air and food

Sample matrix	Sample preparation	Assay procedure	Limit of detection	Reference
Air	Draw air through impinger containing aqueous pararosaniline; treat with acidic pararosaniline and sodium sulfite	Spectro-metry	10 $\mu g/m^3$	Georghiou *et al.* (1993)
	Draw air through PTFE filter and impingers, each treated with sodium bisulfite solution; develop colour with chromotropic acid and sulfuric acid; read absorbance at 580 nm	Spectro-metry	0.5 μg/sample	NIOSH (1994a) [Method 3500]
	Draw air through solid sorbent tube treated with 10% 2-(hydroxymethyl) piperidine on XAD-2; desorb with toluene	GC/FID	1 μg/sample	NIOSH (1994b) [Method 2541]
		GC/FID & GC/MS	2 μg/sample	NIOSH (1994c) [Method 2539]
		GC/NSD	20 $\mu g/m^3$	Occupational Safety and Health Administration (1990a) [Method 52]
	Draw air through impinger containing hydrochloric acid/2,4-di-nitrophenylhydrazine reagent and isooctane; extract with hexane/di-chloromethane	HPLC/UV	2 $\mu g/m^3$	Environmental Protection Agency (1988) [Method TO5]
	Draw air through a glassfibre filter impregnated with 2,4-dinitrophenyl-hydrazine; extract with acetonitrile	HPLC/UV	15 $\mu g/m^3$	Deutsche Forschungs-gemeinschaft (1993) [Method 1]
	Draw air through silica gel coated with acidified 2,4-dinitrophenyl-hydrazine reagent	HPLC/UV	2 $\mu g/m^3$ (0.6–123 $\mu g/m^3$)	Environmental Protection Agency (1999c); INRS (2003) [Method TO11A]
	Draw air through a cartridge containing silica gel coated with 2,4-dinitrophenylhydrazine; extract with acetonitrile	HPLC/UV	0.07 $\mu g/m^3$	Sandner *et al.* (2001)
	Draw air through a cartridge containing silica gel coated with 2,4-dinitrophenylhydrazine; extract with acetonitrile	HPLC/UV	0.07 μg/ sample	NIOSH (2003a) [Method 2016]

Table 1 (contd)

Sample matrix	Sample preparation	Assay procedure	Limit of detection	Reference
	Expose passive monitor containing bisulfite-impregnated paper; desorb with deionized water; acidify; add chromotropic acid; read absorbance at 580 nm	Chromo-tropic acid test	0.14 $\mu g/m^3$	Occupational Safety and Health Administration (1990b) [Method ID-205]
	Collect gases with portable direct-reading instrument; compare spectra with references	FTIRS	0.49 $\mu g/m^3$	NIOSH (2003b) [Method 3800]
Dust (textile or wood)	Draw air through inhalable dust sampler containing a PVC filter; extract with distilled water and 2,4-dinitrophenylhydrazine/acetonitrile	HPLC/UV	0.08 $\mu g/$ sample	NIOSH (1994d) [Method 5700]
Food	Distil sample; add 1,8-dihydroxy-naphthalene-3,6-disulfonic acid in sulfuric acid; purple colour indicates presence of formaldehyde	Chromo-tropic acid test	NR	AOAC (2003) [Method 931.08]
	Distil sample; add to cold sulfuric acid; add aldehyde-free milk; add bromine hydrate solution; purplish-pink colour indicates presence of formaldehyde	Hehner-Fulton test	NR	AOAC (2003) [Method 931.08]

FTIRS, Fourier transform infrared spectrometry; GC/FID, gas chromatography/flame ionization detection; GC/MS, gas chromatography/mass spectrometry; GC/NSD, gas chromatography/nitrogen selective detection; HPLC/UV, high-performance liquid chromatography/ultraviolet detection; NR, not reported; PTFE, polytetrafluoroethylene; PVC, polyvinyl chloride

1.2   Production and use

1.2.1   *Production*

Formaldehyde has been produced commercially since 1889 by the catalytic oxidation of methanol. Various specific methods were used in the past, but only two are widely used currently: the silver catalyst process and the metal oxide catalyst process (Bizzari, 2000; Reuss *et al.*, 2003; Gerberich & Seaman, 2004).

The silver catalyst process is conducted in one of two ways: (i) partial oxidation and dehydrogenation with air in the presence of silver crystals, steam and excess methanol at 680–720 °C and at atmospheric pressure (also called the BASF process; methanol conversion, 97–98%); and (ii) partial oxidation and dehydrogenation with air in the presence of crystalline silver or silver gauze, steam and excess methanol at 600–650 °C (primary conversion of methanol, 77–87%); the conversion is completed by distilling the product and recycling the unreacted methanol. Carbon monoxide, carbon dioxide, methyl formate and formic acid are by-products (Bizzari, 2000; Reuss *et al.*, 2003; Gerberich & Seaman, 2004).

In the metal oxide (Formox) process, methanol is oxidized with excess air in the presence of a modified iron–molybdenum–vanadium oxide catalyst at 250–400 °C and atmospheric pressure (methanol conversion, 98–99%). By-products are carbon monoxide, dimethyl ether and small amounts of carbon dioxide and formic acid (Bizzari, 2000; Reuss *et al.*, 2003; Gerberich & Seaman, 2004).

Paraformaldehyde, a solid polymer of formaldehyde, consists of a mixture of poly-(oxymethylene) glycols [$HO–(CH_2O)_n–H$; $n = 8–100$]. The formaldehyde content is 90–99%, depending on the degree of polymerization, the value of n and product specifications; the remainder is bound or free water. As a convenient source of formaldehyde for certain applications, paraformaldehyde is prepared commercially by the concentration of aqueous formaldehyde solutions under vacuum in the presence of small amounts of formic acid and metal formates. An alternative solid source of formaldehyde is the cyclic trimer of formaldehyde, 1,3,5-trioxane, which is prepared commercially by strong acid-catalysed condensation of formaldehyde in a continuous process (Bizzari, 2000; Reuss *et al.*, 2003; Gerberich & Seaman, 2004).

Available information indicates that formaldehyde was produced by 104 companies in China, 19 companies in India, 18 companies in the USA, 15 companies each in Italy and Mexico, 14 companies in Russia, 11 companies each in Brazil and Japan, eight companies each in Canada and Germany, seven companies each in China (Province of Taiwan), Malaysia and the United Kingdom, six companies each in Argentina and Spain, five companies in Belgium, four companies each in Colombia, France, Iran, the Netherlands and Thailand, three companies each in Chile, Israel, Poland, Portugal, the Republic of Korea, Sweden, Turkey and the Ukraine, two companies each in Australia, Austria, Ecuador, Egypt, Pakistan, Peru, Romania and Serbia and Montenegro, and one company each in Algeria, Azerbaijan, Bulgaria, Denmark, Estonia, Finland, Greece, Hungary, Indonesia, Ireland, Lithuania, Norway, Saudi Arabia, Singapore, Slovakia, Slovenia, South Africa, Switzerland, Uzbekistan and Venezuela (Chemical Information Services, 2004).

Available information indicates that paraformaldehyde was produced by eight companies in China, four companies each in Germany and India, three companies each in Russia and the USA, two companies each in China (Province of Taiwan), Iran, Mexico and Spain and one company each in Canada, Egypt, Israel, Italy, Japan, the Netherlands, the Republic of Korea, Romania, Saudi Arabia and the United Kingdom (Chemical Information Services, 2004).

Available information indicates that 1,3,5-trioxane was produced by three companies in Germany, two companies each in China, India and the USA and one company in Poland (Chemical Information Services, 2004).

Production of formaldehyde in selected years from 1983 to 2000 and in selected countries is shown in Table 2. Worldwide capacity, production and consumption of formaldehyde in 2000 are shown in Table 3.

Table 2. Production of 37% formaldehyde in selected regions (thousand tonnes)

Country or region	1983	1985	1990	1995	2000
North America					
Canada	256	288	288	521	675
Mexico	79	106	118	139	136
USA	2520[a]	2663	3402	3946	4650
Western Europe[b]	3757	3991	4899	5596	6846[c]
Japan	1089	1202	1444	1351	1396

From Bizzari (2000)
[a] Data for 1980
[b] Includes Austria, Belgium, Denmark, Finland, France, Germany, Greece, Ireland, Italy, the Netherlands, Norway, Portugal, Spain, Sweden, Switzerland and the United Kingdom
[c] Data for 1999

1.2.2 Use

Worldwide patterns of use for formaldehyde in 2000 are shown in Table 4. The most extensive use of formaldehyde is in the production of resins with urea, phenol and melamine, and of polyacetal resins. Formaldehyde-based resins are used as adhesives and impregnating resins in the manufacture of particle-board, plywood, furniture and other wood products; for the production of curable moulding materials (appliances, electric controls, telephones, wiring services); and as raw materials for surface coatings and controlled-release nitrogen fertilizers. They are also used in the textile, leather, rubber and cement industries. Further uses are as binders for foundry sand, stonewool and glasswool mats in insulating materials, abrasive paper and brake linings (WHO, 1989; IARC, 1995; Reuss *et al.*, 2003; Gerberich & Seaman, 2004).

Another major use of formaldehyde is as an intermediate in the synthesis of other industrial chemical compounds, such as 1,4-butanediol, trimethylolpropane and neopentyl glycol, that are used in the manufacture of polyurethane and polyester plastics, synthetic resin coatings, synthetic lubricating oils and plasticizers. Other compounds produced from formaldehyde include pentaerythritol, which is used primarily in raw materials for surface coatings and explosives, and hexamethylenetetramine, which is used as a cross-linking agent for phenol–formaldehyde resins and explosives. The complexing agents, nitrilotriacetic acid (see IARC, 1990a) and ethylenediaminetetraacetic acid, are derived from formaldehyde and are components of some detergents. Formaldehyde is used for the production of 4,4′-methylenediphenyl diisocyanate (see IARC, 1979), which is a constituent of polyurethanes that are used in the production of soft and rigid foams, as adhesives and to bond particle-board (WHO, 1989; IARC, 1995; Reuss *et al.*, 2003; Gerberich & Seaman, 2004).

Polyacetal plastics produced by the polymerization of formaldehyde are incorporated into automobiles to reduce weight and fuel consumption, and are used to make functional

Table 3. World supply and demand for 37% formaldehyde in 2000 (thousand tonnes)

Country/region	Production	Consumption
North America		
Canada	675	620
Mexico	136	137
USA	4 650	4 459
South and Central America[a]	638	636
Western Europe[b]	7 100	7 054
Eastern Europe[c]	1 582	1 577
Middle East[d]	454	438
Japan	1 396	1 395
Africa[e]	102	102
Asia		
China	1 750	1 752
Indonesia	891	892
Malaysia	350	350
Republic of Korea	580	580
Other[f]	789	795
Australia and New Zealand	304	304
Total	21 547	21 091

From Bizzari (2000)

[a] Includes Argentina, Brazil, Chile, Colombia, Ecuador, Peru, Uruguay and Venezuela

[b] Includes Austria, Belgium, Denmark, Finland, France, Germany, Greece, Ireland, Italy, the Netherlands, Norway, Portugal, Spain, Sweden, Switzerland and the United Kingdom

[c] Includes Bulgaria, the Czech Republic, Hungary, Lithuania, Poland, Romania, Russia, Slovakia, Slovenia, the Ukraine and Yugoslavia

[d] Includes Iran, Israel, Saudi Arabia and Turkey

[e] Includes Algeria, Nigeria, South Africa and Tunisia

[f] Includes Bangladesh, Cambodia, China (Province of Taiwan), Democratic People's Republic of Korea, India, Laos, Myanmar, Pakistan, the Philippines, Singapore, Sri Lanka, Thailand and Viet Nam

components of audio and video electronic equipment. Formaldehyde is also the basis for products that are used to manufacture dyes, tanning agents, precursors of dispersion and plastics, extraction agents, crop protection agents, animal feeds, perfumes, vitamins, flavourings and drugs (WHO, 1989; Reuss et al., 2003).

Formaldehyde itself is used to preserve and disinfect, for example, human and veterinary drugs and biological materials (viral vaccines contain 0.05% formalin as an inactivating agent), to disinfect hospital wards and to preserve and embalm biological specimens. Formaldehyde and medications that contain formaldehyde are also used in dentistry (Lewis, 1998). Formaldehyde is used as an antimicrobial agent in many cosmetics products,

Table 4. Worldwide use patterns (%) of formaldehyde in 2000

Region or country	Use (million tonnes)	UFR	PFR	PAR	MFR	BDO	MDI	PE	HMTA	TMP	Other[a]
USA	4.5	24.2	16.6	12.7	3.1	11.2	6.8	5.0	2.6		17.8[b]
Canada	0.62	51.3	32.3		3.2			12.9			
Mexico	0.14	70.8	11.7		5.1				11.7		0.7
South and Central America[c]	0.64	55.8	18.9		7.9		1.6	10.8			5.0
Western Europe[d]	7.1	44.4	8.6	7.1	7.5	6.7	5.4	5.4	2.0	2.1	10.9
Eastern Europe[e]	1.6	71.5	5.1		3.2			4.4	8.8		6.9
Africa[f]	0.10	70.6	14.7		7.8						6.9
Middle East[g]	0.43	75.1	4.6		14.8						5.5
Japan	1.4	12.3	7.7	32.9	4.8	2.1	8.4	6.7	2.2	2.2	20.7[h]
Asia[i]	4.4	54.2	9.8	8.4	8.7			5.8	2.9		10.2
Oceania[j]	0.30	67.4	12.2		20.4						

From Bizzari (2000)

UFR, urea–formaldehyde resins; PFR, phenol–formaldehyde resins; PAR, polyacetal resins; MFR, melamine–formaldehyde resins; BDO, 1,4-butane-diol; MDI, 4,4′-diphenylmethane diisocyanate; PE, pentaerythritol; HMTA, hexamethylenetetramine; TMP, trimethylolpropane

[a] Not defined

[b] Including chelating agents, trimethylolpropane, trimethylolethane, paraformaldehyde, herbicides, neopentyl glycol, pyridine chemicals, nitroparaffin derivatives, textile treating and controlled-release fertilizer

[c] Includes Argentina, Brazil, Chile, Colombia, Ecuador, Peru, Uruguay and Venezuela

[d] Includes Austria, Belgium, Denmark, Finland, France, Germany, Greece, Ireland, Italy, the Netherlands, Norway, Portugal, Spain, Sweden, Switzerland and the United Kingdom

[e] Includes Bulgaria, the Czech Republic, Hungary, Lithuania, Poland, Romania, Russia, Slovakia, Slovenia, the Ukraine and Yugoslavia

[f] Includes Algeria, Nigeria, South Africa and Tunisia

[g] Includes Iran, Israel, Saudi Arabia and Turkey

[h] Including 6.4% for paraformaldehyde

[i] Includes Bangladesh, Cambodia, China, China (Province of Taiwan), Democratic People's Republic of Korea, India, Indonesia, Laos, Malaysia, Myanmar, Pakistan, the Philippines, Republic of Korea, Singapore, Sri Lanka, Thailand and Viet Nam

[j] Includes Australia and New Zealand

including soaps, shampoos, hair preparations, deodorants, lotions, make-up, mouthwashes and nail products (Cosmetic Ingredient Review Expert Panel, 1984; Reuss *et al.*, 2003).

Formaldehyde is also used directly to inhibit corrosion, in mirror finishing and electroplating, in the electrodeposition of printed circuits and in the development of photographic films (Reuss *et al.*, 2003).

Paraformaldehyde is used in place of aqueous solutions of formaldehyde, especially when the presence of water interferes, e.g. in the plastics industry for the preparation of phenol, urea and melamine resins, varnish resins, thermosets and foundry resins. Other uses include the synthesis of chemical and pharmaceutical products (e.g. Prins reaction, chloromethylation, Mannich reaction), the production of textile products (e.g. for crease-resistant finishes), the preparation of disinfectants and deodorants (Reuss *et al.*, 2003) and in selected pesticide applications (Environmental Protection Agency, 1993).

1.3   Occurrence

Formaldehyde is a gaseous pollutant from many outdoor and indoor sources. Outdoors, major sources of formaldehyde include power plants, manufacturing facilities, incinerators and automobile exhaust emissions. Forest fires and other natural sources of combustion also introduce formaldehyde into the ambient air. Other than in occupational settings, the highest levels of airborne formaldehyde have been detected indoors where it is released from various building materials, consumer products and tobacco smoke. Formaldehyde may be present in food, either naturally or as a result of contamination (Suh *et al.*, 2000).

Natural and anthropogenic sources of formaldehyde in the environment, and environmental levels in indoor and outdoor air, water, soil and food have been reviewed (WHO, 1989; IARC, 1995; ATSDR, 1999).

1.3.1   *Natural occurrence*

Formaldehyde is ubiquitous in the environment; it is an endogenous chemical that occurs in most life forms, including humans. It is formed naturally in the troposphere during the oxidation of hydrocarbons, which react with hydroxyl radicals and ozone to form formaldehyde and other aldehydes as intermediates in a series of reactions that ultimately lead to the formation of carbon monoxide and dioxide, hydrogen and water. Of the hydrocarbons found in the troposphere, methane is the single most important source of formaldehyde. Terpenes and isoprene that are emitted by foliage react with hydroxyl radicals to form formaldehyde as an intermediate product. Because of their short half-life, these sources of formaldehyde are important only in the vicinity of vegetation. Formaldehyde is one of the volatile compounds that are formed in the early stages of decomposition of plant residues in the soil, and occurs naturally in fruit and other foods (WHO, 1989; IARC, 1995).

An overview of the formation and occurrence of formaldehyde in living organisms has been reported (Kalász, 2003). The reader is referred to Section 4.1 for a discussion of blood levels of endogenously formed formaldehyde in humans.

1.3.2   *Occupational exposure*

Estimates of the number of persons who are occupationally exposed to formaldehyde worldwide are not available. However, an estimate of the number of people who were exposed in the European Union in the early 1990s is available from the International Information System on Occupational Exposure to Carcinogens (more commonly referred to as CAREX) (Kauppinen *et al.*, 2000). Approximate numbers of persons who were exposed to levels of formaldehyde above 0.1 ppm [0.12 mg/m^3] are presented by major industry sector in Table 5. While these are not precise estimates, they do indicate that exposure to formaldehyde, at least at low levels, may occur in a wide variety of industries.

Three main sets of circumstances may lead to occupational exposure to formaldehyde. The first is related to the production of aqueous solutions of formaldehyde (formalin) and their use in the chemical industry, e.g. for the synthesis of various resins, as a preservative in medical laboratories and embalming fluids and as a disinfectant. A second set is related to its release from formaldehyde-based resins in which it is present as a residue and/or through their hydrolysis and decomposition by heat, e.g. during the manufacture of wood products, textiles, synthetic vitreous insulation products and plastics. In general, the use of phenol–formaldehyde resins results in much lower emissions of formaldehyde than that of urea- and melamine-based resins. A third set of circumstances is related to the pyrolysis or combustion of organic matter, e.g. in engine exhaust gases or during firefighting.

(a)   *Manufacture of formaldehyde, formaldehyde-based resins and other chemical products*

Concentrations of formaldehyde measured in the 1980s during the manufacture of formaldehyde and formaldehyde-based resins are summarized in Table 6. More recent data were not available to the Working Group.

Mean levels during the manufacture of formaldehyde were below 1 ppm [1.2 mg/m^3]. These workers may also be exposed to methanol (starting material), carbon monoxide, carbon dioxide and hydrogen (process gases) (Stewart *et al.*, 1987).

The reported mean concentrations in the air of factories that produce formaldehyde-based resins vary from < 1 to > 10 ppm [< 1.2 to > 12.3 mg/m^3]. There are obvious differences between factories (the earliest measurements date from 1979) but no consistent seasonal variation. Chemicals other than formaldehyde to which exposure may occur depend on the types of resin manufactured: urea, phenol, melamine and furfural alcohol are the chemicals most commonly reacted with liquid formaldehyde (formalin). Some processes require the addition of ammonia, and alcohols are used as solvents in the production of liquid resins (Stewart *et al.*, 1987).

Table 5. Approximate number of workers exposed to formaldehyde above background levels (0.1 ppm) in the European Union, 1990–93

Industry	Estimate
Manufacture of furniture and fixtures, except primarily of metal	179 000
Medical, dental, other health and veterinary services	174 000
Manufacture of wearing apparel, except footwear	94 000
Manufacture of wood and wood and cork products, except furniture	70 000
Personal and household services	62 000
Construction	60 000
Manufacture of textiles	37 000
Iron and steel basic industries	29 000
Manufacture of fabricated metal products, except machinery	29 000
Manufacture of other non-metallic mineral products	23 000
Manufacture of machinery, except electrical	20 000
Manufacture of industrial chemicals	17 000
Manufacture of other chemical products	17 000
Manufacture of plastic products not classified elsewhere	16 000
Agriculture and hunting	16 000
Manufacture of paper and paper products	13 000
Printing, publishing and allied industries	13 000
Wholesale and retail trade and restaurants and hotels	13 000
Manufacture of transport equipment	11 000
Manufacture of electrical machinery, apparatus and appliances	10 000
Manufacture of footwear	9 000
Manufacture of glass and glass products	8 000
Research and scientific institutes	7 000
Non-ferrous metal basic industries	6 000
Manufacture of leather and products of leather or of its substitutes	6 000
Beverage industries	4 000
Manufacture of instruments, photographic and optical	4 000
Other manufacturing industries	3 000
Food manufacturing	3 000
Crude petroleum and natural gas production	2 000
Manufacture of rubber products	4 000
Financing, insurance, real estate and business services	3 000
Education services	2 000
Sanitary and similar services	2 000
Services allied to transport	2 000
Manufacture of miscellaneous products of petroleum and coal	1 000
Other industries	2 000
Total (all industries)	971 000

From Kauppinen *et al.* (2000); CAREX (2003)

Table 6. Concentrations of formaldehyde in the workroom air in formaldehyde and resin manufacturing plants

Industry and operation	No. of measurements	Mean[a] (ppm [mg/m³])	Range (ppm [mg/m³])	Year	Reference
Special chemical manufacturing plant (USA)	8	NR	< 0.03–1.6 [0.04–2.0]	NR	Blade (1983)
Production of formaldehyde (Sweden)	9	0.3 [0.3]	NR	1980s	Rosén et al. (1984)
Resin manufacture (Sweden)	22	0.5 [0.6]	NR	1980s	Rosén et al. (1984)
Formaldehyde manufacture (USA)				1983	Stewart et al. (1987)
Plant no. 2, summer	15	0.6[b] [0.7]	0.03–1.9 [0.04–2.3]		
Plant no. 10, summer	9	0.7[b] [0.9]	0.6–0.8 [0.7–1.0]		
Resin manufacture (USA)				1983–84	Stewart et al. (1987)
Plant no. 1, summer	24	3.4[b] [4.2]	0.2–13.2 [0.3–16.2]		
Plant no. 6, summer[c]	6	0.2[b] [0.3]	0.1–0.2 [0.1–0.3]		
Plant no. 7, summer	9	0.2[b] [0.3]	0.1–0.3 [0.1–0.4]		
Plant no. 7, winter	9	0.6[b] [0.7]	0.4–0.9 [0.5–1.1]		
Plant no. 8, summer[c,d]	13	0.4[b] [0.7]	0.2–0.8 [0.3–1.0]		
Plant no. 8, winter[c,d]	9	0.1[b] [0.1]	0.1–0.2 [0.1–0.3]		
Plant no. 9, summer[c,d]	8	14.2[b] [17.5]	4.1–30.5 [5.0–37.5]		
Plant no. 9, winter	9	1.7[b] [2.1]	1.1–2.5 [1.4–3.1]		
Plant no. 10, summer[d]	23	0.7[b] [0.9]	0.3–1.2 [0.4–1.5]		
Chemical factory producing formaldehyde and formaldehyde resins (Sweden)	62	0.2 [0.3]	0.04–0.4 [0.05–0.5]	1979–85	Holmström et al. (1989a)
Resin plant (Finland)					Heikkilä et al. (1991)
Furan resin production	3	2.3 [2.9]	1.0–3.4 [1.3–4.2]	1982	
Maintenance	4	2.9 [3.6]	1.4–5.5 [1.8–6.9]	1981	
Urea–formaldehyde resin production	7	0.7 [0.9]	0.6–0.8 [0.7–1.1]	1981	

NR, not reported
[a] Arithmetic mean unless otherwise specified
[b] Mean and range of geometric means
Some of the results were affected by the simultaneous occurrence in the samples (Stewart et al., 1987) of:
[c] phenol (leading to low values)
[d] particulates that contained nascent formaldehyde (leading to high values).

No measurements of exposure to formaldehyde in other chemical plants where it is used, e.g. in the production of pentaerythritol, hexamethylenetetramine or ethylene glycol, were available to the Working Group.

(b)   Histopathology and disinfection in hospitals

Formalin is commonly used to preserve tissue samples in histopathology laboratories. Concentrations of formaldehyde are sometimes high, e.g. during tissue disposal, preparation of formalin and changing of tissue processor solutions (Belanger & Kilburn, 1981). The usual mean concentration during exposure is approximately 0.5 ppm [0.6 mg/m^3]. Other agents to which pathologists and histology technicians may be exposed include xylene (see IARC, 1989a), toluene (see IARC, 1989b), chloroform (see IARC, 1987c) and methyl methacrylate (see IARC, 1994a) (Belanger & Kilburn, 1981). Concentrations of airborne formaldehyde in histopathology laboratories and during disinfection in hospitals are presented in Table 7.

Levels of formaldehyde were measured in 10 histology laboratories using area samplers for 1–4 h for a study of neurobehavioural and respiratory symptoms. Concentrations of formaldehyde in areas where tissue specimens were prepared and sampled were 0.25–2.3 mg/m^3 (Kilburn et al., 1985). In two studies in Israel, pathology staff were divided into two groups: those who had low exposure (mean, 0.5 mg/m^3), which included laboratory assistants and technicians, and those who had high exposure (mean, 2.8 mg/m^3), which included physicians and hospital orderlies, based on 15-min samples (Shaham et al., 2002, 2003). Another study by the same group [it is not clear whether these are the same data or not] reported 15-min area measurements of 1.7–2.0 mg/m^3 and personal measurements of 3.4–3.8 mg/m^3 during exposure (Shaham et al., 1996a,b).

Formaldehyde has also been used extensively in hospitals for disinfection (IARC, 1995; see Table 7).

(c)   Embalming and anatomy laboratories

Formaldehyde is used as a tissue preservative and disinfectant in embalming fluids (Table 7). Some parts of bodies that are to be embalmed are also cauterized and sealed with a hardening compound that contains paraformaldehyde powder. The concentration of formaldehyde in the air during embalming depends on its content in the embalming fluid, the type of body, ventilation and work practices; mean levels are approximately 1 ppm [1.2 mg/m^3]. Embalming of a normal intact body usually takes approximately 1 h. Disinfectant sprays are occasionally used, and these may release small amounts of solvent, such as isopropanol (Williams et al., 1984). Methanol is used as a stabilizer in embalming fluids, and concentrations of 0.5–22 ppm [0.7–28.4 mg/m^3] have been measured during embalming. Low levels of phenol have also been detected in embalming rooms (Stewart et al., 1992).

Skisak (1983) measured levels of formaldehyde in the breathing zone at dissecting tables and in the ambient air in a medical school in the USA for 12 weeks. Concentrations of > 1.2 mg/m^3 formaldehyde were found in 44% of the breathing zone samples and

Table 7. Concentrations of formaldehyde in the workroom air of mortuaries, hospitals and laboratories

Industry and operation (location) / Type of sample	No. of measurements	Mean [a] (ppm [mg/m³])	Range (ppm [mg/m³])	Year	Reference
Histopathology laboratories					
Pathology laboratory (Sweden)	13	0.5 [0.7]	NR	1980s	Rosén et al. (1984)
Histology laboratory, tissue specimen preparation and sampling (USA)	NR	NR	0.2–1.9 [0.25–2.3]	NR	Kilburn et al. (1985)
Pathology laboratories (Germany)	21	0.5 [b] [0.6]	< 0.01–1.2 [< 0.01–1.6]	1980–88	Triebig et al. (1989)
Hospital laboratories (Finland)	80	0.5 [0.6]	0.01–7.3 [0.01–9.1]	1981–86	Heikkilä et al. (1991)
Histology laboratory (Israel)				NR	Shaham et al. (1996a,b)
Area samples	NR	NR	1.4–1.6 [1.7–2.0]		
Personal samples	NR	NR	2.8–3.1 [3.4–3.8]		
Teaching laboratory (USA)	16	0.3 [0.4]	max., < 2 [< 2.5]	NR	Tan et al. (1999)
Pathology laboratories (Turkey)	10	NR		NR	Burgaz et al. (2001)
Histology laboratory (Israel)	NR			NR	Shaham et al. (2002)
Laboratory assistants/technicians (15 min)		0.4 [0.5]	0.04–0.7 [0.05–0.9]		
Physicians and orderlies (15 min)		2.2 [2.8]	0.7–5.6 [0.9–7.0]		
Disinfection in hospitals					
Cleaning hospital floors with detergent containing formaldehyde (Italy) / Personal samples (38–74 min)	4	0.18 [0.22]	0.15–0.21 [0.18–0.26]	NR	Bernardini et al. (1983)
Disinfection of dialysis clinic (USA) / Personal samples (37–63 min)	7	0.6 [0.8]	0.09–1.8 [0.12–2.2]	1983	Salisbury (1983)
Disinfecting operating theatres (Germany)	43	0.4 [c] [0.5]	0.04–1.4 [0.05–1.7]	NR	Elias (1987)
Bedrooms in hospital (Germany)	14	0.05 [0.06]	< 0.01–0.7 [< 0.01–0.9]	1980–88	Triebig et al. (1989)
Disinfecting operating theatres (Germany) [d]				NR	Binding & Witting (1990)
3% cleaning solution	43	0.8 [1.1]	0.01–5.1 [0.01–6.3]		
0.5 % cleaning solution	26	0.2 [0.2]	0.01–0.4 [0.01–0.5]		
Disinfection in hospitals (Finland)	18	0.1 [0.1]	0.03–0.2 [0.04–0.3]	1981–86	Heikkilä et al. (1991)

Table 7 (contd)

Industry and operation (location) Type of sample	No. of measurements	Mean[a] (ppm [mg/m³])	Range (ppm [mg/m³])	Year	Reference
Embalming					
Embalming, six funeral homes (USA)	NR	0.7 [0.9]	0.09–5.3 [0.1–6.5]	NR	Kerfoot & Mooney (1975)
Autopsy service (USA)[d]				NR	Coldiron et al. (1983)
Personal samples	27	1.3[c] [1.7]	0.4–3.3 [0.5–4.0]		
Area samples	23	4.2 [5]	0.1–13.6 [0.1–16.7]		
Museum, taxidermy (Sweden)	8	0.2 [0.3]	NR	1980s	Rosén et al. (1984)
Embalming, seven funeral homes				1980	Williams et al. (1984)
Intact bodies (personal samples)	8	0.3 [0.4]	0.18–0.3 [0.2–0.4]		
Autopsied bodies (personal samples)	15	0.9 [1.1]	0–2.1 [0–2.6]		
Embalming, 23 mortuaries (USA)	NR	1.1 [1.4]	0.03–3.2 [0.04–3.9]	NR	Lamont Moore & Ogrodnik (1986)
8-h TWA		0.2 [0.2]	0.01–0.5 [0.01–0.6]		
Autopsy (Finland)	5	0.7 [0.8]	< 0.1–1.4 [< 0.1–1.7]	1981–86	Heikkilä et al. (1991)
Embalming (USA)				NR	Stewart et al. (1992)
Personal samples	25	2.6 [3.2]	0.3–8.7 [0.4–10.7]		
Area 1	25	2.0 [3.0]	0.2–7.5 [0.3–9.2]		
Area 2	25	2.2 [2.7]	0.3–8.2 [0.3–10.0]		
Embalming (Canada)				NR	Korczynski (1994)
Intact bodies (personal samples)	24	0.6 [0.8]	0.1–4.6 [0.1–5.6]		
Autopsied bodies (personal samples)	24	0.6 [0.8]	0.09–3.3 [0.1–4.1]		
Area samples	72	0.5 [0.6]	0.04–6.8 [0.05–8.4]		
Funeral home, embalming (USA)				NR	Korczynski (1996)
Area samples	4	NR	< 0.1–0.15 [< 0.1–0.19]		
Personal samples	4	0.16 [0.19]	NR		
Anatomy laboratories					
Anatomy laboratory, dissecting (USA) Personal samples	54	NR	0.3–2.6 [0.4–3.2]	NR	Skisak (1983)

Table 7 (contd)

Industry and operation (location) / Type of sample	No. of measurements	Mean[a] (ppm [mg/m³])	Range (ppm [mg/m³])	Year	Reference
Anatomy laboratory, dissecting (USA)				1982–83	Korky (1987)
Laboratory	NR	NR	7–16.5 [8.6–20.3]		
Stock room	NR	NR	2.0–2.6 [2.4–3.2]		
Public hallway	NR	NR	max., < 1 [< 1.2]		
Anatomical theatre (Germany)	29	1.1[b] [1.4]	0.7–1.7 [0.9–2.2]	1980–88	Triebig et al. (1989)
Anatomy laboratory, dissecting (USA)				NR	Akbar-Khanzadeh et al. (1994)
Personal samples (1.2–3.1 h)	32	1.2 [1.5]	0.07–2.9 [0.09–3.6]		
Personal samples (TWA)	NR	0.4 [0.5]	0.09–0.95 [0.11–1.17]		
Area samples (2.5 min)	13	1.4 [1.7]	0.9–1.8 [1.1–2.2]		
Area samples (TWA)	2	1.7 [2.0]	1.0–2.3 [1.2–2.8]		
Anatomy laboratory, dissecting (USA)				NR	Akbar-Kahnzadeh & Mlynek (1997)
Personal samples	44	1.9 [2.3]	0.3–4.5 [0.4–5.5]		
Area samples	76	1.0 [1.2]	0.6–1.7 [0.7–2.1]		
Anatomy laboratory, dissecting (China)	25	0.4 [0.5]	0.06–1.04 [0.07–1.28]	NR	Ying et al. (1997, 1999)
Anatomy laboratory, dissecting (China)	NR	2.4 [2.9]	NR	NR	He et al. (1998)
Anatomy/histology laboratory, dissecting	48	3.0 [3.7]	0.2–9.1 [0.2–11.2]	NR	Kim et al. (1999)
Anatomy laboratory, dissecting (Austria)	NR	0.22 [0.27]	0.11–0.33 [0.13–0.41]	NR	Wantke et al. (2000)
Two locations in a room over 4 weeks	NR	0.12 [0.15]	0.06–0.22 [0.07–0.27]	NR	Wantke et al. (1996b)
Anatomy laboratory, dissecting (Turkey)	NR	NR	max., < 4 [< 5]	NR	Burgaz et al. (2001)
Anatomy laboratory, dissecting (USA)	15	0.9 [1.1]	0.3–2.6 [0.3–3.1]	NR	Keil et al. (2001)
Biology laboratory, dissecting (Canada)				NR	Dufresne et al. (2002)
Laboratory 1	18	0.20 [0.25]	0.08–0.62 [0.11–0.76]		
Laboratory 2	18	0.51 [0.63]	0.3–1.2 [0.3–1.5]		
Anatomy laboratory, dissecting (Japan)	NR	NR	0.11–0.62 [0.14–0.76]	NR	Tanaka et al. (2003)

NR, not reported; TWA, time-weighted average
[a] Arithmetic means unless otherwise specified
[b] Median
[c] Mean of arithmetic means
[d] 8-h TWA

11 ambient air samples; the levels in breathing zone samples were in the range of 0.4–3.2 mg/m³, and 50% of the samples contained 0.7–1.2 mg/m³.

Korky *et al.* (1987) studied the dissecting facilities at a university in the USA during the 1982–83 academic year. Airborne concentrations of formaldehyde were 7–16.5 ppm [8.6–20.3 mg/m³] in the laboratory, 1.97–2.62 ppm [2.4–3.2 mg/m³] in the stockroom and < 1 ppm [< 1.2 mg/m³] in the public hallway.

Concentrations of formaldehyde in the breathing zone of two embalmers in the USA were measured during the embalming of an autopsied body, which generally results in higher exposures than that of non-autopsied bodies. The average was 0.19 mg/m³ [duration of measurement not provided] (Korczynski, 1996).

Samples (1–2-h) taken in an anatomy/histology laboratory in the Republic of Korea for a cross-sectional study of serum antibodies showed concentrations of formaldehyde that ranged from 0.19 to 11.25 mg/m³ with a mean of 3.74 mg/m³ (Kim *et al.*, 1999).

In a cross-sectional study of immunoglobulin (Ig)E sensitization in Austria, concentrations of formaldehyde were measured in two locations in a dissection room for the full period that students were present. The mean level was 0.15 mg/m³ (Wantke *et al.*, 1996a,b). The windows were open and the ventilation was working continuously. In a second study in the same laboratories, medical students were exposed to an average indoor concentration of 0.27 mg/m³ formaldehyde (Wantke *et al.*, 2000).

Levels of formaldehyde measured in anatomy laboratories in China for a cytogenetic study averaged 0.51 mg/m³ over a 3-h period; the peak occurred while cadavers were being dissected (Ying *et al.*, 1997, 1999).

A cross-sectional study on the cytogenetic effects of formaldehyde on anatomy students in China found personal exposures of 2.92 mg/m³ (He *et al.*, 1998).

In a study of respiratory function, 34 personal samples and short-term area samples were collected in a gross anatomy laboratory in the USA. The mean concentration of formaldehyde in the room was 1.53 mg/m³ during the 1.2–3.1-h dissecting period. The direct-reading short-term area samples (2.5-min) averaged 1.68 mg/m³. Eight-hour time-weighted average (TWA) personal exposures ranged from 0.11 to 1.17 mg/m³, with a mean of 0.52 mg/m³ (96% of subjects were exposed to levels of formaldehyde above the 0.38 mg/m³ ceiling, and the 8-h TWA exposure of 3% of them was above 0.94 mg/m³) (Akbar-Khanzadeh *et al.*, 1994). A subsequent study of respiratory function was conducted in the same laboratory because, among other reasons, the concentration of formaldehyde in the embalming solution was increased. The mean concentration of formaldehyde in the personal samples was 2.31 mg/m³ (duration, 2.5 h) (Akbar-Khanzadeh & Mlynek, 1997). In the same laboratory, area measurements were taken in the centre of and at various locations in the room over a 16-week period; each measurement lasted for the time the students were active during a session (3–4 h per day). The average concentration in the centre of the room was 1.13 mg/m³ (15 measurements) (Keil *et al.*, 2001). Breathing zone concentrations were expected to be higher because of the proximity of the students to the cadaver during dissection. Although the room had mechanical air supply and exhaust systems, the ventilation system served the entire building and intake air was contaminated with formaldehyde.

The concentration of formaldehyde in the air in pathology and anatomy laboratories in Turkey did not exceed 2 and 4 mg/m^3, respectively [no other information available], when measured in a study of cytogenetic responses (Burgaz *et al.*, 2001).

In a study of two biological laboratories in Canada where dissection of animal specimens was performed, 3-h personal samples showed mean concentrations of 0.25 mg/m^3 and 0.63 mg/m^3 formaldehyde, respectively (Dufresne *et al.*, 2002). The first laboratory had a general mechanical ventilation system, whereas the second had no ventilation system.

Measurements in an anatomy class in Japan rose to 0.76 mg/m^3 after 10 min of class; 30 min later, the formaldehyde concentration had decreased to 0.14 mg/m^3 (Tanaka *et al.*, 2003).

(*d*)   *Manufacture of wood products and paper*

Exposure to formaldehyde may occur in several sectors of the wood-related industries because of the use of formaldehyde-based resins. Table 8 summarizes the concentrations of formaldehyde observed in the wood product and pulp and paper industries.

Exposure to formaldehyde is typically monitored by measuring its gaseous form; slight additional exposure may occur through the inhalation of formaldehyde bound to wood dust, although this was considered to be negligible in one study (Gosselin *et al.*, 2003). For example, at a plant in the USA that constructed products made of particle-board, measurements were taken for 4.5 h at the sawing operation. A back-up impinger was positioned behind an inhalable dust sampler or a closed-face cassette to capture both dust-bound and gaseous formaldehyde. Levels of formaldehyde gas behind the inhalable dust sampler averaged [132 μg/m^3 (standard deviation [SD], 14 μg/m^3; four samples)] and those of bound formaldehyde from inhalable dust averaged [11 μg/m^3 (SD, 4 μg/m^3; 12 samples)]. Respective measurements for the closed cassettes averaged [147 μg/m^3 (SD, 9 μg/m^3; four samples)] and [8 μg/m^3 (SD, 2 μg/m^3; 12 samples)] (Kennedy *et al.*, 1992).

(i)   *Veneer and plywood mills*

Plywood consists of three or more veneers glued together or a core of solid wood strips or particle-board with veneered top and bottom surfaces. The dried panels may also be patched or spliced by applying a liquid formaldehyde-based adhesive to the edges, pressing the edges together and applying heat to cure the resin. To produce panels, veneers are roller- or spray-coated with formaldehyde-based resins, then placed between unglued veneers. The plywood industry has used formaldehyde-based glues in assembling of plywood for over 50 years. Before the introduction of formaldehyde-based resins in the 1940s, soya bean and blood–albumen adhesives were used, and cold pressing of panels was common. Exposure to formaldehyde from resins may occur among workers during the preparation of glue, during splicing, patching, sanding and hot-pressing operations and among nearby workers. Urea-based resins release formaldehyde more readily during curing than phenol-based resins; however, improvements in the formulation of resins have reduced exposures.

Table 8. Concentrations of formaldehyde in the workroom air of plywood mills, particle-board mills, furniture factories, other wood product plants, paper mills and the construction industry

Industry and operation (location) / Type of sample	No. of measurements	Mean[a] (ppm [mg/m³])	Range (ppm [mg/m³])	Year	Reference
Plywood mills					
Plywood production (Sweden)	47	0.3 [0.4]	NR	1980s	Rosén et al. (1984)
Plywood mills (Finland)					Kauppinen (1986)
Glue preparation, short-term	15	2.2 [2.7]	0.6–5.0 [0.7–6.2]	1965–74	
Glue preparation, short-term	19	0.7 [0.9]	0.1–2.3 [0.1–2.8]	1975–84	
Assembling	32	1.5 [1.9]	< 0.1–4.4 [< 0.1–5.4]	1965–74	
Assembling	55	0.6 [0.7]	0.02–6.8 [0.03–8.3]	1975–84	
Hot pressing	41	2.0 [2.5]	< 0.1–7.7 [< 0.1–9.5]	1965–74	
Hot pressing	43	0.5 [0.6]	0.06–2.1 [0.07–2.6]	1975–84	
Sawing of plywood	5	0.5 [0.6]	0.3–0.8 [0.4–1.0]	1965–74	
Sawing of plywood	12	0.1 [0.1]	0.02–0.2 [0.03–0.3]	1975–84	
Coating of plywood	7	1.0 [1.2]	0.5–1.8 [0.6–2.2]	1965–74	
Coating of plywood	28	0.3 [0.4]	0.02–0.6 [0.03–0.7]	1975–84	
Plywood panelling manufacture (USA)				1983–84	Stewart et al. (1987)
Plant no. 3, winter	27	0.2[b] [0.3]	0.08–0.4 [1.0–0.5]		
Plant no. 3, summer	26	0.1[b] [0.1]	0.01–0.5 [0.01–0.6]		
Plywood mill (Indonesia)	40	0.6 [0.8]	0.2–2.3 [0.3–2.8]	NR	Malaka & Kodama (1990)
Plywood factory (Italy)				NR	Ballarin et al. (1992)
Warehouse	3	0.3 [0.4]	0.1–0.5 [0.2–0.6]		
Shearing press	8	0.08 [0.1]	0.06–0.11 [0.08–0.14]		
Plywood mill (Finland)				1996–97	Mäkinen et al. (1999)
Personal samples					
Patching	6	0.06 [0.07]	0.02–0.08 [0.03–0.10]		
Feeding of drying machine	6	0.05 [0.06]	0.01–0.12 [0.01–0.15]		
Forklift driving	6	0.06 [0.07]	0.02–0.16 [0.02–0.20]		
Scaring	6	0.11 [0.14]	0.06–0.20 [0.07–0.24]		
Assembly (machine I)	4	0.24 [0.30]	0.08–0.66 [0.10–0.81]		
Assembly (machine II)	6	0.12 [0.15]	0.08–0.22 [0.10–0.27]		
Hot pressing (machine I)	5	0.11 [0.13]	0.07–0.19 [0.08–0.23]		

Table 8 (contd)

Industry and operation (location) Type of sample	No. of measurements	Mean[a] (ppm [mg/m³])	Range (ppm [mg/m³])	Year	Reference
Glue preparation	2	0.12 [0.15]	0.06–0.19 [0.07–0.23]		Fransman *et al.* (2003)
Finishing (puttying)	4	0.07 [0.09]	0.06–0.11 [0.07–0.14]		
Carrying plywood piles	2	0.05 [0.06]	0.04–0.06 [0.05–0.07]		
Finishing (sanding)	2	0.04 [0.05]	0.01–0.06 [0.01–0.07]		
Plywood mill (New Zealand)				[2000]	
Dryers	14	0.06[b] [0.07]	GSD, [3.2]		
Composers	2	0.02[b] [0.03]	GSD, [1.0]		
Pressing	5	0.13[b] [0.16]	GSD, [2.7]		
Finishing end	1	0.03[b] [0.04]	NA		
Particle- and other board mills					
Particle-board production (Sweden)	21	0.3 [0.4]	NR	1980s	Rosén *et al.* (1984)
Medium-density fibre board (Sweden)	19	0.2 [0.3]	NR	1980s	Rosén *et al.* (1984)
Particle-board mills (Finland)					Kauppinen & Niemelä (1985)
Glue preparation	10	2.2 [2.7]	0.3–4.9 [0.4–6.0]	1975–84	
Blending	10	1.0 [1.2]	0.1–2.0 [0.1–2.5]	1965–74	
Blending	8	0.7 [0.9]	< 0.1–1.4 [< 0.1–1.7]	1975–84	
Forming	26	1.7 [2.1]	< 0.5–4.6 [< 0.6–5.7]	1965–74	
Forming	32	1.4 [1.7]	0.1–4.8 [0.1–5.9]	1975–84	
Hot pressing	35	3.4 [4.2]	1.1–9.5 [1.4–11.7]	1965–74	
Hot pressing	61	1.7 [2.1]	0.2–4.6 [0.25–5.7]	1975–84	
Sawing	17	4.8 [5.9]	0.7–9.2 [0.9–11.3]	1965–74	
Sawing	36	1.0 [1.2]	< 0.1–3.3 [< 0.1–4.1]	1975–84	
Coating	7	1.0 [1.2]	0.5–1.8 [0.6–2.2]	1965–74	
Coating	12	0.4 [0.5]	0.1–1.2 [0.1–1.5]	1975–84	
Chip-board production (Germany)	24	1.5 [1.9]	< 0.01–8.4 [< 0.01–10]	1980–88	Triebig *et al.* (1989)
Particle-board mill (Indonesia)	9	2.4 [3.0]	1.2–3.5 [1.5–4.3]	NR	Malaka & Kodama (1990)
Block-board mill (Indonesia)	6	0.5 [0.6]	0.4–0.6 [0.5–0.7]	NR	Malaka & Kodama (1990)

Table 8 (contd)

Industry and operation (location) / Type of sample	No. of measurements	Mean[a] (ppm [mg/m³])	Range (ppm [mg/m³])	Year	Reference
Oriented strand board plant (Canada)				1990s	Herbert et al. (1995)
Debarking	5	≤ 0.05 [0.06]	NR		
Pre-heat conveyor	5	≤ 0.05 [0.06]	NR		
Post-heat press conveyor	5	≤ 0.05 [0.06]	NR		
Packaging/storage	5	≤ 0.05 [0.06]	NR		
Fibreboard, sawing and sanding (United Kingdom)				1990s	Chung et al. (2000)
Standard MDF (Caberwood)					
Gaseous form	5	0.06 [0.07]	0.04–0.07 [0.05–0.09]		
Extracted from dust	6	0.08 [0.10]	0.06–0.11 [0.07–0.13]		
Moisture resistant (Medite MR)					
Gaseous form	5	0.05 [0.06]	0.01–0.10 [0.01–0.12]		
Extracted from dust	6	0.10 [0.13]	0.04–0.14 [0.05–0.17]		
Zero added formaldehyde (Medite ZF)					
Gaseous form	6	0.04 [0.04]	0.02–0.06 [0.03–0.07]		
Extracted from dust	6	0.03 [0.04]	0.02–0.06 [0.03–0.07]		
Medite exterior grade (Medex)					
Gaseous form	6	0.03 [0.04]	0.01–0.07 [0.01–0.08]		
Extracted from dust	6	0.04 [0.05]	0.04–0.06 [0.05–0.07]		
Furniture factories					
Furniture factories (Sweden) Varnishing with acid-cured varnishes	32	0.7 [0.9]	NR	1980s	Rosén et al. (1984)
Furniture factories (Finland)				1975–84	Priha et al. (1986)
Feeding painting machine	14	1.1 [1.4]	0.3–2.7 [0.4–3.3]		
Spray painting	60	1.0 [1.2]	0.2–4.0 [0.3–5.0]		
Spray painting assistance	10	1.0 [1.2]	0.2–1.6 [0.3–2.0]		
Curtain painting	18	1.1 [1.4]	0.2–6.1 [0.3–7.5]		
Before drying of varnished furniture	34	1.5 [1.8]	0.1–4.2 [0.1–5.2]		
After drying of varnished furniture	14	1.4 [1.7]	0.2–5.4 [0.3–6.6]		

Table 8 (contd)

Industry and operation (location) Type of sample	No. of measurements	Mean[a] (ppm [mg/m³])	Range (ppm [mg/m³])	Year	Reference
Cabinet-making (Canada)	48	NR	max., < 0.1 [< 0.1]	NR	Sass-Kortsak et al. (1986)
Furniture factories, surface finishing with acid curing paints (Sweden)				NR	Alexandersson & Hedenstierna (1988)
Paint mixer/supervisor	6	0.2 [0.3]	0.1–0.4 [0.2–0.5]		
Mixed duties on the line	5	0.4 [0.5]	0.3–0.5 [0.3–0.6]		
Assistant painters	3	0.5 [0.6]	0.2–0.7 [0.2–0.9]		
Spray painters	10	0.4 [0.5]	0.1–1.1 [0.2–1.3]		
Feeder/receiver	13	0.2 [0.3]	0.1–0.8 [0.1–0.9]		
Furniture factories (Finland)				1981–86	Heikkilä et al. (1991)
Glueing	73	0.3 [0.4]	0.07–1.0 [0.09–1.2]		
Machining in finishing department	9	0.3 [0.4]	0.1–0.9 [0.1–1.1]		
Varnishing	150	1.1 [1.4]	0.1–6.3 [0.1–7.9]		
Manufacture of furniture (Denmark)				NR	Vinzents & Laursen (1993)
Painting	43	0.16 [0.20][b]	GSD, [2.25]		
Glueing	68	0.12 [0.15][b]	GSD, [2.87]		
Wood-working shops (Egypt)				1990s	Abdel Hameed et al. (2000)
Ventilated workshop	14	0.42 [0.52]	0.28–0.54 [0.34–0.66]		
Unventilated workshop	14	0.64 [0.79]	0.48–0.84 [0.59–1.03]		
Other wood product plants					
Glueing in wood industry (Sweden)	65	0.2 [0.3]	NR	1980s	Rosén et al. (1984)
Parquet plant (Finland)				1981	Heikkilä et al. (1991)
Machining	3	0.3 [0.4]	0.16–0.5 [0.2–0.6]		
Varnishing	5	0.8 [1.0]	0.2–1.4 [0.3–1.7]		
Production of wooden structures (Finland)				1981–86	Heikkilä et al. (1991)
Glueing	36	0.7 [0.8]	0.07–1.8 [0.1–2.2]		
Machining	19	0.4 [0.4]	0.1–0.8 [0.1–0.9]		
Manufacture of wooden bars (Finland)				1983	Heikkilä et al. (1991)
Glueing	33	0.6 [0.7]	0.2–1.9 [0.2–2.4]		
Machining	7	1.2 [1.5]	0.2–2.2 [0.3–2.7]		

Table 8 (contd)

Industry and operation (location) Type of sample	No. of measurements	Mean[a] (ppm [mg/m³])	Range (ppm [mg/m³])	Year	Reference
Match mill, impregnation of matchbox parts (Finland) Short-term	2	2.0 [2.5]	1.9–2.1 [2.3–2.6]	1963	Finnish Institute of Occupational Health (1994)
Wooden container mill, glueing and sawing (Finland)	6	0.3 [0.4]	0.2–0.4 [0.3–0.5]	1961	Finnish Institute of Occupational Health (1994)
Paper mills					
Laminated paper production (Sweden)	23	0.3 [0.4]	NR	1980s	Rosén et al. (1984)
Manufacture of offset paper (Sweden)	8	0.2 [0.2]	NR	1980s	Rosén et al. (1984)
Lamination and impregnation of paper with melamine and phenol resins (USA)				1983	Stewart et al. (1987)
Plant no. 6, summer[c,d]	53	0.7[b] [0.9]	< 0.01–7.4 [< 0.01–9.1]		
Plant no. 6, winter[d]	39	0.3[b] [0.4]	0.05–0.7 [0.06–0.9]		
Paper mill (Finland)				1975–84	Heikkilä et al. (1991)
Coating of paper	30	0.7 [0.9]	0.4–31 [0.5–39]		
Gum paper production	4	0.4 [0.5]	0.3–0.6 [0.3–0.8]		
Impregnation of paper with amino resin	6	3.1 [3.9]	0.5–13 [0.6–16]		
Impregnation of paper with phenol resin	20	0.1 [0.1]	0.05–0.3 [0.06–0.4]		
Paper mill (Finland)					Finnish Institute of Occupational Health (1994)
Glueing, hardening, lamination and rolling of special paper	12	0.9 [1.1]	0.3–2.5 [0.4–3.1]	1971–73	
Impregnation of paper with phenol resin, partly short-term	38	7.4 [9.1]	< 1.0–33.0 [< 1.1–40.6]	1968–69	
Paper storage, diesel truck traffic	5	0.3 [0.4]	0.2–0.4 [0.25–0.5]	1969	
Pulp and paper industries (12 countries)				1950–94	Korhonen et al. (2004)
Pulping, refining of stock (8 mills)	25	0.5 [0.6]	0–3.1 [0–3.8]		
Newsprint and uncoated paper machine (2 mills)	7	0.15 [0.18]	0.04–0.46 [0.05–0.57]		
Fine and coated paper machine (6 mills)	51	1.1 [1.4]	0.01–9.9 [0.01–12.2]		

Table 8 (contd)

Industry and operation (location) Type of sample	No. of measurements	Mean[a] (ppm [mg/m³])	Range (ppm [mg/m³])	Year	Reference
Paperboard machine (1 mill)	8	0.5 [0.6]	0.2–2.2 [0.2–2.7]		
Paper/paperboard machine from more than one of above categories (24 mills)	228	0.4 [0.5]	0–6.6 [0–8.1]		
Calendering or on-machine coating (10 mills)	166	4.2 [5.2]	0–50 [0–61.5]		
Winding, cutting and grading (17 mills)	111	0.2 [0.3]	0–1.1 [0–1.4]		
Recycled paper industry (12 countries)					
Re-pulping of waste paper (2 mills)	8	0.2 [0.3]	0.05–0.4 [0.06–0.5]		
Construction industry					
Insulating buildings with urea–formaldehyde foam (Sweden)	6	0.1 [0.2]	NR	1980s	Rosén et al. (1984)
Insulating buildings with urea–formaldehyde foam (USA)	66	1.3[e] [1.6]	0.3–3.1 [0.4–3.8]	NR	WHO (1989)
Varnishing parquet with urea–formaldehyde varnish (Finland)	10	2.9 [3.6]	0.3–6.6 [0.4–8.1]	1976	Heikkilä et al. (1991)
Varnishing parquet with urea–formaldehyde varnish (Finland)	6	4.3 [5.3]	2.6–6.1 [3.2–7.5]	1987	Riala & Riihimäki (1991)
Sawing particle-board at construction site (Finland)	5	< 0.5 [< 0.6]	NR	1967	Finnish Institute of Occupational Health (1994)

GSD, geometric standard deviation; NA, not applicable; NR, not reported
[a] Arithmetic mean unless otherwise specified
[b] Geometric mean
Some of the results in the Stewart et al. (1987) study were affected by the simultaneous occurrence in the samples of:
[c] phenol (leading to low values)
[d] particulates that contained nascent formaldehyde (leading to high values).
[e] Mean of arithmetic means

Recent studies conducted in these industries in Finland and New Zealand (Mäkinen *et al.*, 1999; Fransman *et al.*, 2003) found mean concentrations of formaldehyde to be less than 0.5 mg/m³. In contrast, mean levels of 2 ppm [2.5 mg/m³] have been observed historically in some operations in the Finnish industry (Kauppinen, 1986).

(ii)   *Manufactured board mills*

Both phenol–formaldehyde and urea–formaldehyde resins are used in mills that produce particle- and other manufactured boards, including oriented strand boards and medium-density fibre boards. Phenolic resins are more liable to be used for panels that are destined for applications that require durability under adverse conditions, while urea-based resins are used for less demanding, interior applications. Melamine–formaldehyde resins may also be used to increase durability, but rarely are because they are more expensive. Exposure to formaldehyde and other resin constituents is possible during the mixing of glues, the laying of mat and hot-pressing operations.

Herbert *et al.* (1995) and Chung *et al.* (2000) found levels of formaldehyde below 0.2 mg/m³ in recent studies in Canada and the United Kingdom, respectively, in oriented strand-board and fibre-board plants. Mean exposures greater than 1 ppm [1.2 mg/m³] have been observed in the past in particle- and chip-board mills (Kauppinen & Niemelä, 1985; Triebig *et al.*, 1989; Malaka & Kodama, 1990).

(iii)   *Furniture factories*

Furniture varnishes may contain acid-cured urea–formaldehyde resins dissolved in organic solvents. In Finland, workers were exposed to an average level of about 1 ppm [1.23 mg/m³] formaldehyde in most facilities (Priha *et al.*, 1986; Heikkilä *et al.*, 1991).

In a recent study in wood-working shops in Egypt, the levels of formaldehyde were found to average 0.42 and 0.64 ppm [0.52 and 0.79 mg/m³] in ventilated and unventilated workplaces, respectively (Abdel Hameed *et al.*, 2000). [The origin of the formaldehyde was not stated.]

(iv)   *Paper mills*

Some paper mills produce special products that are coated with formaldehyde-based phenol, urea or melamine resins. Coating agents and other chemicals used in paper mills may also contain formaldehyde as a bactericide.

As part of an IARC international epidemiological study of workers in the pulp and paper industry, measurements were carried out in the production departments of paper and paperboard mills and recycling plants in 12 countries. The highest exposures were observed during calendering or on-machine coating (Korhonen *et al.*, 2004).

(*e*)   *Building and construction industry*

Exposure to formaldehyde may also occur in the construction industry (Table 8). Specialized construction workers who varnish wooden parquet floors may have relatively high exposure. The mean levels of formaldehyde in the air during varnishing with urea–formaldehyde varnishes ranged between 2 and 5 ppm [2.5–6.2 mg/m³]. One coat of varnish takes only about 30 min to apply (Riala & Riihimäki, 1991), but the same worker may apply five or even 10 coats per day. Other chemical agents to which parquetry workers are usually exposed include wood dust from sanding (see IARC, 1995) and solvent vapours from varnishes, putties and adhesives. Operations that may have resulted in exposure to formaldehyde in the building trades are insulation with urea–formaldehyde foam and machining of particle-board, but these have now largely been discontinued. Various levels of formaldehyde have been measured during insulation with urea–formaldehyde foam, but exposure during handling and sawing of particle-board seems to be consistently low. Formaldehyde may be released when synthetic vitreous fibre-based insulation is applied to hot surfaces, i.e. high-temperature insulation in power plants, due to decomposition of the phenol–formaldehyde binder at temperatures > 150 °C (International Labour Office, 2001) (see also under (*f*)).

(*f*)   Manufacture of textiles and garments

The use of formaldehyde-based resins to produce crease-resistant fabrics began in the 1950s. The early resins contained substantial amounts of extractable formaldehyde: over 0.4% by weight of fabric. The introduction of dimethyloldihydroxyethyleneurea resins in 1970 reduced the levels of free formaldehyde in fabrics to 0.15–0.2%. Since then, methylation of dimethyloldihydroxyethyleneurea and other modifications of the resin have decreased the level of formaldehyde gradually to 0.01–0.02% (Elliott *et al.*, 1987). Some flame-retardants contain agents that release formaldehyde (Heikkilä *et al.*, 1991). The cutting and sewing of fabrics release low levels of textile dust, and small amounts of chlorinated organic solvents are used to clean spots. Pattern copying machines may emit ammonia and dimethylthiourea in some plants (Elliott *et al.*, 1987). Finishing workers in textile mills may also be exposed to textile dyes, flame-retardants, carrier agents, textile-finishing agents and solvents (see IARC, 1990b).

Measurements of formaldehyde in the air of textile mills are summarized in Table 9. In the late 1970s and 1980s, levels of formaldehyde in the garment industry averaged 0.2–2 ppm [0.25–2.5 mg/m^3]. However, exposures in the past were generally higher, probably because of the higher content of free formaldehyde in fabrics. For example, the concentrations of formaldehyde were reported to have been 0.9–2.7 ppm [1.1–3.3 mg/m^3] in a post-cure garment manufacturing plant and 0.3–2.7 ppm [0.4–3.3 mg/m^3] in eight other garment manufacturing plants in the USA in 1966 (Elliott *et al.*, 1987). Goldstein (1973) reported that concentrations of formaldehyde in cutting rooms decreased from over 10 ppm [12 mg/m^3] in 1968 to less than 2 ppm [2.4 mg/m^3] in 1973 as a result of improvements in the processes of resin treatment. The mean formaldehyde concentration in air increased from 0.1 to 1.0 ppm [0.12 to 1.23 mg/m^3] in a study in the USA when the formaldehyde content of the fabric increased from 0.015 to 0.04% (Luker & Van Houten, 1990). Measurements from the late 1980s onwards indicate lower levels, usually averaging 0.1–0.2 ppm [0.12–0.25 mg/m^3].

Full-shift personal (for 5.7–6.4 h; eight samples) and area (for 6.3–7.3 h; 12 samples) measurements were taken at a pre-cured permanent-press garment manufacturing plant in

Table 9. Concentrations of formaldehyde in the workroom air of textile mills and garment factories

Industry and operation (location) Type of sample	No. of measurements	Mean[a] (ppm [mg/m³])	Range or SD in ppm [mg/m³]	Year	Reference
Textile mills					
Textile plants (Finland)				1975–78	Nousiainen & Lindqvist (1979)
Finishing department, mixing	8	0.8 [1.1]	< 0.2–>5 [< 0.2–> 6]		
Crease-resistant treatment	52	0.4 [0.5]	< 0.2–>3 [< 0.2–> 4]		
Finishing department (excluding crease-resistant and flame-retardant treatment)	17	0.3 [0.4]	max., 1.3 [1.5]		
Flame-retardant treatment	67	1.9 [2.5]	< 0.2–>10 [< 0.2–> 11]		
Fabric store	6	0.8 [1.1]	0.1–1.3 [0.1–1.6]		
Textile mills (Sweden)				1980s	Rosén et al. (1984)
Crease-resistant treatment	29	0.2 [0.2]	NR		
Flame-retardant treatment	2	1.2 [1.5]	NR		
Garment factories					
Manufacture from crease-resistant cloth (USA)	181	NR	< 0.1–0.9 [< 0.1–1.1]	NR	Blade (1983)
Manufacture of shirts from fabric treated with formaldehyde-based resins (USA)	326	~0.2 [~0.25]	< 0.1–0.4 [< 0.1–0.5]	1980s	Elliott et al. (1987)
Garment industry (Finland)				1981–86	Heikkilä et al. (1991)
Handling of leather	3	0.1 [0.1]	0.02–0.1 [0.03–0.1]		
Pressing	32	0.2 [0.3]	0.02–0.7 [0.03–0.9]		
Sewing	15	0.1 [0.1]	0.02–0.3 [0.03–0.3]		
Sewing plant (USA)				NR	Luker & Van Houten (1990)
Processing of 0.04% formaldehyde fabric	9	1.0 [1.2]	0.5–1.1 [0.6–1.4]		
Processing of 0.015% formaldehyde fabric	9	0.1 [0.1]	< 0.1–0.2 [< 0.1–0.3]		
Garment manufacturing (USA)				NR	Echt & Burr (1997)
Sewers, cutters and bundlers					
Personal samples					
8-h TWA	8	0.21 [0.26]	0.18–0.23 [0.22–0.28]		
Area samples	8	0.16 [0.19]	0.14–0.17 [0.17–0.21]		
8-h TWA	8	0.24 [0.30]	0.17–0.30 [0.21–0.37]		
8-h TWA	8	0.21 [0.26]	0.16–0.25 [0.20–0.31]		

Table 9 (contd)

Industry and operation (location) Type of sample	No. of measurements	Mean[a] (ppm [mg/m^3])	Range or SD in ppm [mg/m^3]	Year	Reference
Cut and spread				NR	Kennedy et al. (1992)
Formaldehyde gas (inhalable dust)	6	0.03	SD, 0.01		
Bound formaldehyde (inhalable dust)	6	< 0.01	SD, < 0.01		
Formaldehyde gas (total dust)	6	0.04	SD, 0.01		
Bound formaldehyde (total dust)	6	< 0.01[b]	SD, < 0.01		
Turn and ticket					
Formaldehyde gas (inhalable dust)	6	< 0.01	SD, < 0.01		
Bound formaldehyde (inhalable dust)	6	< 0.01	SD, < 0.01		
Formaldehyde gas (total dust)	6	0.03	SD, 0.01		
Bound formaldehyde (total dust)	6	< 0.01	SD, < 0.01		
Retail dress shops (USA)	NR	NR	0.1–0.5 [0.1–0.6]	1959	Elliott et al. (1987)
Fabric shops (Finland)	3	0.17 [0.21]	0.12–0.24 [0.15–0.30]	1985–87	Priha et al. (1988)
Fabric stores (USA)	77	0.14 [0.17]	0.03–0.28 [0.04–0.34]	NR	McGuire et al. (1992)
24-h area samples					
Independent stores	33	0.10 [0.13]	0.03–0.28 [0.04–0.34]		
Chain stores	44	0.19 [0.24]	0.09–0.27 [0.11–0.33]		

NR, not reported; SD, standard deviation
[a] Arithmetic mean
[b] Five samples with non-detectable levels

the USA. Levels of exposure to formaldehyde for sewers, cutters and bundlers ranged from 0.22 to 0.28 mg/m³ (8-h TWA, 0.17–0.21 mg/m³). Area measurements of formaldehyde at cutting, sewing, pressing, spreading and receiving (storage) locations ranged from 0.21 to 0.37 mg/m³ (8-h TWA; 0.20–0.31 mg/m³). Full-shift (for 5.8–6.4 h; eight samples) personal measurements of formaldehyde in inhalable dust showed levels of up to 29 µg/mg dust; settled dust samples showed concentrations of 0.7 and 0.8 µg/mg dust (Echt & Burr, 1997). In another garment production facility in the USA, formaldehyde gas and formalde-hyde bound to dust were detected at levels of 26–36 µg/m³ and 0.2–0.7 µg/m³, respectively (Kennedy *et al.*, 1992).

The use of formaldehyde-based resin to finish textiles and some garments may also result in exposure in retail shops. Measurements in dress shops in the USA in the 1950s showed levels up to 0.5 ppm [0.62 mg/m³] (Elliott *et al.*, 1987). The air in three Finnish fabric shops in the 1980s contained 0.15–0.3 mg/m³ formaldehyde (Priha *et al.*, 1988). In fabric stores in the USA that were monitored by placing samplers on a shelf in the store for 24 h, the average concentration of formaldehyde was 0.17 mg/m³ (McGuire *et al.*, 1992).

(g)   Foundries

Formaldehyde-based resins are commonly used as core binders in foundries (Table 10). Urea–formaldehyde resin is usually blended with oleoresin or phenol–formaldehyde resin and mixed with sand to form a core, which is then cured by baking in an oven or by heating from inside the core box (hot-box method). The original hot-box binder was a mixture of urea–formaldehyde resin and furfuryl alcohol (commonly referred to as furan resin). Furan resins were then modified with phenol to produce urea–formaldehyde/furfuryl alcohol, phenol–formaldehyde/furfuryl alcohol and phenol–formaldehyde/urea–formaldehyde resins.

The mean concentrations of formaldehyde measured during core-making and opera-tions following core-making in the 1980s in Sweden and Finland were usually below 1 ppm [1.2 mg/m³]; however, measurements made before 1975 suggest that past expo-sures may have been considerably higher (Heikkilä *et al.*, 1991). Many other chemicals occur in foundries, e.g. silica (see IARC, 1987d) and other mineral dusts, polycyclic aro-matic hydrocarbons (see IARC, 1983), asbestos (see IARC, 1987e), metal fumes and dusts, carbon monoxide, isocyanates (see IARC, 1986), phenols (see IARC, 1989c), organic solvents and amines (see IARC, 1999). These exposures have been described in a previous monograph (IARC, 1984).

(h)   Synthetic vitreous fibre production

Formaldehyde resins are commonly used to bind man-made vitreous fibre products. Measurements of formaldehyde in the air of plants manufacturing synthetic vitreous fibres are summarized in Table 10.

Measurements in glasswool and stonewool plants in the 1980s showed mean concen-trations of 0.1–0.2 ppm [0.12–0.25 mg/m³] formaldehyde. Very high levels were measured

Table 10. Concentrations of formaldehyde in the workroom air of foundries and during the manufacture of synthetic vitreous fibres and plastics

Industry and operation (location) Type of sample	No. of measurements	Mean[a] (ppm [mg/m³])	Range (ppm [mg/m³])	Year	Reference
Foundries					
Foundry (Sweden)				1980s	Rosén et al. (1984)
Hot-box method	5	1.5 [1.9]	NR		
Moulding	17	0.1 [0.1]	NR		
Foundries (Sweden)				NR	Åhman et al. (1991)
Moulders and core-maker handling furan resin sand 8-h TWA	36	0.1 [0.1]	0.02–0.22 [0.02–0.27]		
Foundries (Finland)				Before 1975	Heikkilä et al. (1991)
Core-making	43	2.8 [3.4]	<0.1–>10 [<0.1–>11]		
Core-making	17	0.3 [0.4]	0.02–1.4 [0.03–1.8]	1981–86	
Casting	10	0.2 [0.2]	0.02–0.2 [0.03–0.8]	1981–86	
Moulding	25	0.3 [0.4]	0.04–2.0 [0.05–2.5]	1981–86	
Synthetic vitreous fibre plants					
(Sweden)				1980s	Rosén et al. (1984)
Production	16	0.15 [0.19]	NR		
Form pressing	4	0.16 [0.20]	NR		
(Finland)				1981–86	Heikkilä et al. (1991)
Production	36	0.20 [0.25]	0.02–1.5 [0.03–1.7]		
Form pressing	24	0.09 [0.11]	0.01–0.3 [0.01–0.4]		
Fibrous glass manufacturing plant (USA)				NR	Milton et al. (1996)
Fixed location workers (n = 17)	97	0.07; 0.05[b]	GSD, 4.0		
Forming attendant (n = 2)	11	0.07; 0.03[b]	GSD, 8.2		
Forming attendant leader (n = 3)	18	0.09; 0.07[b]	GSD, 1.9		
Binder water leader (n = 1)	4	0.05; 0.01[b]	GSD, 10.9		
Binder water operator (n = 1)	6	0.06; 0.05[b]	GSD, 2.1		
Pipefitter (n = 1)	5	0.05; 0.05[b]	GSD, 1.4		
Forehearth operator (n = 6)	35	0.07; 0.05[b]	GSD, 4.4		
Curing oven machine operator (n = 3)	18	0.08; 0.07[b]	GSD, 1.7		

Table 10 (contd)

Industry and operation (location) Type of sample	No. of measurements	Mean[a] (ppm [mg/m^3])	Range (ppm [mg/m^3])	Year	Reference
Mobile workers (n = 20)	< 100	0.03; 0.02[b]	GSD, 3.1	1983–84	Stewart et al. (1987)
Crew (packaging) (n = 2)	12	0.02; 0.01[b]	GSD, 4.1		
Washwater tender (n = 1)	3	0.04; 0.04[b]	GSD, 1.5		
Mechanical repair (n = 7)	35	0.02; 0.01[b]	GSD, 3.4		
Electrician (n = 5)	25	0.03; 0.02[b]	GSD, 3.1		
Sheet metal worker (n = 2)	10	0.03; 0.02[b]	GSD, 2.7		
Welder (n = 2)	10	0.04; 0.03[b]	GSD, 2.6		
Pipefitter (n = 1)	5	0.03; 0.02[b]	GSD, 1.9		
Plastics production					
Production of moulded plastic products (USA)				1981–86	Heikkilä et al. (1991)
Plant no. 8, phenol resin, summer	10	0.5[b] [0.6]	0.1–0.9 [0.1–1.1]		
Plant no. 9, melamine resin, summer	13	9.2[b] [11.3]	< 0.01–26.5 [< 0.01–32.6]		
Moulding compound manufacture (USA)					
Plant no. 9, winter	9	2.8[b] [3.4]	0.04–6.7 [0.05–8.2]		
Plant no. 9, summer[c]	18	38.2[b] [47.0]	9.5–60.8 [11.7–74.8]		
Plant no. 1, winter	12	1.5[b] [1.8]	0.9–2.0 [1.1–2.1]		
Plant no. 1, summer	24	9.7[b] [11.9]	3.8–14.4 [4.7–17.7]		
Plant no. 8, winter	13	0.3[b] [0.4]	0.07–0.7 [0.09–0.9]		
Plant no. 7, summer	43	0.3[b] [0.4]	0.05–0.6 [0.06–0.8]		
Plant no. 2, summer	15	6.5[b] [8.0]	0.3–20.6 [0.4–25.3]		
Plastics production (Finland)					
Casting of polyacetal resin	10	0.3 [0.4]	0.06–0.7 [0.08–0.8]		
Casting of urea–formaldehyde resin	4	0.4 [0.5]	0.2–0.5 [0.3–0.6]		
Casting of other plastics	29	< 0.1 [< 0.1]	< 0.1–0.2 [< 0.1–0.3]		
Plastics manufacturing (Canada)				NR	Tikuisis et al. (1995)
Polyethylene extrusion	9	NR	max., [< 0.12]		

GSD, geometric standard deviation; NR, not reported; TWA, time-weighted average
[a] Arithmetic mean unless otherwise specified
[b] Geometric mean
[c] Some of the results were affected by the simultaneous occurrence in the samples of particulates that contained formaldehyde (leading to high values).

occasionally in factories close to cupola ovens and hardening chambers (Heikkilä et al., 1991). Other exposures in man-made vitreous fibre production have been described in a previous monograph (IARC, 2002).

Personal measurements of maintenance and production workers were taken in a fibreglass insulation manufacturing plant. The average level of exposure to formaldehyde for all fixed location workers (basement workers, forehearth operators and curing oven operators; 17 samples) was 0.07 mg/m^3. The mean of the measurements for all mobile workers (packaging crew, washwater tender, mechanical repairer, electrician, sheet metal workers, welder and pipefitter; 20 samples) was 0.03 mg/m^3. No measurement was below the limit of detection (Milton et al., 1996).

(i)   Plastics production

Formaldehyde-based plastics are used in the production of electrical parts, dishware and various other plastic products (Table 10).

The concentrations of formaldehyde measured in such industries have usually been < 1 ppm [1.2 mg/m^3], but much higher exposures may occur. Plastic dust and fumes may be present in the atmospheres of moulded plastic product plants, and exposures in these facilities are usually considerably higher than those in facilities where the products are used. The mean concentration of formaldehyde was > 1 ppm in many plants in the USA where moulding compounds were used. Some workers may have been exposed to pigments, lubricants and fillers (e.g. historically, asbestos and wood flour) that were used as constituents of moulding compounds (Stewart et al., 1987).

An experimental scenario was created in Canada to evaluate thermal decomposition products that are emitted from the extrusion of polyethylene into a variety of products. Eight-hour area samples, collected at worst-case locations at typical operator locations, and 8-h personal samples were collected. All levels of formaldehyde were below 0.12 mg/m^3 (Tikuisis et al., 1995).

(j)   Firefighters

Measurements of the exposure of firefighters to formaldehyde are given in Table 11. One study measured personal exposures to formaldehyde outside a self-contained breathing apparatus (if worn) while fighting fires in two cities in the USA. Formaldehyde was detected in six of 24 samples. Concentrations ranged from 0.1 to 8.3 ppm [0.12–10.2 mg/m^3], with a second highest concentration of 3.3 ppm [4.1 mg/m^3] (Brandt-Rauf et al., 1988). In another study in the USA, levels of formaldehyde ranged from the limit of detection (0.13 mg/m^3) to 9.8 mg/m^3 during knockdown (when the main body of the fire is brought under control), and formaldehyde was detected in 73% of the samples, from the limit of detection to 0.5 mg/m^3, during overhaul (searching for and extinguishing hidden fires) for 22 fires (Jankovic et al., 1991). Exposure levels inside the self-contained breathing masks ranged from the limit of detection to 0.4 mg/m^3. Two of the measurements during knockdown exceeded the 15-min short-term exposure limit (STEL) of 2.5 mg/m^3.

Table 11. Concentrations of formaldehyde during firefighting and exposure to engine exhausts

Industry and operation (location) Type of sample	No. of measurements	Mean[a] (ppm [mg/m³])	Range (ppm [mg/m³])	Year	Reference
Firefighting					
City fire (USA)	24	0.55 [0.68][b]	0.1–8.3 [0.1–10.2][b]	1986	Brandt-Rauf et al. (1988)
City fire (USA)	22 fires			NR	Jankovic et al. (1991)
Knockdown[c]		NR	ND–8 [ND–9.8]		
Overhaul[c]		NR	ND–0.4 [ND–0.5]		
Inside mask		NR	ND–0.3 [ND–0.4]		
Wildland fire (USA)	5	0.05 [0.06]	0.02–0.07 [0.02–0.09]	1990	Reh et al. (1994)
Wildland fire (USA)	30	0.13 [0.16]	0.04–0.3 [0.05–0.4]	1989	Materna et al. (1992)
City fire (USA)	96	0.25 [0.31]	0.02–1.2 [0.02–1.5]	1998	Bolstad-Johnson et al. (2000)
Engine exhaust					
Chain-sawing (Sweden)	NR	0.05 [0.06]	0.02–0.11 [0.03–0.13]	NR	Hagberg et al. (1985)
Chain-sawing (Finland) 8-h TWA	NR	< 0.1 [< 0.1]	< 0.1–0.5 [< 0.1–0.6]	NR	Heikkilä et al. (1991)
Automobile garage Personal samples	53	0.03 [0.04]	NR	NR	Zhang et al. (2003)

ND, not detected; NR, not reported; TWA, time-weighted average
[a] Arithmetic mean
[b] Excluding 18 values noted as 0
[c] See text for definitions

A comprehensive study that monitored air was conducted to characterize exposures of firefighters during 25 structure fires. Exposures of firefighters during overhaul, when they look for hidden fire inside attics, ceilings and walls often without respiratory protection, were measured. Ceiling values for formaldehyde (National Institute for Occupational Safety and Health [NIOSH]; 0.1 ppm [0.12 mg/m^3]) were exceeded at 22 fires (Bolstad-Johnson *et al.*, 2000).

Limited studies of exposure to aldehydes that is related to forest and wildland fires indicate lower exposures. Formaldehyde was detected in all 30 samples collected during a study of wildland fires. Concentrations ranged from 0.048 to 0.42 mg/m^3; the mean was 0.16 mg/m^3 (Materna *et al.*, 1992). A smaller study by NIOSH also detected formaldehyde in each of five samples collected during wildfire. Concentrations ranged from 0.02 to 0.07 ppm [0.02–0.09 mg/m^3] and the mean was 0.05 ppm [0.06 mg/m^3] (Reh *et al.*, 1994).

(k)   Automobile and engine exhausts

Engine exhausts are a source of exposure to formaldehyde (see Section 1.3.3; Table 11).

Maître *et al.* (2002) evaluated individual airborne exposures to gaseous and particulate pollutants of a group of policemen who worked close to traffic in the centre of Grenoble, France. Personal active air samples were collected during the workshifts of eight policemen in summer and winter during the occurrence of a thermal inversion phenomenon for 4 days at each period. Stationary air samples were taken in the policemen's work area during the same period. The median concentration of the personal samples for formaldehyde was 14 μg/m^3 in the summer and 21 μg/m^3 in the winter.

Zhang *et al.* (2003) examined whether work in an automobile garage and tobacco smoke can significantly affect personal exposure to a number of important carbonyl compounds, including formaldehyde. The study was carried out on 22 garage workers (nine smokers and 13 nonsmokers) and 15 non-garage workers (four smokers and 11 nonsmokers). Daily exposure was estimated using 48-h integrated measurements of breathing zone concentrations. The mean formaldehyde concentrations were: 40.6 μg/m^3 for smoking garage workers, 41.1 μg/m^3 for nonsmoking garage workers, 34.6 μg/m^3 for smoking non-garage workers and 30.2 μg/m^3 for nonsmoking non-garage workers (total range, 14.1–80.1 μg/m^3).

(l)   Offices and public buildings

Concentrations of formaldehyde in offices and public buildings (museums, geriatric homes) are given in Table 12.

In Australia, measurements of formaldehyde over 3–4 days were found to average 0.03 mg/m^3 in conventional offices and 1.4 mg/m^3 in portable office buildings (Dingle *et al.*, 2000).

Exposure measurements were taken for an epidemiological study of nasal symptoms in a Swedish office building that had recently been painted with low-emitting products [the

Table 12. Concentrations of formaldehyde in offices and miscellaneous other workplaces

Industry and operation (location) Type of sample	No. of measurements[a]	Mean (ppm [mg/m³])[a]	Range (ppm [mg/m³])[a]	Year	Reference
Offices					
Offices (USA)	25	80.0[b] µg/m³	NR	1981–84	Shah & Singh (1988)
Non-industrial office workplaces and restaurants (Brazil)	12	20.4 µg/m³	4.7–60.7 µg/m³	1993	Miguel et al. (1995)
Four offices on several floors of an office building (Brazil)	11	40 µg/m³	12.2–99.7 µg/m³	1995	Brickus et al. (1998)
Offices (Sweden)				1995–96	Wieslander et al. (1999a)
Recently painted with low-emitting paint	NR	18 µg/m³	16–20 µg/m³		
Three months later	NR	8 µg/m³	7–10 µg/m³		
Control (at the time and 3 months later)	NR	8 µg/m³	8–9 µg/m³		
Offices (Australia)				NR	Dingle et al. (2000)
Conventional offices (18 sites)	NR	27 µg/m³	12–96 µg/m³		
Portable office buildings (20 sites)	40	1400 µg/m³	516–2595 µg/m³		
Six office buildings (USA)	[72]	1.7–13.3 µg/m³[c]	NR	1996–97	Reynolds et al. (2001)
Five office buildings (Taiwan, China)	54	140–1190 µg/m³[d]	NR	NR	Wu et al. (2003)
8-h average during working time from measurements conducted continuously ≥ 24 h					
Miscellaneous					
Coal coking plant (former Czechoslovakia)	NR	0.05[e] [0.06]	< 0.01–0.25 [< 0.01–0.3]	NR	Mašek (1972)
Pitch coking plant (former Czechoslovakia)	NR	0.4[e] [0.5]	0.05–1.6 [0.07–2.0]	NR	Mašek (1972)
Electrical machinery manufacture (Finland)				1977–79	Niemelä & Vainio (1981)
Soldering	47	< 0.1 [< 0.1]	NR		
Lacquering and treatment of melamine plastics	8	0.35 [0.4]	NR		
Rubber processing (USA)	NR	NR	0.4–0.8 [0.5–0.98]	1975	IARC (1982)
Painting with bake-drying paints (Sweden)	13	< 0.1 [< 0.1]	NR	1980s	Rosén et al. (1984)
Abrasive production (Sweden)	20	0.2 [0.3]	NR	1980s	Rosén et al. (1984)

Table 12 (contd)

Industry and operation (location) Type of sample	No. of measurements	Mean (ppm [mg/m^3])[a]	Range (ppm [mg/m^3])[a]	Year	Reference
Sugar mill (Sweden)				1980s	Rosén et al. (1984)
Preservation of sugar beets	26	0.4 [0.5]	NR		
Fur processing	16	NR	0.8–1.6 [1.0–2.0]	1980s	Rosén et al. (1984)
8-h TWA					
Photographic film manufacture (USA)				1983–84	Stewart et al. (1987)
Plants no. 4 and 5, summer	49	0.1[c] [0.1]	< 0.01–0.4 [< 0.01–0.5]		
Plants no. 4 and 5, winter	29	0.3[c] [0.4]	0.02–0.9 [0.03–1.1]		
Agriculture (Finland)					Heikkilä et al. (1991)
Handling of fodder	NR	NR	0.02–0.4 [0.03–0.5]	1982	
Disinfection of eggs	11	2.6 [3.2]	0.2–7.8 [0.3–9.6]	1981–86	Heikkilä et al. (1991)
Metalware plant, bake painting (Finland)	18	0.3 [0.4]	0.03–0.7 [0.04–0.9]	1981–86	Heikkilä et al. (1991)
Print (Finland)				1981–86	Heikkilä et al. (1991)
Development of photographs	11	0.04 [0.05]	0.02–0.1 [0.03–0.13]		
Malt barley production (Finland)				1981	Heikkilä et al. (1991)
Preservation of malt barley	6	0.7 [0.9]	0.4–1.5 [0.5–1.8]		
Photographic laboratories (Finland)	10	0.07 [0.09]	0.02–0.3 [0.03–0.40]	1981–86	Heikkilä et al. (1991)
Fish hatchery (USA)				NR	Lee & Radtke (1998)
Treating fish eggs (6 sites)	6	0.02 [0.02]	0.006–0.038 [0.007–0.05]		
8-h TWA					

NR, not reported; TWA, time-weighted average

[a] Arithmetic mean unless otherwise specified; values in ppm [mg/m^3], unless stated otherwise

[b] Median

[c] Range of geometric means

[d] Range of arithmetic means

[e] Mean of arithmetic means

recency was not identified but appeared to be within a few months]. The measurements taken at that time showed average levels of formaldehyde of 18 $\mu g/m^3$ (range, 16–20 $\mu g/m^3$); those taken 3 months later averaged 8 $\mu g/m^3$ (range, 7–10 $\mu g/m^3$) (Wieslander *et al.*, 1999a). The latter were equivalent to the levels found in the same office complex in an area that had not been redecorated (mean, 8–9 $\mu g/m^3$).

Laser-jet printers have been found to be a source of formaldehyde, as a result of the ozonolysis reactions of volatile organic compounds emitted from the toner powder (Wolkoff *et al.*, 1992; Tuomi *et al.*, 2000). In a study in an office environment in Finland (Tuomi *et al.*, 2000), the emission rate of formaldehyde of three printers that used traditional corona-discharge technology (dating from approximately 1990) ranged from 9 to 46 $\mu g/m^3$, whereas a newer technology printer did not produce detectable levels of formaldehyde.

In another study in Sweden, average levels of formaldehyde in four geriatric homes ranged from 2 to 7 $\mu g/m^3$ (Wieslander *et al.*, 1999b).

(m)   Miscellaneous

Formaldehyde is used in agriculture as a preservative for fodder and as a disinfectant (Table 12). For example, fodder was preserved with a 2% formalin solution several times per year from the late 1960s until the early 1980s on farms in Finland. As the air concentration during preservation was < 0.5 ppm [0.6 mg/m^3], the annual mean exposure was probably very low. Formaldehyde gas is also used 5–10 times a year to disinfect eggs in brooding houses. The concentration of formaldehyde in front of the disinfection chamber immediately after disinfection was as high as 7–8 ppm [8.6–9.8 mg/m^3], but annual exposure from this source probably remains very low (Heikkilä *et al.*, 1991).

One worker in each of six different fish hatcheries in the USA was monitored once over the 15–90-min period it took to treat fish eggs with a formalin solution to control infection. Concentrations ranged from not quantifiable to 1 mg/m^3. Area measurements during treatment were < 0.062–0.84 mg/m^3, and 8-h TWAs were reported to be < 0.01–0.05 mg/m^3 (mean, 0.02 mg/m^3) (Lee & Radtke, 1998).

Formaldehyde is also used or formed during many other industrial operations, such as treatment of fur and leather, preservation of barley and sugar beets, coal and pitch coking, rubber processing and production of abrasives (Table 12). Some of these activities may entail heavy exposure. For example, treatment of furs with formaldehyde resulted in the highest exposure to formaldehyde of all jobs and industries studied in a large Swedish survey in the early 1980s. The 8-h TWA concentration of formaldehyde was assessed to be 0.8–1.6 ppm [1.0–2.0 mg/m^3] and high peak exposures occurred many times per day (Rosén *et al.*, 1984).

Heating of bake-drying paints and soldering may release some formaldehyde in plants where metalware and electrical equipment are produced, but the measured concentrations are usually well below 1 ppm [1.2 mg/m^3] (Rosén *et al.*, 1984).

The mean concentrations of formaldehyde measured during the coating of photographic films and during development of photographs are usually well below 1 ppm [1.2 mg/m^3]

(Table 12). Methanol, ethanol, acetone and ammonia are other volatile agents that may occur in film manufacturing facilities (Stewart *et al.*, 1987).

Formaldehyde has been found consistently in spacecraft atmospheres at concentrations that exceed the 180-day spacecraft maximum allowable concentration of 0.05 mg/m^3. The source is thought to be hardware off-gassing and possibly leakage from experiments that involve fixatives. Small amounts could also be present from human metabolism and exhalation (James, 1997).

1.3.3   *Ambient (outdoor) air*

Measurements of indoor and outdoor levels of formaldehyde have been generated in many countries for several decades. Standard sampling and analytical methodologies are sufficiently sensitive to detect formaldehyde in most samples of ambient (outdoor) air. Concentrations of formaldehyde in urban, suburban and rural areas are presented in Table 13.

Although formaldehyde is a natural component of ambient air, anthropogenic sources usually contribute most to the levels of formaldehyde in populated regions, since ambient levels are generally < 1 µg/m^3 in remote areas. For example, in the unpopulated Eniwetok Atoll in the Pacific Ocean, a mean of 0.5 µg/m^3 and a maximum of 1.0 µg/m^3 formaldehyde were measured in outdoor air (Preuss *et al.*, 1985). Other authors have reported similar levels in remote, unpopulated areas (De Serves, 1994; IARC, 1995; Environment Canada/ Health Canada, 2001).

Outdoor air concentrations of formaldehyde in urban environments are more variable and depend on local conditions. They are usually in the range of 1–20 µg/m^3 (Preuss *et al.*, 1985; IARC, 1995; Jurvelin, 2001). Urban air concentrations in heavy traffic or during severe inversions can range up to 100 µg/m^3 (Báez *et al.*, 1995; IARC, 1995; Williams *et al.*, 1996; de Andrade *et al.*, 1998).

A major source of formaldehyde in urban air is incomplete combustion of hydrocarbon fuels, especially from vehicle emissions (Vaught, 1991; Pohanish, 2002). Combustion processes account directly or indirectly for most of the formaldehyde that enters the atmosphere, particularly from engines that are not equipped with catalytic converters (WHO, 1989; Pohanish, 2002). In the USA, emissions of formaldehyde from automobiles were estimated to be about 277 million kg each year just prior to the introduction of the catalytic converter in 1975 (Environmental Protection Agency, 1976) and to have decreased since (Zweidinger *et al.*, 1988). In Mexico, a comparison of exhaust emissions from light-duty vehicles in the early 1990s showed a 10–30-fold decrease in emissions of formaldehyde from vehicles that were equipped with a catalytic converter compared with those with no catalyst (Schifter *et al.*, 2001). In contrast, emissions of formaldehyde from automobile exhaust have been reported to have risen again with the introduction of oxygenated fuels (Kirchstetter *et al.*, 1996). Gaffney *et al.* (1997) found that, in Albuquerque (NM, USA), the introduction of oxygenated fuels was associated with higher ambient air levels of formaldehyde during the winter, the season during which these fuels were used. Levels of

Table 13. Occurrence of formaldehyde in outdoor (ambient) air

Country	Location/region	Settings	Sampling period	No. of samples	Mean concentration or range of means ($\mu g/m^3$)[a]	Range ($\mu g/m^3$)[a]	Comments	Reference
Algeria	Algiers	Urban	2000–01	10	12.7	5.2–27.1		Cecinato et al. (2002)
	Ouargla	Urban		4	4.0	2.6–5.2		
	Algiers	Suburban		14	11.9	6.0–21.2		
Austria	Exelberg	Semi-rural	1986–87	21	6.4–13.4 ppb	NR	Measured in July and August	Puxbaum et al. (1988)
	Raasdorf	Semi-rural		18	6.6–11.1 ppb	NR	Measured in July and August	
	Schoeneben	Rural		20	4.0–8.9 ppb	NR	Measured in September	
Brazil	São Paulo and Rio de Janeiro	Urban	1993	12	10.7	4.0–27.7	Measured outside non-industrial office workplaces and restaurants	Miguel et al. (1995)
	Salvador, Bahia	Urban	NR	68	2.9–80 ppb	1.3–88 ppb	Collected at six sites around the city	de Andrade et al. (1998)
	Rio de Janeiro	Rural	1995	37	1.2–1.5 ppb	0.2–4.6 ppb	Collected at two sites in rural area	Brickus et al. (1998)
		Urban		11	14.5 ppb	7.1–21.0 ppb	Measured outside of an office building	
	São Paulo	Urban	1999	37	16.4–18.0 ppb / 10.7–13.1 ppb / 9.8–10.7 ppb	1.1–46.3 ppb / 1.2–28.3 ppb / 2.7–38.1 ppb	Collected in winter at two sites: Morning / Midday / Evening	Montero et al. (2001)
	São Paulo	Urban	1997	11	5.0 ppb	1.4–9.7 ppb	Measured in February during use of alcohol fuel	Nguyen et al. (2001)
	Theobroma	Rural	1995	15	12.8 ppb daytime, 16.5 ppb nighttime, 8.6 ppb	5–25 ppb	Measured during 1 week of an open agricultural and silvicultural biomass burning period	Reinhardt et al. (2001)
	Rio de Janeiro	Urban	2000	13	10.8	NR	Collected from May to November during morning commute	Grosjean et al. (2002)
	Rio de Janeiro	Urban	1998–2001	28	13.7 ppb	1.5–54.3 ppb	Measured on a high traffic street in the downtown area	Corrêa et al. (2003)

Table 13 (contd)

Country	Location/region	Settings	Sampling period	No. of samples	Mean concentration or range of means (μg/m^3)[a]	Range (μg/m^3)[a]	Comments	Reference
Canada	Ontario	Rural	1988	49 / 47	1.6 ppb / 1.8 ppb	0.6–4.4 ppb / 0.7–4.2 ppb	Dorset site / Egbert site	Shepson *et al.* (1991)
	Alert, Nunavut	Remote	1992	NR	0.48 / NR	0.04–0.74 / 0.12–0.86	Polar night / Sunlit period	De Serves (1994)
	Nova Scotia	Remote	1993	108	NR	< 0.6–4.2	Summer measurements	Tanner *et al.* (1994), cited in Environment Canada/Health Canada (2001)
	Six provinces	Various	1989–98	NR / NR / NR	NR / NR / NR	ND–27.5 / ND–12.0 / ND–9.9	Measured at eight urban sites / Measured at two suburban sites / Measured at six rural sites	Environment Canada (1999), cited in Environment Canada/Health Canada (2001)
		Rural	1995–96 Spring Summer Winter	NR	NR	max., 3.0 / max., 1.7 / max., 4.4	Near a forest product plant	Environment Canada (1997), cited in Environment Canada/Health Canada (2001)
	Prince Rupert, BC	Urban, residential, and industrial areas	1994–95	96	0.7–3.9	0.08–14.7	Collected from the roofs at four sites	Environment Canada/Health Canada (2001)
	Various	Urban and suburban	1990–98	2819	3.3 (2.8)[b]		Four urban and four suburban sites from the National Air Pollution Survey programme	Liteplo & Meek (2003)

Table 13 (contd)

Country	Location/region	Settings	Sampling period	No. of samples	Mean concentration or range of means ($\mu g/m^3$)[a]	Range ($\mu g/m^3$)[a]	Comments	Reference
China	Hong Kong	Urban	1997–2000	182	3.6–4.2 4.8–5.1	0.6–10 1.9–11	Residential and commercial Residential, commercial and light industrial	Sin et al. (2001)
	Hong Kong	Urban	1999–2000	41	4.1 5.9 2.6	1.0–11.3 NR NR	Overall average (12 months) Summer average (May–August) Winter average (November–February)	Ho et al. (2002)
	Guangzhou	Urban	2002	25	12.4	6.4–29.0	Measured outside a hotel in the evening on 7 consecutive days	Feng et al. (2004)
Denmark	Copenhagen	Urban	1994	37	2.6 ppb	0.2–6.4 ppb	Winter measurements (February)	Granby et al. (1997)
	Lille Valby	Semi-rural		18	0.9 ppb	0.1–2.8 ppb	Winter measurements (February)	
				28	0.8 ppb	0.3–1.8 ppb	Spring measurements (April)	
	Lille Valby	Semi-rural	1995	244	1.2 ppb	0.1–4.7 ppb	Measured in May–July	Christensen et al. (2000)
Egypt	Cairo	Urban	1999	98 49 49	33 ppb 29 ppb 37 ppb	SD, 8.6 SD, 7.1 SD, 9.5	Residential area Spring Summer	Khoder et al. (2000)
France	Grenoble	Urban	1995	NR	NR	2–18 ppb	Measured during 1 week in May	Ferrari et al. (1998)
	Paris	Urban and semi-urban	1985	NR	2–32 ppb	NR	Measured at one urban site and three rural sites with some urban influence	Kalabokas et al. (1988)

Table 13 (contd)

Country	Location/region	Settings	Sampling period	No. of samples	Mean concentration or range of means (µg/m³)[a]	Range (µg/m³)[a]	Comments	Reference
Germany	Mainz-Finthen	Semi-rural	1979	14	1.9 ppb	0.7–5.1 ppb	Measured during July–October	Neitzert & Seiler (1981)
	Deuselbach	Rural		14	1.7 ppb	0.4–3.8 ppb	Measured during November	
	The Alps	Rural	1991	NR	1.3 ppb	0.4–3.3 ppb	Measurement at summit of Wank mountain in October	Slemr & Junkermann (1992)
	Schauinsland	Rural	1992	22	1.0 ppb	0.4–2.3 ppb	Measured continuously over 11 days	Slemr et al. (1996)
Hungary	Budapest	Urban	1987–89	185	14.9 ppb 34.6 ppb	ND–58 ppb 7–176 ppb	Measured at downtown site Measured at the border of downtown with a possible local emission source	Haszpra et al. (1991)
Italy	Rome	Urban	1994–95	56 57	17.0 ppb 11.2 ppb	8.8–27.7 ppb 8.2–17.0 ppb	Measured in summer 1994 Measured in winter 1995	Possanzini et al. (1996)
	Milan	Urban	1998–99	NR	NR 5.9 8.0–15.7	4.1–53.4 NR NR	Winter measurements (six sites) Rural-industrial (one site) Urban (five sites)	Andreini et al. (2000)
Japan	Takasaki	Urban	1984	38	NR	2.5–11.4 ppb	Measured during July and August	Satsumabayashi et al. (1995)
	Osaka	Urban	1997	NR	1.9 ppb	0.1–4.3 ppb	Measured in October–December	Nguyen et al. (2001)
	Nagoya	NR	1998	37	5.8[c]	GSD, 1.5	Measured in February	Sakai et al. (2004)
Lithuania	Kaunas	NR	1998	NR	3.1	1.4–5.3	Measured at 12 municipal monitoring sites	Maroziene & Grazuleviciene (2002)
Mexico	Mexico City	Urban	1993	48	35.5 ppb	5.9–110 ppb	Measured at the University of Mexico campus	Báez et al. (1995)
	Mexico City and Xalapa	Urban	1996–98	145[d]	4–32	2–63	Measured outside two houses, three museums and two offices	Báez et al. (2003)

Table 13 (contd)

Country	Location/region	Settings	Sampling period	No. of samples	Mean concentration or range of means $(\mu g/m^3)^a$	Range $(\mu g/m^3)^a$	Comments	Reference
Norway	Drammen	Urban	1994–97 1998–2000	974 973	8.9 2.9	NR NR	Reduction of mean levels attributed to increase in vehicles with catalysts	Hagen et al. (2000); Oftedal et al. (2003)
South Africa	Cape Point	Semi-rural	1979	5	0.5 ppb	0.2–1.0 ppb	Measured during December	Neitzert & Seiler (1981)
Spain	Madrid	Urban	1996	NR	9.0	4.7–20	Air sampling in September–October from 8 h to 16 h	García-Alonso & Pérez-Pastor (1998)
Sweden	Uppsala	Urban	1998	27	1.3ᶜ	GSD, 1.8	Measured in February–May near 22 houses and five apartments	Sakai et al. (2004)
Taiwan, China	Taipei	Urban	1999	NR	7.2–9.8 ppb	range of max., 20.6–34.8 ppb	Measured from February–June at five locations	Mathew et al. (2001)
United Kingdom	London	Urban	1991–92	9 7	19.2 ppb 7.4 ppb	ND–98 ppb 0.8–13.5 ppb	West London, residential area North London, residential area	Williams et al. (1996)
USA	Country-wide	Various Urban Suburban Rural	1975–85	629 332 281 12	8.3 ppb (4.1 ppb)ᵇ 6.5 ppbᵇ 2.7 ppbᵇ 2.7 ppbvᵇ	NR NR NR NR	All sites combinedᵉ	Shah & Singh (1988)ᶠ
	Atlanta, GA	Urban	1992	217	2.7–3.0 ppb	max., 8.3 ppb	Measured at four locations during July and August	Grosjean et al. (1993)
	Albany, NY	Semi-urban	1991	NR	NR	0.6–3.7 ppb	Measured during October	Khwaja (1995)
	Boston, MA	Residential	1993	8	3.1 ppb	0–3.1 ppb	Winter measurements, outside four residences	Reiss et al. (1995)
				18	2.6 ppb	1.2–5.9 ppb	Summer measurements, outside nine residences	

Table 13 (contd)

Country	Location/region	Settings	Sampling period	No. of samples	Mean concentration or range of means (μg/m³)ᵃ	Range (μg/m³)ᵃ	Comments	Reference
USA (contd)	Denver, CO	Urban	1987–91	NR	3.9 ppb 2.3 ppb 2.7 ppb	NR NR NR	Measured in winter Measured in spring Measured in summer	Anderson et al. (1996)
	Los Angeles, CA	Urban	1993	32	5.3 ppb	1.4–10.6 ppb	Measured during the smog season (September)	Grosjean et al. (1996)
		Rural			0.8 ppb	0.7–1.0 ppb	Background location	
	Eniwetok Atoll	Remote	1980	7	0.4 ppb	max., 0.8 ppb	South Pacific	Preuss et al. (1985)
	Minnesota	Mixed	1991–99	2494	1.7 (1.37)ᵇ	< 0.05–21	Collected at 25 sites throughout the state for varying periods of time	Pratt et al. (2000)
	New York City, NY	Urban	1999	36 36	2.1 5.3		Winter measurements Summer measurements	Kinney et al. (2002)
	Los Angeles County, CA	Semi-urban	1999–2000	69	7.2 ppb	4.3–14.0 ppb		Delfino et al. (2003)
	California	Urban	1990–2002	NR	2.0–4.3	NR	Range of annual averages	California Air Resources Board (2004)

GSD, geometric standard deviation; NR, not reported; SD, standard deviation
ᵃ Unless otherwise specified
ᵇ Median
ᶜ Geometric mean
ᵈ Number of indoor and outdoor measurements combined (see Table 14)
ᵉ Includes urban, suburban, rural, remote and source-dominated sources.
ᶠ Data collected from literature searches, direct contacts with individuals and organisations, reports, computer tapes and direct electronic transfers

formaldehyde in vehicle emissions in 1994 were found to increase by 13% within 2 months after the average oxygen content of fuels sold in the San Francisco Bay (CA, USA) area increased from 0.3 to 2.0% by weight (Kirchstetter *et al.*, 1996). In the Denver (CO, USA) area, use of oxygenated fuels was associated with a 20–75% increase in ambient air levels of formaldehyde, although nearly all ambient air measurements remained below 6 $\mu g/m^3$ (Spitzer, 1997). Local air concentrations as high as 35.4, 41.8 and 44.2 $\mu g/m^3$ have been reported inside vehicles, in parking garages and at service stations, respectively (Spitzer, 1997).

Formaldehyde was detected (detection limit, 0.05 $\mu g/m^3$) in 3810 of 3842 24-h samples from rural, suburban and urban areas in Canada that were collected at 16 sites in six provinces surveyed from August 1989 to August 1998 (Environment Canada, 1999, cited in Environment Canada/Health Canada, 2001). Concentrations ranged from below the detection limit to a maximum of 27.5 $\mu g/m^3$ for eight urban sites, a maximum of 12.03 $\mu g/m^3$ for two suburban sites and a maximum of 9.88 $\mu g/m^3$ for six rural sites. Long-term (1 month–1 year) mean concentrations for the rural sites ranged from 0.78 to 8.76 $\mu g/m^3$. Monthly mean concentrations were highest during the summer, but there was no apparent long-term trend in concentrations of formaldehyde at these sites over this 9-year period (Environment Canada/Health Canada, 2001).

In addition to primary emissions of formaldehyde in vehicle exhaust, secondary formation of formaldehyde by oxidation of alkenes in the atmosphere is also an important source (Altshuller, 1993; Seila *et al.*, 2001). Patterns of diurnal and seasonal variation in levels of formaldehyde and formaldehyde:acetaldehyde ratios have led to the suggestion that natural sources of alkenes add significantly to anthropogenic emissions, particularly during the summer months (Gaffney *et al.*, 1997; Viskari *et al.*, 2000). Photo-oxidation is also a primary degradation pathway for formaldehyde in the atmosphere, with an estimated half-life in the range of a few hours (ATSDR, 1999).

1.3.4   *Residential indoor air*

The occurrence of formaldehyde in indoor air in private housing and public settings is summarized in Table 14.

Levels of formaldehyde in indoor air are often higher by one order of magnitude or more than those outdoors. The concentrations in dwellings depend on the sources of formaldehyde that are present, the age of the source materials, ventilation, temperature and humidity. Indoor sources include pressed wood products (e.g. plywood, particle-board), some insulation materials, carpets, paints and varnishes, clothing and fabrics, cooking, tobacco smoke and the use of formaldehyde as a disinfectant (Gammage & Gupta, 1984; IARC, 1995; Dingle *et al.*, 2000; Hodgson *et al.*, 2000, 2002; Jurvelin, 2003). Off-gassing of urea–formaldehyde foam insulation and particle-board has been reported historically to be a major source of formaldehyde in some dwellings.

In a study on indoor emissions of formaldehyde, quasi steady-state emission rates of formaldehyde from new carpets were measured in a large-scale environmental chamber

Table 14. Occurrence of formaldehyde in indoor air in residential and public settings

Country	Location/region	Sampling period	No. of samples	Mean concentration or range of means (μg/m³)[a]	Range (μg/m³)[a]	Comments	Reference
Residential							
Australia	Victoria	1994–95	NR	12.6 ppb[b] 13.8 ppb[b] 11.3 ppb[b] 11.4 ppb[b]	< 0.3–105 < 0.3–108 < 0.3–108	Eighty households Bedroom Living-room Kitchen	Garrett et al. (1997, 1999)
Austria	Burgenland, Carinthia and Styria	1988–89	234 apartments	< 30–100 ppb 100–500 ppb > 500 ppb		Measured in 33% of the apartments Measured in 48% of the apartments Measured in 19% of the apartments	Koeck et al. (1997)
Canada	Quebec City, QC	NR	28 3 34 6	7.3 9.2 8.2 9.9	max., 20.2 max., 19.7 max., 23.4 max., 19.5	Basement, with combustion appliance Basement, without combustion appliance Ground floor, with combustion appliance Ground floor, without combustion appliance	Lévesque et al. (2001)
	Various	1989–95	151	35.9 (29.8[b])	NR	Pooled data from five studies at various locations	Liteplo & Meek (2003)
Egypt	Cairo	1999	294 147 147	89 ppb 100 ppb 100 ppb 87.6 ppb 105.6 ppb	35–192 ppb 30–213 ppb 28–225 ppb NR NR	Seven apartments Kitchen Bedroom Living room Measured in spring Measured in summer	Khoder et al. (2000)
France	Paris	2001	61 61 61	21.7[c] 24.2[c] 24.5[c]	NR NR NR	Sixty-one dwellings in Paris and suburbs Kitchen Living room Bedroom	Clarisse et al. (2003)
Hungary		1998	123	17.5	0.6–56.7	Homes in six medium-sized cities	Erdei et al. (2003)

Table 14 (contd)

Country	Location/region	Sampling period	No. of samples	Mean concentration or range of means (μg/m³)ᵃ	Range (μg/m³)ᵃ	Comments	Reference
Japan	Country-wide	1998–2001	1642	120 (95.7ᵇ)	max., 979	From 1422 homes distributed throughout the country	Park & Ikeda (2003)
	NR	2000	171	110 ppb / 120 ppb	20–872 ppb / 11–840 ppb	Rooms from 81 houses / Active DNPH method / Detector tube method	Azuma et al. (2003)
	Niigata Prefecture	1999	104	NR	0–740	Data from figure; 29% greater than 100 μg/m³	Sakaguchi & Akabayashi (2003)
	Nagoya	1998	37	17.6ᶜ	max., 73	Dwelling factors and airborne concentrations were also compared	Sakai et al. (2004)
Mexico	Mexico City and Xalapa	1996–98	50ᵈ	37–47	12–81	Measured in two houses	Báez et al. (2003)
Sweden	Uppsala	1998	27	8.3ᶜ	max., 19	Dwelling factors and airborne concentrations were also compared	Sakai et al. (2004)
United Kingdom	London	1991–92	17 / 40	15.0 ppb / 3.4 ppb	ND–93.1 ppb / ND–10.3 ppb	West London, residential area / North London, residential area	Williams et al. (1996)
USA	San Francisco Bay Area, CA	1984	48 / 45	41 ppb / 36 ppb	NR / NR	Kitchen / Main bedroom	Sexton et al. (1986)
	Various	1981–84	273	44.0ᵇ	NR	Mixed locations	Shah & Singh (1988)ᵉ
	Colorado	1992–93	9	26ᵈ / 49ᵈ	8–66 / 33–81	Prior to occupancy / After 5 months of occupancy	Lindstrom et al. (1995)
	Boston, MA	1993	14 / 26	11.1 ppb / 16.1 ppb	6.0–16.1 ppb / 5.9–53.8 ppb	Winter measurements, four residences / Summer measurements, nine residences	Reiss et al. (1995)
	Louisiana	NR	419	460	ND–6600	Measured in 53 houses (75% urban, 25% rural); also measured seasonal differences	Lemus et al. (1998)

Table 14 (contd)

Country	Location/ region	Sampling period	No. of samples	Mean concentration or range of means ($\mu g/m^3$)[a]	Range ($\mu g/m^3$)[a]	Comments	Reference
USA (contd)	East and South-East	1997–98	4 7	34 ppb[d] 36 ppb[d]	21–47 ppb 14–58 ppb	Manufactured houses Site-built houses	Hodgson et al. (2000)
	Florida	2000	NR	94.9	NR	New manufactured house	Hodgson et al. (2002)
	New York City, NY	1999	38 41	12.1 20.9	NR NR	Winter measurements Summer measurements	Kinney et al. (2002)
Public settings							
China	Hotel ballroom	2002	28	29.7	26.3–63.0	Measured in four hotel ballrooms in the evening on 7 consecutive days	Feng et al. (2004)
Italy	Library	1995–96	16	32.7	1.7–67.8	Sixteen libraries at the University of Modena; 10 samples with detectable levels	Fantuzzi et al. (1996)
Mexico	Museum	1996–98	60[d]	11–34	4–59	Three museums	Báez et al. (2003)
Sweden	Hospital	1997	4	5	2–7	Geriatric hospitals built in 1925, 1985, 1993 and 1994	Wieslander et al. (1999b)
	Primary school	1993, 1995	48	9.5	3–16	Twelve randomly selected primary schools	Norbäck et al. (2000)

ND, not detected; NR, not reported
[a] Unless stated otherwise
[b] Median
[c] Geometric mean
[d] Number of indoor and outdoor measurements combined (see Table 13)
[e] Data collected from literature searches, direct contacts with individuals and organisations, reports, computer tapes and direct electronic transfers

(Hodgson *et al.*, 1993). The emission rates in single samples were 57.2 and 18.2 $\mu g/m^2/h$ at 24 and 168 h, respectively, after the start of each experiment. Similar results were observed in a Swedish study in which indoor levels of formaldehyde were found to be higher in homes that had wall-to-wall carpeting (Norbäck *et al.*, 1995).

The release of formaldehyde and volatile organic compounds from newly painted indoor surfaces was investigated in a sample of 62 dwellings in Uppsala, Sweden, in 1991–92. Concentrations of formaldehyde were significantly increased in dwellings where wood paint had been used, but were not related to other types of painting. Wall-to-wall carpeting and wood painting made approximately equal contributions of 13 $\mu g/m^3$ and 16 $\mu g/m^3$ formaldehyde, respectively (Wieslander *et al.*, 1997). The adsorption of formaldehyde to dust particles on wipe samples from homes and offices was investigated to evaluate the extent to which such particles could act as carriers for volatile pollutants and contribute to exposure to formaldehyde. A person exposed to an ambient concentration of 1 ppm [1.2 mg/m^3] formaldehyde would inhale about 1 mg/h formaldehyde vapour when breathing normally (15 L/min). In the presence of 1 mg/m^3 dust (that contains 10 ng/mg formaldehyde based on analysis of the dust samples), the amount of particle-associated formaldehyde inhaled would be approximately 10 ng/h, i.e. five orders of magnitude lower (Rothenberg *et al.*, 1989). The dose of particle-associated formaldehyde to the lower respiratory tract is predicted to be at least four orders of magnitude smaller than the vapour-phase dose to the upper respiratory tract. [The Working Group noted that the conditions of this investigation are also relevant to industrial environments.]

Data on concentrations of formaldehyde in residential indoor air from five studies conducted in Canada between 1989 and 1995 were examined (Health Canada, 2000). Despite differences in sampling mode and duration (i.e. active sampling for 24 h or passive sampling for 7 days), the distribution of concentrations was similar in the five studies. The median, arithmetic mean, 95th percentile and 99th percentile concentrations of the pooled data (151 samples) were 29.8, 35.9, 84.6 and 116 $\mu g/m^3$, respectively (Health Canada, 2000). Similar concentrations have been measured in non-workplace indoor air in other countries.

Personal 48-h exposures of 15 randomly selected participants as well as microenvironment concentrations in each participant's residence and workplace were measured for 16 carbonyl compounds, including formaldehyde, during the summer and autumn of 1997 as part of the Air Pollution Exposure of Adult Urban Populations in Europe (EXPOLIS) study in Helsinki, Finland. The mean personal exposure concentration of formaldehyde was 21.4 ppb [26.3 $\mu g/m^3$]; the mean indoor residential concentration was 33.3 ppb [41.0 $\mu g/m^3$]; the mean outdoor residential concentration was 2.6 ppb [3.2 $\mu g/m^3$]; and the mean workplace concentration was 12.0 ppb [14.8 $\mu g/m^3$] (Jurvelin *et al.*, 2003).

In earlier studies summarized by Preuss *et al.* (1985), the mean concentrations in conventional homes with no urea–formaldehyde foam insulation were 25–60 $\mu g/m^3$. Since the late 1970s, many studies have reported formaldehyde levels in 'mobile homes' (caravans) (see, for example, the review of Gammage & Travis, 1989). The levels appear to decrease as the mobile home ages, with a half-life of 4–5 years (Preuss *et al.*, 1985). In the early 1980s, mean concentrations of 0.4 ppm [0.5 mg/m^3] and individual values as high as several parts per million were measured in new mobile homes. As a result of new standards and regulations established in the mid-1980s for building materials and voluntary reductions by the manufacturers, concentrations of formaldehyde in mobile homes have decreased to approximately 0.1 ppm [0.12 mg/m^3] or less (Gammage & Travis, 1989; Sexton *et al.*, 1989; Gylseth & Digernes, 1992; Lehmann & Roffael, 1992).

Formaldehyde may also occur in indoor air through the degradation of other organic compounds. Naturally occurring unsaturated hydrocarbons, such as limonene and pinene (which may also be released from consumer products), anthropogenic compounds, such as 4-vinylcyclohexene (an emission from carpet padding), and other alkenes that are commonly found in indoor air have been found to produce formaldehyde via their initial reaction with ozone (Zhang *et al.*, 1994; Weschler & Shields, 1996). Reiss *et al.* (1995) estimated that the effective average rate of emissions of formaldehyde from this process in four residences in Boston (MA, USA) was about three times higher in the summer than in the winter.

In a study conducted at the Inhalation Toxicology Research Institute, release rates of formaldehyde were measured for six types of consumer product (Pickrell *et al.*, 1983, 1984). Release rates calculated per unit surface area (μg/m^2 per day) were used to rank the products in the following order: pressed wood products >> clothes ~ insulation products ~ paper products > fabric > carpet. Release rates from pressed wood products ranged from below the limit of detection for an exterior plywood to 36 000 μg/m^2 per day for some panelling. Other release rates were 15–550 μg/m^2 per day for articles of new clothing that had not previously been washed, 52–620 μg/m^2 per day for insulation products, 75–1000 μg/m^2 per day for paper plates and cups, from below the limit of detection to 350 μg/m^2 per day for fabrics and from below the limit of detection to 65 μg/m^2 per day for carpets.

In a follow-up study that was performed as a result of changes in product manufacturing processes, many of these release rates were re-investigated (Kelly *et al.*, 1999). Release rates of formaldehyde were reported to range typically from 9 to 1578 μg/m^2/h for a variety of bare urea–formaldehyde wood products, from 1 to 461 μg/m^2/h for coated urea–formaldehyde wood products, from 42 to 214 μg/m^2/h for permanent press fabrics, from 4 to 50 μg/m^2/h for decorative laminates, from 16 to 32 μg/m^2/h for fibreglass products and from 4 to 9 μg/m^2/h for bare phenol–formaldehyde wood products (Kelly *et al.*, 1999). Paper grocery bags and towels had emission rates of < 0.5 and < 0.6 μg/m^2/h, respectively. For wet products, the emission rates were: latex paint, 326–854 μg/m^2/h; fingernail hardener, 178 000–354 000 μg/m^2/h; nail polish, 20 700 μg/m^2/h; and commercially applied urea–formaldehyde floor finish, 1 050 000 and 421 000 μg/m^2/h for base and topcoats, respectively (Kelly *et al.*, 1999).

1.3.5   *Other exposures*

According to the Environmental Protection Agency Toxics Release Inventory (TRI), in 2001, approximately 9500 tonnes of formaldehyde were released into the environment from 800 domestic manufacturing and processing facilities in the USA. This number represents the sum of all releases of formaldehyde to air (4800 tonnes), water (160 tonnes), soil (70 tonnes) and underground injection wells (4500 tonnes). The TRI data should be used with caution because not all facilities are required to report releases of formaldehyde into the environment (National Library of Medicine, 2004).

Cigarette smoke has been reported to contain levels of a few to over 100 µg formaldehyde per cigarette (IARC, 2004). A 'pack-a-day' smoker may inhale as much as 0.4–2.0 mg formaldehyde (IARC, 1995; ACGIH® Worldwide, 2003).

Cosmetic products that contain formaldehyde, formalin and/or paraformaldehyde may come into contact with hair (e.g. shampoos and hair preparations), skin (deodorants, bath products, skin preparations and lotions), eyes (mascara and eye make-up), oral mucosa (mouthwashes and breath fresheners), vaginal mucosa (vaginal deodorants) and nails (cuticle softeners, nail creams and lotions). Use of aerosol products (e.g. shaving creams) may result in potential inhalation of formaldehyde (Cosmetic Ingredient Review Expert Panel, 1984). A Swedish study on indoor emissions reported that oil-based skin care products that are known to contain formaldehyde precursors (donors) still release formaldehyde into the air after storage for 1 year (Karlberg *et al.*, 1998).

Formaldehyde occurs naturally in foods, and foods may be contaminated as a result of fumigation (e.g. grain), cooking (as a combustion product) and release from formaldehyde resin-based tableware (WHO, 1989). It has been used as a bacteriostatic agent in some foods, such as cheese (Restani *et al.*, 1992). Fruit and vegetables typically contain 3–60 mg/kg, milk and milk products contain about 1 mg/kg, meat and fish contain 6–20 mg/kg and shellfish contain 1–100 mg/kg. Drinking-water generally contains < 0.1 mg/L (WHO, 1989).

Formaldehyde can also be emitted into indoor air during the cooking of fish. Amounts of formaldehyde that formed in a headspace when various kinds of fish flesh were heated to 200 °C ranged from 0.48 µg/g for mackerel to 5.31 µg/g for sardine (Yasuhara & Shibamoto, 1995). Free formaldehyde was found in fish at levels ranging from 1.4 to 40.3 ppm [1.7 to 49.6 mg/m³]; the high levels were attributed to the processes used to freeze the fish products (Nielsen, 2002). When cooking oils are heated to high temperatures (240–280 °C) that are typical of Chinese wok cooking, several volatile mutagenic organic compounds are released, including formaldehyde. Emissions of formaldehyde from several cooking oils (rapeseed, canola, soya bean, peanut) ranged from 23 to 71 µg/L (Shields *et al.*, 1995).

Composting of household waste was also found to generate formaldehyde (Eitzer *et al.*, 1997). [Composting may also be of concern for occupational exposures.]

In some regions, mosquito coils are burned in residences for mosquito control. In a study of the combustion products from two common brands of mosquito coil, formaldehyde was generated at a level of approximately 2–4 mg/g of mosquito coil, which would result in air concentrations in the range of 0.16–0.40 ppm [0.19–0.49 mg/m³] (Chang & Lin, 1998).

Formaldehyde has been used as a chemical germicide to control bacterial contamination in water distribution systems and in the dialysis fluid pathways of artificial kidney machines. In addition, formaldehyde has been used to disinfect hollow fibre dialysers (artificial kidneys) that are reprocessed and re-used only by the same patient (Centers for Disease Control, 1986).

When formalin-sterilized dialysers were rinsed by the technique used in many dialysis centres in the 1970s, undesirable concentrations of formaldehyde were found in the apparatuses at the start of dialysis. When the technique was modified by passing part of the saline through the blood compartment immediately before connection and discarding the saline left in the dialyser at the time of connection, the concentration of formaldehyde infused into the patient fell to below 2 µg/mL. However, the dialysers still contained up to 13 mg formaldehyde which leached slowly during simulated dialysis. Some residual formaldehyde was found in several components of the dialyser, but the majority was contained in the cellulose membrane (Lewis et al., 1981).

Stragier et al. (1995) studied the influence of the type of disinfecting agent used on the necessary rinsing time and rebound release after rinsing re-used dialysers. The rinsing time required to reach undetectable levels of disinfecting agent was longest for formaldehyde and the rebound release 30 min after completion of rinsing was the highest for formaldehyde.

In the USA, the proportion of dialysis centres that use formaldehyde to reprocess dialysers decreased from 94 to 31% during 1983–2000 (Tokars et al., 2000).

1.4   Regulations and guidelines

Occupational exposure limits and guidelines for formaldehyde are presented in Table 15. International regulations and guidelines related to emissions of and exposures to formaldehyde in occupational settings, indoor air and building materials have been reviewed (IARC, 1995; Paustenbach et al., 1997; ATSDR, 1999).

The European Union has adopted a Directive that imposes concentration limits for formaldehyde and paraformaldehyde in cosmetics. These substances are permitted at a maximal concentration of 0.2% by weight or volume (expressed as free formaldehyde) in all cosmetic formulations except nail hardeners, oral hygiene products and aerosol dispensers. Nail hardeners and oral hygiene products may contain maximal concentrations of 5 and 0.1%, respectively, whereas formaldehyde and paraformaldehyde are prohibited for use in aerosol dispensers (except for foams). Labels of cosmetic products are required to list formaldehyde and paraformaldehyde as ingredients when the concentration of either exceeds 0.05% (Cosmetic Ingredient Review Expert Panel, 1984; European Commission, 1990).

The Food and Drug Administration (2003) in the USA identifies formaldehyde: as a secondary direct food additive that is permitted in food for human consumption; for use as a preservative in defoaming agents; as an indirect food additive for use only as a component of adhesives; as an indirect food additive for use only as paper and paperboard

Table 15. Occupational exposure standards and guidelines for formaldehyde

Country or region	Concentration (mg/m^3) [ppm]	Interpretation	Carcinogen classification
Australia	1.2 [1]	TWA	2; Sen
	2.5 [2]	STEL	
Belgium	0.37 [0.3]	Ceiling	
Brazil	2 [1.6]	Ceiling	
China	0.5	Ceiling	
Canada			
Alberta	2.5 [2]	Ceiling	
Ontario	0.37 [0.3]	Ceiling	
Quebec	2.5 [2]	Ceiling	A2[a]
Denmark	0.4 [0.3]	STEL	L, K
Finland	0.37 [0.3]	TWA	
	1.2 [1]	Ceiling	
France	0.6 [0.5]	TWA	
	1.2 [1]	STEL	
Germany	0.37 [0.3]	TWA (MAK)	4; Sh; I
		STEL	
	0.7 [0.6]	Ceiling	
	1.2 [1]		
Hong Kong	0.37 [0.3]	Ceiling	A2[b]
Ireland	2.5 [2]	TWA	
	2.5 [2]	STEL	
Japan	0.6 [0.5]	TWA	2A
Malaysia	0.37 [0.3]	Ceiling	
Mexico	2.5 [2]	Ceiling	A2[b]
Netherlands	1.2 [1]	TWA	
	2.5 [2]	STEL	
New Zealand	1.2 [1]	Ceiling	A2[b]
Norway	0.6 [0.5]	TWA	Ca[c]; Sen
	1.2 [1]	Ceiling	
Poland	0.5	TWA	
	1	STEL	
South Africa	2.5 [2]	TWA	
	2.5 [2]	STEL	
Spain	0.37 [0.3]	STEL	
Sweden	0.6 [0.5]	TWA	Ca[d]; Sen
	1.2 [1]	Ceiling	
Switzerland	0.37 [0.3]	TWA	Sen
	0.74 [0.6]	STEL	
United Kingdom (MEL)	2.5 [2]	TWA	
	2.5 [2]	STEL	

Table 15 (contd)

Country or region	Concentration (mg/m³) [ppm]	Interpretation	Carcinogen classification
USA			
ACGIH (TLV)	0.37 [0.3]	Ceiling	A2[b]; Sen
NIOSH (REL)	0.02 [0.016]	TWA	Ca[d]
	0.12 [0.1]	Ceiling	
OSHA (PEL)	0.9 [0.75]	TWA	Ca[d]
	2.5 [2]	STEL	

From Arbejdstilsynet (2002); Health & Safety Executive (2002); Työsuojelu-säädöksiä (2002); ACGIH® Worldwide (2003); Deutsche Forschungsgemein-schaft (2003); Suva (2003); INRS (2005)
I, local irritant; K, carcinogenic; L, substance with ceiling value; MEL, maximum exposure limit; PEL, permissible exposure limit; REL, recommended exposure limit; Sen, sensitizer; Sh, skin sensitizer; STEL, short-term exposure limit; TLV, threshold limit value; TWA, time-weighted average; 2, probable human carcinogen; 2A, probably carcinogenic to humans (IARC classification); 4, carcinogenic potential with no or little genotoxicity
[a] A2: carcinogenic effects suspected in humans
[b] A2: suspected human carcinogen
[c] Ca: potential cancer-causing agent
[d] Ca: Substance is carcinogenic.

components; as an indirect food additive for use as a preservative in textile and textile fibre polymers; as an indirect food additive for use as an adjuvant in animal glue; and, under specified conditions, as an animal drug and in the manufacture of animal feeds.

Guidelines for levels of formaldehyde in ambient air in living spaces have been set in several countries and range from 0.05 to 0.4 ppm [0.06–0.5 mg/m³], with a preference for 0.1 ppm [0.12 mg/m³] (Lehmann & Roffael, 1992).

Some European countries have established maximum limits for emissions of formalde-hyde from particle-boards, other wood products, furniture and insulation foam: for instance, Denmark, Finland and Sweden have set a maximum of 0.15 mg/m³, measured in a test room of 225 L under standard conditions; in France, the content of formaldehyde that arises from walls insulated with urea–formaldehyde foam should not exceed 0.2 ppm (European Union, 1989).

In the USA, all plywood and particle-board materials that are bonded with a resin system or coated with a surface finish that contains formaldehyde cannot exceed the following formaldehyde emission levels when installed in manufactured homes, as expressed as air concentrations using standard conditions: plywood materials and particle-board flooring products (including urea–formaldehyde-bonded particle-board), 0.25 mg/m³; particle-board materials and medium-density fibre-board, 0.37 mg/m³ (Composite Panel Association, 1999, 2002; Department of Housing and Urban Development, 2003).

2.   Studies of Cancer in Humans

2.1   Cohort studies

More than 25 cohort studies have examined the association between formaldehyde and cancer. Since the previous IARC monograph in 1994 (IARC, 1995), three of these have been updated, and six new studies have been published. The following review divides the studies into those that concern professionals (e.g. pathologists, anatomists and embalmers) and those that concern industrial workers (e.g. formaldehyde producers, formaldehyde resin makers, plywood and particle-board manufacturers, garment workers and workers in the abrasives industry). This division was also made in the previous IARC monograph because of differences between these studies with regard to their findings, the nature of the exposure to formaldehyde and the potential for exposures to other carcinogens or other factors that might confound the findings.

The following discussion is focused largely on the results for sites that may come into direct contact with airborne formaldehyde (cancers of the respiratory tract including cancers of the trachea, bronchus and lung, laryngeal cancer, sinonasal cancer, nasopharyngeal cancer, oral cancer and other pharyngeal cancers) and on leukaemia and brain cancer, for which excess mortality has been reported in several studies.

2.1.1   *Cohorts of industrial workers*

Key study features and findings from the cohort and nested case–control studies of industrial workers are summarized chronologically in Table 16, based on the year of publication of the first report of the cohort. Studies have been conducted on workers who were exposed to formaldehyde in the chemical, garment, fibreglass, iron, wood-working, plastics and paper, pulp and plywood industries. Several of these cohort studies have recently been updated, and the results presented below are largely limited to the updated data, grouped by industry.

(*a*)   *The National Cancer Institute (NCI) Cohort*

Blair *et al.* (1986, 1990a) at the NCI, USA, conducted the largest of the cohort studies, which included over 25 000 workers (88% men) who had first been employed before 1966 in one of 10 industrial facilities in the USA. These facilities manufactured formaldehyde (three plants), formaldehyde resins (six plants), moulding compounds (six plants), moulded plastic products (two plants), photographic films (two plants) and plywood (one plant). Among all of the workers, 11% were considered to be unexposed.

This study included workers from facilities that were also included in studies by Marsh (1982), Wong (1983) and Liebling *et al.* (1984) and in a case–control study by Fayerweather

Table 16. Cohort studies of industrial workers exposed to formaldehyde

Reference, location, years of study	Cohort description Type of analysis (cohort size)	Exposure assessment	Organ site (ICD code)[a]	No. of cases/deaths	SMR (95% CI)	Comments
Coggon et al. (2003), United Kingdom, 1941–2000 (update of Acheson et al., 1984a; Gardner et al., 1993)	Chemical factories that used or produced formaldehyde Standardized mortality (14 014 men)	Level of exposure (background, low, moderate, high); among highly exposed, time period and duration of exposure	All cancers	1511 deaths	1.10 (1.04–1.16)	
			Nasopharynx	1 death	NR	2.0 expected
			Nose and nasal sinuses	2 deaths	0.87 (0.11–3.14)	Two additional cases identified from registry that could not be used in the analysis
			Lymphohaematopoietic	NR	NR	
			Leukaemia	31 deaths	0.91 (0.47–1.59)	
			Mouth (ICD-9, 143–145)	6 deaths	1.28 (0.47–2.78)	
			Lung	594 deaths	1.22 (1.12–1.32)	Increased risk among highly exposed (1.58; 95% CI, 1.40–1.78); inverse trend with duration of exposure
			Brain and central nervous system	30 deaths	0.85 (0.57–1.21)	
Hauptmann et al. (2003, 2004), USA, 1966–94 (update of Blair et al., 1986, 1987)	Manufacturer of formaldehyde, formaldehyde resins, moulding compounds, moulded plastic products, photographic films and plywood Standardized mortality (25 619 workers; 22 493 men, 3126 women)	Duration; quantitative estimates of cumulative, average and highest peak exposure	All cancers	1723 deaths	0.90 (0.86–0.95)	15-year lag for solid cancers; 2-year lag for lymphohaematopoietic cancers
			Nasopharynx	8 deaths	2.10 (1.05–4.21)	The authors noted that the exact CI is 0.91–4.14; statistically significant trend with highest peak exposure; weaker trends observed with duration of, cumulative and average exposures
			Nose and nasal sinuses	3 deaths	1.19 (0.38–3.68)	
			Lymphohaematopoietic	161 deaths	0.80 (0.69–0.94)	
			Leukaemia	65 deaths	0.85 (0.67–1.09)	Statistically significant trend with peak exposure, particularly for myeloid leukaemia; weaker trend with average exposure; no trend with duration of or cumulative exposure
			Buccal cavity	49 deaths	1.01 (0.77–1.34)	
			Lung	641 deaths	0.97 (0.90–1.05)	
			Brain and central nervous system	43 deaths	0.92 (0.68–1.23)	

Table 16 (contd)

Reference, location, years of study	Cohort description Type of analysis (cohort size)	Exposure assessment	Organ site (ICD code)[a]	No. of cases/ deaths	SMR (95% CI)	Comments
Bertazzi et al. (1986, 1989), Italy, 1959–86	Formaldehyde resin makers Standardized mortality (1332 men)	Duration of exposure, latency, age at employment, year of employment, time since beginning of employment	All cancers	62 deaths	1.23 [0.94–1.58][b]	Mortality was close to expected when local rates were used as the referent (1.00 [95% CI, 0.64–1.49])
			Nasopharynx	NR	NR	
			Nasal cavity	0 deaths	NA	SMR with local rates as the referent, 1.43 [95% CI, 0.57–2.95]
			Lymphohaematopoietic	7 deaths	1.77 [0.71–3.65][b]	
			Leukaemia	NR	NR	
			Buccal cavity/pharynx	NR	NR	
			Lung	24 deaths	1.56 [1.00–2.32]	
			Brain	NR	NR	
Edling et al. (1987a), Sweden, 1955–83	Abrasives industry Standardized mortality, standardized incidence (521 male blue-collar workers)	None (area measurements)	All cancers	24 inc. cases	0.84 [0.54–1.25][c]	All cancer mortality SMR, 0.93 [95% CI, 0.54–1.49]
			Nasopharynx	1 inc. case	NR	
			Nasal cavity	0 inc. cases	NA	
			Lymphohaematopoietic	4 inc. cases	NR	
			Leukaemia	0 inc. cases	NA	
			Buccal cavity	0 inc. cases	NA	
			Lung	2 inc. cases	0.57 [0.07–2.06]	
			Brain and central nervous system	1 inc. case	NR	
Pinkerton et al. (2004), USA, 1955–98 (update of Stayner et al., 1988)	Garment industry Standardized mortality (11 039 workers; 2015 men, 9024 women)	Duration, time since first exposure, year of first exposure	All cancers	608 deaths	0.89 (0.82–0.97)	0.96 expected
			Nasopharynx	0 deaths	NA	0.16 expected
			Nasal cavity	0 deaths	NA	
			Lymphohaematopoietic	59 deaths	0.97 (0.74–1.26)	
			Leukaemia	24 deaths	1.09 (0.70–1.62)	
			Myeloid leukaemia	15 deaths	1.44 (0.80–2.37)	Statistically significant excess among workers with both ≥ 10 years of exposure and ≥ 20 years since first exposure (SMR, 2.43; 95% CI, 0.98–5.01)
			Buccal cavity/pharynx	4 deaths	1.33 (0.36–3.41)	
			Lung	147 deaths	0.98 (0.82–1.15)	
			Brain and central nervous system	19 deaths	1.09 (0.66–1.71)	

Table 16 (contd)

Reference, location, years of study	Cohort description Type of analysis (cohort size)	Exposure assessment	Organ site (ICD code)[a]	No. of cases/ deaths	SMR (95% CI)	Comments
Andjelkovich et al. (1995), USA, 1960–89	Foundry workers Standardized mortality (3929 men with potential exposure)	Exposed/ unexposed; none, low, medium and high exposure	All cancers	127 deaths	0.99 (0.82–1.17)	
			Nasopharynx	0 deaths	NA	
			Nasal cavity	0 deaths	NA	
			Lymphohaematopoietic	7 deaths	0.59 (0.23–1.21)	
			Leukaemia	2 deaths	0.43 (0.05–1.57)	
			Buccal cavity/pharynx	6 deaths	1.31 (0.48–2.86)	
					1.16 (0.20–6.51)[d]	
			Lung	51 deaths	1.20 (0.89–1.58)	
					0.59 (0.28–1.20)[d]	
			Brain and central nervous system	2 deaths	0.62 (0.07–2.23)	
Hansen & Olsen (1995, 1996), Denmark	Workers from companies with a history of use or manufacture of formaldehyde Standardized proportionate incidence (eligible cancer cases: 2041 men, 1263 women diagnosed in 1970–84)	Low (white-collar) and above baseline (blue-collar)	ICD-7	*Men*		
			Nasopharynx	4 cases	1.3 (0.3–3.2)	Risk increased among more highly exposed workers with (SPIR, 5.0; 95% CI, 0.5–13.4) or without (SPIR, 3.0; 95% CI, 1.4–5.7) exposure to wood dust
			Nasal cavity	13 cases	2.3 (1.3–4.0)	
			Lymphohaematopoietic Leukaemia (204)	NR 39 cases	NR 0.8 (0.6–1.6)	Risk not increased among more highly exposed
			Buccal cavity/pharynx	23 cases	1.1 (0.7–1.7)	Risk not increased among more highly exposed
			Lung	410 cases	1.0 (0.9–1.1)	
			Brain and nervous system (193)	54 cases	1.1 (0.9–1.5)	Risk not increased among more highly exposed
				Women		
			Nasal cavity	4 cases	2.4 (0.6–6.0)	
			Lymphohaematopoietic Leukaemia	NR 21 cases	NR 1.2 (0.7–1.8)	
			Lung	108 cases	1.2 (0.96–1.4)	
			Brain and nervous system (193)	39 cases	1.2 (0.8–1.6)	

Table 16 (contd)

Reference, location, years of study	Cohort description Type of analysis (cohort size)	Exposure assessment	Organ site (ICD code)[a]	No. of cases/ deaths	SMR (95% CI)	Comments
Chiazze et al. (1997), USA, 1951–91	Fibreglass manufacturing plant workers Standardized mortality and nested case–control (4631 men and women)	Cumulative exposure	All cancers	96 deaths	0.94 (0.77–1.15)[b]	Analysis restricted to 2933 white men
			Nasopharynx	NR	NR	
			Nasal cavity	NR	NR	
			Lymphohaematopoietic	5 deaths	0.46 (0.15–1.08)	
			Leukaemia	1 death	0.24 (0.006–1.36)	
			Buccal cavity/pharynx	2 deaths	0.70 (0.08–2.52)	
			Lung	47 deaths	1.26 (0.93–1.68)	Excess risk for lung cancer reduced when local rates were used (SMR, 1.17; 95% CI, 0.86–1.55); positive trend in case–control study with cumulative exposure to formaldehyde among smokers
			Brain and nervous system	6 deaths	1.48 (0.54–3.23)	
Stellman et al. (1998), USA, 1982–88	Workers in the American Cancer Society CPS-II study employed in wood-related occupations or who reported exposure to wood dust Retrospective cohort mortality (45 399 men, of whom 387 reported exposure to formaldehyde)	Dichotomous (yes/no) with and without employment in a wood occupation	All cancers	367 deaths	0.98 (0.86–1.12)	
			Formaldehyde alone	367 deaths	0.98 (0.86–1.12)	
			Formaldehyde + wood	14 deaths	1.61 (0.95–2.72)	
			Nasopharynx	NR	NR	
			Nasal cavity	NR	NR	
			Lymphohaematopoietic			
			Formaldehyde alone	28 deaths	1.22 (0.84–1.77)	
			Formaldehyde + wood	3 deaths	3.44 (1.11–10.68)	
			Leukaemia			
			Formaldehyde alone	12 deaths	0.96 (0.54–1.71)	
			Formaldehyde + wood	2 deaths	5.79 (1.44–23.25)	
			Buccal cavity/pharynx	NR	NR	
			Lung			
			Formaldehyde alone	104 deaths	0.93 (0.73–1.18)	
			Formaldehyde + wood	7 deaths	2.63 (1.25–5.51)	
			Brain (ICD-9, 191)	NR	NR	

Table 16 (contd)

Reference, location, years of study	Cohort description Type of analysis (cohort size)	Exposure assessment	Organ site (ICD code)[a]	No. of cases/ deaths	SMR (95% CI)	Comments
Marsh et al. (2001); Youk et al. (2001), USA, 1945–92	Fibreglass workers Standardized mortality and nested case–control (32 000 men and women, 22% of person–years exposed to formaldehyde)	Duration of, cumulative and average exposure	All cancers	2243 deaths	0.98 (0.94–1.02)[b]	SMR was reduced and no longer significant when local rates were used (SMR, 1.06; 95% CI, 1.00–1.14); a statistically significant excess among formaldehyde-exposed workers observed in the case–control study (smoking-adjusted odds ratio, 1.61; 95% CI, 1.02–2.56); no significant trend with duration of or cumulative exposure; some evidence for a trend with average exposure
			Nasopharynx	NR	NR	
			Nasal cavity	NR	NR	
			Lymphohaematopoietic	199 deaths	0.92 (0.80–1.06)	
			Leukaemia	NR	NR	
			Buccal cavity/pharynx	63 deaths	1.07 (0.82–1.37)	
			Lung	838 deaths	1.17 (1.09–1.25)	
			Brain and central nervous system	50 deaths	0.78 (0.58–1.03)	

Nested case–control studies

Reference, location, years of study	Characteristics of cases and controls	Exposure assessment	Organ site/exposure category	No. of cases (exposed)	Odds ratio (95% CI)	Comments
Bond et al. (1986), USA, 1944–80	308 male incident cases of lung cancer from a cohort of 19 608 employees at a chemical company; two controls per case matched on race, year of birth (5 years) and year of first employment	Exposure profile developed based on work history at the company	Lung			Formaldehyde was not assessed in great detail.
			No lag period	(9)	0.62 (0.29–1.34)	
			Lag period ≥ 15 years	(4)	0.31 (0.11–0.86)	

Table 16 (contd)

Reference, location, years of study	Characteristics of cases and controls	Exposure assessment	Organ site/exposure category	No. of cases (exposed)	Odds ratio (95% CI)	Comments
Ott et al. (1989), USA, 1940–78	Deaths identified within a cohort of 29 139 male workers at two chemical manufacturing facilities and a research and development centre; five controls per case selected from cohort and frequency-matched by decade of first employment	Use of formaldehyde in department where subjects worked	*Ever exposed* Non-Hodgkin lymphoma Multiple myeloma Non-lymphocytic leukaemia Lymphocytic leukaemia	52 (2) 20 (1) 39 (2) 18 (1)	2.0 1.0 2.6 2.6	Number of controls overall by exposure status and confidence intervals not given; adjustment for age was evaluated but dropped due to substantial change in risk estimates.
Partanen et al. (1990), Finland, 1957–80 (updated from Partanen et al., 1985)	136 male incident cases* from a cohort of 7307 workers in 35 particle-board, plywood and formaldehyde glue factories and sawmills who entered the factories in 1944–66; three controls per case selected randomly among the same cohort, matched by year of birth, alive at the time of diagnosis of the corresponding case	Plant- and time-specific job–exposure matrices; work history based on factory registers, interviews of factory personnel and questionnaires to study subjects or relatives	All cancers combined* Ever exposed Peak exposure Dustborne formaldehyde Lung Ever exposed Peak exposure Dustborne formaldehyde	136 (20) (7) (14) 118 (18) (7) (12)	1.40 (0.72–2.74)[e] 0.95 (0.30–3.05)[e] 1.37 (0.66–2.82)[e] 1.25 (0.60–2.60)[e] 1.10 (0.31–3.85)[e] 1.13 (0.51–2.52)[e]	Adjusted for vital status; adjustment for cigarette smoking did not affect the results. *Tongue, mouth, pharynx, nose and nasal sinuses, larynx and lung/trachea (ICD-7 141, 143–8, 160–1, 162,0–1)

CI, confidence interval; ICD, international classification of diseases; inc., incident; NA, not applicable; NR, not reported; SMR, standardized mortality ratio; SPIR, standardized proportionate incidence ratio

[a] The ICD code is only mentioned when the organ site studied is different from that in the other studies.
[b] The authors presented results using either the national population or the local population as the referent. The results presented here are based on the national population.
[c] Data on cancer incidence and mortality were presented. The results in this column are for cancer incidence.
[d] Relative risk of medium- plus high-exposed groups versus unexposed, adjusted for race, smoking and exposure to silica
[e] 90% confidence interval

et al. (1983). For the purposes of this review, the results from these earlier studies were considered to be subsumed by the NCI study. In the earlier follow-up (Blair *et al.*, 1986), the NCI study had found an excess of lung cancer in white men in comparison with the national population of the USA, but the excess did not appear to increase with increasing cumulative exposure to formaldehyde. Several investigators performed re-analyses of the results on lung cancer (Robins *et al.*, 1988; Sterling & Weinkam, 1988, 1989a,b; Marsh *et al.*, 1992a,b, 1994; Sterling & Weinkam 1994, 1995; Callas *et al.*, 1996). The re-analyses by Sterling and Weinkam (1988, 1989a,b, 1994, 1995) did suggest a relationship between cumulative exposure and mortality from lung cancer, although their first two reports were found to have errors (Blair & Stewart, 1989; Sterling & Weinkam, 1989b). A positive exposure–response relationship between cumulative exposure to formaldehyde and lung cancer was not suggested in the re-analyses by Robins *et al.* (1988), Marsh *et al.* (1992a,b, 1994) or Callas *et al.* (1996). The results from these re-analyses are superseded by the most recent findings in the NCI cohort, which are described below.

The cohort that was originally followed for vital status through to 1980 was recently updated by Hauptmann *et al.* (2003, 2004) through to 1994. This study included a comprehensive evaluation of historical levels of exposure to formaldehyde and of other potentially confounding exposures (Stewart *et al.*, 1986; Blair & Stewart, 1990). Time-dependent estimates were developed for duration of exposure (years), average exposure (parts per million [ppm]), cumulative exposure (ppm–years) and highest peak exposure (ppm) to formaldehyde. Concomitant exposure to particulates that contained formaldehyde was also assessed. Expected numbers of deaths were estimated using the person–years method and age-, race- and sex-specific rates for the general population in the USA; log-linear Poisson regression models were used to analyse the relationship between the various measures of exposure to formaldehyde and cancer mortality. In the analyses, exposures to formaldehyde were lagged by 2 years for lymphatic and haematopoetic neoplasms and by 15 years for solid cancers. Potential confounding by age, calendar time, sex, race and pay category (Poisson regression only) was controlled for in the analyses. In addition, potential confounding was evaluated for duration of exposure to each of 11 other substances (i.e. antioxidants, asbestos, carbon black, dyes and pigments, hexamethylenetetramine, melamine, phenol, plasticizers, urea, wood dust and benzene) and for duration of work as a chemist or laboratory technician.

Based on comparisons with the national population, mortality from all cancers was lower than expected in the unexposed (376 deaths; standardized mortality ratio [SMR], 0.76; 95% confidence interval [CI], 0.69–0.84) and, but to a lesser extent, in the population exposed to formaldehyde (1723 deaths; SMR, 0.90; 95% CI, 0.86–0.95) (Hauptmann *et al.*, 2004). Decreased mortality was observed in both groups for lymphohaematopoietic neoplasms (exposed: 161 deaths; SMR, 0.80; 95% CI, 0.69–0.94; unexposed: 17 deaths; SMR, 0.62; 95% CI, 0.39–1.00) (Hauptmann *et al.*, 2003) and solid tumours (exposed: 1580 deaths; SMR, 0.91; 95% CI, 0.87–0.96; unexposed: 341 deaths; SMR, 0.78; 95% CI, 0.70–0.86) (Hauptmann *et al.*, 2004).

A statistically significant exposure–response relationship was observed between peak exposure to formaldehyde and all lymphatic and haematopoietic neoplasms (p_{trend} = 0.002) in the Poisson regression analysis. (The trend tests presented here and subsequently were based on analyses that were restricted to the exposed workers.) This relationship was largely due to a strong exposure–response relationship for leukaemia (p_{trend} = 0.004) and, to a lesser extent, for Hodgkin disease (p_{trend} = 0.04). The relationship was stronger for myeloid leukaemia (p_{trend} = 0.009) than for the other histological subtypes of leukaemia. The relative risk for the highest category of peak exposure ($\geq$ 4.0 ppm) was 2.46 (29 deaths; 95% CI, 1.31–4.62) for all leukaemia and 3.46 (14 deaths; 95% CI, 1.27–9.43) for myeloid leukaemia. Weaker and statistically non-significant exposure–response relationships were observed with average intensity of exposure for leukaemia (p_{trend} = 0.24) and myeloid leukaemia (p_{trend} = 0.09). There was little evidence for a relationship between cumulative exposure or duration of exposure and risk for either leukaemia or myeloid leukaemia (Hauptmann *et al.*, 2003). [The Working Group noted the contrast between the findings from the person–years analysis, which did not reveal an excess of leukaemia, and the Poisson regression analysis which demonstrated a significant exposure–response relationship between peak exposure and leukaemia. The Working Group also noted that Poisson regression, which uses internal analysis, is less prone to confounding by socioeconomic status and other factors.]

Based on eight cases, a significant excess mortality from nasopharyngeal cancer was observed among formaldehyde-exposed workers in comparison with the national population (SMR, 2.10; 95% CI, 1.05–4.21). A highly statistically significant (p_{trend} < 0.001) exposure–response relationship was observed between peak exposure to formaldehyde and risk for nasopharyngeal cancer in the Poisson regression analysis. All exposed cases were in the highest category of peak exposure, and the relative risk was 1.83. This analysis excluded one case which, according to cancer registry data, had been misclassified as nasopharyngeal cancer. Weaker exposure–response relationships were observed between nasopharyngeal cancer and average, cumulative and duration of exposure (p_{trend} = 0.07, 0.03 and 0.15, respectively).

Three cases of cancer of the nose and nasal cavity were observed in the exposed group, which were slightly in excess of the expected (SMR, 1.19; 95% CI, 0.38–3.68). A total of 49 deaths from cancer of the buccal cavity occurred among exposed subjects, which was as expected with respect to mortality in the national population in the USA. Relative risks for the highest exposure categories of average intensity, peak and cumulative exposure were elevated (relative risks, 1.89, 1.83 and 1.74, respectively), but trends were not significant or only of borderline significance (p_{trend} = 0.50, 0.07 and 0.37, respectively). No consistent positive association was observed for cancer of the larynx for any of the exposure metrics and the number of deaths (23) was as expected with respect to mortality in the national population. Combination of cancers of the nasopharynx, mouth, salivary gland, nasal cavity and larynx (upper respiratory tract) resulted in increasing relative risks with increasing average intensity (a twofold significantly elevated relative risk in the highest exposure category compared with the low exposure category; p_{trend} = 0.12 among the exposed only) and with peak exposure, but not with cumulative exposure or duration of exposure. Mortality from lung cancer was slightly lower than expected among the formaldehyde-exposed group (641 deaths; SMR, 0.97; 95% CI, 0.90–1.05). No evidence of a positive relationship between mortality from lung cancer and any of the exposure measures was observed. In fact, mortality from lung cancer appeared to decrease with duration of exposure (p_{trend} = 0.03) and with cumulative exposure (p_{trend} = 0.14) to formaldehyde (Hauptmann *et al.*, 2004). [The Working Group noted that the strengths of this study included its relatively large number of workers, long period of follow-up and the high quality of the exposure assessment.]

Marsh and Youk (2004) re-analysed the updated data from the NCI cohort (Hauptmann *et al.*, 2003). In addition to reproducing the results presented by Hauptmann *et al.* (2003), three further analyses were performed in relation to risk for mortality from leukaemia. Using the cut-off points for exposure categories defined in Hauptmann *et al.* (2003), exposure category-specific SMRs, based on mortality rates for the national population, increased with increasing peak and average intensity of exposure for all leukaemias combined and for myeloid leukaemia; the SMRs for myeloid leukaemia ranged from 0.43 and 0.71 in the lowest exposed category of peak and average intensity, respectively, to 1.42 and 1.45 in the highest category of these metrics. Findings were similar when regional mortality rates were used. The use of alternative cut-off points for average intensity of exposure, in order to achieve similar numbers of deaths from all leukaemias combined in each exposed category, resulted in relative risk estimates similar to those observed by Hauptmann *et al.* (2003). Analyses of duration of time worked in the highest peak category did not generally indicate higher risks among those who had experienced high peaks for a longer time.

Marsh *et al.* (1996) studied one plant (in Wallingford, CT) that was also included in the NCI cohort study (Hauptmann *et al.*, 2003). They enumerated the cohort independently and conducted their own exposure assessment, but their general approach was similar. More recently, Marsh *et al.* (2002) analysed mortality through to 1998 and exposure through to 1995 for the 7328 workers (82% white men) who were employed during 1941–84. Overall, vital status was determined for 98% of the cohort and cause of death for 95% of 2872 deaths. The majority of subjects (54%) had worked for less than 1 year at the plant. More than 1300 workers (18%) had been employed for more than 10 years. The updated exposure assessment used the same methods as the earlier study (Marsh *et al.*, 1996), and included an examination of data on sporadic measurements from the period 1965–87 and the use of protective equipment. The analysis evaluated malignancies of the upper and lower respiratory tract. Compared with local county mortality rates, SMRs were elevated for cancers of the nasopharynx (seven deaths; SMR, 5.00; 95% CI, 2.01–10.30), all pharynx (22 deaths; SMR, 2.23; 95% CI, 1.40–3.38), all buccal cavity and pharynx (31 deaths; SMR, 1.52; 95% CI, 1.03–2.15), nasal sinus (three deaths; SMR, 3.06; 95% CI, 0.63–8.93), larynx (13 deaths; SMR, 1.59; 95% CI, 0.84–2.71) and lung (262 deaths; SMR, 1.21; 95% CI, 1.06–1.36). SMRs for nasopharyngeal cancer based on local county rates increased monotonically with cumulative exposure to formaldehyde (no death; SMR, 0; 95% CI, 0–15.41 for unexposed; one death; SMR, 3.97; 95% CI, 0.10–22.10 for

> 0–< 0.004 ppm–years; three deaths; SMR, 5.89; 95% CI, 1.22–17.22 for 0.004–0.219 ppm–years; and three deaths; SMR, 7.51; 95% CI, 1.55–21.93 for ≥ 0.22 ppm–years). In a case–control study of pharyngeal cancer nested in the cohort, deaths from cancer of the oropharynx (five), nasopharynx (seven), hypopharynx (three) and unspecified pharynx (seven) were compared with 67 controls matched on race, sex, age and year of birth (within 2 years) with respect to occupational exposure to formaldehyde, and additional information on occupational and non-occupational exposures was obtained by telephone interviews, partly with next of kin [proportion of next-of-kin interviews not reported]. Based on exact conditional logistic regression, relative risks for the combined group of pharyngeal cancers, adjusted for tobacco smoking and years of employment in the factory, increased with increasing duration of exposure to formaldehyde and particularly with increasing duration of exposure to levels of formaldehyde > 0.2 ppm, but not with average intensity of exposure or cumulative exposure. Separate analyses for nasopharyngeal cancer were not presented due to small numbers.

[The earliest year of entry into this cohort was earlier than that in the NCI cohort, the cohort was enumerated independently from the NCI cohort and exposures were assessed separately using measurements and other information provided by the company but not those made by an industrial hygienist for the NCI study. The exposure estimates were generally about 10 times lower than those reported in Hauptmann *et al.* (2003, 2004). Marsh *et al.* (2002) suggested that this difference was because Hauptmann *et al.* (2003, 2004) used data from several plants to estimate exposure in each plant, whereas Marsh *et al.* (2002) based the assessment only on the plant under study. However, this suggestion is incorrect (Blair & Stewart, 1990). All data considered in the exposure estimates in a given plant in the Hauptmann *et al.* (2003, 2004) study were only from that plant.]

(b)   *Garment workers: The National Institute for Occupational Safety and Health (NIOSH) Cohort*

Stayner *et al.* (1985, 1988) at NIOSH, USA, conducted a proportionate mortality study and a retrospective cohort study of mortality of garment workers exposed to formaldehyde. The cohort study included approximately 11 000 predominantly female (82%) workers from three facilities that manufactured shirts from fabrics that were treated with formaldehyde resins to impart permanent press characteristics. Workers who were included in the cohort study had worked for at least 3 months after the time that formaldehyde-treated fabrics were introduced into the process, which was 1959 in two of the facilities and 1955 in the third. Time-weighted 8-h geometric mean exposure levels in different departments in the three plants were found to range from 0.09 to 0.20 ppm at the time the study was initiated. Continuous air monitoring suggested no substantial peaks. Historical exposure levels were not available; however, exposure levels are believed to have been substantially higher in the earlier years of the study because the methods of treatment with formaldehyde resin have been steadily improved over time to reduce the amount of free formaldehyde in the fabrics. Exposure measurements reported at other facilities before 1970 ranged from 0.3 to 10 ppm (Stayner *et al.*, 1988) (see Section 1.3.2(*f*)). The investigators reported finding no evidence that other potentially carcinogenic exposures were present at the study facilities. Follow-up of the cohort for vital status, which was originally through to 1982, was recently extended to 1998 (Pinkerton *et al.*, 2004). Life-table methods that applied national and state rates were used. The results from analyses were similar for the cancer sites of a-priori interest when both national and state rates were used. Life-table analyses that used a multiple cause-of-death approach (Steenland *et al.*, 1992) were also conducted. Poisson regression models were used to analyse the relationship between duration of exposure and risk for cancer.

Mortality from all cancers (608 deaths; SMR, 0.89; 95% CI, 0.82–0.97) was shown to be significantly lower than that expected based upon comparisons with the national population. The observed numbers of cases of respiratory cancer (152 deaths; SMR, 0.98; 95% CI, 0.83–1.14) and of cancer of the brain and central nervous system (19 deaths; SMR, 1.09; 95% CI, 0.66–1.71) were found to be close to expectation. Mortality from buccal cancer, which was found to be elevated (four deaths; SMR, 3.53; 95% CI, 0.96–9.02) in the original study (Stayner *et al.*, 1988), was only slightly elevated (four deaths; SMR, 1.33; 95% CI, 0.36–3.41) in the updated study (Pinkerton *et al.*, 2004). No cases of nasopharyngeal (0.96 expected) or nasal (0.16 expected) cancer were observed. A slight excess of mortality from leukaemia (24 deaths; SMR, 1.09; 95% CI, 0.70–1.62) was observed, which was a certain degree higher for myeloid leukaemia (15 deaths; SMR, 1.44; 95% CI, 0.80–2.37). The excess mortality from myeloid leukaemia was greatest among workers who were first exposed during the earliest years of the study (before 1963) when exposures to formaldehyde were presumably higher (11 deaths; SMR, 1.61 [95% CI, 0.80–2.88]), among workers with 10 or more years of exposure (eight deaths; SMR, 2.19 [95% CI, 0.95–4.32]) and among workers with 20 or more years since first exposure (13 deaths; SMR, 1.91 [95% CI, 1.02–3.27]). A greater than twofold excess in mortality from myeloid leukaemia was observed among workers with both more than 10 years of exposure and 20 or more years since first exposure to formaldehyde (seven deaths; SMR, 2.43; 95% CI, 0.98–5.01). In contrast to leukaemia, the risk for respiratory cancer decreased with duration of employment and time since first exposure. [The Working Group noted that strengths of this study were the apparent absence of other potentially confounding carcinogenic exposures in the workplace and the long follow-up.]

(c)   *Chemical industry workers*

Acheson *et al.* (1984a) assembled a large cohort of workers from six chemical facilities in the United Kingdom, and Coggon *et al.* (2003) reported the findings from an update of the vital status of the cohort to 2000. The cohort included approximately 14 000 workers who had been employed after 1937 and before 1965, at a time when formaldehyde was used or produced, and personnel records at the plants were believed to be complete. Jobs were classified into one of five categories of exposure to formaldehyde, i.e. background, low, moderate, high or unknown. No exposure measurements were available before 1970. Based on the later measurements and workers' recall of irritant symptoms, it was estimated that the TWA exposure concentrations corresponded to: background, < 0.1 ppm; low exposure, 0.1–0.5 ppm; moderate exposure, 0.6–2.0 ppm; and high exposure, > 2.0 ppm. Person–years and Poisson regression analyses were conducted. An adjustment for local geographical variations in mortality was made in some analyses, which entailed multi-plying the expected deaths by SMRs for the area in which the plant was located.

Mortality was elevated to some extent for all cancers (1511 deaths; SMR, 1.10; 95% CI, 1.04–1.16), and this was more pronounced among workers who had ever worked in a job that was classified as entailing high exposure to formaldehyde (621 deaths; SMR, 1.31; 95% CI, 1.21–1.42). This excess mortality was largely attributable to a statistically significant excess of mortality from cancers of the stomach (150 deaths; SMR, 1.31; 95% CI, 1.11–1.54) and lung (594 deaths; SMR, 1.22; 95% CI, 1.12–1.32). The excess of mortality from lung cancer was greatest among men who had high exposure (272 deaths; SMR, 1.58; 95% CI, 1.40–1.78). The excess incidence of lung cancer among the highly exposed decreased with adjustment for local rates, although it remained statistically signi-ficant (SMR, 1.28; 95% CI, 1.13–1.44). Mortality from lung cancer was higher among workers who were highly exposed before 1965 when levels of exposure to formaldehyde would be expected to be higher (243 deaths; SMR, 1.61; 95% CI, 1.41–1.82). Mortality from lung cancer demonstrated a non-significant inverse relationship with the number of years worked in high-exposure jobs (p_{trend} = 0.13) and showed no trend with time since first employment in a job that entailed high exposure (p_{trend} = 0.93).

A statistically non-significant excess mortality from pharyngeal cancer was observed (15 deaths; SMR, 1.55; 95% CI, 0.87–2.56), which was to some degree greater among highly exposed workers (six deaths; SMR, 1.91; 95% CI, 0.70–4.17). One death from naso-pharyngeal cancer was observed where 2.0 were expected; two cases of sinonasal cancer were observed where 2.3 were expected, but neither individual was highly exposed. A review of tumour registry data identified two additional cases of sinonasal cancer, both in individuals who were highly exposed, but it was not possible to determine the expected number of incident cases because of limitations in the tumour registry system. Slight excess mortality, based on a small number of cases, was observed in men who had had high expo-sure for cancers of the tongue (three deaths; SMR, 1.91; 95% CI, 0.39–5.58) and mouth (two deaths; SMR, 1.32; 95% CI, 0.16–4.75). Mortality from cancer of the brain and central nervous system and from leukaemia was lower than expected among the entire cohort (SMRs, 0.85 and 0.91, respectively) and among the high-exposure group (SMRs, 0.63 and 0.71, respectively). [The Working Group noted that this study probably included a substantial number of workers who had relatively high exposures: 4000 workers had ever worked in jobs that were classified as entailing exposures greater than 2 ppm. The Working Group also noted the long follow-up. However, there was a lack of exposure measurements before 1970, and this may have led to some misclassification of exposures.]

Bond *et al.* (1986) conducted a case–control study in a cohort of 19 608 men who had been employed for 1 year or longer at a large chemical production facility in Texas, USA, between 1940 and 1980, which included all 308 workers who had died from lung cancer and 588 controls chosen at random from among men in the same cohort. Two series of controls, individually matched to cases on race, year of birth (± 5 years) and year of first employment, were selected: one among men who were still alive when the matched subjects died of lung cancer, and one among men who had died ≤ 5 years after the matched subjects. Exposures (ever or never) to 171 chemical and physical agents, including formaldehyde, were assessed by an industrial hygienist on the basis of a review of documentation on the subject's employment history at the facility and industrial hygiene records; six exposures, not including formaldehyde, were assessed in greater detail. Only nine men who had lung cancer (3%) were judged ever to have been exposed to formaldehyde, and a negative association was seen between this exposure and mortality from lung cancer (not adjusted for other exposure variables), with an odds ratio of 0.62 (95% CI, 0.29–1.34); incorporation into the analysis of a 15-year minimal latency gave an odds ratio of 0.31 (95% CI, 0.11–0.86).

(d) Fibreglass workers

Marsh *et al.* (2001) updated and expanded an earlier cohort study of mortality of workers who had been employed at any of 10 fibreglass manufacturing plants in the USA that had been previously studied by Enterline *et al.* (1987). The study included over 32 000 workers who had been employed for at least 1 year between 1945 and 1978 in one of the 10 study facilities. The cohort was expanded to include women, workers who had been employed after the original 1963 end date and workers from additional worksites; the vital status of the cohort was established until the end of 1992. In addition to expanding and updating the cohort, the study introduced new information on potential exposures to several known and potential carcinogens other than fibreglass (asbestos, arsenic, asphalt, epoxy, polycyclic aromatic hydrocarbons, phenolics, silica, styrene and urea), including formaldehyde. Exposure to formaldehyde was the most common exposure [22% of the person–years] after respirable fibres [28% of the person–years] in the study. The median exposure to formaldehyde for the cohort was 0.066 ppm and ranged from 0.03 to 0.13 ppm in the different plants. Person–years methods were used to analyse the mortality of the cohort in comparison with both national population and local death rates. Overall cancer mortality was slightly lower than expected in comparison with both national (2243 deaths; SMR_{US}, 0.98; 95% CI, 0.94–1.02) and local rates (SMR_{local}, 0.94; 95% CI, 0.90–0.98). A statistically significant excess of mortality from respiratory cancer was observed for the whole cohort when national rates were used (874 deaths; SMR_{US}, 1.16; 95% CI, 1.08–1.24), which was weaker and of borderline significance ($p = 0.05$) when local rates were used as a referent (SMR_{local}, 1.06; 95% CI, 1.00–1.14). This excess was largely attributable to an excess mortality from cancers of the trachea, bronchus and lung (838 deaths; SMR_{US}, 1.17; 95% CI, 1.09–1.25; SMR_{local}, 1.07; 95% CI, 1.00–1.14).

The association of respiratory cancer with specific exposures was examined in a nested case–control study in which the cases were male members of the cohort who had died from respiratory tumours during 1970–92 (Marsh *et al.*, 2001; Stone *et al.*, 2001; Youk *et al.*, 2001). Each case was randomly matched with a control who had the same date of birth to within 1 year, who was at risk during 1970–92 and who was alive and at risk at the age when the case died. Smoking histories were ascertained through telephone interviews with the subjects themselves or a proxy. Complete data were available for 502 of 713 matched pairs, and unmatched cases and controls were combined with the matched set nearest in age (at the time of death of the case). Thus, the analysis was based on 631 cases and 570 controls. Of the cases, 96% had been diagnosed with carcinoma of the trachea, bronchus or lung. Individual exposures in the matched set to formaldehyde, respirable fibres and silica before the age at which the case died were estimated from industrial hygiene data using a job–exposure matrix that took into account time period, plant and department. Analysis was performed using conditional logistic regression with adjustment for smoking. In a first analysis (Youk *et al.*, 2001), nine different configurations of time lag and window of exposure were examined for average intensity of exposure and cumulative exposure. When exposure was not weighted in relation to the time of case death, the odds ratio for ever exposure to formaldehyde was 1.61 (95% CI, 1.02–2.56) and a similar risk estimate was obtained when a 5-year lag was applied (odds ratio, 1.62; 95% CI, 1.04–2.54). Otherwise, however, the risk estimates for ever exposure were lower, and there were no clear trends with cumulative or average intensity of exposure (which for most subjects were < 2 ppm–years and < 0.14 ppm, respectively).

This analysis was then extended by application of a conditional logistic regression model that adjusted for exposure to respirable fibres as well as tobacco smoking, and used piecewise linear functions (linear splines) with knots at the deciles of the distributions of exposure in the cases. Cumulative exposure to formaldehyde was not significantly associated with increased risk in any of the models examined, but there was a suggestion of increased risk (of borderline statistical significance) with average intensity of exposure at the upper end of the range (Stone *et al.*, 2001). [The Working Group noted that exposures to formaldehyde in this cohort of fibreglass workers appeared to be lower than those in the studies of industrial and textile workers reviewed earlier in this section.]

Chiazze *et al.* (1997) conducted a retrospective cohort study of mortality of 4631 workers at a fibreglass manufacturing plant in Anderson, SC, USA. This included a nested case–control study for lung cancer (47 cases) which collected information from interviews on tobacco smoking, socioeconomic factors and a historical reconstruction of several exposures at the plant, including formaldehyde. Controls for this analysis were individuals in the cohort who had not died from lung cancer, or from suicide or homicide (for ethical reasons). The controls were matched to the cases based on year of birth (± 2 years) and survival to the end of follow-up or death (± 2 years). Person–years methods of analysis were used to analyse the cohort study, and conditional logistic regression was used to analyse the case–control study. Cumulative exposure to formaldehyde was the only exposure in the case–control analysis to exhibit a positive relationship with risk for lung cancer. Among smokers only, lung cancer was elevated in the highest (> 1000 ppm–days; odds ratio, 2.07; 95% CI, 0.17–25.5) and next to highest (100–999 ppm–days; odds ratio, 1.72; 95% CI, 0.57–5.23) cumulative exposure groups, but these excesses were based on a small number of cases and were statistically non-significant.

(e)   *Woodworkers*

Partanen *et al.* (1985) conducted a case–control study in a cohort of 3805 male production workers who had been employed for at least 1 year in one of three particle-board factories, seven plywood factories, eight sawmills and one formaldehyde glue factory between 1944 and 1966. Of these, 57 men were declared to the Finnish Cancer Registry as having cancer of the respiratory tract (including at least 51 cases of lung cancer), oral cavity or pharynx in 1957–80. Three controls were selected at random from the same cohort and were individually matched to the case by year of birth. Plant- and time-specific job–exposure matrices were constructed for 12 chemicals, including formaldehyde (Kauppinen & Partanen, 1988), and were combined with the work histories of the subjects to yield several indicators of exposure; supplementary information on tobacco smoking was collected for 68% of cases and 76% of controls, by means of a postal questionnaire, from study subjects or their relatives. A slight, non-significant increase in risk for all cancers combined was seen among workers who had had any exposure to at least 0.1 ppm (0.12 mg/m^3) formaldehyde in contrast to workers who had had no exposure to formaldehyde, which yielded an odds ratio of 1.44 [95% CI, 0.6–3.5]; an odds ratio of 1.27 [95% CI, 0.5–3.5] was obtained when a minimal latency of 10 years before diagnosis was assumed. No significant association was found with other indicators of exposure to formaldehyde (mean level of and cumulative exposure, repeated peak exposures and 'formaldehyde in wood dust'). Adjustment for cigarette smoking did not change the overall results.

In an expansion of the study to include a total of 35 Finnish factories and 7307 woodworkers who had been employed during 1944–65, Partanen *et al.* (1990) identified 136 newly diagnosed cases of cancer of the respiratory tract (118 lung cancers, 12 laryngeal cancers and one sinonasal cancer), oral cavity (four cases) and pharynx (one case) from the files of the Finnish Cancer Registry for 1957–82. The additional factories were mainly involved in construction carpentry and furniture manufacture. Three controls were provided for each new cancer case, and exposure to formaldehyde and 11 other occupational agents was assessed by the same methods as those described in the initial study (Partanen *et al.*, 1985; Kauppinen & Partanen, 1988). Of 20 cases who had had any exposure to formaldehyde (odds ratio, 1.4 [95% CI, 0.6–3.1]), 18 were cancers of the lung (odds ratio, 1.3 [95% CI, 0.5–3.0]) and two were cancers at other sites (odds ratio, 2.4 [95% CI, 0.3–18]). Adjustment for tobacco smoking reduced the odds ratios to 1.1 for all cancers combined and to 0.7 for lung cancer separately and rendered the odds ratio for cancers at other sites unassessable. The unadjusted odds ratios for all cancer cases were 1.5 [95% CI, 0.7–3.6] for an estimated mean level of formaldehyde of 0.1–1 ppm [0.12–1.23 mg/m^3] and 1.0 [95% CI, 0.1–8.2] for > 1 ppm, in comparison with no exposure. Other indicators of exposure to formaldehyde, which included an estimate of cumulative exposure and duration of exposure to peak levels > 2 ppm [2.46 mg/m^3], showed similarly inconsistent dose–response relationships, i.e. the lowest risks in the highest exposure categories. Allowance for a minimal latency of 10 years further reduced the risk estimates for the subgroups who had had the presumed highest exposures to odds ratios generally below 1.0.

[The Working Group noted that there were too few cancers at sites other than the lung to allow a meaningful analysis; consequently, this was essentially a study of lung cancer.]

Stellman *et al.* (1998) studied mortality among workers exposed to wood dust in the American Cancer Society's Cancer Prevention Study. From the original cohort of over half a million men, sufficient data were available for 362 823 who were included in the study. Of these, 45 399 reported either employment in a wood-related occupation or exposure to wood dust. As part of the investigation, data were also collected on self-reported exposure to formaldehyde, and incidence density ratios according to exposure were derived for death from each of several cancers during 6 years of follow-up. This analysis adjusted for age and for smoking habits. In comparison with men who had never been employed in a wood-working occupation and who did not report regular exposure to wood dust, those who had been wood-workers and who reported exposure to formaldehyde had elevated mortality from lung cancer (seven deaths; relative risk, 2.63; 95% CI, 1.25–5.51) and leukaemia (two deaths; relative risk, 5.79; 95% CI, 1.44–23.25). In men exposed to formaldehyde who had not worked in wood-related occupations, the corresponding risk estimates for lung cancer and leukaemia were 0.93 (95% CI, 0.73–1.18) based on 104 deaths and 0.96 (95% CI, 0.54–1.71) based on 12 deaths, respectively. Results for sinonasal and nasopharyngeal cancers were not reported. [The Working Group noted that this study should be given little weight in the evaluation because of the small number of formaldehyde-exposed workers and the limitations in the subjective exposure assessment for formaldehyde.]

(f)   Iron foundry workers

Andjelkovich *et al.* (1990) studied a cohort of 8147 men who had been employed for 6 months or longer at an iron foundry in the USA. In a nested case–control study (Andjelkovich *et al.*, 1994), the case group comprised all members of the cohort who died from primary lung cancer during 1950–89 and were ascertained from various sources. They included 200 men in whom lung cancer was certified as the underlying cause of death, 13 in whom it was a contributory cause and seven who died from carcinomatosis with a primary lung tumour that was confirmed from hospital records or through the local cancer registry. Ten controls were selected for each case by incidence density sampling; they were of the same race and had attained at least the same age as their matched case. Just over half of the controls (52.2%) were still alive at the end of the follow-up period. In total, 50.9% of cases and controls were white. Exposure to silica (high, medium or low) and formaldehyde (high, medium, low or none) was classified by means of a job–exposure matrix based on industrial hygiene data, walk-through surveys, job description, knowledge of the tasks performed in a job and reports in the scientific literature. [In the analysis reported, exposure to formaldehyde was dichotomized as some versus none; no data were provided on the probable levels of airborne concentrations.] Data on tobacco smoking (yes or no) were available for 75.5% of cases and 68.6% of a random subset of two controls per case and were obtained from various sources including the subject himself, his next of kin, plant medical records, hospital medical records and death certificates. Analysis was performed using conditional logistic regression with and without the inclusion of lag periods. Overall, 25% each of cases and controls were classed as having been exposed to formaldehyde. After adjustment for tobacco smoking, birth cohort (< 1915 versus ≥ 1915) and cumulative exposure to silica (partitioned to four levels at the quartiles), the odds ratio for unlagged exposure to formaldehyde was 1.31 (95% CI, 0.83–2.07); with the incorporation of increasing lag periods, this risk estimate decreased progressively to 0.84 (95% CI, 0.44–1.60) for a 20-year lag. Risk estimates were little affected by the inclusion of tobacco smoking in the regression models, and there was no evidence of an interaction between formaldehyde and smoking. [The Working Group noted that data to support this statement were not shown.]

The relation of formaldehyde to risk for cancer was examined further in a subset of 3929 men from the full cohort who had worked in jobs that entailed potential exposure to formaldehyde for at least 6 months between January 1960 and May 1987 (Andjelkovich *et al.*, 1995). The mortality of this group was compared with that of the national population (by the person–years method), with that of an internal reference population of 2032 cohort members who had worked during the same period in jobs that did not entail exposure to formaldehyde and with that of an occupational referent population assembled by the NCI and NIOSH, using Poisson regression analysis. Cumulative exposure to formaldehyde and silica was estimated for each worker based on detailed occupational histories and evaluation of job-specific exposure levels by an occupational hygienist. Smoking status was ascertained for 65.4% of the exposed subcohort and 55.1% of the unexposed control subcohort. In the follow-up through to 1989 and in comparison with national death rates, mortality from all cancers was close to that expected in both the formaldehyde-exposed (127 deaths; SMR, 0.99; 95% CI, 0.82–1.17) and unexposed (95 deaths; SMR, 0.97; 95% CI, 0.79–1.19) populations. In both the exposed and unexposed subcohorts, a statistically non-significant excess of mortality from cancers of the buccal cavity and pharynx (exposed: six deaths; SMR, 1.31; 95% CI, 0.48–2.86; unexposed: five deaths; SMR, 1.69; 95% CI, 0.54–3.95) and lung cancer (exposed: 51 deaths; SMR, 1.20; 95% CI, 0.89–1.58; unexposed: 38 deaths; SMR, 1.19; 95% CI, 0.84–1.63) was observed. Mortality from cancers of the lung, buccal cavity and pharynx was not found to increase with cumulative exposure in the Poisson regression analysis. Mortality from laryngeal cancer (two deaths; SMR, 0.98; 95% CI, 0.11–3.53), cancer of the brain and central nervous system (two deaths; SMR, 0.62; 95% CI, 0.07–2.23) and leukaemia (two deaths; SMR, 0.43; 95% CI, 0.05–1.57) was lower than expected among the exposed.

(g)   Other chemical workers and plastics manufacturers

A study of mortality among workers at a formaldehyde resin plant in Italy (Bertazzi *et al.*, 1986) included 1332 male workers who had ever been employed for at least 30 days between the launch of the plant in 1959 and 1980. Follow-up for vital status was extended from 1980 to 1986 in a second study (Bertazzi *et al.*, 1989). Work histories of past employees were reconstructed from interviews with retired workers, current workers and foremen. Actual or reconstructed work histories were available for all but 16.5% of the cohort. Job mobility was low, and 79% of the workers had held a single job throughout their career. On the basis of their work histories, workers were placed into one of three categories: exposed to formaldehyde, exposed to compounds other than formaldehyde and exposure unknown. Individual exposures could not be estimated, but the mean concentrations in fixed area samples that were taken between 1974 and 1979 were 0.2–3.8 mg/m^3 [0.2–3.1 ppm]. SMRs were calculated using the person–years methods to estimate expected numbers based on national and local mortality rates, and were adjusted for age and calendar time. A deficit of lung cancer was observed among workers who had been exposed to formaldehyde; six cases of lung cancer were observed and 8.7 were expected. Excess mortality from lymphatic and haematopoietic neoplasms was observed among formaldehyde-exposed workers based on only three deaths (SMR, 1.73 [95% CI, 0.36–5.06]). During the first follow-up (Bertazzi *et al.*, 1986), no nasal cancer was recorded (0.03 expected).

Ott *et al.* (1989) evaluated data from a nested case–control study within a cohort of 29 139 men who had been employed in two chemical manufacturing facilities and a research and development centre. Cases were subjects who had died between 1940 and 1978 from non-Hodgkin lymphoma (52 cases), multiple myeloma (20 cases), non-lympho-cytic leukaemia (39 cases) and lymphocytic leukaemia (18 cases); information on death certificates was used to determine cause of death. Five controls per case were selected from the total employee cohort and were frequency-matched to cases by decade of first employ-ment and duration of survival after first employment. Potential exposure to several chemicals, including formaldehyde, was assessed based on use of the chemical in the work area or in an activity in which the subject was involved at a specific time. Because adjust-ment for age did not substantially change the risk estimates, crude odds ratios were presented. Odds ratios for ever versus never exposed to formaldehyde for non-Hodgkin lymphoma (two exposed cases), multiple myeloma (one exposed case), non-lymphocytic (two exposed cases) and lymphocytic (one exposed case) leukaemia were 2.0, 1.0, 2.6 and 2.6, respectively. [The Working Group noted that confidence intervals were not provided and could not be calculated because the number of exposed controls was not given.]

Dell and Teta (1995) conducted a retrospective cohort study of mortality of 5932 male employees at a plastics manufacturing and research and development facility in Bound Brook, NJ, USA. Workers who were included in the cohort had worked for at least 7 months between 1946 and 1967 at the facility where they had been exposed to a number of chemi-cals, including asbestos, polyvinyl chloride and formaldehyde. The cohort was followed for vital status through to 1988. Only 111 of the cohort members had held jobs that involved potential exposure to formaldehyde. Person–years methods were applied in which national and state mortality rates were used as the referent. The analysis was stratified by whether workers were paid hourly or were salaried, by duration of employment with lag intervals of 0, 10 and 15 years and by time since first employment. Mortality for all cancers was close to expected (using national rates) among hourly workers (334 deaths; SMR, 1.02; 95% CI, 0.92–1.14). Excess mortality was observed among hourly workers for cancers of the pancreas (25 deaths; SMR, 1.46; 95% CI, 0.95–2.16), lung (124 deaths; SMR, 1.10; 95% CI, 0.92–1.31) and other parts of the respiratory system (five deaths; SMR, 3.73; 95% CI, 1.21–8.70). The excess mortality from cancers of other parts of the respiratory system was entirely due to an excess mortality from pleural mesothelioma, which was most probably attributable to exposure to asbestos. An excess of mortality from lung cancer (4 observed, 1.1 expected) was noted among 57 workers who had been exposed to formaldehyde in the hexamethylenetetramine process. No cases of nasal or nasopharyngeal cancer were observed. [The Working Group and the authors noted that, because of its small size, this study was relatively uninformative with regard to formaldehyde.]

(h)   Abrasives industry

Cancer mortality and incidence among workers in the abrasives industry in Sweden was evaluated by Edling *et al.* (1987a) in plants that manufactured grinding wheels and employed abrasives bound with formaldehyde resins. The levels of formaldehyde were reported to be 0.1–1.0 mg/m^3. A cohort of 911 workers (211 women in administration and production and 700 men, of whom 521 were blue-collar workers) who had been employed for at least 5 years between 1955 and 1983 was followed for mortality through to 1983 and for cancer incidence through to 1981, yielding 79 deaths and 24 incident cancers. Deaths and morbidity that occurred at the age of 75 years or older were excluded because of concerns about diagnostic validity. Person–years methods were used to generate expected numbers based on rates for the general population, stratified for age, calendar year and sex. No significant excesses of mortality or morbidity were seen among male blue-collar workers, administrative personnel or among women. All cancer mortality (17 deaths; SMR, 0.93 [95% CI, 0.54–1.49]) and incidence (24 cases; standardized incidence ratio (SIR), 0.84 [95% CI, 0.54–1.25]) were slightly lower than expected. Lung cancer incidence was lower than expected (two cases; SIR, 0.57 [95% CI, 0.07–2.06]). No cases of leukaemia, or nasal or buccal cancer were observed. One case of nasopharyngeal cancer and one of cancer of the nervous system were reported.

(i)   Mixed industrial exposures

Hansen and Olsen (1995) conducted a standardized proportionate cancer incidence study of workers in Denmark. Individuals who were born between 1897 and 1964 and had been diagnosed with cancer between 1970 and 1984 were identified from the Danish Cancer Registry. Employment histories were established through linkage to the Supplementary Pension Fund, which began in 1964. A total of 91 182 men who had cancer, who met the study criteria and who had records in the Supplementary Pension Fund were identified. The companies in which individuals worked were identified by the Fund and the use of formaldehyde by these companies was retrieved from the Danish Product Register. Cancer patients whose longest work experience after 1964 was at one of the companies that used formaldehyde and was at least 10 years before the date of diagnosis were regarded as being potentially exposed to formaldehyde. White-collar workers were assumed to have low exposure, blue-collar workers were assumed to have high exposure and workers with a missing job title were assumed to have unknown exposure to formaldehyde. [The Working Group noted that this may not be a very reliable means of classifying workers with regard to exposure.] Blue-collar cases who had worked in wood and furniture companies and carpentry enterprises or had worked as a cabinet maker, joiner or carpenter were classified as having potential exposure to wood dust. A parallel study included 73 423 women with incident cancer and records of the Supplementary Pension Fund (Hansen & Olsen, 1996). Standardized proportionate incidence of cancer ratios (SPICR) were estimated using age-, sex- and calender period-specific proportions among all employees in Denmark as the reference. A statistically significant excess of mortality from cancer of the nasal cavity and paranasal sinuses (SPICR, 2.3; 95% CI, 1.3–4.0) was observed among male workers who were potentially exposed to formaldehyde, based on 13 cases. Among women, the SPICR was 2.4 (95% CI, 0.6–6.0), based on four cases. The excess mortality from nasal cancer observed in men was more pronounced among blue-collar workers who were exposed to formaldehyde only (nine cases; SPICR, 3.0; 95% CI, 1.4–5.7) or who had co-exposure to formaldehyde and wood dust (two cases; SPICR, 5.0; 95% CI, 0.5–13.4). The observed number of cases was close to expected for cancers of the buccal cavity and pharynx (23 cases; SPICR, 1.1; 95% CI, 0.7–1.7), nasopharynx (four cases; SPICR, 1.3; 95% CI, 0.3–3.2), brain and nervous system (54 cases; SPICR, 1.1; 95% CI, 0.9–1.5), larynx (32 cases; SPICR, 0.9; 95% CI, 0.6–1.2) and lung (410 cases; SPICR, 1.0; 95% CI, 0.9–1.1) and for leukaemia (39 cases; SPICR, 0.8; 95% CI, 0.6–1.6). No cancer site showed risk estimates that were significantly different from unity among women.

2.1.2   *Cohort and proportionate mortality studies of professional groups*

Pathologists, anatomists, embalmers and funeral directors have been studied because they use formaldehyde as a tissue preservative. Investigations of these occupations have several methodological problems. The use of national statistics to generate expected numbers may bias estimates of relative risks downwards for some cancers and upwards for others because some of these groups have a higher socioeconomic level than the general population; only a few investigations included a special referent population that was designed to diminish potential socioeconomic confounding. None of these studies presented the data necessary to adjust for tobacco use. Since anatomists and pathologists in the USA generally smoke less than the general population (Sterling & Weinkam, 1976), estimates of relative risks for smoking-related cancers will be artificially low. Without adjustments, the biases introduced by socioeconomic factors and tobacco smoking may be strong enough to preclude any possibility of detecting an excess occurrence of tobacco-related cancers. This may be less of a problem for embalmers, however, because their smoking habits may not differ from those of the general population (Sterling & Weinkam, 1976). In no study were risk estimates developed by level of exposure, and in only a few studies were risks evaluated by duration of exposure. When exposure estimates are not presented in the following text, they were not provided in the original study. Non-differential error in exposure assessment, which occurs when the measures of exposure are about equally inaccurate for study subjects who do and do not have the cancer of interest, diminishes the chances of uncovering an underlying association, as it biases estimates of the relative risk towards the null. Key study features and findings from the cohort and proportionate mortality studies of professional groups are summarized in Table 17 by subgroups of profession.

(a)   *Cohort of British pathologists and medical technicians*

Harrington and Shannon (1975) evaluated the mortality of pathologists and medical laboratory technicians in Great Britain in 1975. A total of 2079 members of the Royal College of Pathologists and the Pathological Society who were alive in 1955 were enrolled and followed for vital status through to 1973. The Council for Professions Supplementary to Medicine enabled the identification of 12 944 technicians. Ten of the pathologists who died and 20 of the medical technicians who died were women, but the number of women included in the cohort was not provided. Expected numbers of deaths were calculated from sex-, 5-year calendar period- and 5-year age group-specific rates for England and Wales or Scotland. A deficit in mortality from cancer was observed in both pathologists (40 observed, 66.9 expected) and medical technicians (37 observed, 59.8 expected). The SMR for lymphatic and haematopoietic cancer was significantly elevated among pathologists (eight deaths [SMR, 2.00; 95% CI, 0.86–3.94]), but not among technicians (three deaths [SMR, 0.55; 95% CI, 0.11–1.59]). No excess incidence of leukaemia was observed in either group. The SMRs for cancers at other sites were all below 1.0.

The study of British pathologists was extended and expanded by Harrington and Oakes (1984), who added new entrants and traced new and previously studied subjects from 1974 through to 1980. The population now included 2307 men and 413 women. SMRs were calculated using expected rates based on age-, sex- and calendar time-specific data from England and Wales. The SMR for all cancers among men was 0.61 (32 deaths [95% CI, 0.42–0.86] and that among women was 1.41 (seven deaths [95% CI, 0.57–2.90]). Mortality from brain cancer was significantly elevated among men (four deaths; SMR, 3.33 [95% CI, 0.91–8.53] $p < 0.05$), but not among women. No cases of nasal or nasal sinus cancer were observed, but the expected number was small (0.12). Mortality from lung cancer among men was significantly lower than expected (nine deaths; SMR, 0.41 [95% CI, 0.19–0.78]). Mortality from leukaemia and other lymphatic and hematopoetic neoplasms was close to that expected [men and women combined: three deaths; SMR, 0.92; 95% CI, 0.18–2.68].

This cohort was further evaluated by Hall *et al.* (1991), who extended follow-up of mortality from 1980 through to 1986 and added new members of the Pathological Society, which resulted in 4512 individuals available for study (3069 men and 803 women in England and Wales; 409 men in Scotland; and 231 members from Northern Ireland and women from Scotland for whom corresponding reference rates were not available). Sex-specific SMRs were based on expected rates for England and Wales or Scotland (for men only), as appropriate, and were adjusted for age (5-year groups) and calendar time. The SMRs for all causes of death were all considerably below 1.0: men from England and Wales, 0.43 (176 deaths; 95% CI, 0.37–0.50); women from England and Wales, 0.65 (18 deaths; 95% CI, 0.38–1.03); and men from Scotland, 0.50 (29 deaths; 95% CI, 0.34–0.72). The SMRs for cancers at all sites were 0.40 (44 deaths; 95% CI, 0.29–0.54) and 0.59 (nine

Table 17. Cohort and proportionate mortality studies of cancer in professionals exposed to formaldehyde

Reference, country, years of study	Study population, design (study size)	Exposure assessment	Organ site	No. of cases/deaths	SMR^a (95% CI)	Comments
British pathologists and medical technicians						
Hall et al. (1991), United Kingdom, 1974–87 (update of Harrington & Oakes, 1984, plus new members since 1973)	Pathologists, SMR (4512 men and women) [sex distribution not reported]	None	All cancers	53 deaths	0.45 (0.34–0.59)	Data presented for men and women from England and Wales (n = 3872)
			Nasopharynx	NR	NR	
			Nasal cavity	NR	NR	
			Lymphohaematopoietic	10 deaths	1.44 (0.69–2.65)	
			Leukaemia	4 deaths	1.52 (0.41–3.89)	
			Lung	9 deaths	0.19 (0.09–0.36)	
			Brain and central nervous system	6 deaths	2.18 (0.80–4.75)	
Anatomists and pathologists in the USA						
Stroup et al. (1986), USA, 1925–79	Anatomists, SMR (2239 men)	Duration	All cancers	118 deaths	0.64 (0.53–0.76)	
			Nasopharynx	NR	NR	
			Nasal cavity	0 deaths	(0.0–7.2)	0.5 expected
			Lymphohaematopoietic	18 deaths	1.2 (0.7–2.0)	
			Lymphoma	2 deaths	0.7 (0.1–2.5)	
			Leukaemia	10 deaths	1.5 (0.7–2.7)	
			Chronic myeloid leukaemia	3 deaths	8.8 (1.8–25.5)	Analysis limited to 1969–79
			Other lymphatic tissue	6 deaths	2.0 (0.7–4.4)	
			Buccal cavity/pharynx	1 death	0.2 (0.0–0.8)	
			Lung	12 deaths	0.3 (0.1–0.5)	No trend with duration
			Brain and central nervous system	10 deaths	2.7 (1.3–5.0)	Trend with duration
Logue et al. (1986), USA, 1962–77	Pathologists, SMR (5585 men)	None	Nasopharynx	NR	NR	Rate of buccal cavity/pharyngeal cancer was twice as high among pathologists than among radiologists.
			Nasal cavity	NR	NR	
			Lymphohaematopoietic	NR	0.48 (NR)	
			Leukaemia	NR	1.06 (NR)	
			Buccal cavity/pharynx	NR	0.71 (NR)	
			Respiratory system	NR	0.24 (p < 0.01)	

Table 17 (contd)

Embalmers and funeral directors

Reference, country, years of study	Study population, design (study size)	Exposure assessment	Organ site	No. of cases/deaths	SMR[a] (95% CI)	Comments
Walrath & Fraumeni (1983), New York, USA, 1925–80	Embalmers and embalmers/funeral directors, PMR/PCMR (1132 white men)	Time since first licence, age at first licence	All cancers	243 deaths	1.00	PCMR
			Nasopharynx	NR	NR	0.5 expected
			Nasal cavity	0 deaths	NA	PMR
			Lymphohaematopoietic	25 deaths	1.21	PCMR
			Lympho- and reticulosarcoma	5 deaths	0.82	PCMR
			Other lymphatic cancers	6 deaths	1.23	PMR
			Leukaemia	12 deaths	1.19	PCMR
			Myeloid leukaemia	6 deaths	[1.5]	PMR
			Buccal cavity/pharynx	8 deaths	1.03	PCMR; 0 deaths from nasopharyngeal cancer
				7 deaths	2.01	PMR, embalmers only
				1 death	0.28	PMR, funeral directors
			Lung	70 deaths	1.11	PCMR (+ two deaths from pleural cancer)
			Brain and central nervous system	9 deaths	1.38	PCMR
				6 deaths	2.34	PMR, embalmers only, $p < 0.05$
				3 deaths	0.93	PMR, funeral directors
Walrath & Fraumeni (1984), California, USA, 1925–80	Embalmers, PMR/PCMR (1007 white men)	Duration	All cancers	205 deaths	1.00	PCMR; $p < 0.05$ for PMR
			Nasopharynx	NR	NR	trend with duration
			Nasal cavity	0 deaths	NA	0.6 expected
			Lymphohaematopoietic	19 deaths	1.22	PMR
			Lympho- and reticulosarcoma	3 deaths	[1.0]	PMR
			Leukaemia	12 deaths	1.40	PCMR; $p < 0.05$ for PMR; trend with duration
			Myeloid leukaemia	6 deaths	[1.50]	PMR
			Buccal cavity/pharynx	8 deaths	0.99	PCMR, inverse trend with duration; 0 deaths from nasopharyngeal cancer
			Lung	41 deaths	0.87	PCMR, no trend with duration
			Brain	9 deaths	1.68	PCMR; $p < 0.05$ for PMR; no trend with duration

Table 17 (contd)

Reference, country, years of study	Study population, design (study size)	Exposure assessment	Organ site	No. of cases/deaths	SMR[a] (95% CI)	Comments
Levine et al. (1984), Canada, 1950–77	Embalmers, SMR (1413 men)	None	All cancers	58 deaths	0.87 [0.66–1.12]	
			Nasopharynx	NR	NR	
			Nasal cavity	0 deaths	NA	0.2 expected
			Lymphohaematopoietic	8 deaths	1.23 [0.53–2.43]	
			Leukaemia	4 deaths	[1.60] [0.44–4.10]	
			Buccal cavity/pharynx	1 death	[0.48] [0.01–2.65]	Histological type not mentioned
			Lung	19 deaths	0.94 [0.57–1.47]	
			Brain and central nervous system	3 deaths	[1.15] [0.24–3.37]	
Hayes et al. (1990), USA, 1975–85	Embalmers/funeral directors, PMR (3649 white men, 397 non-white men)	None	All cancers	900 deaths	1.07 (1.01–1.15)	White
				102 deaths	1.08 (0.87–1.31)	Non-white
			Nasopharynx	3 deaths	1.89 (0.39–5.48)	White
				1 death	4.00 (0.10–22.3)	Non-white
			Nasal cavity	0 deaths	NA	White and non-white, 1.7 expected
			Lymphohaematopoietic	100 deaths	1.31 (1.06–1.59)	White
				15 deaths	2.41 (1.35–3.97)	Non-white
			Lympho- and reticulosarcoma	11 deaths	1.08 (0.54–1.93)	White
				1 death	1.89 (0.05–10.5)	Non-white
			Lymphatic leukaemia	5 deaths	0.57 (0.19–1.33)	White
				2 deaths	2.99 (0.36–10.7)	Non-white
			Myeloid leukaemia	23 deaths	1.61 (1.02–2.41)	White
				1 death	1.06 (0.02–5.93)	Non-white
			Other and unspecified leukaemia	17 deaths	2.08 (1.21–3.34)	White
				3 deaths	4.92 (1.01–14.36)	Non-white
			Buccal cavity/pharynx	26 deaths	1.19 (0.78–1.74)	White
				4 deaths	1.25 (0.34–3.20)	Non-white
			Lung	285 deaths	0.97 (0.86–1.09)	White
				23 deaths	0.75 (0.47–1.13)	Non-white men
			Brain and central nervous system	24 deaths	1.23 (0.80–1.84)	White
				0 deaths	NA	Non-white, 0.8 expected

CI, confidence interval; NA, not applicable; NR, not reported; PCMR, proportionate cancer mortality ratio; PMR, proportionate mortality ratio; SMR, standardized mortality ratio
[a] Unless otherwise stated

deaths; 95% CI, 0.27–1.12) among men from England and Wales and Scotland, respectively, and 0.95 (nine deaths; 95% CI, 0.43–1.80) among women from England and Wales. No significant excess was seen for cancer at any site. Non-significant excess mortality occurred for brain cancer (six deaths; SMR, 2.40; 95% CI, 0.88–5.22) and lymphatic and haematopoietic cancer (nine deaths; SMR, 1.42; 95% CI, 0.65–2.69) among men from England and Wales, breast cancer (four deaths; SMR, 1.61; 95% CI, 0.44–4.11) among women from England and Wales and prostatic cancer (two deaths; SMR, 3.30; 95% CI, 0.39–11.8) among men from Scotland.

(b)   Anatomists and pathologists in the USA

Stroup *et al.* (1986) evaluated mortality among members of the American Association of Anatomists. A total of 2317 men had joined the Association between 1888 and 1969; because only 299 women had joined during this period, they were not included. Ninety-eight of the men were excluded because they had died, moved or were lost to follow-up before 1925, which resulted in a final study size of 2239. Follow-up of the cohort for vital status was accomplished from the date the person joined the association until 1979. The expected numbers of deaths were calculated from age-, race-, sex- and calendar time-specific rates for the general population of the USA for the period 1925–79 or for male members of the American Psychiatric Association, a population that should be similar to anatomists with regard to socioeconomic status, in 1900–69. In comparison with the general population, the cohort showed a very large 'healthy worker effect', with SMRs of 0.65 for all causes (738 deaths) and 0.64 (118 deaths; 95% CI, 0.53–0.76) for cancer at all sites. Excess mortality was observed for cancers of the brain and central nervous system (10 deaths; SMR, 2.7; 95% CI, 1.3–5.0), leukaemia (10 deaths; SMR, 1.5; 95% CI, 0.7–2.7) and lymphatic tissues other than lymphosarcoma, reticulosarcoma, Hodgkin disease and leukaemia (six deaths; SMR, 2.0; 95% CI, 0.7–4.4). The risk for brain cancer increased with duration of membership, from 2.0 for < 20 years to 2.8 for 20–39 years and to 7.0 for ≥ 40 years; no such pattern was seen for lung cancer or leukaemia. Of the 10 deaths from leukaemia, five were myeloid and the SMR for chronic myeloid leukaemia was statistically significantly elevated (three deaths; SMR, 8.8; 95% CI, 1.8–25.5) in the period 1969–79 for which cell type-specific mortality rates were available. The SMRs were below 1.0 for lung cancer (12 deaths; SMR, 0.3; 95% CI, 0.1–0.5) and oral and pharyngeal cancer (one death; SMR, 0.2; 95% CI, 0.0–0.8). No death from nasal cancer occurred (0.5 expected). When compared with members of the American Psychiatric Association, anatomists had deficits in mortality from lung cancer (seven deaths; SMR, 0.5; 95% CI, 0.2–1.1) and leukaemia (three deaths; SMR, 0.8; 95% CI, 0.2–2.9), but they still had an excess mortality from brain cancer (nine deaths; SMR, 6.0; 95% CI, 2.3–15.6).

Logue *et al.* (1986) evaluated mortality among 5585 members of the College of American Pathologists listed in the Radiation Registry of Physicians. The cohort was established by enrolling members between 1962 and 1972 and following them up through to 1977. Direct comparisons were made between the mortality rates of pathologists and a cohort of 4418 radiologists and used the Mantel-Haenszel procedure with adjustment for age and calendar time for large categories of death (e.g. all cancers). Indirect comparisons that used mortality rates for white men in the USA in 1970 as the referent were also performed to compute SMRs. The age-adjusted mortality rate for all cancers was found to be slightly lower in pathologists than in radiologists (1.37 versus 1.51 per 1000 person–years). Based on comparisons with the national population, a deficit in mortality was observed among pathologists for cancers of the buccal cavity and pharnyx (SMR, 0.71) and respiratory system (SMR, 0.24) and for lymphatic and haematopoietic neoplasms other than leukaemia (SMR, 0.48). Mortality from leukaemia was slightly elevated (SMR, 1.06) among pathologists. [The number of deaths for each cancer site was not reported.] However, the age-adjusted mortality rate for leukaemia was higher among radiologists than among pathologists (0.15 versus 0.10 per 1000 person–years). [Confidence intervals were not reported and could not be estimated since observed and expected numbers of deaths were not reported.]

(c)   Embalmers and funeral directors

Walrath and Fraumeni (1983) used licensing records from the New York State (USA) Department of Health, Bureau of Funeral Directing and Embalming to identify 1678 embalmers who had been licensed between 1902 and 1980 and who had died between 1925 and 1980. Death certificates were obtained for 1263 (75%) decedents (1132 white men, 79 non-white men, 42 men of unknown race and 10 women); proportionate mortality ratios (PMRs) and proportionate cancer mortality ratios (PCMRs) were calculated for white men and non-white men on the basis of age-, race-, sex- and calendar time-specific proportions in the general population. Observed and expected numbers were generally not provided for non-white men, but it was indicated that there was a significant excess mortality from cancers of the larynx (two deaths) and lymphatic and haematopoietic system (three deaths) in this group. Among white men, the PCMR was 1.00 (243 deaths) for all cancers combined. PCMRs for specific cancers were 1.03 (eight deaths) for buccal cavity and pharynx, 1.11 (70 deaths) for lung, 1.38 (nine deaths) for brain, 1.21 (PMR; 25 deaths) for lymphatic and haematopoietic system, 0.82 (five deaths) for lymphosarcoma and reticulosarcoma (ICD-8 200) and 1.19 (12 deaths) for leukaemia. Six of the leukaemia deaths (4.1 expected) were from myeloid leukaemia [PMR, 1.5]. No deaths occurred from cancer of the nasal sinuses or nasopharynx. There was little difference in PMRs by time since first licence. The subjects who were recruited had been licensed as either embalmers or as both embalmers and funeral directors. Mortality patterns were analysed separately for the two groups because the authors assumed that persons who were licensed only as embalmers would have had more exposure to formaldehyde than embalmers who were also funeral directors. The PMR for cancer of the brain and central nervous system was significantly increased among people who were licensed only as embalmers (six deaths; PMR, 2.34; $p < 0.05$) but not among those who also were licensed as a funeral director (three deaths; PMR, 0.93). A difference was also observed for mortality from cancer of the buccal cavity and pharynx: the PMR for embalmers was 2.01 (seven deaths) and that for embalmers/funeral directors was 0.28 (one death). Neoplasms of the lymphatic and haematopoietic system were only elevated among individuals who were licensed as both an embalmer and funeral director (16 deaths; PMR, 1.39).

Walrath and Fraumeni (1984) used the records of the California (USA) Bureau of Funeral Directing and Embalming to examine proportionate mortality among embalmers who had first been licensed in California between 1916 and 1978. They identified 1109 embalmers who died between 1925 and 1980, comprised of 1007 white men, 39 non-white men, 58 white women and five non-white women. Only mortality of white men was analysed. PMRs and PCMRs were calculated using age-, race-, sex- and calendar year-specific proportions from the general population of the USA. Total cancer mortality was significantly greater than that expected (205 deaths; PMR, 1.21 for all cancers combined). Also, a statistically significant excess of proportionate mortality was observed for cancers of the colon (30 deaths; PMR, 1.87), prostate (23 deaths; PMR, 1.75), brain and central nervous system (nine deaths; PMR, 1.94) and leukaemia (12 deaths; PMR, 1.75). The magnitude of these excesses was reduced and no longer statistically significant in the PCMR analyses (Table 17). Mortality from cancers of the buccal cavity and pharynx was slightly elevated in the PMR analysis (eight deaths; PMR, 1.31) but not in the PCMR analysis (PCMR, 0.99). Mortality from lung and pleural cancers was close to expected in both the PMR (41 observed, 42.9 expected; PMR, 0.96) and PCMR (0.87) analyses. There was no death from cancer of the nasal passages (0.6 expected). Mortality from leukaemia was found to be increased predominantly among embalmers who had had a licence for 20 or more years (eight deaths; PMR, 2.21). Six of the 12 cases of leukaemia were of the myeloid type [PMR, 1.5].

Mortality among 1477 male embalmers who had been licensed by the Ontario (Canada) Board of Funeral Services between 1928 and 1957 was evaluated by Levine *et al.* (1984). The cohort was followed for mortality from the date of first licence through to 1977. Expected numbers of deaths were derived from the mortality rates for men in Ontario in 1950–77, adjusted for age and calendar year. Since mortality rates for Ontario were not available before 1950, person–years and deaths in the cohort before that time were excluded from the analysis, which left 1413 men known to be alive in 1950. Mortality from all cancers was observed to be slightly lower than expected (58 deaths; SMR, 0.87 [95% CI, 0.66–1.12]). A small and statistically non-significant excess in mortality was observed for cancers of the lymphatic and haematopoietic system (eight deaths; SMR, 1.23 [95% CI, 0.53–2.43]) and leukaemia (four deaths [SMR, 1.60; 95% CI, 0.44–4.10]). Mortality from cancers of the buccal cavity and pharynx (one death [SMR, 0.48; 95% CI, 0.01–2.65]), lung (19 deaths; SMR, 0.94 [95% CI, 0.57–1.47]) and brain (three deaths [SMR, 1.15; 95% CI, 0.24–3.37]) was close to or lower than expected. No death from cancer of the nose, middle ear or sinuses was observed (0.2 expected).

Hayes *et al.* (1990) identified 6651 deceased embalmers/funeral directors from the records of licensing boards and state funeral directors' associations in 32 states and the District of Columbia and from the vital statistics offices of nine states and New York City in the USA between 1975 and 1985. Death certificates were received for 5265. Exclusion of 449 decedents included in previous studies of embalmers in New York (Walrath &

Fraumeni, 1983) and California (Walrath & Fraumeni, 1984), 376 subjects who probably did not work in the funeral industry, eight subjects of unknown race or age at death and 386 women left 4046 male decedents available for analysis (3649 whites and 397 non-whites). PMRs and PCMRs were calculated on the basis of expected numbers from race- and sex-specific groups of the general population, adjusted for 5-year age and calendar-time categories. The PMR for all cancers was 1.07 (900 deaths; 95% CI, 1.01–1.15) for whites and 1.08 (102 deaths; 95% CI, 0.87–1.31) for non-whites. The PMRs for specific cancers were: buccal cavity and pharynx (whites: 26 deaths; PMR, 1.19; 95% CI, 0.78–1.74; non-whites: four deaths; PMR, 1.25; 95% CI, 0.34–3.20), nasopharynx (whites: three deaths; PMR, 1.89; 95% CI, 0.39–5.48; non-whites: one death; PMR, 4.00; 95% CI, 0.10–22.3), nasal sinuses (whites and non-whites: 0 observed, 1.7 expected), lung (whites: 285 deaths; PMR, 0.97; 95% CI, 0.86–1.09; non-whites: 23 deaths; PMR, 0.75; 95% CI, 0.47–1.13), brain and central nervous system (whites: 24 deaths; PMR, 1.23; 95% CI, 0.80–1.84; non-whites: 0 observed, 0.8 expected) and lymphatic and haematopoietic system (whites: 100 deaths; PMR, 1.31; 95% CI, 1.06–1.59; non-whites: 15 deaths; PMR, 2.41; 95% CI, 1.35–3.97). The risks for cancers of the lymphatic and haematopoietic system and brain and central nervous system did not vary substantially by licensing category (embalmer versus funeral director), by geographical region, by age at death or by source of data on mortality. Among the lymphatic and haematopoietic cancers, the PMRs were significantly elevated for myeloid leukaemia (both groups combined: 24 deaths; PMR, 1.57; 95% CI, 1.01–2.34) and other and unspecified leukaemia (both groups combined: 20 deaths; PMR, 2.28; 95% CI, 1.39–3.52); non-significant excesses of mortality were observed for several other histological types.

2.1.3   *Other cohort studies*

In a study of users of various medicinal drugs based on computer-stored hospitalization records of the outpatient pharmacy at the Kaiser–Permanente Medical Center in San Francisco (CA, USA), Friedman and Ury (1983) evaluated cancer incidence in a cohort of 143 574 pharmacy users from July 1969 through August 1973 and followed them up to the end of 1978. The number of cases among users of specific drugs was compared with the number expected on the basis of rates for all pharmacy users, adjusted for age and sex. Since many analyses were performed (56 cancers and 120 drugs, for 6720 combinations), chance findings would be expected. Five cancers were associated with use of formaldehyde solution (topically for warts) (morbidity ratio, 0.8 [95% CI, 0.3–2.0]). The morbidity ratio for lung cancer was significantly elevated (four cases; morbidity ratio, 5.7 [95% CI, 1.6–15]) for people who used formaldehyde. Information on tobacco smoking was not provided. [The Working Group noted the short period of follow-up, the small number of cases and the lack of detailed information on exposure that made this study largely uninformative.]

Several studies have evaluated risk for cancer in haemodialysis patients who may have been potentially exposed to formaldehyde (see Section 1.3.2). [The Working Group considered these studies to be largely uninformative since some patients with chronic renal failure receive immunosuppressive drugs, which are known to increase their risk for cancer, and because these studies are generally small, have short follow-up and provide limited or no information on exposures to formaldehyde.]

2.2   Case–control studies

Case–control studies have been used to examine the association between exposure to formaldehyde and various cancers. For rare tumours such as sinonasal and nasopharyngeal cancer, they have the potential to provide greater statistical power than can normally be achieved in cohort studies. Against this advantage, however, must be set the difficulties in assessing exposure to formaldehyde retrospectively in community-based studies. This requirement is usually addressed through expert evaluation of job histories by an occupational hygienist, or through the use of a job–exposure matrix. For a chemical such as formaldehyde, however, these methods tend to lack specificity when applied to the general population. Thus, the subjects who are classed as having been exposed to formal-dehyde in community-based case–control studies usually have lower exposures on average than those in occupational cohorts that are specially selected for investigation because they are known to experience high exposures. Exposures to formaldehyde were assessed in some studies by asking study subjects whether they had been exposed to formaldehyde. This use of self-reported exposures is of questionable validity and in particular may lead to recall bias.

2.2.1   *Cancers of the nasal cavity and paranasal sinuses*

The study design of and results from case–control studies on cancers of the nasal cavity, paranasal sinuses, nasopharynx and hypopharynx associated with exposure to formaldehyde are summarized in Table 18.

With the purpose of investigating the carcinogenic effects of exposure to wood dust, Hernberg *et al.* (1983a) conducted a joint Nordic case–control study of 167 patients in Finland, Sweden and most of Denmark in whom primary malignant tumours of the nasal cavity and paranasal sinuses had been diagnosed between July 1977 and December 1980 and 167 country-, age- and sex-matched controls who had been diagnosed with cancers of the colon and rectum. The study subjects represented 58% of all cancers identified at these anatomical sites; the exclusions were due to early deaths or to non-responding or missing controls. Information on the occupations and tobacco smoking habits of the study subjects was obtained by standardized telephone interview. None of the cases or controls had worked in the particle-board or plywood industry or in the production of formal-dehyde or formaldehyde-based glues. No association was found between sinonasal cancer and other occupations in which exposure to formaldehyde was considered to be most probable. A total of 18 cases and six controls had worked in 'painting, lacquering and glueing', a category that the authors considered may have entailed minimal exposure to

Table 18. Case–control studies of cancers of the nasal cavity, paranasal sinuses, nasopharynx and hypopharynx

Reference, study location, years of study	Organ site (ICD code)	Characteristics of cases	Characteristics of controls	Exposure assessment	Exposure categories	Relative risk (95% CI)	Adjustment for potential confounders	Comments
Hernberg et al. (1983a), Denmark, Finland, Sweden, 1977–80	Nasal cavity and parasinuses (160.0–160.9; ICD revision not given)	167 patients [sex distribution not reported] with primary malignant tumours	167 patients with cancer of the colon and rectum, matched by country, sex and age	Employment in particle-board or plywood industry Painting, lacquering and glazing	Yes/no Yes/no	0 cases, 0 controls 18 cases, 6 controls		Concomitant exposure of 15 cases to wood dust
Brinton et al. (1984), USA, 1970–80	Nasal cavity and parasinuses (ICD-8 160.0, 160.2–160.5, 160.8–160.9)	160 (93 men, 67 women), including 86 squamous-cell carcinomas and 24 adenocarcinomas or adenoid cystic carcinomas; 61 in nasal cavity, 71 in maxillary sinus and 28 other sinus or overlapping sites	290 (178 hospital controls, 112 death certificate controls); hospital controls were required to be alive for living cases; death certificate controls were identified for deceased cases; matched on age, sex, race and county of residence	Telephone interviews with subjects or next of kin included a checklist of industries and self-reported exposures including formaldehyde.	*Men and women combined* Unexposed Exposed	1.0 0.35 (0.1–1.8)	Adjusted for sex; control for tobacco use did not change results.	Formaldehyde exposure assessment was self-reported; only 33% of cases and 39% of controls were interviewed directly; for the remainder, exposures relied on recall of next of kin.
Olsen et al. (1984), Denmark, 1970–82	Nasal cavity, nasal sinuses (160.0, 160.2, 160.9) and nasopharynx (146) (ICD revision not given)	754 incident patients [sex distribution not reported] selected from the Danish Cancer Registry including 488 carcinomas of the nasal cavity and sinuses and 266 carcinomas of the nasopharynx	2465 patients with cancers of the colon, rectum, prostate and breast; frequency-matched by sex, age (± 5 years) and year of diagnosis (± 5 years); 4.2% of men and 0.1% of women exposed to formaldehyde	Record linkage with pension fund with compulsory membership; job title from Central Pension Registry; exposure assessed blindly as certain, probable, unlikely, unknown	*Sinonasal* *Industries and occupations with certain exposure to formaldehyde* Ever exposed Unexposed to wood dust Exposed to wood dust Exposure for > 10 years before diagnosis Unexposed to wood dust Exposed to wood dust Adjusted for wood dust *Industries and occupations with certain or possible exposure* Men Women *Nasopharynx*	2.8 (1.8–4.3) 1.8 (0.7–4.9) 3.5 (2.2–5.6) 3.1 (1.8–5.4) 1.5 (0.4–5.3) 4.1 (2.3–7.3) 1.6 (0.7–3.6) 0.7 (0.3–1.7) 2.6 (0.3–21.9)	Unadjusted Unadjusted	Data for sinonasal cancer reported for men only

Table 18 (contd)

Reference, study location, years of study	Organ site (ICD code)	Characteristics of cases	Characteristics of controls	Exposure assessment	Exposure categories	Relative risk (95% CI)	Adjustment for potential confounders	Comments
Hayes et al. (1986a), Netherlands, 1978–81	Nasal cavity and accessory sinuses (ICD-9 160.0, 160.2–160.5)	91 male patients histologically confirmed, alive or deceased	195 age-stratified random sample of living men resident in the Netherlands in 1982 or deceased in the Netherlands in 1980	Taking into account job history, time period and potential frequency of exposure, exposure was classified into 10 groups independently by two occupational hygienists (assessment A and B)	*Any exposure to formaldehyde* Assessment A Assessment B *No or little exposure to wood dust* Assessment A Assessment B *Moderate to high exposure to wood dust* Assessment A Assessment B *Squamous-cell carcinoma only* Assessment A Assessment B	 2.5 (1.5–4.3)[a] 1.9 (1.2–3.0)[a] 2.5 [1.0–5.9] 1.6 [0.8–3.1] 1.9 [0.6–6.5] NR 3.0 [1.2–7.8] 1.9 [0.9–4.1]	Standardized for age in 10-year groups; control for usual number of cigarettes smoked did not modify the results. No or little exposure to wood dust	Relative risk for adeno-carcinoma for those ever employed in the wood and paper industry, 11.3 (90% CI, 4.0–35.1); moderate increase associated with increase in level of exposure to formaldehyde with no concomitant exposure to wood dust
Olsen & Asnaes (1986), Denmark, 1970–82	Nasal cavity, paranasal sinuses (160.0, 160.2–160.9) and naso-pharynx (146) (ICD revision not given)	759 (509 men, 250 women) histologically confirmed cancers of the nasal cavity and para-nasal sinuses (466 cases; 310 men, 156 women) and nasopharynx (293 cases; 199 men, 94 women)	2465 patients with cancers of the colon, rectum, prostate and breast frequency-matched by sex, age (± 5 years) and year of diagnosis (± 5 years); 4.2% of men and 0.1% of women exposed to formaldehyde	Record linkage with pension fund with compulsory membership; job title from Central Pension Registry; exposure assessed blindly as certain, probable, unlikely, unknown	*Likely or possible exposure to formaldehyde ≥ 10 years before diagnosis* Squamous-cell carcinoma (215) Adenocarcinoma (39)	 2.4 (0.8–7.4) 1.8 (0.5–6.0)	Adjusted for exposure to wood dust	Data presented for men for cancer of the nasal cavity and paranasal sinuses; no association observed with naso-pharyngeal cancer

Table 18 (contd)

Reference, study location, years of study	Organ site (ICD code)	Characteristics of cases	Characteristics of controls	Exposure assessment	Exposure categories	Relative risk (95% CI)	Adjustment for potential confounders	Comments
Vaughan *et al.* (1986a), USA, 1979–83	Nasal cavity (160) and pharynx (146–149) (ICD revision not given)	285 incident cases [sex distribution not reported] identified by the local Cancer Surveillance System, aged 20–74 years, including oro- and hypopharynx (205), nasopharynx (27) and sinuses (53)	552 identified by random-digit dialling	Job-exposure linkage system, resulting in four categories: high, medium, low and background	*Sinonasal* Low exposure Medium or high exposure Highest exposure score *Nasopharynx* Low exposure Medium or high exposure Highest exposure score *Oro-/hypopharynx* Low exposure Medium exposure High exposure Highest exposure score	*Sinonasal* 0.8 (0.4–1.7) 0.3 (0.0–1.3) 0.3 (0.0–2.3) *Nasopharynx* 1.2 (0.5–3.3) 1.4 (0.4–4.7) 2.1 (0.6–7.8) *Oro-/hypopharynx* 0.8 (0.5–1.4) 0.8 (0.4–1.7) 0.6 (0.1–2.7) 1.5 (0.7–3.0)	Age, sex, cigarette smoking and alcohol consumption	
Vaughan *et al.* (1986b), USA, 1979–83	Nasal cavity (160) and pharynx, (146–149) (ICD revision not given)	285 incident cases [sex distribution not reported] identified by the local Cancer Surveillance System, aged 20–74 years, including oro- and hypopharynx (205), nasopharynx (27) and sinuses (53)	552 identified by random-digit dialling	Residential exposure: residential history since 1950	*Sinonasal* Mobile home Particle-board at home 1–9 years ≥ 10 years *Nasopharynx* Mobile home 1–9 years ≥ 10 years Particle-board at home 1–9 years ≥ 10 years *Oro-/hypopharynx* Mobile home 1–9 years ≥ 10 years Particle-board at home 1–9 years ≥ 10 years	*Sinonasal* 0.6 (0.2–1.7) 1.8 (0.9–3.8) 1.5 (0.7–3.2) *Nasopharynx* 2.1 (0.7–6.6) 5.5 (1.6–19.4) 1.4 (0.5–3.4) 0.6 (0.2–2.3) *Oro-/hypopharynx* 0.9 (0.5–1.8) 0.8 (0.2–2.7) 1.1 (0.7–1.9) 0.8 (0.5–1.4)	Sex, age, cigarette smoking and alcohol consumption Cigarette smoking and race Sex, age, cigarette smoking and alcohol consumption	

Table 18 (contd)

Reference, study location, years of study	Organ site (ICD code)	Characteristics of cases	Characteristics of controls	Exposure assessment	Exposure categories	Relative risk (95% CI)	Adjustment for potential confounders	Comments
Rousch et al. (1987), USA, 1935–75	Nasal cavity and sinuses, and naso-pharynx (ICD code not given)	198 men with sinonasal cancer and 173 with nasopharyngeal cancer registered at the Connecticut Tumor Registry	605 men who died during the same period, selected by random sampling without matching or stratification	Job title, industry, specific employment, year of employment, obtained from death certificates and city directories	*Sinonasal*	0.8 (0.5–1.3)	Age and calendar period	
					Probably exposed for most of working life			
					Plus exposure ≥ 20 years before death	1.0 (0.5–1.8)		
					Plus exposure to high level for some years	1.0 (0.5–2.2)		
					Plus exposure to high level ≥ 20 years before death	1.5 (0.6–3.9)		
					Nasopharynx	1.0 (0.6–1.7)		
					Probably exposed for most of working life			
					Plus exposure ≥ 20 years before death	1.3 (0.7–2.4)		
					Plus exposure to high level for some years	1.4 (0.6–3.1)		
					Plus exposure to high level ≥ 20 years before death	2.3 (0.9–6.0)		

Table 18 (contd)

Reference, study location, years of study	Organ site (ICD code)	Characteristics of cases	Characteristics of controls	Exposure assessment	Exposure categories	Relative risk (95% CI)	Adjustment for potential confounders	Comments
Luce et al. (1993), France, 1986–88	Nasal cavity and parasinuses (ICD-9 160.0, 160.2–160.9)	207 cases (167 men, 40 women): 59 men and 18 women with squamous-cell carcinomas, 82 men and five women with adenocarcinomas and 25 men and 17 women with other histology	409 from two sources: 323 hospital cancer controls (15 sites) frequency-matched by age and sex; 86 proposed by cases, matched by age (± 10 years), sex and residence	Industrial hygienist review of structured job interview, classifying exposure by frequency, concentration and duration; computation of cumulative exposure level and lifetime average level	*Squamous-cell carcinoma* Possibly exposed Probably or definitely Average level ≤ 2 Average level > 2 Duration ≤ 20 years Duration > 20 years Cumulative level ≤ 30 > 30	**Men** 0.96 (0.38–2.42) 0.70 (0.28–1.73) 1.32 (0.54–3.24) 1.09 (0.48–2.50) 0.76 (0.29–2.01) 1.26 (0.54–2.94) 0.68 (0.27–1.75)	Adjusted for age, exposure to wood dust and exposure to glues and adhesives	Adjustment for usual cigarette use or for smoking history did not change results.
					Adenocarcinoma Possibly exposed Probably or definitely Average level ≤ 2 Average level > 2 Duration ≤ 20 years Duration > 20 years Cumulative level ≤ 30 30–60 > 60	1.28 (0.16–10.42) 4.15 (0.96–17.84) 5.33 (1.28–22.20) 1.03 (0.18–5.77) 6.86 (1.69–27.80) 1.13 (0.19–6.90) 2.66 (0.38–18.70) 6.91 (1.69–28.23)		Most cases of adenocarcinomas exposed to both formaldehyde wood dust; very large odds ratio (288) for wood dust; therefore, there is concern about the possibility of incomplete adjustment for wood dust in these results.
					Other histology Possibly exposed Probably or definitely Average level ≤ 2 Average level > 2 Duration ≤ 20 years Duration > 20 years Cumulative level ≤ 30 > 30	0.81 (0.15–4.36) 1.67 (0.51–5.42) 3.04 (0.95–9.70) 2.82 (0.94–8.43) 1.62 (0.48–5.51) 2.18 (0.65–7.31) 2.21 (0.73–6.73)		

Table 18 (contd)

Reference, study location, years of study	Organ site (ICD code)	Characteristics of cases	Characteristics of controls	Exposure assessment	Exposure categories	Relative risk (95% CI)	Adjustment for potential confounders	Comments
West et al. (1993), Philippines [study years not reported]	Nasopharynx (ICD code not given)	104 incident cases (76 men, 28 women) histologically confirmed	104 hospital controls matched for sex, age and hospital ward type; 101 community controls matched for sex, age and neighbourhood	Occupation classified as likely or unlikely to involve exposure to formaldehyde; duration of exposure; 10-year lag period; years since first exposure; age at start of exposure	< 15 years ≥ 15 years < 15 years (10-year lag) ≥ 15 years (10-year lag) Age ≥ 25 years at first exposure Age < 25 years at first exposure First exposure < 25 years before diagnosis First exposure ≥ 25 years before diagnosis	2.7 (1.1–6.6) 1.2 (0.5–3.2) 1.6 (0.6–3.8) 2.1 (0.7–6.2) 1.2 (0.5–3.3) 2.7 (1.1–6.6) 1.3 (0.6–3.2) 2.9 (1.1–7.6)	Years since first exposure to dust and/or exhaust fumes	
Gustavsson et al. (1998), Sweden, 1988–91	Oro- and hypopharynx (ICD-9 146, 148)	545 incident male cases among residents of two regions, aged 40–79 years [including at least 124 cases of pharyngeal cancer]	641 selected by stratified random sampling; frequency-matched to cases by age (10–15-year groups) and region	Work history reviewed by occupational hygienist; occupations coded by intensity and probability of exposure	Ever exposed	1.01 (0.49–2.07)	Age, region, alcohol, consumption and smoking habits	
Armstrong et al. (2000), Malaysia, (Selagor and Federal Territory), 1987–92	Nasopharyngeal squamous-cell carcinoma (ICD code not given)	282 Chinese men and women from four centres (prevalent and incident cases) [no information on age distribution]	One Chinese control selected by multistage area sampling per case; matched by age and sex	Structured in-home interviews; occupational exposures assessed by a job-exposure matrix	Any (unadjusted) Any (adjusted)	1.24 (0.67–2.32) 0.71 (0.34–1.41)	Diet and tobacco use	Mixture of prevalent (42%) and incident (58%) cases

Table 18 (contd)

Reference, study location, years of study	Organ site (ICD code)	Characteristics of cases	Characteristics of controls	Exposure assessment	Exposure categories	Relative risk (95% CI)	Adjustment for potential confounders	Comments
Laforest et al. (2000), France, 1989–91	Hypopharynx (squamous-cell) (ICD code not given)	201 men with confirmed histology from 15 hospitals [no information on age]	296 male patients with other (selected) primary tumours from the same or nearby hospitals; recruited 1987–91; matched by age	Structured in-person interviews; occupational exposures assessed with a job–exposure matrix earlier developed	Ever exposed	1.35 (0.86–2.14)	Age, tobacco smoking, alcohol consumption, coal dust and asbestos	
					Probability of exposure (%)			
					<10	1.08 (0.62–1.88)		
					10–50	1.01 (0.44–2.31)		
					>50	3.78 (1.50–9.49)		
					Duration (years)			
					<7	1.09 (0.50–2.38)		
					7–20	1.39 (0.74–2.62)		
					>20	1.51 (0.78–2.92)		
					Cumulative level			
					Low	1.03 (0.51–2.07)		
					Medium	1.57 (0.81–3.06)		
					High	1.51 (0.74–3.10)		
					Exclusion of subjects with exposure probability < 10%			
					Ever exposed	1.74 (0.91–3.34)		
					Duration (years)			
					<7	0.74 (0.20–2.68)		
					7–20	1.65 (0.67–4.08)		
					>20	2.70 (1.08–6.73)		
					Cumulative level			
					Low	0.78 (0.11–5.45)		
					Medium	1.77 (0.65–4.78)		
					High	1.92 (0.86–4.32)		

Table 18 (contd)

Reference, study location, years of study	Organ site (ICD code)	Characteristics of cases	Characteristics of controls	Exposure assessment	Exposure categories	Relative risk (95% CI)	Adjustment for potential confounders	Comments
Vaughan et al. (2000), USA (Connecticut, metropolitan Detroit, Iowa, Utah, Washington), 1987–93	Epithelial nasopharyngeal carcinoma: epithelial NOS (801x–804x), undifferentiated or non-keratinizing (8020–1, 8072–3, 8082) and squamous-cell (805x–808x, except 8072–3)	196 men and women [sex distribution not reported] from five cancer registries, aged 18–74 years	244 population-based selected by random digit dialling; frequency-matched by sex, cancer registry and age (5-year groups)	Structured telephone interviews; occupational exposures assessed by a job-exposure matrix	Ever exposed	1.3 (0.8–2.1)	Age, sex, race, centre, cigarette use, proxy status and education	Data presented for any potential exposure (possible, probable or definite); not influenced by a 10-year lag period or adding wood dust exposure to models
					Max. exposure (ppm)			
					< 0.1	1.4 (0.8–2.4)		
					0.1–0.5	0.9 (0.4–2.3)		
					> 0.5	1.6 (0.3–7.1)		
					p for trend	0.57		
					Duration (years)			
					1–5	0.8 (0.4–1.6)		
					6–17	1.6 (0.7–3.4)		
					≥ 18	2.1 (1.0–4.5)		
					p for trend	0.070		
					Differentiated squamous-cell and epithelial NOS only			
					Ever exposed	1.6 (1.0–2.8)		
					Duration (years)			
					1–5	0.9 (0.4–2.1)		
					6–17	1.9 (0.9–4.4)		
					≥ 18	2.7 (1.2–6.0)		
					p for trend	0.014		
					Cumulative exposure (ppm–years)			
					0.05–0.4	0.9 (0.4–2.0)		
					> 0.4–1.10	1.8 (0.8–4.1)		
					> 1.10	3.0 (1.3–6.6)		
					p for trend	0.033		

Table 18 (contd)

Reference, study location, years of study	Organ site (ICD code)	Characteristics of cases	Characteristics of controls	Exposure assessment	Exposure categories	Relative risk (95% CI)	Adjustment for potential confounders	Comments
Hildesheim et al. (2001) Taiwan, China, 1991–94	Nasopharynx; > 90% non-keratinizing and undifferentiated and remainder squamous-cell carcinomas (ICD code not given)	375 histologically confirmed hospital cases (31% women), aged < 75 years	325 community controls, individually matched on sex, age (5 years) and district of residence	Structured in-person interviews; occupational exposures assessed by an industrial hygienist; blood specimen was tested for anti-EBV antibodies.	Ever exposed *Duration* 1–10 years >10 years *p* for trend *Cumulative exposure* < 25 ≥ 25 *p* for trend	1.4 (0.93–2.2) 1.3 (0.69–2.3) 1.6 (0.91–2.9) 0.08 1.3 (0.70–2.4) 1.5 (0.88–2.7) 0.10	Age, sex, education and ethnicity	Observations were not influenced by adding wood dust exposure to models; in a sub-analysis restricted to 360 cases and 94 controls seropositive for at least one type of antibody against EBV, the association between exposure to formaldehyde and nasopharyngeal cancer appeared somewhat stronger.
Berrino et al. (2003), France, Italy, Spain, Switzerland, 1979–82	Hypopharynx and epilarynx (ICD code not given)	100 men, incident cases histologically confirmed from six centres, aged ≤ 55 years	819 men from the general local population of each centre; age- and sex-stratified	Structured in-person interviews; occupational exposures assessed by an expert panel using a previously established job-exposure matrix	*Probability of exposure* Possible Probable and certain	1.3 (0.6–2.6) 0.5 (0.1–1.8)	Age, centre, tobacco use, alcohol consumption, diet, socio-economic status, asbestos, PAHs, chromium, arsenic, wood dust, solvents, other dusts and gases	[The credibility of the negative finding is limited because formaldehyde was the agent for which the validity of the job-exposure matrix was lowest.]

CI, confidence interval; EBV, Epstein-Barr virus; ICD, international code of diseases; NOS, not otherwise specified; PAHs, polycyclic aromatic hydrocarbons

[a] 90% confidence interval

formaldehyde; when workers exposed to wood dust were excluded, more controls than cases had been exposed (three cases, six controls). [The Working Group noted that the study was not designed to address exposure to formaldehyde and that all the cases in Denmark were also included in the study of Olsen *et al.* (1984).]

In a case–control study conducted in four hospitals in North Carolina and Virginia, USA, in 1970–80, 193 men and women who had primary malignancies of the nasal cavity and sinuses were identified (Brinton *et al.*, 1984). Two hospital controls who were alive at the date of the interview were selected for each living patient and matched on hospital, year of admission, age, sex, race and administrative area; for deceased patients, two similarly matched controls were chosen: one patient who had attended the same hospital but who was not necessarily alive at the date of the interview, and one deceased person who was identified from records of the state vital statistics offices. Patients who had cancer of the buccal cavity and pharynx, nasal cavity, middle ear and accessory sinuses, larynx and oesophagus and patients who had various nasal disorders were excluded from the control group. Telephone interviews were completed for 160 of the nasal cancer patients (83%) and 290 of the controls (78%), either directly with the patients themselves (33% of cases and 39% of controls) or with their next of kin. Occupational exposures were assessed by the interviewee's recall in response to a checklist of exposures, including formaldehyde. Exposure to formaldehyde was reported for two nasal cancer patients (one man and one woman), to yield an odds ratio of 0.35 (95% CI, 0.1–1.8). [The Working Group noted that the exposure assessment was limited as it relied on self-reports and, furthermore, that a high proportion of interviews were with next of kin. The informativeness of the study was further limited by the small number of exposed subjects.]

In a population-based study in Denmark (Olsen *et al.*, 1984), 488 men and women in whom cancer of the sinonasal cavities had been diagnosed during the period 1970–82 and reported to the national cancer registry were matched to 2465 controls for sex, age and year of diagnosis, who were selected from all patients in whom cancer of the colon, rectum, prostate or breast had been diagnosed during the same period. Histories of exposure to formaldehyde, wood dust and 10 other specified compounds or industrial procedures were assessed by industrial hygienists who were unaware of the case or control status of the study subjects, on the basis of individual employment histories obtained from a national pension scheme in operation since 1964. The industrial hygienists classified subjects according to whether they had definitely or probably been exposed, had not been exposed or had undetermined exposure to individual compounds during 1964–82. Of the controls, 4.2% of men and 0.1% of women had held occupations that presumably entailed exposure to formaldehyde. The odds ratios for definite exposures to formaldehyde (unadjusted for any other occupational exposure and using the no exposure category as the reference level) were 2.8 (95% CI, 1.8–4.3) for men and 2.8 (95% CI, 0.5–14) for women. Further results were not presented for women. Adjustment for exposure to wood dust reduced the risk estimate for men to 1.6, which was no longer significant. Only five men in the group of 33 workers with definite exposure to formaldehyde had not been exposed to wood dust. Probable exposure to formaldehyde was associated with a slightly increased risk for sinonasal cancer in men (odds ratio, 1.2; 95% CI, 0.8–1.7). [The Working Group noted that the employment histories of study subjects were restricted to 1964 or later and that the study was limited by the fact that the industries that used formaldehyde in Denmark in this study seemed to be dominated by exposure to wood dust, which makes assessment of the separate effect of exposure to formaldehyde on the risk for sinonasal cancer difficult.]

A re-analysis was performed (Olsen & Asnaes, 1986) in which data on 215 men with squamous-cell carcinoma and 39 with adenocarcinoma of the sinonasal cavities were exa-mined separately. An odds ratio (adjusted for exposure to wood dust) of 2.3 (95% CI, 0.9–5.8) for squamous-cell carcinoma was found for 13 cases who had ever been exposed to formaldehyde; of these, four had not been exposed to wood dust, which gave an odds ratio of 2.0 (95% CI, 0.7–5.9). Introduction of a 10-year lag period into the analysis yielded odds ratios of 2.4 (95% CI, 0.8–7.4) and 1.4 (95% CI, 0.3–6.4), respectively. The analysis revealed an association between exposure to wood dust and adenocarcinoma (odds ratios for any exposure, 16.3; 95% CI, 5.2–50.9) but only a weak association with squamous-cell carcinoma (odds ratio, 1.3; 95% CI, 0.5–3.6). For the 17 cases of adenocarcinoma in men who had ever been exposed to formaldehyde, the odds ratio, after adjustment for exposure to wood dust, was 2.2 (95% CI, 0.7–7.2), and that among men who had been exposed 10 or more years before diagnosis was 1.8 (95% CI, 0.5–6.0); however, only one man who had an adenocarcinoma had been exposed to formaldehyde alone. [The Working Group noted a concern that possibly incomplete adjustment for confounding from exposure to wood dust in the assessment of the risk for adenocarcinoma could explain the weak association observed with exposure to formaldehyde, but also noted that the assessment of risk for squamous-cell carcinoma was unlikely to have been affected because squamous-cell carci-noma was not clearly associated with exposure to wood dust.]

From an examination of medical records in the six major institutions in the Netherlands for surgical and radiographic treatment of tumours of the head and neck, Hayes et al. (1986a) identified 116 men, aged 35–79 years, in whom a histologically confirmed epithelial cancer of the nasal cavity or paranasal sinuses had been diagnosed during 1978–81. The cases were frequency-matched on age with 259 population controls who were chosen randomly from among living male residents of the Netherlands in 1982 (in a ratio of 2:1 for all patients) and from among deceased men in 1980 (in an approximate ratio of 1:1 for dead cases). Detailed histories, including information on exposure to a selected list of substances in the workplace and subjects' tobacco smoking habits, were obtained by personal interview of study subjects or their next of kin, with a participation of 78% for 91 case patients and 75% for 195 controls. Independently of one another, two industrial hygienists (A and B) reviewed job histories and graded possible exposure to formaldehyde. Exposure to wood dust was assessed similarly by one hygienist. At least some potential occupational exposure to formaldehyde was considered to have occurred for 23% of all study subjects by assess-ment A and for 44% by assessment B; among 224 subjects with little or no exposure to wood dust, exposure to formaldehyde was considered by assessments A and B to have occurred in 15 and 30%, respectively. For 62 subjects who were classed as having moderate or high exposure to wood dust, there was a weak association with exposure to formaldehyde as assessed by hygienist A (odds ratio, 1.9 [95% CI, 0.6–6.5]), but no odds ratio could be derived for exposure as assessed by hygienist B. For the 224 subjects who had little or no exposure to wood dust, the odds ratios for exposure to formaldehyde were 2.5 [95% CI, 1.0–5.9] (hygienist A) and 1.6 [95% CI, 0.8–3.1] (hygienist B). When the analysis was restricted to 45 cases of squamous-cell carcinoma of the paranasal sinuses who had little or no exposure to wood dust, the odds ratios for high exposure to formaldehyde were 3.1 [95% CI, 0.7–13.5] (hygienist A) and 2.4 [95% CI, 0.9–6.1] (hygienist B). [The Working Group noted that a greater proportion of case patients than controls were deceased (36% versus 14%) and variable numbers of next of kin were interviewed; furthermore, 10% of controls but none of the case patients were interviewed by telephone. The Group noted, however, that, although assessments A and B differed, both gave positive results.]

Vaughan *et al.* (1986a) conducted a population-based case–control study in a 13-county area in western Washington State, USA. The study included incident cases of sino-nasal and pharyngeal cancer that were identified from a cancer registry that was reported to identify 98–99% of the cancers in the study area. Cases eligible for study were between the ages of 20 and 74 years and had a date of diagnosis between 1979 and 1983 for sino-nasal cancer, and from 1980 to 1983 for pharyngeal cancer. Control subjects were identified by random-digit dialling and were frequency-matched to be similar in age and sex as the cases. Medical, tobacco smoking, alcohol use, residential and occupational histories were collected in a telephone interview with study subjects or their next of kin. Of the 415 cases eligible for study, 59 could not be located or were deceased with no known next of kin and 61 were not interviewed due to physician or subject refusal. Of the 295 cases who were successfully interviewed, 10 did not meet the eligibility requirements of the study, resulting in 285 cases being included in the analysis (53 sinonasal, 27 nasopharyngeal and 205 oro- or hypopharyngeal cancers). Approximately half of the case interviews were with their next of kin. Of a total of 690 persons eligible as controls, 573 were interviewed; 21 of these were excluded because they did not meet the eligibility requirements of the study, which resulted in 552 controls being available for analysis. [Although not explicitly stated, it appears that none of the interviews of the controls were by proxy.] Occupational exposure to formaldehyde was assessed by means of a job–exposure linkage system in which each job within each industry was classified according to the likelihood of exposure (unlikely, possible or probable). Those jobs that were defined as probably exposed were further classified into high or low exposure intensity. These two measures of exposure were then combined into a summary variable that resulted in the following four levels: (1) high (probable exposure to high levels), (2) medium (probable exposure to low levels), (3) low (possible exposure at any level) and (4) background. For the analysis, an estimate of the duration of exposure and the maximum exposure level (low, medium or high) reached in any job was developed for each individual. A cumulative exposure score was also developed by combining the information on duration and level of exposure. Unconditional logistic regression was used for the analysis in which age, sex and other potential confounders were controlled for when necessary. The odds ratios for sinonasal cancer,

adjusted for sex, age, cigarette smoking and alcohol consumption, decreased with increasing exposure by all of the measures. The odds ratios observed were: 0.8 (95% CI, 0.4–1.7)
for low and 0.3 (95% CI, 0.0–1.3) for medium or high maximum exposure level attained;
0.7 (95% CI, 0.3–1.4) for 1–9 years and 0.4 (95% CI, 0.1–1.9) for ≥ 10 years of exposure;
and 0.5 (95% CI, 0.1–1.6) for 5–19 and 0.3 (95% CI, 0.0–2.3) for ≥ 20 units of the exposure
score. [The number of exposed cases could not be determined for these analyses.] An analysis was also performed in which the exposure score was estimated at 16 years before the
date of diagnosis for the case and 16 years before the date of interview for the controls (i.e.
lagged by 16 years). Lagging the exposures in this way resulted in no cases in the high
exposure group, and did not produce interpretable findings. [The Working Group noted that
the different proportions of interviews conducted with next of kin of cases and controls
may have affected the odds ratios.]

Vaughan *et al.* (1986b) also explored the relationships between these types of tumour
and residential exposure to formaldehyde. Living in a mobile home and the presence of
urea–formaldehyde foam insulation, particle-board or plywood in residences were taken as
indirect measures of residential exposure. Five of the patients with sinonasal cancer had
lived in a mobile home (odds ratio, 0.6; 95% CI, 0.2–1.7), all for fewer than 10 years; 25
had lived in residences constructed with particle-board or plywood, which yielded odds
ratios of 1.8 (95% CI, 0.9–3.8) for periods of < 10 years and 1.5 (95% CI, 0.7–3.2) for
≥ 10 years. The risks associated with exposure to formaldehyde foam insulation could not
be estimated, because of low exposure frequencies.

Roush *et al.* (1987) reported on a population-based case–control study of 371 men registered at the Connecticut (USA) Tumor Registry with a diagnosis of sinonasal cancer (198
cases) or nasopharyngeal cancer (173 cases), who had died of any cause in Connecticut in
1935–75, and 605 male controls who had died during the same period and were selected
randomly from the files of Connecticut death certificates, without stratification or matching.
Information on the occupations of the study subjects was derived from death certificates and
from annual city directories; the latter were consulted 1, 10, 20, 25, 30, 40 and 50 years
before death, when available. Odds ratios for occupation–cancer relationships based on
occupational information obtained from death certificates were similar to the corresponding
odds ratios based on city directory information in two previous studies. Each occupation
held by case patients and controls was assessed by an industrial hygienist (blinded to
case–control status) with regard to the likelihood (none, possibly, probably, definitely) and
level (0, < 1 ppm, ≥ 1 ppm) of workplace exposure to formaldehyde, and study subjects were
subsequently categorized into one unexposed and four exposed groups according to degrees
of probable exposure to formaldehyde. For sinonasal cancer, the odds ratio, adjusted for age
at death, year of death and number of jobs reported, was 0.8 (95% CI, 0.5–1.3) for those who
had probably been exposed to some level of formaldehyde for most of their working life
compared with all others. In order to evaluate high short-term exposures, the odds ratio for
those who fulfilled the more restricted exposure criteria of being probably exposed to some
level for most of their working life and probably exposed to high levels for some years was
1.0 (95% CI, 0.5–2.2) and, for those who had probably been exposed to some level for most

of their working life and probably exposed to high levels at some point 20 or more years before death, the odds ratio was 1.5 (95% CI, 0.6–3.9).

Luce *et al.* (1993) conducted a case–control study of men and women who had primary malignancies of the nasal cavities and paranasal sinuses and were diagnosed in one of 27 hospitals in France between January 1986 and February 1988. Three hundred and three cases were identified; 57 had died and, of the remaining 246 cases, 32 could not be located or were too ill and seven refused to participate. Histological confirmation was available in the medical records of all but one of the remaining 207 case patients. Four hundred and forty-three control subjects were selected by frequency matching for age and sex among patients in whom another cancer had been diagnosed during the same period at the same or a nearby hospital (340 subjects) or from a list of names of healthy individuals provided by the cases (103 subjects). Sixteen could not be located or were too ill and 18 declined to participate, which left 409 controls for analysis. Occupational exposures to formaldehyde and 14 other substances or groups of substances were assessed by an industrial hygienist on the basis of information that was obtained during a personal interview at the hospital (for the cancer patients) or at home (for the healthy controls) on job histories, a number of pre-defined occupational exposures, socioeconomic variables and tobacco smoking habits. Study subjects were classified according to the likelihood of exposure to each of the suspected determinants of sinonasal cancer and were grouped into one of four categories: none, possible, probable or definite exposure; the latter two were further split into a number of subgroups according to three levels and calendar periods of exposure and combinations thereof. For formaldehyde, a cumulative index was calculated from the levels and duration of exposure, as well as lifetime occupational exposure. Among men, 36% of the controls and 55% of the cases were classified as potentially exposed to formaldehyde. The risks associated with exposure to formaldehyde were reported for men only. For the 59 cases who had squamous-cell carcinoma, odds ratios (adjusted for age and exposure to wood and glue) were 1.26 (95% CI, 0.54–2.94) and 0.68 (95% CI, 0.27–1.75) for the index categories of lower and higher cumulative exposure among the probable/definite exposure group. Similar patterns were evident by lifetime average level and duration of exposure. Among the 82 cases of adenocarcinoma, 67 were in the probable/definite exposure group. Odds ratios (adjusted for age and exposure to wood and glue) categorized into three levels of the cumulative exposure index were 1.13 (95% CI, 0.19–6.90), 2.66 (95% CI, 0.38–18.70) and 6.91 (95% CI, 1.69–28.23), respectively. However, most (71/82) of the formaldehyde-exposed cases of adenocarcinoma had also been exposed to wood dust, and the odds ratio for being exposed to wood dust and formaldehyde versus neither was very large (odds ratio, 692; 95% CI, 91.9–5210). Only four cases of adenocarcinoma were classified as exposed to formaldehyde but not wood dust (odds ratio, 8.1; 95% CI, 0.9–72.9). [The Working Group noted that residual confounding by exposure to wood dust may have occurred.]

2.2.2   *Nasopharyngeal carcinoma*

The study design of and results from case–control studies of the association of expo-sure to formaldehyde with cancer of the nasopharynx are summarized in Table 18.

The study by Olsen *et al.* (1984) (described in detail in Section 2.2.1) also evaluated the risk of exposure to formaldehyde among 266 men and women who had been diagnosed with nasopharyngeal cancer. The odds ratio, unadjusted for other occupational exposures, for exposure to formaldehyde was 0.7 (95% CI, 0.3–1.7) for men and 2.6 (95% CI, 0.3–21.9) for women.

The association between nasopharyngeal carcinoma and exposure to formaldehyde was also examined in the population-based case–control study in 13 counties of Washington State conducted by Vaughan *et al.* (1986a,b) (described in Section 2.2.1). The odds ratios increased slightly with all of the measures of occupational exposure examined in this study. The observed odds ratios in the analysis of the maximum exposure level achieved were: 1.2 (seven exposed cases; 95% CI, 0.5–3.3) for low exposure and 1.4 (four exposed cases; 95% CI, 0.4–4.7) for medium or high exposures; 1.2 (eight exposed cases; 95% CI, 0.5–3.1) for 1–9 years and 1.6 (three exposed cases; 95% CI, 0.4–5.8) for ≥ 10 years of exposure; and 0.9 (three exposed cases; 95% CI, 0.2–3.2) for 5–19 units and 2.1 (three exposed cases; 95% CI, 0.6–7.8) for ≥ 20 units of the cumulative exposure score. When a lag period of 15 years or more was introduced into the analysis, the odds ratio associated with the highest cumu-lative exposure score to formaldehyde was unchanged (two exposed cases; odds ratio, 2.1; 95% CI, 0.4–10). An association was found between living in a mobile home and risk for nasopharyngeal cancer, with odds ratios of 2.1 (four exposed cases; 95% CI, 0.7–6.6) for < 10 years and 5.5 (four exposed cases; 95% CI, 1.6–19.4) for ≥ 10 years of residence. An analysis was performed that considered the joint effect of occupational exposure and residence in a mobile home. Subjects were considered to be occupationally exposed in this analysis if they had a cumulative exposure score of 5 or more. A relatively strong association was observed among individuals who were exposed occupationally and had ever lived in a mobile home compared with those who had neither exposure (odds ratio, 6.7; 95% CI, 1.2–38.9), although this finding was based on only two cases and seven controls with joint exposure.

In the study by Roush *et al.* (1987) (described in Section 2.2.1), the odds ratios for men with nasopharyngeal cancer were presented in the following categories: those who had probably been exposed to some level for most of their working life; those who had probably been exposed to some level for most of their working life and probably been exposed to high levels for some years; and those who had probably been exposed to some level for most of their working life and probably been exposed to high levels at some point 20 or more years before death. The odds ratios were, respectively, 1.0 (95% CI, 0.6–1.7), 1.4 (95% CI, 0.6–3.1) and 2.3 (95% CI, 0.9–6.0).

The etiology of nasopharyngeal carcinoma was studied in the Philippines; both viral (Hildesheim *et al.*, 1992) and non-viral (West *et al.*, 1993) risk factors were addressed. West *et al.* (1993) conducted a case–control study of 104 histologically confirmed cases of nasopharyngeal carcinoma in Rizal Province, where the incidence rates of this tumour (4.7/100 000 men and 2.6/100 000 women) were intermediate between those in China and those in western countries. The cases (100% response rate) were identified at the Philippines General Hospital, as were 104 hospital controls (100% response rate), who were matched to cases on sex, age and type of hospital ward; 101 community controls (77% response rate), who were matched on sex, age and neighbourhood, were also available. Hospital controls were selected from the rosters of patients who were present on the same day that a suspected case was confirmed by biopsy; patients who had disorders that were possibly linked to dietary patterns were excluded (gastrointestinal cancer, peptic ulcer, chronic cirrhosis, gallbladder disease). Community controls were asked to participate on the basis of their living in a house close to that of their matched case. A personal interview included questions on tobacco smoking and areca nut habits, diet, sociodemographic variables and occupational history. An industrial hygienist classified each job held by the study subjects as likely or unlikely to involve exposure to formaldehyde, solvents, exhaust fumes, wood dust, dust in general and pesticides, and combined the classification with information on period and duration of employment in such occupations. Since the findings on occupational exposures did not differ when hospital and community controls were considered separately, only results from the comparison of cases versus all controls are shown. Four exposure indices were established for each subject: total duration, duration lagged by 10 years, number of years since first exposure and age at first exposure. The risk for nasopharyngeal carcinoma was associated with exposure to formaldehyde; the odds ratios, adjusted for the effects of dusts and exhaust fumes and other suspected risk factors, were 1.2 (12 exposed cases; 95% CI, 0.41–3.6) for subjects who were first exposed < 25 years before diagnosis and 4.0 (14 exposed cases; 95% CI, 1.3–12.3) for those who were first exposed ≥ 25 years before diagnosis. In the subgroup of subjects who were first exposed to formaldehyde ≥ 25 years before diagnosis and first exposed to dust and/or exhaust fumes ≥ 35 years before diagnosis, an odds ratio of 15.7 (95% CI, 2.7–91.2) was found relative to people who were not exposed to either factor [numbers exposed not given]. The odds ratio for an overall exposure of ≥ 15 years (eight exposed cases; odds ratio, 1.2; 95% CI, 0.48–3.2) was lower than that for a duration of < 15 years (19 exposed cases; odds ratio, 2.7; 95% CI, 1.1–6.6). However, when exposure was lagged by 10 years, those exposed for ≥ 15 years showed an odds ratio of 2.1 (eight exposed cases; 95% CI, 0.70–6.2). Subjects who were first exposed before the age of 25 years had an odds ratio of 2.7 (16 exposed cases; 95% CI, 1.1–6.6), while the odds ratio for those who were first exposed at age 25 or more years was 1.2 (11 exposed cases; 95% CI, 0.47–3.3). Subjects who reported daily use of anti-mosquito coils had a 5.9-fold (95% CI, 1.7–20.1) increase in risk compared with those who reported never using coils in a model that adjusted for potential confounders (West *et al.*, 1993). [The Working Group noted that formaldehyde has been reported to occur in the smoke released from anti-mosquito coils (see Section 1), and that the authors did not control for the presence of Epstein-Barr viral (EBV) antibodies, which showed a strong association with nasopharyngeal cancer (odds ratio, 21) in the study of Hildesheim *et al.* (1992).]

A study from Malaysia investigated nasopharyngeal cancer based on cases that were ascertained through records of histologically confirmed diagnoses at four centres that had a radiotherapy unit (Armstrong *et al.*, 2000). In total, 530 Chinese cases of squamous-cell carcinomas of the nasopharynx who had resided in the study area for at least 5 years were diagnosed between 1 January 1987 and 30 June 1992. Among these, only 282 (53%) were included in the study (69% men), since 121 (23%) had died, 63 (12%) could not be located, four (1%) were too ill to participate and 60 (11%) refused to participate. One control with no history of cancer of the head, neck or the respiratory system was selected from the Chinese population who had resided for at least 5 years in the study area and matched to each case by sex and age (within 3 years). Information on exposures (complete residential and occupational history, alcohol and tobacco use and consumption of 55 food items at age 10 and 5 years before diagnosis) of cases and controls was obtained by structured in-home interviews by trained interviewers. Occupational history included job description, work performed, calendar time, machines, tools and substances used, size and type of workplace, and exposure to dusts, smoke, gases and chemicals. [It appears that additional questionnaires that collected more detailed information on some jobs were also used.] Exposure to 22 agents, which were selected for their ability to deposit on or be absorbed into the nasopharynx, was identified by job, calendar years, frequency (days per week) and duration (hours per day). Jobs were coded using the official Malaysian classification scheme. Four levels of exposure (none, low, medium and high) were established. [It was not clear whether the exposure assessment was made using a job–exposure matrix approach or on an individual level, because both approaches are referenced.] Dermal exposure was considered. The proportion of study participants with exposure to formaldehyde was 9.9% of cases and 8.2% of controls. For any versus no occupational exposure to formaldehyde, the odds ratio for both sexes combined was 1.24 (95% CI, 0.67–2.32) and 0.71 (95% CI, 0.34–1.43) after adjustment for diet and tobacco use. No dose–response relationship appeared with increasing duration of formaldehyde exposure.

In a multicentred, population-based case–control study from five cancer registries in the USA, associations between occupational exposure to formaldehyde and wood dust and nasopharyngeal cancer were investigated (Vaughan *et al.*, 2000). At four of the five registries, the investigators identified cases diagnosed between 1 April 1987 and 30 June 1991, while case ascertainment at the fifth registry was extended for an additional 2 years. Eligible cases were men and women aged 18–74 years who had any histological type of nasopharyngeal cancer. Interviews were completed for 231 of the 294 eligible cases identified, and included 44 (19%) that were conducted with the next of kin (usually the spouse). The 196 cases who had epithelial cancers were further classified into three histological subgroups: differentiated squamous-cell (118 cases), undifferentiated or non-keratinizing (54 cases) or epithelial not otherwise specified (24 cases). Controls were identified by random-digit dialling and were frequency-matched by age (5-year age groups), sex and cancer registry. Among 324 eligible controls, 246 were interviewed (76%), two of whom were excluded because they had no telephone, which left 244 controls for analysis; for three controls, the interview was conducted with the next of kin. Experienced interviewers from each of the five cancer registries conducted structured telephone interviews with the study subjects, which included questions on demographic background, previous medical conditions and use of medication, family history of cancer, use of alcohol and tobacco, and a lifetime history of occupational and chemical exposures, including those to formaldehyde and wood dust. For each job that had been held for at least 6 months, information was collected on job title, typical activities within the job, the type of industry and the dates at which employment began and ended. Industrial hygienists blindly assessed exposure to formaldehyde and wood dust on a job-by-job basis for each subject, based on all the available information. For each job held, both the probability (none or unlikely, possible, probable, definite) of exposure to formaldehyde and a related estimated concentration of exposure to formaldehyde (low, moderate, high) which represented an 8-h TWA were assigned. Cut-off points for analyses by duration and cumulative exposure were based on the 50th and 75th percentiles among exposed controls. The proportion of subjects who were potentially exposed to formaldehyde was 40.3% of cases compared with 32.4% of controls. For persons who were ever exposed occupationally to formaldehyde versus those who were unexposed, the odds ratio adjusted for age, sex, race, cancer registry, cigarette use, next-of-kin status and education for all epithelial nasopharyngeal cancer was 1.3 (95% CI, 0.8–2.1); for the histological subcategories of undifferentiated and non-keratinizing, differentiated squamous-cell and epithelial not otherwise specified, the odds ratios were 0.9 (95% CI, 0.4–2.0), 1.5 (95% CI, 0.8–2.7) and 3.1 (95% CI, 1.0–9.6), respectively. There was no consistent pattern of association or trend in risk with estimated maximum exposure concentration for all histological types combined. A trend of increasing risk was seen with increasing duration of exposure (p_{trend} = 0.07). The odds ratio for persons who had worked at least 18 years in jobs with potential exposure was 2.1 (95% CI, 1.0–4.5). Further analyses were conducted that excluded cancers of undifferentiated and non-keratinizing histology. The adjusted odds ratio by estimated probability of exposure to formaldehyde was 1.6 (95% CI, 1.0–2.8) for ever having held a job classified as 'possible, probable or definite', 2.1 (95% CI, 1.1–4.2) for 'probable or definite' and 13.3 (95% CI, 2.5–70) for 'definite'. Within the group classified with 'possible, probable or definite' exposure to formaldehyde, the subgroups with duration of exposure of 1–5 years, 6–17 years and over 18 years had odds ratios of 0.9 (95% CI, 0.4–2.1), 1.9 (95% CI, 0.9–4.4) and 2.7 (95% CI, 1.2–6.0), respectively, and the p_{trend} value for a dose–response relationship was 0.014. A similar dose–response pattern within this group was seen for estimated cumulative exposure (p_{trend} = 0.033). When the group was restricted to subjects with probable or definite exposure, the significance of trends lessened with respect to duration of exposure (p = 0.069) and cumulative exposure (p = 0.13). When a 10-year lag period was included, the overall findings remained similar. Moreover, the odds ratios for exposure to formaldehyde were essentially unaffected by adding exposure to wood dust to the models.

Hildesheim *et al.* (2001) investigated the associations between occupational exposure to formaldehyde, wood dust and organic solvents and risk for nasopharyngeal cancer. Incident cases (< 75 years) with histologically confirmed diagnoses were identified from two hospitals in Taipei, China (Province of Taiwan). Of 378 eligible cases that were identified,

375 agreed to participate in the study. About one third (31%) of the cases were women. One control with no history of nasopharyngeal cancer was matched to each case with respect to age (5 years), sex and district of residence. In total, 87% of eligible controls agreed to participate, which left 325 controls for the analysis. All study participants were interviewed by trained interviewers (nurses). Cases were interviewed at the time of biopsy and before treatment. The interviews obtained information on sociodemographic characteristics, diet, cigarette smoking and betel-quid chewing, residential and medical history and a complete occupational history for all jobs that had been held for at least 1 year since the age of 16 years. Living mothers were interviewed about the childhood diet of study participants. Data on occupational history were reviewed blindly by an industrial hygienist. Standard industrial and occupational classification codes were assigned to each job. Each code was assigned a classification (10 levels) for probability and intensity of exposure to formaldehyde, wood dust and organic solvents. In total, 156 of 2034 jobs (7.7%) were classified as entailing exposure to formaldehyde. Blood specimens were collected from 369 cases and 320 controls, and serum was tested for various antibodies against EBV, which is known to be associated with nasopharyngeal cancer. After adjustment for age, sex, education and ethnicity, the odds ratio (both sexes combined) for ever exposure to formaldehyde was 1.4 (95% CI, 0.93–2.2). The odds ratios for ≤ 10 years and > 10 years of exposure to formaldehyde were 1.3 (95% CI, 0.69–2.3) and 1.6 (95% CI, 0.91–2.9), respectively. Those exposed for > 20 years had an odds ratio of 1.7 (95% CI, 0.77–3.5), but the trend for ≤ 10, 10–20, and > 20 years of exposure did not reach statistical significance. The odds ratios by estimated cumulative exposure (intensity × duration) gave a similar pattern. The observed associations were not substantially affected by additional adjustment for exposure to wood dust or organic solvent. In the sub-analyses that were restricted to 360 cases and 94 controls who were seropositive for at least one of five antibodies against EBV, the association between exposure to formaldehyde and nasopharyngeal cancer appeared to be stronger to some extent. Thus, the odds ratio of ever versus never having been exposed was 2.7 (95% CI, 1.2–6.2). However, no clear dose–response pattern was observed with increasing duration of exposure or estimated cumulative exposure.

2.2.3   *Cancers of the oro- and hypopharynx*

The study design of and results from case–control studies of the association of exposure to formaldehyde with cancer of the oro- and hypopharynx are summarized in Table 18.

The association between oro- and hypopharyngeal cancer and exposure to formaldehyde was examined in the population-based case–control study by Vaughan *et al.* (1986a,b) (described in detail in Section 2.2.1). Evidence for a weak trend in the odds ratios was observed with the number of years of occupational exposure to formaldehyde (odds ratio, 0.6; 95% CI, 0.3–1.0 for 1–9 years; odds ratio, 1.3; 95% CI, 0.7–2.5 for ≥ 10 years) and the exposure score (odds ratio, 0.6; 95% CI, 0.3–1.2 for 5–19 units; odds ratio, 1.5; 95% CI, 0.7–3.0 for ≥ 20 units), but not with the maximum exposure level attained (odds ratio, 0.8; 95% CI, 0.5–1.4 for low; odds ratio, 0.8; 95% CI, 0.4–1.7 for medium; odds ratio, 0.6; 95% CI, 0.1–2.7 for high). No association was observed between risk for oro- and hypopharyngeal cancer and living in a mobile home (odds ratio, 0.9; 95% CI, 0.5–1.8 for 1–9 years; odds ratio, 0.8; 95% CI, 0.2–2.7 for ≥ 10 years), or duration of living in residences with internal construction or renovation using particle-board or plywood (odds ratio, 1.1; 95% CI, 0.7–1.9 for 1–9 years; odds ratio, 0.8; 95% CI, 0.5–1.4 for ≥ 10 years).

Gustavsson *et al.* (1998) carried out a case–control study of histologically verified squamous-cell carcinoma of the oral cavity, pharynx, larynx and oesophagus among men aged 40–79 years who were born in Sweden and were resident in two regions of the country. Between 1 January 1988 and 31 January 1991, the investigators sought to identify all incident cases of these tumours in the study population through weekly reports from departments of otorhinolaryngology, oncology and surgery, supplemented by information from regional cancer registries. Cases identified incidentally at autopsy were excluded. The referents were selected by stratified random sampling from population registers, and were frequency-matched to the cases for region and age in 10- or 15-year age groups. All subjects were interviewed by one of two nurses (the cases were mostly interviewed in hospital and the referents mainly at home), who used a structured questionnaire to obtain information on smoking, oral snuff use, alcohol consumption and lifetime history of jobs held for > 1 year. The work histories were reviewed by an occupational hygienist who was blind to the case or referent status of the subject, and were coded for intensity and probability of exposure to 17 agents, including formaldehyde; 9.4% of the referents were classed as exposed. An index of cumulative exposure was derived from the product of the probability, intensity and duration of exposure across the entire work history. Exposure histories were available for 90% of the 605 cases identified (including 138 who had pharyngeal cancer) and for 85% of the 756 referents. [The exact number of cases of pharyngeal cancer included in study was not reported.] Unconditional logistic regression was used to estimate incidence rate ratios adjusted for region, age (in 10- or 15-year bands), average alcohol intake over the past 5 years (four levels) and smoking status (current, former or never). The incidence rate ratio for pharyngeal cancer and formaldehyde was 1.01 (95% CI, 0.49–2.07) based on 13 exposed cases.

A case–control study of incident male cases of hypopharyngeal and laryngeal squamous-cell cancers was conducted at 15 hospitals in France between 1 January 1989 and 30 April 1991 (Laforest *et al.*, 2000). Initially, 664 such patients were identified, but 21% of cases from the combined group were excluded due to health problems, death before interview, refusal, being non-alcohol drinkers or because they could not be contacted, which left 201 cases of hypopharyngeal cancer for analysis. Potential controls were male patients with primary cancers at other sites who were selected from the same or nearby hospitals as the cases, were recruited between 1987 and 1991 and were frequency-matched to the cases by age. Of the 355 controls who were initially identified, 59 [17%] were excluded for similar reasons as the cases. Specially trained occupational physicians interviewed the study subjects on demographic characteristics, alcohol consumption, use of tobacco and lifetime occupational history. Each job was coded with respect to occupation and industry, and occupational exposures, including formaldehyde, were assessed using a previously developed job–exposure matrix to estimate the probability and level of exposure. An index of cumulative exposure was derived for each subject based on the product of probability, level and duration of exposure in each job. Altogether, [29%] of controls and [41%] of the cases of hypopharyngeal cancer were classified as ever having been exposed to formaldehyde. The age-, asbestos-, coal dust-, alcohol- and smoking-adjusted odds ratio for ever versus never exposure to formaldehyde was 1.35 (95% CI, 0.86–2.14). There was a trend of increasing odds ratios with increasing probability of exposure to formaldehyde (p_{trend} < 0.005); a probability of exposure of over 50% showed an odds ratio of 3.78 (95% CI, 1.50–9.49). No significant trends were noted by duration of exposure or estimated cumulative exposure. After exclusion of study subjects who had a probability of exposure to formaldehyde of less than 10%, the odds ratio increased with duration of exposure (p_{trend} < 0.04) and with cumulative level of exposure (p_{trend} < 0.14). [The Working Group noted that the controls were interviewed at a later date than cases and did not necessarily come from the same hospital, and that interviewers were not blind to the case–control status, although they were not aware of the study hypotheses.]

A case–control study of incident laryngeal and hypopharyngeal cancer was conducted during 1979–82 in six centres in four European countries (Berrino *et al.*, 2003). An attempt was made to include all incident cases from the centres, and 304 cases of hypopharyngeal cancer (including the epilarynx) were included. The participation rate varied by centre from 70 to 92%. Initially, the purpose of the study was to investigate the association between alcohol consumption, use of tobacco and diet and cancer at the two sites. An age- and sex-stratified random sample of controls was selected from the general population from each centre with an average participation rate of 74%. Information on alcohol consumption, tobacco smoking, diet and all jobs held for at least 1 year after 1944 was obtained by in-person interviews at the hospital before the treatment of cases; controls were interviewed at home. A panel of occupational physicians, industrial hygienists and chemical engineers assessed blindly the probability of exposure to 16 industrial chemicals, including formaldehyde. Among persons younger than 55 years [for whom a lifelong complete job history was available], the odds ratio for hypopharyngeal cancer (100 cases) adjusted for age, centre, tobacco use, alcohol consumption, socioeconomic status, diet and exposure to potential chemical confounders was 1.3 (95% CI, 0.6–2.6) in the group that was possibly exposed versus those who were never exposed and 0.5 (95% CI, 0.1–1.8) in the group that was probably and certainly exposed versus those who were never exposed to formaldehyde. [It is unclear whether controls were all from the catchment populations of the hospitals at which the cases were diagnosed. In research outside this study to evaluate the job–exposure matrix used, it was found that its performance for formaldehyde was poor. Any resultant misclassification of exposures would be expected to bias risk estimates towards unity.]

2.2.4   *Cancers of the lung and larynx*

The study design of and results from case–control studies of the association of cancers of the lung and larynx with exposure to formaldehyde are summarized in Table 19.

Andersen *et al.* (1982) conducted a case–control study in Denmark of doctors (79 men and five women) for whom a notification of lung cancer had been made in the files of the nationwide Danish Cancer Registry during the period 1943–77. Three control subjects per case, matched individually on sex and age, were selected at random from among individuals on official lists of Danish doctors. Information on postgraduate specialization and places of work during the professional career of cases and controls was obtained from medical directories and supplementary files at the Danish Medical Society. Potential exposure to formaldehyde was assumed to be associated with working in pathology, forensic medicine and anatomy. None of the doctors who had lung cancer had specialized in any of these fields, but one control doctor was a pathologist. Eight male case patients and 23 controls had been employed at some time in pathology, forensic medicine or anatomy, to give an odds ratio of 1.0 (95% CI, 0.4–2.4).

Fayerweather *et al.* (1983) reported on a case–control study of mortality from cancer among chemical workers in eight plants in the USA where formaldehyde was manufactured or used. A total of 493 active or pensioned men were known to have died from cancer during 1957–79, but 12 were excluded from the study because their work histories were unavailable. The remaining 481 men were individually matched on age, pay class, sex and date of first employment to 481 controls selected from among employees who had been on the company's active pay rolls during the last year of employment of the corresponding case. The cases included 181 lung cancers and eight laryngeal cancers. The work histories of both case and control subjects were ascertained principally from personnel records, but also from medical records and interviews with colleagues; a job–exposure matrix was used to classify jobs according to the nature and level of exposure to formaldehyde that they entailed into three categories: 'continuous-direct', 'intermittent' or 'background'. Smoking histories were obtained for about 90% of subjects, primarily by interviewing living co-workers. Of the 481 cases, 142 (30%) had had potential exposure to formaldehyde. The data were analysed by latency period, duration of exposure, exposure level and frequency, cumulative exposure index, age at and year of death and age at and year of first exposure. In none of the analyses was the relative risk for lung cancer significantly greater than 1.0 ($p > 0.05$). When a cancer induction period of 20 years was allowed for, 39 subjects with lung cancer and 39 controls had potentially been exposed to formaldehyde; the odds ratios were 1.20 [95% CI, 0.6–2.8] and 0.79 [95% CI, 0.4–1.6] for subgroups with < 5 years and ≥ 5 years of exposure, respectively.

In a population-based case–control study, Coggon *et al.* (1984) used death certificates to obtain information on the occupations of all men under the age of 40 years in England and Wales who had died from bronchial carcinoma during 1975–79. These were compared with controls who had died from any other cause, and who were matched for sex, year of death, local authority district of residence and date of birth (within 2 years). Of 598 cases

Table 19. Case–control studies of cancers of the lung and larynx

Reference, study location, years of study	Organ site (ICD code)	Characteristics of cases	Characteristics of controls	Exposure assessment	Exposure categories	Relative risk (95% CI)	Adjustment for potential confounders	Comments
Andersen et al. (1982), Denmark, 1943–77	Lung	84 doctors (79 men, five women) registered in Denmark who died of lung cancer	252 randomly selected from official list of Danish doctors, matched on sex and age	Information on postgraduate specialization and professional career employment	Ever employed in pathology, forensic medicine or anatomy	1.0 (0.4–2.4)		Both cases and controls were medical doctors.
Fayerweather et al. (1983), USA, 1957–79	Lung and larynx	Active or pensioned employees (all men) who died of cancer (181 lung, eight larynx)	189 employees matched on sex, age, pay class and date at first employment, selected from annual payroll roster among employees active during the case's last year of employment	Job–exposure matrix to classify exposure according to frequency and intensity (continuous/ direct, intermittent, background) based on personnel and medical records and interviews with colleagues	Lung <5 years ≥5 years	1.20 [0.6–2.8] 0.79 [0.4–1.6]	Tobacco smoking	Analysis included a latency period of 20 years between exposure and disease.
Coggon et al. (1984), United Kingdom, 1975–79	Lung (bronchial carcinoma)	598 men ≤ 40 years old who died of bronchial carcinoma in England and Wales	1180 men who had died from any other cause, matched by year of death, district of residence and date of birth (± 2 years)	Job–exposure matrix based on classification coding in three categories (none, low, high) of exposure	All exposed occupations Occupations with high exposure	1.5 (1.2–1.8) 0.9 (0.6–1.4)		$p < 0.001$

Table 19 (contd)

Reference, study location, years of study	Organ site (ICD code)	Characteristics of cases	Characteristics of controls	Exposure assessment	Exposure categories	Relative risk (95% CI)	Adjustment for potential confounders	Comments
Gérin et al. (1989), Canada, 1979–85	Lung (oat-cell carci-noma; squamous-cell carci-noma; adeno-carcinoma; others including unspecified)	857 men aged 35–70 years resident in the area of Montréal	1523 men with cancer at other sites (cancer controls) and 533 men selected from electoral list (population controls), stratified by age	Semi-structured questionnaire on lifetime work history; exposure profile developed based on proba-bility, frequency, concentration and duration of expo-sure and period of first exposure	Cancer controls Ever Short Long–low Long–medium Long–high Population controls Ever Short Long–low Long–medium Long–high	0.8 (0.6–1.0) 0.8 (0.6–1.2) 0.5 (0.3–0.8) 1.0 (0.7–1.4) 1.5 (0.8–2.8) 0.8 (0.6–1.1) 1.0 (0.6–1.8) 0.5 (0.3–0.8) 0.9 (0.5–1.6) 1.0 (0.4–2.4)	Age, ethnic group, socio-economic status, cigarette smoking, dirtiness of job and various other potential confounders	Increased relative risk for adeno-carcinoma of the lung with long exposure to high concentration
Wortley et al. (1992), United Kingdom, 1983–87	Larynx (ICD-0 161.0–161.9)	235 [sex distribution not given] identified through local cancer surveillance system	547 identified by random-digit dialling selected to be similar in age and same sex	In-person interview; job-exposure matrix based on both likelihood and degree of exposure	Peak Low Medium High Duration < 1 year 1–9 years ≥ 10 years Exposure scores < 5 5–19 ≥ 20	1.0 (0.6–1.7) 1.0 (0.4–2.1) 2.0 (0.2–19.5) 1.0 0.8 (0.4–1.3) 1.3 (0.6–3.1) 1.0 1.0 (0.5–2.0) 1.3 (0.5–3.3)	Age, tobacco smoking, alcohol drinking and education	
Brownson et al. (1993), USA, 1986–91	Lung	429 white women aged 30–84 years, former or never smokers	1021 women selected from state driver's licence files (< 65 years old) or health care roster (≥ 65 years old), group- matched for age	Telephone and in-person interview	Ever exposed	0.9 (0.2–3.3)	Age and history of previous lung disease	All exposed cases and controls were lifelong non-smokers.

Table 19 (contd)

Reference, study location, years of study	Organ site (ICD code)	Characteristics of cases	Characteristics of controls	Exposure assessment	Exposure categories	Relative risk (95% CI)	Adjustment for potential confounders	Comments
Gustavsson *et al.* (1998), Sweden, 1988–91	Larynx (ICD-9 161)	157 male incident cases aged 40–79 years	641 selected by stratified random sampling; frequency-matched to cases by age (10–15-year groups) and region	Work history reviewed by occupational hygienist; occupations coded by intensity and probability of exposure	Ever exposed	1.45 (0.83–2.51)	Region of incidence, age, alcohol intake and tobacco smoking status	
Laforest *et al.* (2000), France, 1989–91	Larynx (ICD code not given)	296 men with confirmed histology of cancer of the epi-larynx, glottis, supra-glottis, subglottis and larynx unspecified	296 men with other (selected) primary tumours selected from the same or nearby hospitals, recruited in 1987–91, matched by age	Structured in-person interviews; occupational exposures were assessed with a job-exposure matrix developed earlier	Ever exposed	1.14 (0.76–1.70)	Age, tobacco smoking, alcohol drinking and exposure to coal dust	
					Exposure probability			
					< 10%	1.16 (0.73–1.86)		
					10–50%	1.12 (0.55–2.30)		
					> 50%	1.04 (0.44–2.47)		
					Excluding subjects with exposure probability < 10%			
					Ever exposed	1.17 (0.63–2.17)		
					Duration of exposure			
					< 7 years	1.68 (0.60–4.72)		
					7–20 years	0.86 (0.33–2.24)		
					> 20 years	1.14 (0.47–2.74)		
					Cumulative exposure			
					Low	0.68 (0.12–3.90)		
					Medium	1.86 (0.76–4.55)		
					High	0.91 (0.42–1.99)		

Table 19 (contd)

Reference, study location, years of study	Organ site (ICD code)	Characteristics of cases	Characteristics of controls	Exposure assessment	Exposure categories	Relative risk (95% CI)	Adjustment for potential confounders	Comments
Berrino et al. (2003), France, Italy, Spain, Switzerland, 1979–82	Larynx (glottis, supraglottis)	213 male incident cases aged ≤ 55 years	819 men from general local population of each centre, stratified by age	Structured in-person interviews; occupational exposures assessed by an expert panel using a previously established job–exposure matrix	Probability of exposure Possible Probable or definite	1.4 (0.8–2.7) 1.0 (0.4–2.3)	Age, centre, tobacco use, alcohol drinking, diet, socioeconomic status, asbestos, PAHs, chromium, arsenic, wood dust, solvents, other dusts and gases	[The credibility of the negative finding is limited because formaldehyde was the agent for which the validity of the job–exposure matrix was lowest.]
Elci et al. (2003), Turkey, 1979–84	Larynx (ICD-0 161.0–2, –9)	940 male incident cases at Oncology Treatment Center	1519 male patients with malignant or benign pathology	Standardized questionnaire administered at hospital on occupational history; job–exposure matrix	Ever exposed Intensity Low Medium High Probability Low Medium High	1.0 (0.8–1.3) 1.1 (0.8–1.5) 0.5 (0.2–1.3) 0.7 (0.1–7.1) 1.0 (0.7–1.4) 1.1 (0.6–2.2) 1.0 (0.1–11.2)	Age, tobacco use and alcohol drinking	Analysis by subtype of cancer (glottis, supraglottis, other) did not show any elevation of risk. No trend with intensity or probability of exposure

CI, confidence interval; ICD, international code of diseases; PAHs, polycyclic aromatic hydrocarbons who were identified, 582 were matched with two controls and the remainder with one control. Occupations were coded according to the Office of Population Census and Surveys 1970 classification, and a job–exposure matrix was constructed by an occupational hygienist, in which the occupations were grouped according to three levels (high, low and none) of exposure to nine known or putative carcinogens, including formaldehyde. The group of occupations that were classed as entailing exposure to formaldehyde was associated with an elevated odds ratio for bronchial carcinoma of 1.5 (95% CI, 1.2–1.8); for those occupations in which exposure was presumed to be high, the odds ratio was 0.9 (95% CI, 0.6–1.4). [The Working Group noted that information on occupation from death certificates is limited; they also noted the young age of the subjects and the consequent short exposure and latency.]

In a population-based case–control study in the area of Montréal, Canada, 857 men who were diagnosed with histologically confirmed primary lung cancer during 1979–85 were identified (Gérin et al., 1989). Two groups of control subjects were established: one was composed of 1523 men who were diagnosed during the same years as cases with cancers of other organs (oesophagus, stomach, colorectum, liver, pancreas, prostate, bladder, kidney, melanoma and lymphoid tissue) and the other was composed of 533 men who were selected from electoral lists of the Montréal area. Interviews or completed questionnaires that yielded lifelong job history and information on potential non-occupational confounders were obtained from the cancer patients or their next of kin and from the population controls, with response rates of 82% and 72%, respectively. Each job was classified by a group of chemists and hygienists according to the probability, intensity and frequency of exposure to some 300 agents, including formaldehyde. Nearly one-quarter of all men had potentially been exposed to formaldehyde in at least one of the jobs they had held during their working life; however, only 3.7% were considered to be definitely exposed and only 0.2% were considered to have had high exposure, defined as more than 1.0 ppm [1.23 mg/m^3] formaldehyde in the ambient air. Odds ratios, adjusted for age, ethnic group, socioeconomic status, cigarette smoking, the 'dirtiness' of the jobs held and various other potentially confounding workplace exposures, were 0.8 (95% CI, 0.6–1.2) for < 10 years of exposure to formaldehyde, 0.5 (95% CI, 0.3–0.8) for ≥ 10 years of presumed exposure to < 0.1 ppm [0.12 mg/m^3], 1.0 (95% CI, 0.7–1.4) for ≥ 10 years of presumed exposure to 0.1–1.0 ppm [0.12–1.23 mg/m^3] and 1.5 (95% CI, 0.8–2.8) for ≥ 10 years of presumed exposure to > 1.0 ppm formaldehyde compared with controls with other cancers. In comparison with the population controls, the equivalent odds ratios were 1.0 (95% CI, 0.6–1.8), 0.5 (95% CI, 0.3–0.8), 0.9 (95% CI, 0.5–1.6) and 1.0 (95% CI, 0.4–2.4), respectively. Marginally increased risks were seen for subjects with the adenocarcinoma subtype of lung cancer who had had long exposure to a high concentration of formaldehyde, with odds ratios of 2.3 (95% CI, 0.9–6.0) and 2.2 (95% CI, 0.7–7.6) in comparison with the cancer and population control groups, respectively; however, the estimates were based on only seven exposed cases.

Wortley et al. (1992) studied 291 male and female residents aged 20–74 years of a 13-county area of western Washington, USA, in whom laryngeal cancer was diagnosed in

1983–87 and notified to a population-based cancer registry in the area; 81% were success-fully interviewed. Control subjects were identified by random-digit dialling and were selected when similar in age and of the same sex as cases; 80% of eligible subjects were interviewed, which left 547 for analysis. Lifetime histories of occupational, tobacco smoking and alcohol drinking were obtained by personal interview, and each job held for at least 6 months was coded according to the US census codes for industries and occu-pations. A job–exposure matrix was used to classify each job according to the probability and degree of exposure to formaldehyde and five other agents. Summary measures were derived for each subject's lifetime peak exposure, duration of exposure and a score based on both duration and level of exposure. The risk for laryngeal cancer, adjusted for age, smoking and drinking habits and length of education, was not associated with exposure to formaldehyde to a significant degree. The odds ratios were 1.0 (95% CI, 0.6–1.7) for patients with any 'low' exposure, 1.0 (95% CI, 0.4–2.1) for any 'medium' exposure and 2.0 (two exposed cases; 95% CI, 0.2–20) for any 'high' exposure. Odds ratios of 0.8 (95% CI, 0.4–1.3) and 1.3 (95% CI, 0.6–3.1) were seen for exposure for < 10 years and ≥ 10 years and of 1.0 (95% CI, 0.5–2.0) and 1.3 (95% CI, 0.5–3.3) for medium and high formaldehyde score, respectively. [The report suggests that the cases in fact came from only three of the 13 counties, whereas the controls came from the larger area. If this is the case, there may have been important potential for bias.]

A case–control study in Missouri, USA, focused on white women aged 30–84 years, who were lifelong nonsmokers or who had stopped smoking for at least 15 years (Brownson et al., 1993). Incident cases of lung cancer during 1986 to mid-1991 were identified through the local cancer registry; information for inclusion in the study was successfully obtained for 429 (69%) of the 650 eligible subjects. This was achieved through two series of interviews completed either by the subject (42%) or her next of kin, during which questions were asked on demographic characteristics, non-occupational risk factors and 28 occupational risk factors, including formaldehyde. For cases under the age of 65 years, controls were obtained from state drivers' licence files, while controls for older cases were selected from Medicare files, group-matched to the cases for age, with a ratio of approximately 2.2:1. Of 1527 potentially eligible controls, 1021 (73%) completed two interviews similar to those for the cases. Analysis was performed using multiple logistic regression. Three cases and 10 controls, all of whom were lifelong nonsmokers, reported occupational exposure to formaldehyde which, with adjustment for age and history of previous lung disease, gave an odds ratio of 0.9 (95% CI, 0.2–3.3).

A case–control study in Sweden of squamous-cell carcinoma of the upper airways and upper digestive tract (Gustavsson et al., 1998) (described in detail in Section 2.2.3) com-pared 157 men who had laryngeal cancer with 641 referents. After adjustment for region of incidence, age, average alcohol intake over the past 5 years and smoking status, the esti-mated incidence rate ratio for cancer of the larynx in men exposed to formaldehyde was 1.45 (95% CI, 0.83–2.51) based on 23 exposed cases. No dose–response trend was appa-rent for either cumulative exposure or duration of exposure.

A case–control study at 15 hospitals in France (Laforest *et al.*, 2000) (described in detail in Section 2.2.3) included 296 patients with laryngeal cancer. For this disease, comparison with the 296 controls gave an odds ratio (adjusted for age, alcohol consumption, smoking and exposure to coal dust) of 1.14 (95% CI, 0.76–1.70) for exposure to formaldehyde overall. No clear pattern of risk estimates was observed in relation to probability, duration or cumulative levels of exposure.

A case–control study by Berrino *et al.* (2003) at six centres in France, Italy, Spain and Switzerland (described in detail in Section 2.2.3) included 213 cases of laryngeal cancer who were under 55 years of age. No association was found with probable or definite exposure to formaldehyde at levels above the background for the general population (odds ratio, 1.0; 95% CI, 0.4–2.3).

A case–control study of laryngeal cancer in Turkey (Elci *et al.*, 2003) focused on patients who were admitted to the oncology centre of a hospital in Istanbul during 1979–84. Information on occupational history and consumption of alcohol and tobacco was elicited at the time of admission by a trained interviewer using a standardized questionnaire, and a job–exposure matrix was applied to the occupational history to assign probability and intensity of exposure to each of five substances including formaldehyde. After exclusion of women and patients with incomplete information on risk factors or tumour site, 940 of 958 cases were available for analysis (mean age, 52.9 years). These men were compared with 1308 controls who had various cancers that are not thought to have the same causes as carcinoma of the larynx and 211 who had benign pathologies. Analysis was performed using unconditional logistic regression with adjustment for age, use of tobacco (ever versus never) and consumption of alcohol (ever versus never). The odds ratio for any exposure to formaldehyde was 1.0 (95% CI, 0.8–1.3) based on 89 exposed cases. No significant elevation of risk was found for subsets of cases classified by anatomical location of the tumour (supraglottis, glottis, others), and there were no significant trends in risk by intensity or probability of exposure. [It is unclear how completely the occupational information in this study reflected lifetime histories of work.]

2.2.5   *Lymphohaematopoietic malignancies*

The study design of and results from the case–control studies of the association of lymphohaematopoietic malignancies and exposure to formaldehyde are summarized in Table 20.

In the study of Gérin *et al.* (1989) (described in detail in Section 2.2.4) in Montréal, Canada, levels of occupational exposure to formaldehyde of 53 cases of Hodgkin lymphoma and 206 cases of non-Hodgkin lymphoma were compared with those of 2599 cases of other cancers and 533 population controls. Using population controls and adjusting for age, ethnic group, self-reported income, tobacco smoking and dirtiness of jobs held, plus occupational and non-occupational factors that were identified as potential confounders, odds ratios for non-Hodgkin lymphoma were 0.7 (13 exposed cases; 95% CI, 0.3–1.6) for < 10 years of exposure compared with non-exposed and 1.1 (15 exposed cases; 95% CI,

Table 20. Case–control studies of lymphohaematopoietic malignancies

Reference, study location, years of study	Organ site (ICD code)	Characteristics of cases	Characteristics of controls	Exposure assessment	Exposure categories	Relative risk (95% CI)	Adjustment for potential confounders	Comments
Gérin et al. (1989), Canada, 1979–85	Hodgkin lymphoma	53 male incident cases	533 population-based	Lifetime job histories obtained by interview and translated into level of exposure to formaldehyde	Ever	0.5 (0.2–1.4)	Age, ethnic group, self-reported income, tobacco smoking, dirtiness of jobs held and potentially confounding occupational and non-occupational factors	Similar results were obtained when 2599 cases of other cancers were used as control group.
	Non-Hodgkin lymphoma	206 male incident cases			< 10 years duration	0.7 (0.3–1.6)		
					≥ 10 years duration			
					Low[a]	1.1 (0.5–2.2)		
					Medium[a]	1.0 (0.5–2.1)		
					High[a]	0.5 (0.1–1.7)		
Linos et al. (1990), USA (years of study not given)	Leukaemia	578 male incident cases	1245 population-based	Lifetime occupational history obtained	Ever employed in funeral home or crematorium	2.1 [0.4–10.0] based on four exposed cases	Adjusted for age and state of residence	Significantly elevated relative risks of 6.7 and 6.7 for acute myeloid leukaemia and follicular non-Hodgkin lymphoma, but based on small numbers
	Non-Hodgkin lymphoma	622 male incident cases				3.2 [0.8–13.4] based on six exposed cases		
Partanen et al. (1993), Finland, 1957–1982	Leukaemia	12 male cases diagnosed among a cohort of 7307 production workers in wood industry	79 randomly selected from cohort and matched by year of birth and vital status in 1983	Work history from company records complemented for cases only by interviews with plant personnel and questionnaires completed by subjects or next of kin; plant- and period-specific job–exposure matrix	< 3 ppm–months	1.00	Matching factors accounted for by conditional logistic regression	Data collection was more exhaustive for cases than for controls, which could have led to bias. Relative risk for all three outcomes combined did not substantially change when adjusted for wood dust or for solvents.
					≥ 3 ppm–months	1.40 (0.25–7.91) (two exposed cases)		
	Hodgkin disease	Four male cases	21		< 3 ppm–months	1.00		
					≥ 3 ppm–months	NA (one exposed case)		
	Non-Hodgkin lymphoma	Eight male cases	52		< 3 ppm–months	1.00		
					≥ 3 ppm–months	4.24 (0.68–26.6) (four exposed cases)		

Table 20 (contd)

Reference, study location, years of study	Organ site (ICD code)	Characteristics of cases	Characteristics of controls	Exposure assessment	Exposure categories	Relative risk (95% CI)	Adjustment for potential confounders	Comments
West et al. (1995), United Kingdom (years of study not given)	Myelo-dysplastic syndrome	400 (216 men, 184 women) newly diagnosed, resident in study area and aged > 15 years	400 cancer-free patients from out-patient clinics and inpatient wards; matched 1:1 by age (± 3 years), sex, area of residence and hospital and year of diagnosis (± 2 years)	Personal interview on work history and for duration and intensity of exposure to formaldehyde; all questionnaires reviewed by team of experts	> 10 h lifetime exposure of any intensity > 50 h lifetime exposure of medium or high intensity > 2500 h lifetime exposure of medium or high intensity	1.17 [0.51–2.68] 2.33 [0.55–11.35] 2.00 [0.32–15.67]	No adjustment for smoking or other factors	
Tatham et al. (1997), USA, 1984–88	Non-Hodgkin lymphoma and sub-groups	1048 men (185 small-cell diffuse lymphoma, 268 follicular lym-phoma and 526 large-cell diffuse lymphoma) from population-based cancer registries, born 1929–53	1659 selected by random-digit dialling, matched by area of registry and 5-year categories of date of birth	Telephone interview including questions on specific materials which participants may have worked with	Ever exposed All combined Small-cell diffuse Follicular Large-cell diffuse	1.20 (0.86–1.50) 1.40 (0.87–2.40) 0.71 (0.41–1.20) 1.10 (0.79–1.70)	Matching factors, age at diagnosis, year entered the study, ethnicity, education, Jewish religion, never having married, AIDS risk behaviours, use of seizure medication, service in or off the coast of Viet Nam and cigarette smoking	

Table 20 (contd)

Reference, study location, years of study	Organ site (ICD code)	Characteristics of cases	Characteristics of controls	Exposure assessment	Exposure categories	Relative risk (95% CI)	Adjustment for potential confounders	Comments
Blair et al. (2001), USA, 1980–83	Leukaemia and myelo-dysplasia	513 white men, 30 years or older, identified from the Cancer Registry of Iowa and among all men from a surveillance network of hospitals in Minnesota; 214 chronic lymphoid, 132 acute myeloid, 46 chronic myeloid, 13 acute lymphoid, 58 myelodysplasia and 50 others	1087 selected by random-digit dialling from Health Care Financing Administration lists and from state death certificate files, frequency-matched by 5-year age group, vital status at time of interview and state of residence	Personal interviews including lifetime occupational history; formaldehyde assessed in a blinded fashion in terms of probability and intensity, each on a 4-point scale based on job title and industry	Acute myeloid Low-medium High Chronic myeloid Low-medium High Chronic lymphoid Low-medium High Myelodysplasia Low-medium High All combined Low-medium High	 0.9 (0.5–1.6) – (no case) 1.3 (0.6–3.1) 2.9 (0.3–24.5) 1.2 (0.7–1.8) 0.6 (0.1–5.3) 0.8 (0.3–1.9) – (no cases) 1.0 (0.7–1.4) 0.7 (0.2–2.6)	· Matching factors, post-secondary education, hair dye use, tobacco smoking, first degree relative with hematolympho-poietic tumour and agricultural use of pesticides	None of the acute lymphocytic lymphoma cases was exposed.

AIDS, acquired immunodeficiency syndrome; CI, confidence interval; ICD, international code of diseases; NA, not applicable

[a] Average exposure index

0.5–2.2), 1.0 (14 exposed cases; 95% CI, 0.5–2.1) and 0.5 (five exposed cases; 95% CI, 0.1–1.7) for > 10 years of exposure to low, medium and high cumulative levels, respectively. Because there were only eight exposed cases of Hodgkin lymphoma, the odds ratio for ever versus never exposed was calculated to be 0.5 (95% CI, 0.2–1.4). Odds ratios did not differ substantially when cases of other cancers were used as the control group.

In an analysis of the same multi-site case–control study of Gérin *et al.* (1989), Fritschi and Siemiatycki (1996) evaluated risk from occupational exposure to 294 substances, including formaldehyde, with slightly different numbers of cases of Hodgkin lymphoma (54) and non-Hodgkin lymphoma (215) and 23 cases of myeloma. Cases were compared with a pool of 1066 controls that comprised 533 population controls who were selected from electoral lists of the Montréal area and by random-digit dialling and a random sample of 533 of 2357 patients who had other cancers (excluding lung cancer). Results for exposure to formaldehyde were not presented for Hodgkin or non-Hodgkin lymphoma due to a lack of previous evidence of an association, or for myeloma due to the same lack of previous evidence and because fewer than four cases had been exposed.

In a study of 578 male cases of leukaemia, 622 male cases of non-Hodgkin lymphoma and 1245 population-based controls in Iowa and Minnesota (USA), Linos *et al.* (1990) observed elevated risks for both leukaemia (four exposed cases; odds ratio, 2.1 [95% CI, 0.4–10]) and non-Hodgkin lymphoma (six exposed cases; odds ratio, 3.2 [95% CI, 0.8–13.4]) among men who had been employed in funeral homes and crematoria, which indicated some degree of occupational exposure to formaldehyde and other compounds. The risks were particularly high for the acute myeloid subtype of leukaemia (odds ratio, 6.7 [95% CI, 1.2–36]) and the follicular subtype of non-Hodgkin lymphoma (odds ratio, 6.7 [95% CI, 1.2–37]). However, each of these estimates was based on only three exposed cases.

In Finland, Partanen *et al.* (1993) identified eight cases of non-Hodgkin lymphoma, four cases of Hodgkin disease and 12 cases of leukaemia that were diagnosed between 1957 and 1982 and reported to the Finnish Cancer Registry among a cohort of 7307 production workers who were first employed in the wood industry between 1945 and 1963. One to eight referents were matched to each case by year of birth and vital status in 1983 from among cancer-free cohort members, which resulted in a total of 152 referents. Exposure to a number of substances, including formaldehyde, was estimated based on company records and a job–exposure matrix. For cases, but not for controls, job histories were completed by interviews of selected persons at the plants and by questionnaires sent to the cases or their next of kin in 1982–83. Using a 10-year lag interval, subjects were classified as exposed to formaldehyde when their estimated cumulative exposure reached 3 ppm–months. For leukaemia and lymphomas combined, exposure to formaldehyde was associated with an odds ratio of 2.49 (seven exposed cases; 95% CI, 0.81–7.59) based on conditional logistic regression. Adjustment of the analysis for exposure to solvents or for wood dust or exclusion of subjects who were exposed to solvents did not substantially alter the result. Odds ratios for specific cancers were 4.24 (four exposed cases; 95% CI, 0.68–26.6) for non-Hodgkin lymphoma and 1.40 (two exposed cases; 95% CI, 0.25–7.91) for leukaemia. Only one case of Hodgkin disease was exposed and the odds ratio was not calculated. [The Working Group as well as the authors noted the small number of cases and the possibility of bias due to the higher accuracy and completeness in the collection of exposure data for cases compared with controls that most probably resulted in an upward bias of odds ratios for all exposures evaluated. However, the odds ratio for all cancers combined was not elevated for wood dust, terpenes, chlorophenols or engine exhaust.]

West *et al.* (1995) evaluated lifetime exposures through occupation, environment and hobby among 400 patients over 15 years of age who had been newly diagnosed with myelodysplastic syndrome in South Wales, Wessex and West Yorkshire, United Kingdom. Of 635 eligible cases, 28% died before the interview, 3% were too ill, 2% had moved out of the study area and 5% refused to participate. Cancer-free controls were selected from outpatient clinics and inpatient wards of medicine, ear, nose and throat surgery, ortho-paedics and geriatrics and were individually matched to cases by age ($\pm$ 3 years), sex, area of residence and hospital, and year of diagnosis ($\pm$ 2 years). The personal interviews collected, among other information, data on work history and probed study subjects for duration and intensity (low, medium, high) of exposure to more than 70 hazards, including formaldehyde. Lifetime duration of exposure was estimated after consultation with indus-trial chemists and occupational hygienists. A minimal practical background level of expo-sure was set at 10 h in a lifetime, under which people were considered to be unexposed. Odds ratios were calculated as the ratio of discordant pairs and were 1.17 (15 exposed cases [95% CI, 0.51–2.68]) for $\geq$ 10 h lifetime exposure of any intensity versus no expo-sure, 2.33 ([95% CI, 0.55–11.35]) for > 50 h lifetime exposure of medium or high inten-sity versus no exposure and 2.00 ([95% CI, 0.32–15.67]) for > 2500 h lifetime exposure of medium or high intensity versus no exposure.

In a population-based case–control study, Tatham *et al.* (1997) evaluated the risks for subtypes of non-Hodgkin lymphoma with respect to exposure to formaldehyde among 1048 male cases that included 185 cases of small-cell diffuse lymphoma, 268 cases of follicular lymphoma and 526 cases of large-cell diffuse lymphoma who were born between 1929 and 1953, diagnosed between 1984 and 1988 and listed in the population-based cancer registries of the states or cities of Connecticut, Iowa, Kansas, Atlanta, Miami, San Francisco, Detroit or Seattle, USA. Diagnosis was confirmed by a panel of three pathologists. A total of 1659 controls were selected by random-digit dialling and were frequency-matched to cases on area of the registry and 5-year categories of date of birth. Of the 2354 and 2299 eligible cases and controls, respectively, 2073 [88%] and 1910 [83%] were alive and could be inter-viewed, while a further 1025 cases and 251 controls were excluded for various reasons, that included non-confirmation of diagnosis [562 cases], not being a resident in the USA before 1969, a history of acquired immunodeficiency syndrome (AIDS) or related illness, systemic lupus erythematosus, non-AIDS-related immunodeficiency, rheumatoid arthritis or a history of treatment with immunosuppressive drugs, chemotherapy or radiation. Cases and controls were interviewed by telephone on their background characteristics, lifestyle and medical, military and work history. The job history included questions on specific materials with or around which participants may have worked, including formaldehyde. Relative risks were based on conditional logistic regression, stratified for the matching factors (area of registry and date of birth) and adjusted for age at diagnosis, year of entry into the study, ethnicity, education, Jewish religion, never having married, AIDS risk behaviours, use of seizure medication, service in or off the coast of Viet Nam and cigarette smoking. For ever versus never having been exposed to formaldehyde, relative risks were 1.40 (21 exposed cases; 95% CI, 0.87–2.40) for small-cell diffuse lymphoma, 0.71 (17 exposed cases; 95% CI, 0.41–1.20) for follicular lymphoma, 1.10 (46 exposed cases; 95% CI, 0.79–1.70) for large-cell diffuse lymphoma and 1.20 (93 exposed cases; 95% CI, 0.86–1.50) for all cases of non-Hodgkin lymphoma combined. Of all the controls, 130 (7.8%) reported having been exposed to formaldehyde.

Blair *et al.* (2000) evaluated occupational exposure to formaldehyde in a population-based case–control study of leukaemia and myelodysplasia. Cases were identified among white men who were 30 years or older from the Cancer Registry of Iowa (1981–83) and among all men from a surveillance network of hospitals in Minnesota which covered 97% of hospital beds in this area (1980–82). Controls were identified by random-digit dialling, from Health Care Financing Administration lists or from state death certificate files, depending on their age and vital status, and were frequency-matched to cases by 5-year age group, vital status at the time of interview and state of residence. A total of 669 eligible cases was identified, and interviews were conducted with 340 cases of leukaemia and 238 surrogates for deceased subjects and those who were too ill to interview. Cases and controls who lived in four large cities were excluded because the main purpose of the study was to evaluate agricultural risks; furthermore, subjects who had farming as their sole occupation were excluded from this analysis because the incidence of leukaemia has been shown to be elevated among farmers. This left 214 cases of chronic lymphocytic leukaemia, 132 of acute myeloid leukaemia, 46 of chronic myeloid leukaemia, 13 of acute lymphocytic leukaemia, 58 of myelodysplasia and 50 others and 1087 controls. Interviews were conducted in 1981–84 and included a lifetime occupational history with job titles and industries. Exposure to selected substances, including formaldehyde, was assigned by an industrial hygienist in terms of probability and intensity in a blinded fashion, each on a four-point scale (non-exposed, low, medium and high intensity). Odds ratios were based on unconditional logistic regression adjusted for the matching factors and agricultural use of pesticides, post-secondary education, use of hair dyes, tobacco smoking and having a first-degree relative who had a haematolymphopoietic tumour. Compared with no exposure to formaldehyde, odds ratios were 0.9 (14 exposed cases; 95% CI, 0.5–1.6) for low/medium intensity of exposure for acute myeloid leukaemia (no cases with high exposure); 1.3 (seven exposed cases; 95% CI, 0.6–3.1) for low/medium exposure and 2.9 (one exposed case; 95% CI, 0.3–24.5) for high exposure for chronic myeloid leukaemia; 1.2 (29 exposed cases; 95% CI, 0.7–1.8) for low/medium exposure and 0.6 (one exposed case; 95% CI, 0.1–5.3) for high exposure for chronic lymphocytic leukaemia; 0.8 (six exposed cases; 95% CI, 0.3–1.9) for low/medium exposure for myelodysplasia (no cases with high exposure); and 1.0 (61 exposed cases; 95% CI, 0.7–1.4) for low/medium exposure and 0.7 (three exposed cases; 95% CI, 0.2–2.6) for high exposure for all leukaemias and myelo-dysplasia combined. Of the 1087 controls, 128 [11.8%] were estimated to have low/

medium and nine [0.8%] to have high exposure to formaldehyde. None of the cases of acute lymphocytic leukaemia was exposed.

Nisse *et al.* (2001) evaluated the risk for myelodysplastic syndrome among 204 incident cases who were diagnosed during 1991–96 at the University Hospital of Lille (northern France) and 204 controls who were randomly selected from the electoral register and individually matched to cases by size of town of residence, sex and age (± 3 years). Cases who had secondary myelodysplastic syndrome after treatment for cancer and those who were unable to answer the questionnaire were excluded. The questionnaire was the same as that used in the study by West *et al.* (1995) and exposure evaluation was based on the method of Siemiatycki *et al.* (1981). Odds ratios for exposure to formaldehyde were not reported because the 95% CI for the univariate odds ratio for ever versus never having been exposed included 1, or because there were fewer than four exposed subjects.

2.2.6   *Cancers at other sites*

The study design of and results from the case–control studies of exposure to formaldehyde and cancer at sites other than those presented in the above sections are summarized in Table 21, in chronological order. The description of the studies below, in contrast, groups the reports by study population.

Within the Montréal multisite cancer study, the database that was analysed for lung cancer (see Section 2.2.4), Hodgkin disease, non-Hodgkin lymphoma and myeloma (see Section 2.2.5) was also used to study various other cancer sites in relation to exposure to formaldehyde. The results were published in separate reports and are presented below.

In addition to the sites cited above, Gérin *et al.* (1989) (see Section 2.2.4) analysed data for cancer of the oesophagus, stomach, colorectum, liver, pancreas, prostate, urinary bladder and kidney and for melanoma of the skin. Odds ratios were not elevated for any of these cancers.

Siemiatycki *et al.* (1994) conducted an analysis of urinary bladder cancer using a set of 484 pathologically confirmed cases of bladder cancer, 1879 controls who had cancers at other sites, excluding lung and kidney cancers, and 533 population controls. No evidence of an association was found between exposure to formaldehyde and the risk for bladder cancer: odds ratios, adjusted for non-occupational and occupational confounders, were 1.2 (67 exposed cases; 95% CI, 0.9–1.6) for non-substantial exposure and 0.9 (17 exposed cases; 95% CI, 0.5–1.7) for substantial exposure.

Dumas *et al.* (2000) analysed the association between occupational exposure to a large number of substances, occupations and industries and rectal cancer. A total of 257 men, who were aged 35–70 years and diagnosed with a rectal cancer between 1979 and 1985, were compared with 1295 controls who had cancers at sites other than the rectum, lung, colon, rectosigmoid junction, small intestine and peritoneum; adjustments were made for potential non-occupational (age, education, cigarette smoking, beer consumption, body mass index and respondent status) but not for occupational variables. Exposure to formaldehyde was associated with rectal cancer: the odds ratios were 1.2 (36 exposed

Table 21. Case–control studies of cancers at other sites

Reference, study location, years of study	Organ site (ICD code)	Characteristics of cases	Characteristics of controls	Exposure assessment	Exposure categories	Odds ratio (95% CI)	Adjustment for potential confounders	Comments
Gérin et al. (1989), Canada, 1979–85	Oesophagus Stomach Colorectum Liver Pancreas Prostate Bladder Kidney Skin melanoma	Men aged 35–70 years resident in Montréal 107 250 787 50 117 452 486 181 121	Pool of population selected from electoral list, and cancer controls; depending of the cancer site under study, the number of controls varied from 1733 to 2741.	Semi-structural probing interview, assessment of exposures by chemists and industrial hygienists	Short Long-low Long-medium Long-high	No association for any of these sites (most odds ratios very close to 1.0)	Selection of data-based confounders (variables according to each specific cancer), plus age, ethnic group, socio-economic status, cigarette smoking and dirtiness of job	Short and long refer to the duration, and low, medium and high to the intensity of exposure.
Merletti et al. (1991), Italy, 1982–84	Oral cavity or oropharynx	86 male incident cases	Random sample of 385 men, stratified by age, from the files of residents	Full occupational history linked to a job-exposure matrix	Any exposure Probable or definite	1.6 (0.9–2.8) 1.8 (0.6–5.5)	Age, education, area of birth, tobacco smoking and alcohol drinking	Only six exposed cases in the probable or definite exposure group
Goldoft et al. (1993), USA, 1979–89	Melanoma of the nasal cavity or nasopharynx	Nine cases [sex distribution not reported]	Random-digit dialling, frequency-matched on sex and age at diagnosis (controls from Vaughan et al., 1986a,b)	Interview	Living in a residence with foam insulation Occupational exposure Employed in industries with potential exposure[a]	3.57 (0.09–19.8) Obs./exp. 0/0.27 Obs./exp. 0/0.8		
Siemiatycki et al. (1994), Canada, 1979–86	Bladder	484 men aged 35–70 years resident in Montréal	533 population and 1879 cancer controls	See Gérin et al. (1989)	Non-substantial Substantial	1.2 (0.9–1.6) 0.9 (0.5–1.7)	Age, ethnicity, socioeconomic status, tobacco smoking, coffee consumption, status of respondent and other occupational exposures	Results based on pooled controls

Table 21 (contd)

Reference, study location, years of study	Organ site (ICD code)	Characteristics of cases	Characteristics of controls	Exposure assessment	Exposure categories	Odds ratio (95% CI)	Adjustment for potential confounders	Comments
Cantor et al. (1995), USA, 1984–89	Breast (female)	33 509 women with breast cancer as the cause of death	117 794 women who died from non-cancer causes; frequency-matched for age and race	Usual occupation on death certificate linked to a job–exposure matrix, with levels of probability and of intensity of exposure	Exposure levels Low Medium High Low Medium High	*Blacks* 1.14 $p < 0.05$ 0.93 1.20 $p < 0.05$ *Whites* 1.38 $p < 0.05$ 1.30 $p < 0.05$ 1.36 $p < 0.05$	Age at death, socioeconomic status and excluding women with lowest probability of exposure	No trend was observed.
Holly et al. (1996), USA, 1978–87	Uveal melanoma	221 white men aged 20–74 years	447 white men selected by random-digit dialling; matched for area and age	Recall through telephone interviews	Ever	2.9 (1.2–7.0)	Age, number of naevis, eye colour and skin response to exposure to midday summer sun	
Gustavsson et al. (1998), Sweden, 1988–91	Oral cavity and oesophagus (ICD-9 141, 143-5, 150)	250 incident cases among men aged 40–79 years resident in two regions (oral cavity, 128; oesophagus, 122)	641 men selected by stratified random sampling; frequency-matched to cases by age (10–15-year groups) and region	Work history reviewed by occupational hygienist; occupations coded by intensity and probability of exposure	Ever Oral cavity Oesophagus	1.28 (0.64–2.54) 1.90 (0.99–3.63)	Region, age, alcohol consumption and tobacco smoking habits	
Kernan et al. (1999), USA, 1984–93	Pancreas	63 097 persons with pancreatic cancer as the cause of death [sex and race distribution not reported]	252 386 persons who died from non-cancer causes; frequency-matched by state, sex, race and age (5-year groups)	Usual occupation on death certificate linked to a job–exposure matrix, with levels of probability and of intensity of exposure	Exposure level Low Medium High Exposure probability Low Medium High	1.2 (1.1–1.3) 1.2 (1.1–1.3) 1.1 (1.0–1.3) 1.2 (1.1–1.3) 1.2 (1.1–1.3) 1.4 (1.2–1.6)	Age, marital status, residential status, sex and race	No trend was observed; analysis by race and sex also provided

Table 21 (contd)

Reference, study location, years of study	Organ site (ICD code)	Characteristics of cases	Characteristics of controls	Exposure assessment	Exposure categories	Odds ratio (95% CI)	Adjustment for potential confounders	Comments
Dumas et al. (2000), Canada, 1979–85	Rectum	257 men aged 35–70 years resident in Montréal	533 population and 1295 cancer controls	See Gérin et al. (1989)	Any Substantial	1.2 (0.8–1.9) 2.4 (1.2–4.7)	Age, education, cigarette smoking, beer drinking, body mass index and respondent status	Results based on cancer controls and not in accordance with those of Gérin et al. (1989)
Wilson et al. (2004), USA, 1984–89	Salivary gland (ICD-9, 142.0–1, –9)	[2405] persons with cancer of the salivary gland as the cause of death (whites: 1347 men, 890 women; African–Americans: 93 men, 75 women)	[9420] persons who died from non-cancer causes, excluding infectious diseases; frequency-matched for age, race, sex and region	Usual occupation on death certificate linked to a job–exposure matrix, with levels of probability and of intensity of exposure	Mid-high probability and intensity	*White men and women* 1.6 (1.3–2.0) *Black women* 1.9 (0.8–5.1)	Age, marital status and socioeconomic status	High level of diagnosis misclassification suspected

CI, confidence interval; ICD, international code of diseases

[a] Wood-work, furniture manufacture, pulp and paper mill, textile, foundry and smelter

cases; 95% CI, 0.8–1.9) for any exposure and 2.4 (13 exposed cases; 95% CI, 1.2–4.7) for substantial exposure, with an increase in risk by concentration and duration of exposure. [This result contrasts with the findings of Gérin *et al.* (1989), in which none of the odds ratios for colorectal cancer was greater than 1.0 in any of the exposure subgroups, including the highest. These odds ratios were for all colorectal cancers, but the authors stated that "the results for subsites of the colorectum — colon, rectosigmoid and rectum — were essentially similar to those of the entire category".]

A series of systematic case–control analyses of various cancers in relation to exposure to different occupational agents, including formaldehyde, were conducted using death certificates collected from 1984 to 1989 in 24 states of the USA (Cantor *et al.*, 1995; Kernan *et al.*, 1999; Wilson *et al.*, 2004). Death certificates were coded for usual occupation and industry according to the classification designed for the 1980 US census. Individual exposures were derived by linking the occupation–industry codes with a job–exposure matrix that assessed the probability and level of exposure to 31 occupational agents.

Cantor *et al.* (1995) conducted a case–control study of occupational exposure and female breast cancer mortality in the USA. After excluding homemakers, 33 509 cases and 117 794 controls remained. Estimates were adjusted for age at death and socioeconomic status and excluded women who had a low probability of exposure. Exposure to formaldehyde was associated with the risk for breast cancer among white and black women: for whites, odds ratios were 1.14 ($p < 0.05$), 0.93 and 1.2 ($p < 0.05$) for women who had low, medium and high intensity of exposure, respectively; among black women, significantly elevated ($p < 0.05$) odds ratios of 1.38, 1.30 and 1.36 were found for those who had low, medium and high intensity of exposure, respectively [confidence intervals not shown].

Kernan *et al.* (1999) conducted a case–control study of pancreatic cancer. Cases were 63 097 persons who had died from pancreatic cancer in 1984–93. Controls were 252 386 persons who had died from causes other than cancer during the same period. Occupational exposure to formaldehyde was associated with a moderately increased risk for pancreatic cancer for both men and women and for both racial groups (blacks and whites), with odds ratios of 1.2 (95% CI, 1.1–1.3), 1.2 (95% CI, 1.1–1.3), 1.1 (95% CI, 1.0–1.3) for subjects with low, medium and high intensity of exposure, respectively, and 1.2 (95% CI, 1.1–1.3), 1.2 (95% CI, 1.1–1.3) and 1.4 (95% CI, 1.2–1.6) for subjects with low, medium and high probabilities of exposure, respectively. There was no apparent exposure–response pattern with intensity, but the exposure–response relationships by probability of exposure were consistent across each level of exposure intensity.

Using the same database as Cantor *et al.* (1995), Wilson *et al.* (2004) conducted a study of salivary gland cancer. The cases were [2405] persons who had died from salivary gland cancer between 1984 and 1989. Four controls per case, frequency-matched for sex, age, race and region, were selected from among persons who had died during the same period from other causes, excluding infectious diseases (because of a suspected viral etiology of salivary gland cancer); a total of 9420 controls were included. Occupation as coded on the death certificate was available for 95.3% of white and 87.3% of black men and for 45% of white and 30.9% of black women. Among white men and women, an odds ratio, adjusted for age, marital status and socioeconomic status, of 1.6 (95% CI, 1.3–2.0) was observed with 'mid–high' probability and 'mid–high' intensity of exposure to formaldehyde [categories not further defined]. The trend was significant ($p < 0.001$), but there was no dose–response pattern of monotonically increasing risk with increasing intensity and probability of exposure. No association between exposure to formaldehyde and salivary gland cancer was observed among African-American men and women combined. Among African-American women, the adjusted odds ratio for 'mid–high' intensity of exposure was 1.9 (95% CI, 0.8–5.1). No results were given separately for African-American men.

[The Working Group considered that this series of systematic analyses was limited by potential misclassification of some specific cancers when ascertained through death certificates, and by the use of occupation codes from death certificates to assess lifelong occupational exposure to formaldehyde.]

Merletti *et al.* (1991) reported a case–control study of 86 male residents of Turin, Italy, who had a diagnosis of cancer of the oral cavity or oropharynx that was notified to the population-based cancer registry of the city between 1 July 1982 and 31 December 1984, and a random sample of 385 men, stratified by age, who were chosen from files of residents of Turin. The cancers among the cases were: oropharynx (12), tongue (15), floor of the mouth (24), soft palate complex (14), other sites (11) and unspecified sites of the oral cavity (10). Detailed occupational history since 1945 and lifelong histories of tobacco smoking and alcohol drinking were obtained by personal interview. Each job that had been held for at least 6 months was coded according to the International Standard Classification of Occupations and the International Standard Industrial Classification, and a job–exposure matrix for 13 agents (including formaldehyde) which are known or suspected carcinogens of the respiratory tract and three non-specific exposures (dust, gas and solvents) was applied to the occupation–industry code combination of study subjects; the matrix was developed at the IARC for use in a similar study of laryngeal cancer. Study subjects were grouped into three categories of presumed frequency and intensity of exposure to formaldehyde (no, any, probable or definite exposure), with the 'no exposure' group (exposure not higher than that of the general population) as the reference level. Odds ratios were calculated using unconditional logistic regression adjusting for age, tobacco smoking, alcohol drinking, education and place of birth. An association was suggested between cancer of the oral cavity or oropharynx and exposure to formaldehyde, with odds ratios of 1.6 (95% CI, 0.9–2.8) for 'any exposure' and 1.8 (95% CI, 0.6–5.5) for 'probable or definite' exposure; however, only 25 and six cases were exposed, respectively. No relationship was seen with duration of exposure to formaldehyde, with odds ratios of 1.7 for 1–15 years of exposure and 1.5 for ≥ 16 years within the 'any exposure' category, and of 2.1 and 1.4, respectively, within the 'probable or definite' exposure category. Separate results for an association with exposure to formaldehyde were not reported for the 12 men who had oropharyngeal cancer. [The Working Group noted that confounding by tobacco and alcohol could not be excluded from the interpretation of the observed association between exposure to formaldehyde and oral cancer.]

As part of the population-based case–control study of sinonasal cancer by Vaughan *et al.* (1986a,b) (see Section 2.2.1), Goldoft *et al.* (1993) interviewed nine of 14 patients who had been diagnosed with melanoma of the nose or nasopharynx between 1979 and 1989. The frequency of their exposure to formaldehyde was compared with that of the control subjects included in the study of Vaughan *et al.* (1986a,b). One subject had lived in a residence that was insulated with formaldehyde-based foam [0.3 expected]. None of the melanoma patients reported specific occupational exposure to formaldehyde (0.3 expected), and none reported having been employed in industries that would probably entail exposure to formaldehyde (0.8 expected). [The Working Group noted that it was unclear how the expected numbers were calculated.]

Holly *et al.* (1996) conducted a case–control study in the western USA to determine the relation of occupations and chemical exposures to the risk for uveal melanoma. Two hundred and twenty-one white men, aged 20–74 years and referred for treatment to a specialized unit in San Francisco between 1978 and 1987, were included and successfully interviewed. A group of 447 controls were selected by random-digit dialling (white men from the same geographical area and within the same 5-year age group), and 77% were successfully interviewed by telephone. Exposure to chemicals, including formaldehyde, was determined by asking the subjects whether they thought they were ever regularly exposed (at least 3 h per week for at least 6 months) in their jobs, hobbies, leisure or home maintenance. When ever to never having been exposed to formaldehyde was compared, an elevated odds ratio of 2.9 (13 exposed cases; 95% CI, 1.2–7.0), adjusted for potential non-occupational confounders, was found. [The Working Group and the authors noted the potential for recall bias when chemical exposures are ascertained from the subject's memory.]

A case–control study by Gustavsson *et al.* (1998) (see Section 2.2.3) included 128 cases of oral cancer and 122 cases of oesophageal cancer (in addition to cancers of the pharynx and larynx). There was no significant association between exposure to formaldehyde and the risk for oral cancer (14 exposed cases; odds ratio, 1.28; 95% CI, 0.64–2.54), but the risk for cancer of the oesophagus was elevated and bordered on statistical significance (19 exposed cases; odds ratio, 1.90; 95% CI, 0.99–3.63).

2.3   Pooled analysis and meta-analyses

2.3.1   *Pooled analysis*

Luce *et al.* (2002) performed a pooled analysis of data from 12 case–control studies on sinonasal cancer [cancer of the nasal cavity and paranasal sinuses, ICD-9 code 160] that were conducted in China (Zheng *et al.*, 1992), France (Luce *et al.*, 1992, 1993; Leclerc *et al.*, 1994), Germany (Bolm-Audorff *et al.*, 1990), Italy (Merler *et al.*, 1986; Comba *et al.*, 1992a,b; Magnani *et al.*, 1993), the Netherlands (Hayes *et al.*, 1986a,b), Sweden (Hardell *et al.*, 1982) and the USA (Brinton *et al.*, 1984, 1985; Vaughan *et al.*, 1986a; Vaughan, 1989; Vaughan & Davis, 1991). An earlier pooled analysis ('t Mannetje *et al.*, 1999) used data from eight of these 12 studies. As the earlier study is subsumed by the more extensive analysis of Luce *et al.* (2002), results from 't Mannetje *et al.* (1999) are not presented.

The analysis by Luce *et al.* (2002) included data from four (Brinton *et al.*, 1984; Vaughan *et al.*, 1986a; Hayes *et al.*, 1986a; Luce *et al.*, 1993) of the six case–control studies that primarily focused on exposure to formaldehyde that are described in Section 2.2.1, but not those by Olsen *et al.* (1989) or Roush *et al.* (1987). In addition, data were obtained from a further seven studies that were originally designed to address exposures to substances other than formaldehyde (particularly wood dust) and one unpublished study. A total of 195 cases of adenocarcinoma (169 men, 26 women) and 432 cases of squamous-cell carcinoma (330 men, 102 women) were compared with 3136 controls (2349 men, 787 women). The study by Luce *et al.* (1993) in France contributed approximately half of the cases of adenocarcinoma. Cases were diagnosed between 1968 and 1990 and were ascertained from different sources; study subjects were interviewed between 1979 and 1990 using different methods. Studies also varied with respect to the mode of selection of controls and the vital status of subjects at recruitment. Lifetime occupational histories collected in the individual studies were recoded with the occupation and industry codes from International Standard Classifications. These codes and industrial hygiene data were the basis for the development of a job–exposure matrix that provided estimates of the probability (unexposed, 1–10%, 10–50%, 50–90%, > 90%) and intensity (< 0.25 ppm, 0.25–1 ppm, > 1 ppm) of exposure to formaldehyde. Numerical values were assigned to each exposure category, and the job-specific products of the assigned value and duration of employment were summed over each individual's total work history (using 0-, 10- and 20-year lag intervals) to estimate cumulative exposure. For the analysis, the cumulative exposure index was categorized into one of four classes (unexposed and tertiles among controls) that were denoted as no, low, medium and high exposure. Odds ratios were derived by unconditional logistic regression and were stratified by sex and histology with adjustment for age (three categories) and study. In analyses of adenocarcinoma in men, adjustment was also made for wood and leather dust. Tobacco smoking was evaluated as a potential confounder, but was not included in the final models because effect estimates did not change substantially after adjustment. Among subjects exposed to low, medium or high levels of formaldehyde compared with unexposed subjects, estimated odds ratios were 1.2 (43 exposed cases; 95% CI, 0.8–1.8), 1.1 (40 exposed cases; 95% CI, 0.8–1.6) and 1.2 (30 exposed cases; 95% CI, 0.8–1.8) for squamous-cell carcinoma among men; 0.7 (six exposed cases; 95% CI, 0.3–1.9), 2.4 (31 exposed cases; 95% CI, 1.3–4.5) and 3.0 (91 exposed cases; 95% CI, 1.5–5.7) for adenocarcinoma among men; 0.6 (six exposed cases; 95% CI, 0.2–1.4), 1.3 (seven exposed cases; 95% CI, 0.6–3.2) and 1.5 (six exposed cases; 95% CI, 0.6–3.8) for squamous-cell carcinoma among women; and 0.9 (two exposed cases; 95% CI, 0.2–4.1), 0.0 (no cases) and 6.2 (five exposed cases; 95% CI, 2.0–19.7) for adenocarcinoma among women, respectively. Slight increases in these odds ratios were observed with 10- and 20-year lag intervals. Among men, studies were heterogeneous with respect to the effects of exposure to formaldehyde on adenocarcinoma, with a significantly better fit of a model that included interaction terms between exposure effects and study compared with a model with no such interaction terms ($p < 0.01$). [The Working Group noted that this heterogeneity may have led to inappropriately narrow confidence intervals since the analytical model did not account for random effects.] Among men with little or no exposure to wood dust, the odds ratios for adenocarcinoma with high level exposure to formaldehyde was 2.2 (95% CI, 0.8–6.3). [The Working Group considered that, for adenocarcinoma, residual confounding by exposure to wood dust was possible despite the attempts to control for it. This is because of the high degree of correlation between exposure to wood dust and exposure to formaldehyde, and the very strong association between adenocarcinoma and exposure to wood dust. Only 11 male cases of adenocarcinoma who had low, medium or high exposure to formaldehyde were categorized as never having been exposed to wood dust.]

2.3.2 Meta-analyses

(a) Respiratory cancers (Table 22)

In a meta-analysis on the relationship between exposure to formaldehyde and cancer, Blair et al. (1990b) added up the observed and expected numbers of various cancers across 32 cohort and case–control studies. They found no substantially elevated mortality from cancer of the lung or of the nasal nasal cavity for persons who were ever exposed or for those who had a higher level or duration of exposure. For cancer of the nasopharynx, mortality in persons who had a higher level or duration of exposure was elevated 2.1-fold [95% CI, 1.1–3.5] with 13 observed deaths. Among professionals, mortality from leukaemia (SMR, 1.6 [95% CI, 1.3–1.9]) and that from brain cancer (SMR, 1.5 [95% CI, 1.1–1.9]) were elevated. No significant associations were observed for other cancers.

In addition to the studies evaluated by Blair et al. (1990b), a meta-analysis of respiratory cancers by Partanen (1993) included two additional studies (Brinton et al., 1984; Merletti et al., 1991) and two updates (Gallagher et al., 1989; Partanen et al., 1990). The analysis used lagged and confounder-adjusted inputs, whenever available, and derived summary relative risks using a log-Gaussian, fixed effects model. For nasopharyngeal cancer, risk ratios were 1.59 (23 deaths; 95% CI, 0.95–2.65) and 2.74 (11 deaths; 95% CI, 1.36–5.55) for low/medium and substantial level or duration of exposure, respectively. Partanen (1993) found a relative risk for cancer of the nasal cavities and paranasal sinuses of 1.68 (95% CI, 1.00–2.82) for the highest category of exposure, while the corresponding risk calculated by Blair et al. (1990b) was 1.1 [95% CI, 0.7–1.5]. [This discrepancy may be explained by differences in the selection of studies for inclusion in the two meta-analyses or by differences in the way in which exposure categories were defined]. For the combined category of cancers of the oropharynx, lip, tongue, salivary glands and mouth, the aggregated data did not suggest associations with exposure to formaldehyde. Overall, Blair et al. (1990b) and Partanen (1993) were in good agreement with regard to the risks for lung cancer, nasopharyngeal carcinoma and miscellaneous cancers of the upper respiratory tract.

Collins et al. (1997) calculated meta-relative risks for cancers of the lung, nose or nasopharynx based on results from 11 cohort studies, three proportionate mortality studies

Table 22. Summary of results from three meta-analyses on respiratory cancers and exposure to formaldehyde

Level or duration of exposure to formaldehyde	Site							
	Lung		Nose and nasal sinuses		Nasopharynx		Other respiratory	
	O/E	mRR (95% CI)	O/E	mRR (95% CI)	O/E	mRR (95% CI)	O/E	mRR (95% CI)
Any								
Blair et al. (1990b)[a]	[1692/1681]	[1.0 (0.95–1.06)]	[61/58]	[1.0 (0.8–1.3)]	[35/27]	[1.3 (0.9–1.8)]	NR	NR
Partanen (1993)[b,c]	833/752	1.11 (1.03–1.19)	93/78	1.11 (0.81–1.53)	36/21	2.00 (1.36–2.90)	69/57	1.18 (0.87–1.59)
Collins et al. (1997)[d]	2080/2506	1.0 (0.9–1.0)	936/808	1.0 (1.0–1.1)	455/412	1.3 (1.2–1.5)	NR	NR
Low/medium								
Blair et al. (1990b)[a]	514/422	1.2 [1.1–1.3]	38/46	0.8 [0.6–1.1]	30/27	1.1 [0.7–1.6]	NR	NR
Partanen (1993)[b,c]	518/425	1.2 (1.1–1.3)	33/30	1.10 (0.67–1.79)	23/16	1.59 (0.95–2.65)	52/48	1.05 (0.74–1.51)
Substantial								
Blair et al. (1990b)[a]	250/240	1.0 [0.9–1.2]	30/28	1.1 [0.7–1.5]	13/6	2.1 [1.1–3.5]	NR	NR
Partanen (1993)[b,c]	233/216	1.1 (0.95–1.2)	36/21	1.68 (1.00–2.82)	11/4	2.74 (1.36–5.55)	23/20	1.15 (0.64–2.09)

CI, confidence interval; mRR, meta-relative risk; NR, not reported; O/E, observed/expected

[a] Blair et al. (1990b) included the following studies in their analysis: Harrington & Shannon (1975), Petersen & Milham (1980), Jensen & Andersen (1982), Fayerweather et al. (1983), Friedman & Ury (1983), Marsh (1983), Milham (1983), Walrath & Fraumeni (1983), Wong (1983), Acheson et al. (1984a,b), Coggon et al. (1984), Harrington & Oakes (1984), Levine et al. (1984), Liebling et al. (1984), Malker & Weiner (1984), Olsen et al. (1984), Walrath & Fraumeni (1984), Partanen et al. (1985), Stayner et al. (1985), Walrath et al. (1985), Bertazzi et al. (1986), Blair et al. (1986), Bond et al. (1986), Gallagher et al. (1986), Hayes et al. (1986a,b), Logue et al. (1986), Stroup et al. (1986), Vaughan et al. (1986a,b), Blair et al. (1987), Roush et al. (1987), Stayner et al. (1988), Bertazzi et al. (1989), Gérin et al. (1989), Blair et al. (1990a) and Hayes et al. (1990),

[b] The analysis for lung cancer was performed for industrial workers only, as at least some of the data for professionals were confounded by social class.

[c] Partanen (1993) included in his analysis the above studies and: Brinton et al. (1984), Merletti et al. (1991); in addition, Partanen et al. (1985) was updated with Partanen et al. (1990), and Gallagher et al. (1986) was updated with Gallagher et al. (1989).

[d] Collins et al. (1997) included in their analysis the above studies (except for Petersen & Milham (1980), Friedman & Ury (1983), Marsh (1983), Milham (1983), Wong (1983), Acheson et al. (1984a,b), Harrington & Oakes (1984), Liebling et al. (1984), Malker & Weiner (1984), Stayner et al. (1985), Walrath et al. (1985), Gallagher et al. (1986), Logue et al. (1986), Blair et al. (1987, 1990a) and Merletti et al. (1991)) and added the following studies: Hernberg et al. (1983a,b), Olsen & Asnaes (1986), Hall et al. (1991), Matanoski (1991), Chiazze et al. (1993), Gardner et al. (1993), Luce et al. (1993), West et al. (1993), Marsh et al. (1994) and Andjelkovich et al. (1995).

and 15 case–control studies that were published between 1975 and 1995. The analysis did not include all of the studies from the meta-analyses by Blair *et al.* (1990b) and Partanen (1993), but added several studies, most of which were published after 1992. Using a fixed effects model, an overall meta-relative risk for lung cancer of 1.0 (95% CI, 0.9–1.0) was calculated based on 24 studies with 2080 observed cases, but there was substantial hetero-geneity across studies ($p < 0.00001$) which was mainly due to the difference between industrial cohort studies (meta-relative risk, 1.1; 95% CI, 1.0–1.2) and case–control studies (meta-relative risk, 0.8; 95% CI, 0.7–0.9). For nasal cancer, the overall meta-relative risk was 1.0 (95% CI, 1.0–1.1) based on 20 studies with 936 observed cases. Separate analyses by study type gave a meta-relative risk of 0.3 (95% CI, 0.1–0.9) for cohort studies and 1.8 (95% CI, 1.4–2.3) for case–control studies. Meta-relative risks for nasopharyngeal cancer were 1.3 (95% CI, 1.2–1.5) overall based on 12 studies with 455 cases, and 1.6 (95% CI, 0.8–3.0) for cohort studies with reported expected deaths. To address a potential publica-tion bias, all cohort studies were combined and missing expected numbers were estimated based on an approximation of the ratio of deaths from nasopharyngeal and lung cancer from the corresponding ratio observed in another study; this gave a meta-relative risk of 1.0 (95% CI, 0.5–1.8).

(*b*)   *Pancreatic cancer* (Table 23)

Ojajärvi *et al.* (2000) evaluated occupational exposures in relation to pancreatic cancer in a meta-analysis based on 92 studies that represented 161 different exposed populations. Eligible studies had to fulfil certain criteria and had to be agent-specific with direct risk estimates for one or several of 23 agents or for job titles with verified exposures to the agents. Proportionate mortality and incidence studies were excluded. For exposure to formaldehyde, five eligible populations were identified with a meta-relative risk of 0.8 (95% CI, 0.5–1.0), and point estimates of the meta-relative risks for different subsets of the meta-analysis by gender, type of diagnosis and study design ranged from 0.5 to 1.0. There was no evidence of heterogeneity of point estimates between populations. [The studies or populations included in the evaluation of formaldehyde were not clearly identified. The NCI cohort study by Blair *et al.* (1986) (see Section 2.1.1(*a*)) was apparently not included.]

Collins *et al.* (2001a) calculated a meta-relative risk for pancreatic cancer based on results from 14 studies, including eight cohort studies, four proportionate cancer mortality or incidence studies and two case–control studies that were published between 1983 and 1999. Based on a fixed effects model, an overall meta-relative risk of 1.1 (95% CI, 1.0–1.2) was calculated with no substantial heterogeneity across studies ($p = 0.12$). Meta-relative risks by type of job were 0.9 (95% CI, 0.8–1.1) for industrial workers (five studies that included 137 pancreatic cancers), 1.3 (95% CI, 1.0–1.6) for embalmers (four studies that included 88 pancreatic cancers) and 1.3 (95% CI, 1.0–1.7) for pathologists and ana-tomists (three studies that included 60 pancreatic cancers). There was no indication of publication bias. It was mentioned that the two studies that evaluated risk for pancreatic cancer at various exposure levels (Blair *et al.*, 1986; Kernan *et al.*, 1999) did not find monotonically increasing risks with increasing exposure levels. [Four (three cohort

Table 23. Summary of results from meta-analyses of pancreatic cancer and exposure to formaldehyde

	Ojajärvi et al. (2000)[a]		Collins et al. (2001a)[b]		
	Populations	mRR (95% CI)	Studies	No. of cases	mRR (95% CI)
All studies	5	0.8 (0.5–1.0)	14	364	1.1 (1.0–1.2)
Sex					
Men	3	0.8 (0.5–1.3)			
Unspecified or both	2	0.6 (0.3–1.1)			
Histological diagnosis					
Yes	2	0.5 (0.3–0.9)			
No	3	0.9 (0.7–1.3)			
Study type					
Case–control and cohort with internal reference	2	0.5 (0.3–1.6)			
SMR/SIR	3	0.9 (0.7–1.3)			
Cohort			8	132	1.0 (0.8–1.2)
Case–control			2	79	1.0 (0.5–2.0)
PMR/PIR			4	153	1.2 (1.0–1.4)
Type of job					
Industrial			5	137	0.9 (0.8–1.1)
Embalmer			4	88	1.3 (1.0–1.6)
Pathologist and anatomist			3	60	1.3 (1.0–1.7)

CI, confidence interval; mRR, meta-relative risk; PMR/PIR, proportionate mortality ratio/proportionate incidence ratio; SMR/SIR, standardized mortality ratio/standardized incidence ratio
[a] Ojajärvi et al. (2000) studied occupational exposures and pancreatic cancer in 92 studies and 161 different exposed populations. The studies used for their evaluation of formaldehyde are not listed specifically. However, the study by Blair et al. (1986) was apparently not included.
[b] Collins et al. (2001a) included the following studies in their analyses: Walrath & Fraumeni (1983), Levine et al. (1984), Walrath & Fraumeni (1984), Blair et al. (1986), Stroup et al. (1986), Stayner et al. (1988), Gérin et al. (1989), Hayes et al. (1990), Matanoski (1991), Hall et al. (1991), Gardner et al. (1993), Andjelkovich et al. (1995), Hansen & Olsen (1995) and Kernan et al. (1999).

studies and one proportionate incidence study) of the 14 studies included were also referenced in the meta-analysis by Ojajärvi et al. (2000).]

 (*c*) *Leukaemia*

 Collins and Lineker (2004) calculated meta-relative risks for leukaemia based on the results from 12 cohort studies, four proportionate mortality or incidence studies and two case–control studies that were published between 1975 and 2004. Using a fixed effects model, an overall meta-relative risk for leukaemia of 1.1 (95% CI, 1.0–1.2) was calculated based on 287 observed cases with borderline heterogeneity across studies ($p = 0.07$). Separate analyses by study type showed heterogeneity among proportionate mortality or incidence studies (meta-relative risk, 1.2; 95% CI, 1.0–1.5; p-heterogeneity = 0.02), but not among cohort studies (meta-relative risk, 1.0; 95% CI, 0.9–1.2) or among the two case–control studies (meta-relative risk, 2.4; 95% CI, 0.9–6.5). Increased risk was observed in studies of embalmers (meta-relative risk, 1.6; 95% CI, 1.2–2.0) and pathologists and anatomists (meta-relative risk, 1.4; 95% CI, 1.0–1.9), but not among industrial workers (meta-relative risk, 0.9; 95% CI, 0.8–1.0). There was no indication of substantial publication bias. [This meta-analysis did not include the studies by Logue *et al.* (1986), Partanen *et al.* (1993), Stellman *et al.* (1998) or Blair *et al.* (2001). Results from Harrington and Shannon (1975) and Harrington and Oakes (1984) were both included despite overlapping study populations. The Working Group noted that the findings of the meta-analysis would be sensitive to the choice of effect measures based on external rather than internal comparisons from some studies. Also, the analysis did not take into account risk estimates for higher-exposure subgroups or information on exposure–response relationships in the industrial cohort studies.]

3.   Studies of Cancer in Experimental Animals

3.1   Inhalation

3.1.1   *Mouse*

Groups of 42–60 C3H mice [sex and age unspecified] were exposed to concentrations of 0, 50, 100 or 200 mg/m^3 formaldehyde (US Pharmacopeia grade) vapour for 1 h per day, three times a week, ostensibly for 35 weeks. Treatment of mice with the highest concentration was discontinued after the 11th exposure because of severe toxicity, and 36 of the mice exposed to 50 mg/m^3 for 35 weeks were subsequently exposed to 150 mg/m^3 for a further 29 weeks. Surviving animals in the initial groups were killed at 35 weeks and those on extended treatment at 68 weeks. The nasal epithelium was not examined, either grossly or microscopically. There was no evidence of induction of pulmonary tumours at any dose. Basal-cell hyperplasia, squamous-cell metaplasia and atypical metaplasia were seen in the trachea and bronchi of most of the exposed mice but not in untreated controls (Horton *et al.*, 1963). [The Working Group noted the high doses used, the short intervals of exposure, the short duration of the experiment and the lack of pathological examination of the nose.]

Groups of 119–120 male and 120–121 female B6C3F$_1$ mice, 6 weeks of age, were exposed to 0, 2.0, 5.6 or 14.3 ppm [0, 2.5, 6.9 or 17.6 mg/m^3] formaldehyde (> 97.5% pure) vapour by whole-body exposure for 6 h per day on 5 days per week for up to 24 months, followed by a 6-month observation period with no further exposure. Ten males and 10 females from each group were killed at 6 and 12 months, no or one male and 19–20 females at 18 months, 17–41 of each sex at 24 months and 9–16 females at 27 months. Between 0 and 24 months, 78 male and 30 female controls, 77 males and 34 females exposed to 2 ppm formaldehyde vapour, 81 males and 19 females exposed to 5.6 ppm and 82 males and 34 females exposed to 14.3 ppm died; all animals that died or were killed were examined grossly. Thorough histopathological examinations were performed on control and high-dose mice, on multiple sections of the nasal cavity and on all lesions that were identified grossly in the other two groups. Squamous-cell carcinomas occurred in the nasal cavities of 2/17 male mice in the high-dose group that were killed at 24 months. No nasal cavity tumours developed in male mice treated with lower doses of formaldehyde, in females at any dose or among 21 male or 31 female control mice killed at 24 months ($p > 0.05$). A variety of non-neoplastic lesions (such as squamous-cell hyperplasia, squamous-cell metaplasia and dysplasia) were commonly found in the nasal cavities of mice exposed to formaldehyde, particularly at 14.3 ppm (Kerns *et al.*, 1983a,b; Gibson, 1984).

3.1.2   *Rat*

Groups of 119–120 male and 120 female Fischer 344 rats, 7 weeks of age, were exposed to 0, 2.0, 5.6 or 14.3 ppm [0, 2.5, 6.9 or 17.6 mg/m^3] formaldehyde (> 97.5% pure) vapour by whole-body exposure for 6 h per day on 5 days per week for up to 24 months and were then observed for 6 months with no further exposure. Ten males and 10 females from each group were killed at 6 and 12 months, 19–20 of each sex at 18 months, 13–54 at 24 months, 0–10 at 27 months and 0–6 at 30 months. Between 0 and 24 months, six males and 13 females in the control group, 10 males and 16 females exposed to 2 ppm, 19 of each sex exposed to 5.6 ppm and 57 males and 67 females exposed to 14.3 ppm died; all animals that died or were killed were examined grossly. Histopathological examinations were performed on multiple sections of the nasal cavity, on all lesions that were identified grossly and on all major tissues of each organ system (approximately 40 per animal) from control and high-dose rats. The findings for the nasal cavity are summarized in Table 24. While no nasal cavity malignancies were found in rats exposed to 0 or 2.0 ppm formaldehyde, two squa-mous-cell carcinomas (1/119 males and 1/116 females examined) occurred in the group exposed to 5.6 ppm and 107 (51/117 males and 52/115 females examined) in those exposed to 14.3 ppm ($p < 0.001$). Five additional nasal cavity tumours (classified as carcinoma, undifferentiated carcinoma/sarcoma and carcinosarcoma) were identified in rats exposed to 14.3 ppm; two of these tumours were found in rats that also had squamous-cell carcinomas of the nasal cavity. There was a significant overall increase in the incidence of polypoid adenomas in treated animals (males and females combined) when compared with controls ($p = 0.02$, Fisher's exact test). The incidences of polypoid adenomas were marginally significantly elevated in females at the low dose ($p = 0.07$, Fisher's exact test) and in males at the middle dose ($p = 0.06$, Fisher's exact test) (see also Table 24). A variety of non-neo-plastic lesions were commonly found in the nasal cavities of rats exposed to formaldehyde, particularly at 14.3 ppm (Swenberg *et al.*, 1980; Kerns *et al.*, 1983a,b; Gibson, 1984). More

Table 24. Neoplastic lesions in the nasal cavities of Fischer 344 rats exposed to formaldehyde vapour

Lesion	Exposure (ppm)							
	0		2.0		5.6		14.3	
	M	F	M	F	M	F	M	F
No. of nasal cavities examined	118	114	118	118	119	116	117	115
Squamous-cell carcinoma	0	0	0	0	1	1	51[a]	52[a]
Nasal carcinoma	0	0	0	0	0	0	1[b]	1
Undifferentiated carcinoma or sarcoma	0	0	0	0	0	0	2[b]	0
Carcinosarcoma	0	0	0	0	0	0	1	0
Osteochondroma	1	0	0	0	0	0	0	0
Polypoid adenoma	1	0	{ 4	4[c]	6[d]	0	4	1 }[e]

From Kerns *et al.* (1983a)

[a] $p < 0.001$, pair-wise comparisons
[b] One animal in this group also had a squamous-cell carcinoma.
[c] [$p = 0.07$, Fisher's exact test in comparison with female controls]
[d] [$p = 0.06$, Fisher's exact test in comparison with male controls]
[e] [$p = 0.02$, Fisher's exact test in comparison of all treated rats with controls]

than half (57%) of the squamous-cell carcinomas in rats exposed to 14.3 ppm formaldehyde were observed on the anterior portion of the lateral side of the nasoturbinate and the adjacent lateral wall, 25% were located on the midventral nasal septum, 10% on the dorsal septum and roof of the dorsal meatus and a small number (3%) on the maxilloturbinate (Morgan *et al.*, 1986a).

In a study to investigate the carcinogenicity of bis(chloromethyl)ether formed *in situ* in inhalation chambers by mixing formaldehyde and hydrogen chloride gas at high concentrations before introduction into the chamber in order to maximize its formation, 99 male Sprague–Dawley rats, 8 weeks of age, were exposed to a mixture of 14.7 ppm [18.1 mg/m^3] formaldehyde [purity unspecified] vapour and 10.6 ppm [15.8 mg/m^3] hydrogen chloride gas for 6 h per day on 5 days per week for life. The average level of bis(chloromethyl)ether was 1 ppb [4.7 µg/m^3]. Groups of 50 rats were sham-exposed to air or were untreated. The animals were allowed to die naturally and were then necropsied. Histological sections of nasal cavities, respiratory tract, major organs and gross lesions were prepared and examined microscopically. No nasal cancers were found in the controls, but 28 of the treated rats developed tumours of the nasal cavity, 25 of which were squamous-cell carcinomas [$p < 0.001$, Fisher's exact test] and three of which were papillomas. Mortality was greater in the treated group than in controls throughout the experiment; about 50% of the exposed rats were still alive at 223 days, when the first nasal carcinoma was observed. About two-thirds of the exposed rats showed squamous-cell metaplasia of the nasal mucosa; these lesions were not seen in controls (Albert *et al.*, 1982).

In a follow-up study, groups of 99–100 male Sprague-Dawley rats, 9 weeks of age, were exposed for 6 h per day on 5 days per week for life to: (1) 14.3 ppm [17.6 mg/m^3] formaldehyde [purity unspecified] and 10 ppm [14.9 mg/m^3] hydrogen chloride gas mixed before dilution in the exposure chamber to maximize formation of bis(chloromethyl)ether; (2) 14.1 ppm [17.3 mg/m^3] formaldehyde and 9.5 ppm [14.2 mg/m^3] hydrogen chloride gas not mixed before introduction into the exposure chamber; (3) 14.2 ppm [17.5 mg/m^3] formaldehyde vapour alone; (4) 10.2 ppm [15.2 mg/m^3] hydrogen chloride gas alone; or (5) air (sham-exposed controls). A control group of 99 rats was also available. The findings in the nasal cavity are summarized in Table 25. At the end of the experiment, 38 squamous-cell carcinomas of the nasal cavities and 10 papillomas or polyps were observed in rats exposed to formaldehyde alone; none were seen in the controls ($p \le 0.001$, Fisher's exact test). No differences were reported between groups in the incidences of tumours outside the nasal cavity (Albert et al., 1982; Sellakumar et al., 1985).

Table 25. Neoplastic lesions in the nasal cavities of male Sprague-Dawley rats exposed to formaldehyde (HCHO) and/or hydrogen chloride (HCl) vapour

Lesion	Group 1: Premixed HCl (10 ppm) and HCHO (14.3 ppm)	Group 2: Non-premixed HCl (9.5 ppm) and HCHO (14.1 ppm)	Group 3: HCHO (14.2 ppm)	Group 4: HCl (10.2 ppm)	Group 5: Air controls	Colony controls
No. of rats examined	100	100	100	99	99	99
Squamous-cell carcinoma	45	27	38	0	0	0
Adenocarcinoma	1	2	0	0	0	0
Mixed carcinoma	0	0	1	0	0	0
Fibrosarcoma	1	0	1	0	0	0
Aesthesioneuroepithelioma	1	0	0	0	0	0
Papillomas or polyps	13	11	10	0	0	0
Tumours in organs outside the respiratory tract	22	12	10	19	25	24

From Sellakumar et al. (1985)

Nine groups of 45 male Wistar rats [age unspecified], initially weighing 80 g, were exposed to 0, 10 or 20 ppm [0, 12.3 or 25 mg/m^3] formaldehyde [purity unspecified] vapour beginning 1 week after acclimatization. Whole-body exposures for 6 h per day on 5 days per week were continued for 4, 8 or 13 weeks; thereafter, the rats were observed during recovery periods of 126, 122 or 117 weeks, respectively, after which all survivors were killed. All rats were autopsied and examined by gross pathology; histological examination was limited to six cross-sections of the nose of each rat. Hyperplasia and metaplasia of the nasal epithelium were found to persist in rats exposed to formaldehyde. Significant tumour incidences are presented in Table 26. In control rats, the only nasal tumours reported were two squamous-cell carcinomas among 45 rats that were exposed to air for 8 weeks: one was a small tumour found at 130 weeks which appeared to involve a nasolachrymal duct; the second was a large squamous-cell carcinoma in a rat killed at

Table 26. Nasal tumours in male Wistar rats exposed to formaldehyde for 4, 8 or 13 weeks followed by observation up to 126 weeks

Exposure time; no. of rats	Tumour	Dose (ppm [mg/m^2])		
		0	10 [12.3]	20 [25]
4 weeks				
No. of rats		44	44	45
	Polypoid adenoma	0	0	1[a]
	Squamous-cell carcinoma	0	0	1
8 weeks				
No. of rats		45	44	43
	Polypoid adenoma	0	0	1[a]
	Squamous-cell carcinoma	2	1	1
13 weeks				
No. of rats		45	44	44
	Squamous-cell carcinoma	0	1	3[a]
	Cystic squamous-cell carcinoma	0	0	1
	Carcinoma *in situ*	0	0	1[a]
	Ameloblastoma	0	0	1

From Feron *et al.* (1988)
[a] Considered by the authors to be related to exposure to formaldehyde

week 94, which formed a large mass outside the nasal cavity and was thought to have arisen in a nasolachrymal duct or maxillary sinus. The tumours were considered by the authors not to resemble those observed in the rats exposed to formaldehyde. Rats exposed to 10 ppm formaldehyde also had two squamous-cell carcinomas: one was reported to be a small nasolachrymal-duct tumour in a survivor at 130 weeks, and the second occurred largely outside the nasal cavity in association with an abnormal incisor tooth in a rat killed at week 82. Rats exposed to 20 ppm formaldehyde had 10 tumours: polypoid adenomas of the nasal cavity were found in one rat exposed for 4 weeks and killed at 100 weeks and in another rat exposed for 8 weeks and killed at 110 weeks; six were squamous-cell carcinomas, two of which were thought to originate in the nasolachrymal ducts, one of which appeared to be derived from the palate and the three others, all in the group exposed for 13 weeks, appeared to arise from the naso- or maxillo-turbinates and formed large tumours that invaded the bone and subcutaneous tissues. The other two neoplasms observed in treated animals were an ameloblastoma found at week 73 and an exophytic tumour of the nasal septum of doubtful malignancy, which was designated a carcinoma *in situ*, in a rat that died at 81 weeks. The authors concluded that the nasal tumours were induced by formaldehyde only at 20 ppm and at an incidence of 4.5% (six tumours/132 rats) [$p = 0.01$, Fisher's exact test] (Feron *et al.*, 1988). [The Working Group noted that positive findings were made in spite of the short duration of exposure.]

A total of 720 male specific pathogen-free Wistar rats [age unspecified], initially weighing 30–50 g, were acclimatized for 1 week, and then the nasal mucosa of 480 of the rats was severely injured bilaterally by electrocoagulation. One week later, groups of

180 rats were exposed to 0, 0.1, 1.0 or 10 ppm [0, 0.123, 1.23 or 12.3 mg/m³] formaldehyde [purity unspecified] vapour by whole-body exposure for 6 h per day on 5 days per week. Half of the animals (30 undamaged and 60 damaged rats) were exposed for 28 months, and the other half (30 undamaged and 60 damaged rats) were exposed for only 3 months and then allowed to recover for 25 months with no further treatment. All surviving rats were killed at 29 months, autopsied and examined grossly; histological examination was restricted to six cross-sections of the nose of each rat. The neoplastic lesions found in the nasal cavity are summarized in Table 27. A high incidence of nasal tumours (17/58) was found in rats that had damaged noses and were exposed to 10 ppm formaldehyde for 28 months; only one was found in 54 controls [$p < 0.001$; Fisher's exact test]; and only one of the 26 rats that had undamaged noses and were exposed to 10 ppm formaldehyde for 28 months developed a nasal tumour. The tumour incidences in the other groups were low (0–4%). Eight additional squamous-cell carcinomas found in this study that appeared to be derived from the nasolachrymal ducts were excluded from the analysis (Woutersen *et al.*, 1989).

Table 27. Nasal tumours in male Wistar rats that had damaged or undamaged noses and were exposed to formaldehyde vapour for 28 months or 3 months followed by a 25-month recovery period

Exposure time; no. of rats	Tumour	Exposure (ppm [mg/m³])							
		0		0.1 [0.123]		1.0 [1.23]		10.0 [12.3]	
		U	D	U	D	U	D	U	D
28 months									
Effective number		26	54	26	58	28	56	26	58
	Squamous-cell carcinoma	0	1	1	1	1	0	1	15
	Adenosquamous carcinoma	0	0	0	0	0	0	0	1
	Adenocarcinoma	0	0	0	0	0	0	0	1
3 months									
Effective number		26	57	30	57	29	53	26	54
	Squamous-cell carcinoma	0	0	0	2	0	2	1	1
	Carcinoma *in situ*	0	0	0	0	0	0	0	1
	Polypoid adenoma	0	0	0	0	0	0	1	0

From Woutersen *et al.* (1989)
U, undamaged nose; D, damaged nose

In a study to explore the interaction between formaldehyde and wood dust, two groups of 16 female Sprague-Dawley rats, 11 weeks of age, were exposed either to air or to formaldehyde [purity unspecified] at an average concentration of 12.4 ppm [15.3 mg/m³]. Exposures were for 6 h per day for 5 days a week for a total of 104 weeks. At the end of the experiment, surviving animals were killed, and histological sections were prepared from five cross-sections of the nose of each rat. Pronounced squamous-cell metaplasia or metaplasia with dysplasia was observed in 10/16 rats exposed to formaldehyde and in

0/15 controls. One exposed rat developed a squamous-cell carcinoma. Neither the frequency nor the latent periods of induction of tumours outside the nasal cavity differed from those in controls (Holmström *et al.*, 1989b). [The Working Group noted the small numbers of animals used in the study.]

To study the correlation of indices of regional cell proliferation with the sites of formaldehyde-induced nasal squamous-cell carcinomas, five groups of 90 and one (high-dose) group of 147 male Fischer 344 (CDF(F344)CrlBr) rats, 8–9 weeks of age, were exposed to 0, 0.69, 2.05, 6.01, 9.93 or 14.96 ppm [0, 0.84, 2.4, 7.2, 12 or 18 mg/m^3] formaldehyde vapour (produced by thermal depolymerization of paraformaldehyde) by whole-body exposure for 6 h per day on 5 days per week for up to 24 months; six rats per group were killed at 3, 6, 12 and 18 months for interim observation. Histopathological examination of the nasal cavities was performed on all rats. The distribution of the nasal tumours was recorded on diagrams of the nasal passages at 30 selected levels that were designed to permit accurate localization of nasal lesions. In the high-dose group, survival was significantly decreased relative to that in the control group (18.8% versus 35.7%; $p < 0.001$, life-table analysis using the product-limit procedure of Kaplan and Meier; Cox's method for pairwise comparisons). Survival in the other exposure groups was similar to that in controls. According to the authors, formaldehyde induced nasal squamous-cell carcinomas in a highly non-linear fashion: no such tumours were observed after exposure to 2 ppm or lower or in controls; the incidences in the groups exposed to 6.01, 9.93 and 14.96 ppm were 1/90 [1%], 20/90 (22%) and 69/147 (45%) [47% according to the Working Group], respectively. The single nasal tumour found in the 6.01-ppm group was located in the anterior lateral meatus, a region that was predicted to receive a relatively high dose of formaldehyde. The time-to-tumour appearance of nasal squamous-cell carcinomas was 622, 555 and 350 days in the 6.01-, 9.93- and 14.96-ppm groups, respectively. No other type of nasal tumour was found among controls or among animals exposed to the two lowest concentrations. Polypoid adenomas (5/90 (5.6%) and 14/147 (9.5%)), rhabdomyosarcomas (1/90 [1%] and 1/47 [1%]) and adenocarcinomas (1/90 [1%] and 1/147 [1%]) were observed in the nasal cavities of rats exposed to 9.93 and 14.96 ppm, respectively. Formaldehyde-induced non-neoplastic nasal lesions were primarily confined to the transitional and respiratory epithelium of the anterior passages, were only found in the groups exposed to the three highest concentrations and were most severe in the groups exposed to 9.93 and 14.96 ppm. These lesions mainly comprised epithelial hypertrophy, hyperplasia and metaplasia, mixed inflammatory cell infiltrates, turbinate adhesions and, in many high-dose animals, significant distortion and destruction of the nasoturbinate architecture. In rats exposed to 6.01 ppm, non-neoplastic lesions were minimal or absent, and were limited to focal squamous metaplasia in the anterior regions (Monticello *et al.*, 1996).

Four groups of 32 male Fisher 344 rats (F-344/DuCrj), 5 weeks of age, were exposed to 0, 0.3, 2.17 and 14.85 ppm [0, 0.36, 2.6 and 17.8 mg/m^3] formaldehyde [purity unspecified] vapour by whole-body exposure for 6 h per day on 5 days per week for up to 28 months. A group of 32 rats served as unexposed room controls. The formaldehyde vapour was produced from a 37% aqueous formaldehyde solution containing 10%

methanol as an anti-polymerization agent. Rats in the 0-ppm control group were exposed to the same concentration of methanol (4.2 ppm) as those of the high-dose group. At 12, 18 and 24 months, five (randomly selected) animals per group (in the high-dose group, only two animals were alive at 24 months) were killed and examined grossly. At 28 months, all survivors were killed and necropsied. Animals that were found dead or killed *in extremis* also underwent necropsy. Histopathological examinations were performed on five anatomically specified cross-sections of the nose from all animals, on all lesions identified grossly and on other major organs (approximately 23 per animal) [probably all control and all exposed animals, although this was not mentioned specifically]. The total number of animals that died or were killed in moribund condition were 11 room controls and eight, six, 10 and 20 0-ppm control, low-, mid- and high-dose rats, respectively. Mortality rates (calculated by the life-table technique) at 28 months were 59.6% of room controls, 45.5% of 0-ppm controls, 31.8% of the 0.3-ppm group, 55.9% of the 2.17-ppm group and 88.3% of the 14.85-ppm group ($p \leq 0.01$ compared with the 0-ppm group; Fisher's exact test). Gross and microscopic pathological changes attributable to exposure to formaldehyde were found only in the nose. Except for an unclassified sarcoma found in one room control, nasal tumours were seen only in the high-dose group, and included three squamous-cell papillomas, 13 squamous-cell carcinomas ($p \leq 0.01$; Fisher's exact test) and one sarcoma. Grossly, the first nasal tumour was observed in the high-dose group after 13 weeks of exposure. Most of the nasal tumours were located in the incisor teeth and maxillary turbinate regions. Large tumours invaded the subcutis through the nasal bones. Hyperplasia with squamous-cell metaplasia of the nasal epithelium [not further specified] was found only in rats exposed to formaldehyde, the incidences (combined for all animals examined at interim and terminal sacrifices and found dead or killed *in extremis*) of which were 0/32, 0/32, 4/32, 7/32 ($p \leq 0.01$; Fisher's exact test) and 29/32 ($p \leq 0.01$; Fisher's exact test) for the room-control, 0-, 0.3-, 2.17- and 14.96-ppm groups, respectively. Hyperkeratosis of the nasal epithelium was found in 1/32 rats exposed to 2.17 ppm and in 26/32 rats exposed to 14.96 ppm ($p \leq 0.01$; Fisher's exact test); papillary hyperplasia of the nasal epithelium was seen in 2/32 rats in the high-dose group (Kamata *et al.*, 1997).

3.1.3   *Hamster*

A group of 88 male Syrian golden hamsters [age unspecified] was exposed to 10 ppm [12.3 mg/m^3] formaldehyde [purity unspecified] for 5 h a day on 5 days a week for life; 132 untreated controls were available. At necropsy, all major tissues were preserved, and histological sections were prepared from two transverse sections of the nasal turbinates of each animal; longitudinal sections were taken of the larynx and trachea, and all lung lobes were cut through the major bronchus. No tumours of the nasal cavities or respiratory tract were found in either controls or animals exposed to formaldehyde.

In a second study in the same report, 50 male Syrian golden hamsters [age unspecified] were exposed to 30 ppm [36.9 mg/m^3] formaldehyde [purity unspecified] for 5 h once a week for life. A group of 50 untreated hamster served as controls. When the animals died, their respiratory tract tissues were preserved, stained with Wright's stain, rendered semitransparent and evaluated for 'subgross' evidence of tumours. Areas of dense staining of 1 mm or more were scored as tumours. Multiple transverse sections of the nasal turbinates were evaluated similarly. No nasal tumours were observed in control or treated hamsters (Dalbey, 1982).

3.2   Oral administration

Rat

In a study to evaluate the effects of formaldehyde on gastric carcinogenesis induced by oral administration of N-methyl-N'-nitro-N-nitrosoguanidine (MNNG) (see Section 3.4.2), two groups of 10 male Wistar rats, 7 weeks of age, received tap-water for the first 8 weeks of the study. During weeks 8–40, one group was continued on tap-water and the other group received 0.5% formaldehyde [purity unspecified] in the drinking-water. Animals that were still alive at 40 weeks were killed; rats that survived beyond 30 weeks were considered as effective animals for the study. Necropsy was performed on most animals that died and all animals that were killed, and the stomach and other abdominal organs were examined grossly and histologically. Eight of 10 animals that had received formaldehyde in the drinking-water and none of the controls developed forestomach papillomas ($p < 0.01$, Fisher's exact test) (Takahashi *et al.*, 1986).

Wistar rats, obtained at 5 weeks of age and acclimatized for 9 days, were divided into four groups of 70 males and 70 females and were treated for up to 24 months with drinking-water that contained formaldehyde generated from 95% pure paraformaldehyde and 5% water. The mean doses of formaldehyde were 0, 1.2, 15 or 82 mg/kg bw per day for males and 0, 1.8, 21 or 109 mg/kg bw per day for females. Selected animals were killed at 53 and 79 weeks, and all surviving animals were killed at 105 weeks. Thorough necropsies were performed on all animals. Extensive histological examinations were made of animals in the control and high-dose groups; somewhat less extensive examinations were made of animals that received the low and middle doses, but the liver, lung, stomach and nose were examined in each case. Treatment-related atrophy, ulceration and hyper-plastic lesions were found in the forestomachs and glandular stomachs, but the incidence of tumours did not vary notably between groups. Two benign gastric papillomas were observed (one in a male at the low dose and the other in a female control). The authors noted that the other tumours observed were common in this strain of rat and that there was no indication of a treatment-related tumour response (Til *et al.*, 1989).

Two groups of male and female Sprague-Dawley breeder rats, 25 weeks of age, were given 0 (20 males and 20 females) or 2500 (18 males and 18 females) ppm formaldehyde [purity unspecified] in the drinking-water for life. The offspring of these breeders were ini-tially exposed transplacentally to 0 (59 males and 49 females) or 2500 ppm (36 males and 37 females) formaldehyde via their mothers beginning on day 13 of gestation and then received the same levels in the drinking-water for life. [The Working Group noted the lack of information on selection of the offspring.] All animals were necropsied and subjected to histopathological examination. The survival rates in the treated groups were similar to those of controls. According to the authors, the preliminary results of this study showed a slight, statistically non-significant increase in the incidence of leukaemias (including haemolymphoreticular lymphomas) in male and female breeders exposed to formaldehyde. A statistically non-significant increase in the incidence of leukaemias was also reported in the exposed male, but not in the exposed female, offspring (see Table 28). The authors also reported a variety of malignant and benign tumours of the stomach and intestines in the treated animals (see Table 28). Leiomyosarcoma was the most frequent malignant tumour. [The incidence of leiomysarcomas in the intestines was statistically significantly increased in the exposed offspring, both in females and in males and females combined; $p \leq 0.01$, χ^2 test.] This gastrointestinal tumour was exceptionally rare in the historical controls of this laboratory (Soffritti *et al.*, 1989). Concerns about the results by Soffritti *et al.* (1989) and their interpretation were published by Feron *et al.* (1990). One concern was that incidences of leukaemia in untreated Sprague-Dawley rats vary widely and that incidences similar to those seen in the group that received formaldehyde have been reported previously among controls in the same laboratory and in others.

Seven groups of 50 male and 50 female Sprague-Dawley rats, 7 weeks of age, received 10, 50, 100, 500, 1000 or 1500 mg/L formaldehyde (purity > 99.0%; 0.3% methanol as stabilizer; impurities: 0.6 mg/L iron, 0.1 mg/L lead, < 5.0 mg/L sulfur and < 5.0 mg/L chlorine) or 15 mg/L methanol in the drinking-water for 104 weeks. A control group of 100 males and 100 females received tap-water alone. By week 163, all animals had died. The consumption of treated drinking-water decreased in males of the high-dose group and in females of the three highest-dose groups (approximately 30% according to Soffritti *et al.*, 1989). No differences between treated and control animals were observed in food consumption, body weight or survival. Moreover, no treatment-related non-neoplastic changes were detected by gross or histopathological examination. Percentages of animals that had malignant tumours and incidences of major tumours are presented in Table 29. Tumour incidences in the treated groups were compared with those in the untreated control group and statistically significantly increases were found in the number of males that had malignant tumours in the high-dose group, and in the incidences of malignant mammary gland tumours in females in the 1500-mg/L group, of testicular interstitial-cell adenomas in the 1000-mg/L group and of haemolymphoreticular tumours in males in the four highest- and in females in the two highest-dose groups. According to the authors, there was a dose–response relationship [no statistics given] for the increased incidences of haemolymphoreticular tumours. Gastrointestinal leiomyomas and leiomyosarcomas, which are very rare tumours in the strain of rats used, occurred sporadically in some formaldehyde-treated animals but not in controls (Soffritti *et al.*, 2002). [The Working Group performed statistical analyses for trend and incidence in comparison with the methanol-treated group and found that the only statistically significant increases were in the total number of animals that had malignant tumours ($p < 0.01$) and in the incidences of haemolymphoreticular tumours ($p < 0.01$) in high-dose males and of testicular interstitial-cell adenomas ($p < 0.01$)

Table 28. Incidences (%) of leukaemia and tumours (benign and malignant) of the gastrointestinal tract after administration of formaldehyde in the drinking-water to Sprague-Dawley breeder rats and their offspring

Treatment	No. of rats	Leukaemias				Stomach			Intestine		
		Lymphoblastic leukaemias and lymphosarcomas	Immunoblastic lymphosarcomas	Others	Total	Papilloma/ acanthoma/ adenoma	Adeno-carcinoma/ squamous-cell carcinoma	Leiomyo-sarcoma	Adenoma	Adeno-carcinoma	Leiomyo-sarcoma
Breeders (25 weeks old)											
0 ppm											
Male	20	–	–	–	–	–	–	–	–	–	–
Female	20	5.0	–	–	5.0	–	–	–	–	–	–
Male + female	40	2.5	–	–	2.5	–	–	–	–	–	–
2500 ppm											
Male	18	–	5.6	5.6	11.1	–	5.6	–	–	–	–
Female	18	5.6	5.6	–	11.1	5.6	–	–	–	–	–
Male + female	36	2.8	5.6	2.8	11.1	2.8	2.8	–	–	–	–
Offspring											
0 ppm											
Male	59	–	3.4	1.7	5.1	–	–	–	–	–	–
Female	49	–	4.1	2.0	6.1	–	–	–	–	–	–
Male + female	108	–	3.7	1.8	5.5	–	–	–	–	–	–
2500 ppm											
Male	36	2.8	8.2	–	11.1	2.8	2.8	2.8	2.8	2.8	–
Female	37	–	–	–	–	–	2.7	2.7	–	2.7	13.5[a]
Male + female	73	1.4	4.1	–	5.5	1.4	2.8	2.7	1.4	2.7	6.8[a]

From Soffritti et al. (1989)

[a] $p \leq 0.01$; χ^2 test, calculated by the Working Group

Table 29. Percentage of animals that had malignant tumours and incidence of selected types of tumour in a number of organs of Sprague-Dawley rats after administration of formaldehyde in the drinking-water for up to 24 months

Site and type of tumour	Males								Females							
	Formaldehyde dose (mg/L)															
	0	0[a]	10	50	100	500	1000	1500	0	0[a]	10	50	100	500	1000	1500
No. of animals	100	50	50	50	50	50	50	50	100	50	50	50	50	50	50	50
Animals bearing malignant tumours (%)	38	42	28	24	44	48	46	72[b,c]	43	46	40	40	50	38	58	54
Mammary gland																
Adenocarcinoma	1	0	0	0	0	0	0	2	11	14	4	8	16	6	18	22
Fibrosarcoma	0	2	0	0	0	0	0	0	0	0	2	0	4	2	2	0
Liposarcoma	0	0	0	0	2	0	0	0	0	2	0	2	0	4	0	2
Angiosarcoma	0	0	0	0	0	2	0	0	0	0	0	0	0	0	0	0
Total	1	2	0	0	2	2	0	2	11	16	6	10	20	12	20	24[d]
Forestomach																
Leiomyosarcoma	0	0	2	0	0	0	0	0	0	0	0	0	0	0	0	0
Glandular stomach																
Leiomyosarcoma	0	0	0	0	0	0	2	0	0	0	0	0	0	0	0	0
Intestine																
Leiomyoma	0	0	0	0	0	0	0	0	0	0	2	2	0	0	0	6
Leiomyosarcoma	0	0	0	0	0	0	0	4	0	0	0	2	0	0	0	0
Testes																
Interstitial-cell adenoma	10	6	6	12	12	20	24[d,e]	18								
Haemolymphoreticular tissues[f]																
Lymphomas and leukaemias	8	20	8	20	26[b]	24[d]	22[d]	46[b,c,g]	7	10	10	14	16	14	22[d]	20[d]

From Soffritti et al. (2002)

[a] 15 mg/L methanol
[b] $p < 0.01$, χ^2 test, versus untreated controls
[c] [$p < 0.01$, χ^2 test, versus methanol group; calculated by the Working Group]
[d] $p < 0.05$, χ^2 test, versus untreated controls [the Working Group noted that this category is an aggregate of tumours of different cellular origin]
[e] [$p < 0.01$, 2-tail Fisher exact test, versus methanol group; calculated by the Working Group]
[f] Including thymus, spleen and subcutaneous, mesenteric and pancreatic lymph nodes
[g] [$p < 0.01$ for trend, Cochran Armitage; calculated by the Working Group]

in the 1000-mg/L group. There was a statistically significant dose–response relationship for the increased incidences of haemolymphoreticular tumours ($p < 0.01$) in males. The Working Group noted the 'pooling' of lymphomas and leukaemias (designated as haemo-lymphoreticular neoplasias), the lack of reporting of non-neoplastic lesions and the absence of information on incidences of haemolymphoreticular tumours in historical controls.] Preliminary results of this study were published by Soffritti *et al.* (1989). [The Working Group noted that, in spite of the extensive histopathological examinations on which the preliminary data on tumours presented by Soffritti *et al.* (1989) were stated to be based, the reported total number of animals that had haemolymphoreticular neoplasias increased from 79 (Soffritti *et al.*, 1989) to 150 (Soffritti *et al.*, 2002).]

3.3   Dermal application

Mouse

In a study to evaluate the effects of formaldehyde on skin carcinogenesis induced by 7,12-dimethylbenz[*a*]anthracene (DMBA) (see Section 3.4.1), two groups of 16 male and 16 female Oslo hairless mice [age unspecified] received topical applications of 200 μL aqueous solution of 1 or 10% formaldehyde on the skin of the back twice a week for 60 weeks. Animals were observed weekly for skin tumours. All of the animals treated with 10% formaldehyde were necropsied and the brain, lungs, nasal cavities and all tumours of the skin and other organs were examined histologically. Virtually no changes were found in the mice treated with 1% formaldehyde. The 10% dose induced slight epi-dermal hyperplasia and a few skin ulcers. No benign or malignant skin tumours or tumours in other organs were observed in either group (Iversen, 1986). [The Working Group noted that no group treated with water only was included.]

3.4   Administration with known carcinogens and other modifying factors

3.4.1   *Mouse*

Oslo hairless mice [initial number and age unspecified] received a single topical application of 51.2 μg DMBA in 100 μL reagent-grade acetone on the skin of the back. Nine days later, a group of 16 male and 16 female mice received twice-weekly applications of 200 μL 10% formaldehyde in water (technical-grade formalin) on the skin of the back. Another group of 176 mice [sex unspecified] was given no further treatment. Animals were observed weekly for skin tumours for 60 weeks (first group) or 80 weeks (second group). All of the animals treated with 10% formaldehyde were necropsied, and the brain, lungs, nasal cavities and all tumours of the skin and other organs were examined histologically. In the first group, 3/32 mice had lung adenomas and 11/32 (34%) had 25 skin tumours, including three squamous-cell carcinomas and 22 papillomas. In mice that received DMBA alone, 225 skin tumours (including six squamous-cell carcinomas) occurred in 85/176 (48%) animals. Statistical analysis of the results for these two groups showed that formaldehyde significantly enhanced the rate of skin tumour induction ($p = 0.01$, Peto's test), and reduced the latency period for the tumours (Iversen, 1986). [The Working Group noted the incomplete reporting of the tumours in the group of rats treated with DMBA alone.]

3.4.2   Rat

Two groups of 30 and 21 male Wistar rats, 7 weeks of age, received 100 mg/L MNNG in the drinking-water and a standard diet that contained 10% sodium chloride for 8 weeks. Thereafter, the rats received the standard diet and 0 or 0.5% formaldehyde in the drinking-water for a further 32 weeks. Animals still alive at 40 weeks were killed, and rats that survived 30 weeks or more were considered as effective animals for the study. Necropsies were performed on most animals that died and on all animals that were killed at week 40. Malignant tumours of the stomach and duodenum were found in 4/30 (13%) rats that received MNNG and in 5/17 (29%) rats that received both MNNG and formaldehyde [not significant]. Adenocarcinomas of the glandular stomach were found in 4/17 (23.5%) rats that received the combined treatment and in 1/30 rats that received MNNG alone ($p < 0.05$, Fisher's exact test). Papillomas of the forestomach were found in 15/17 rats that received the combined treatment and in 0/30 that received MNNG alone ($p < 0.01$, Fisher's exact test). The incidence of adenomatous hyperplasia of the fundus of the glandular stomach was significantly greater in the group that received the combined treatment (15/17) than in those that received MNNG alone (0/30) ($p < 0.01$, Fisher's exact test) (Takahashi *et al.*, 1986).

Groups of 50 female white non-inbred rats [strain and age not specified] received intra-tracheal injections of one of three doses of benzo[*a*]pyrene as a suspension in 5% albumin in saline once every 2 weeks for 20 weeks (total doses, 0, 0.02, 0.1 or 5.0 mg/animal). One group of 50 female rats served as an untreated control. All benzo[*a*]pyrene-treated groups were then exposed by inhalation to 0, 0.003, 0.03 or 0.3 mg/m³ formaldehyde for 7 h per day on 5 days per week for 12 months. All animals were maintained until natural death, and organs and tissues that were suspected to have developed a tumour were subjected to histological examination. Tumours developed in rats of all 16 groups. Two of 39 effective (survived to the time of the first tumour development) rats in the control group developed reticulosarcomas of the lung and two developed fibroadenomas of the mammary gland. Similar tumours were observed at almost the same incidence in rats exposed to the three doses of formaldehyde alone. The incidence of total tumours in benzo[*a*]pyrene-treated rats was dose-dependent and varied from 13 to 28%. The incidence of lung tumours varied from 9 to 19%. In the mid- and high-dose groups, squamous-cell cysts and carcinomas of the lung were observed as well as lymphatic leukaemia. The tumour response to the combined treatment with benzo[*a*]pyrene and formaldehyde was also dose-dependent. The most prominent and statistically significant increase in the incidence of lung tumours (43%) and all tumours (69%) occurred in rats that were treated with the highest doses of benzo[*a*]pyrene and formaldehyde (5.0 mg and 0.3 mg/m³, respectively). In addition, tumours developed earlier in this group and had greater multiplicity than those in animals that were exposed to benzo[*a*]pyrene or formaldehyde alone. The authors concluded that the combined treatment of rats with benzo[*a*]pyrene and formaldehyde leads to an increase in tumour response which is manifested as an increased incidence of tumours, a reduction in the latency period of tumour development and a broader spectrum of tumours (Yanysheva *et al.*, 1998). [The Working Group noted the very low level of exposure to formaldehyde compared with levels used in other experiments in rats.]

3.4.3   *Hamster*

Groups of male Syrian golden hamsters [age unspecified] were treated in various ways: 50 were exposed by inhalation to 30 ppm [36.9 mg/m^3] formaldehyde [purity unspecified] for 5 h per day once a week for life; 100 hamsters were injected subcutaneously with 0.5 mg *N*-nitrosodiethylamine (NDEA) once a week for 10 weeks and then given no further treatment; 50 hamsters were injected with NDEA once a week for 10 weeks, exposed to 30 ppm formaldehyde for 5 h, 48 h before each injection of NDEA, and then received weekly exposure to 30 ppm formaldehyde for life; and the fifth group of [presumably] 50 hamsters was injected with NDEA once a week for 10 weeks and then exposed to 30 ppm formaldehyde for 5 h per day once a week for life, beginning 2 weeks after the last injection of NDEA. A group of 50 animals served as untreated controls. After the animals had died, the respiratory tract tissues were removed, stained with Wright's stain, rendered semitransparent and evaluated for 'subgross' evidence of tumours. Areas of dense staining greater than 1 mm in 2–3-mm transverse-step sections of nasal turbinates were scored as tumours. No tumours were observed in untreated hamsters or those exposed only to formaldehyde, but 77% of hamsters treated with NDEA alone had tumours at one or more sites in the respiratory tract. Ten or more such lesions from each tissue were examined histologically, and all were found to be adenomas. Lifetime exposure of NDEA-treated hamsters to formaldehyde did not increase the number of tumour-bearing animals. The incidences of nasal tumours in NDEA-treated groups were low (0–2%). The only significant increase was in the multiplicity of tracheal tumours in the group that received formaldehyde concurrently with and subsequent to injections of NDEA compared with that in animals that received NDEA alone ($p < 0.05$, Kolmogorov–Smirnoff test) (Dalbey, 1982).

4. Other Data Relevant to an Evaluation of Carcinogenicity and its Mechanisms

4.1   Absorption, distribution, metabolism and excretion

4.1.1   *Toxicokinetics*

(*a*)   *Humans*

In humans, as in other animals, formaldehyde is an essential metabolic intermediate in all cells. It is produced endogenously from serine, glycine, methionine and choline, and it is generated in the demethylation of *N*-, *O*- and *S*-methyl compounds. It is an essential intermediate in the biosynthesis of purines, thymidine and certain amino acids (Neuberger, 1981).

The endogenous concentration of formaldehyde, determined by GC–MS (Heck *et al.*, 1982), in the blood of human subjects not exposed to formaldehyde was 2.61 ± 0.14 µg/g blood (mean ± standard error [SE]; range, 2.05–3.09 µg/g) (Heck *et al.*, 1985), i.e. about 0.1 mmol/L (assuming that 90% of the blood volume is water and the density of human blood is 1.06 g/cm^3 (Smith *et al.*, 1983)). This concentration represents the total concentration of both free and reversibly bound endogenous formaldehyde in the blood.

The concentration of formaldehyde measured in the blood of six human volunteers immediately after exposure by inhalation to 1.9 ppm [2.3 mg/m^3] for 40 min was 2.77 ± 0.28 µg/g, which did not differ from the pre-exposure concentration due to metabolically formed formaldehyde (see above). The absence of an increase is explained by the fact that formaldehyde reacts rapidly at the site of contact and is swiftly metabolized by human erythrocytes (Malorny *et al.*, 1965), which contain formaldehyde dehydrogenase (FDH) (Uotila & Koivusalo, 1987) and aldehyde dehydrogenase (ALDH) (Inoue *et al.*, 1979).

Overton *et al.* (2001) developed a mathematical model to predict interactions of formaldehyde in the respiratory tract, based on a one-dimensional equation of mass transport to each generation of an adult human, symmetric, bifurcating Weibel-type respiratory tract anatomical model, augmented by an upper respiratory tract. This predicted that over 95% of inhaled formaldehyde would be retained by the respiratory tract and that the flux is over 1000 times higher in the first tracheobronchial region compared with the first pulmonary region with no flux in the alveolar sacs.

A GC method was used to examine the urinary excretion of formate by veterinary medical students who were exposed to low concentrations of formaldehyde, in order to determine whether monitoring of formate is a useful biomarker for human exposure to formaldehyde (Gottschling *et al.*, 1984). The average baseline level of formate in the urine of 35 unexposed subjects was 12.5 mg/L, but this varied considerably both within and among subjects (range, 2.4–28.4 mg/L). No significant changes in concentration were detected over a 3-week period of exposure to formaldehyde at a concentration in air of less than 0.5 ppm [0.61 mg/m^3]. The authors concluded that biological monitoring of formic acid in the urine to determine exposure to formaldehyde is not a feasible technique at this concentration.

(b) Experimental systems

(i) In vivo

The steady-state concentrations of endogenous formaldehyde have been determined by GC–MS (Heck *et al.*, 1982) in the blood of Fischer 344 rats (2.24 ± 0.07 µg/g of blood (mean ± SE)) (Heck *et al.*, 1985) and three rhesus monkeys (2.04 ± 0.40 µg/g of blood; range, 1.24–2.45 µg/g) (Casanova *et al.*, 1988). These concentrations are similar to those measured in humans by the same method (see Section 4.1.1(*a*)). The blood concentrations of formaldehyde immediately after a single exposure of rats to 14.4 ppm [17.6 mg/m^3] (for 2 h) or subacute exposure of monkeys to 6 ppm [7.3 mg/m^3] (for 6 h per day on 5 days per week for 4 weeks) were indistinguishable from those before exposure.

More than 93% of a dose of inhaled formaldehyde was absorbed readily by the tissues of the respiratory tract (Kimbell *et al.*, 2001a). In rats, formaldehyde is absorbed almost entirely in the nasal passages (Chang *et al.*, 1983; Heck *et al.*, 1983). In rhesus monkeys, absorption occurs primarily in the nasal passages but also in the trachea and proximal regions of the major bronchi (Monticello *et al.*, 1989; Casanova *et al.*, 1991). The efficiency and sites of formaldehyde uptake are determined by nasal anatomy, which differs greatly among species (Schreider, 1986). The structure of the nose gives rise to complex airflow patterns, which have been correlated with the location of formaldehyde-induced nasal lesions in both rats and monkeys (Morgan *et al.*, 1991).

The mucocilliary apparatus is an important defence system in the respiratory tract and may provide protection of the underlying epithelium from gases and vapours. Schlosser (1999) performed limiting-case calculations to determine the significance of convective mucus transport and chemical reaction to formaldehyde in rat nasal epithelial mucus. Less than 4.6% of absorbed formaldehyde can be bound to amino groups (serum albumin) after 20 min of exposure; therefore, at the slowest mucus flow rates measured in rats (~1 mm/min), a fluid element of mucus could travel more than 2 cm before binding 5% of the absorbed formaldehyde by which time the element would probably have left the nose (site of toxic response). Given the solubility of formaldehyde in mucus (water) and estimates of total mucus flow, as much as 22–42% of inhaled formaldehyde may be removed by mucus flow.

After exposure by inhalation, absorbed formaldehyde can be oxidized to formate and carbon dioxide or can be incorporated into biological macromolecules via tetrahydro-folate-dependent one-carbon biosynthetic pathways (see Fig. 1). The fate of inhaled formaldehyde was studied in Fischer 344 rats exposed to [^{14}C]formaldehyde (at 0.63 or 13.1 ppm [0.8 or 16.0 mg/m^3]) for 6 h. About 40% of the inhaled ^{14}C was eliminated as

Figure 1. Biological reactions and metabolism of formaldehyde

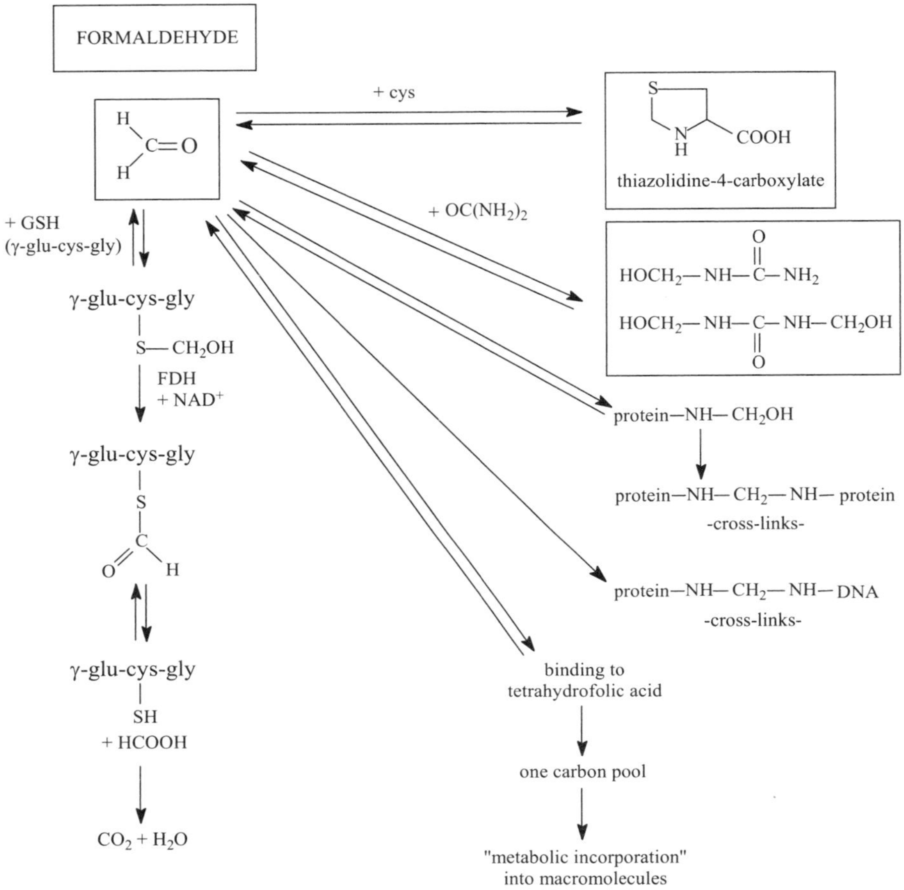

Adapted from Bolt (1987)

expired [^{14}C]carbon dioxide over a 70-h period; 17% was excreted in the urine, 5% was eliminated in the faeces and 35–39% remained in the tissues and carcass. Elimination of radioactivity from the blood of rats after exposure by inhalation to 0.63 ppm or 13.1 ppm [^{14}C]formaldehyde is multiphasic. After inhalation, the terminal half-time of the radioactivity in the plasma was approximately 55 h (Heck *et al.*, 1983). Analysis of the time course of residual radioactivity in plasma and erythrocytes after inhalation or intravenous injection of [^{14}C]formaldehyde or intravenous injection of [^{14}C]formate showed that the radioactivity is due to incorporation of ^{14}C (as [^{14}C]formate) into serum proteins and erythrocytes and subsequent release of labelled proteins and cells into the circulation (Heck *et al.*, 1983). The half-time of formaldehyde in rat plasma after intravenous administration is reported to be approximately 1 min (Rietbrock, 1965).

The fate of [^{14}C]formaldehyde after dermal application to Fischer 344 rats, Dunkin–Hartley guinea-pigs and cynomolgus monkeys was described by Jeffcoat *et al.* (1983). Aqueous formaldehyde was applied to a shaven area of the lower back, and the rodents were placed in metabolism cages for collection of urine, faeces, expired air and [^{14}C]formaldehyde evaporated from the skin. Monkeys were seated in a restraining chair and were fitted with a plexiglass helmet for collection of exhaled [^{14}C]carbon dioxide. The concentrations of ^{14}C in the tissues, blood and carcass of rodents were determined at the end of the experiment. Rodents excreted about 6.6% of the dermally applied dose in the urine over 72 h, while 21–28% was collected in the air traps. It was deduced that almost all of the air-trapped radioactivity was due to evaporation of formaldehyde from the skin, since less than 3% of the radioactivity (i.e. 0.6–0.8% of the applied ^{14}C) was due to [^{14}C]carbon dioxide. Rodent carcass contained 22–28% of the ^{14}C and total blood about 0.1%; a substantial fraction of ^{14}C (3.6–16%) remained in the skin at the site of application. In monkeys, only 0.24% of the dermally applied [^{14}C]formaldehyde was excreted in the urine, and 0.37% was accounted for as [^{14}C]carbon dioxide in the air traps; about 0.015% of the radioactivity was found in total blood and 9.5% in the skin at the site of application. Less than 1% of the applied dose was excreted or exhaled, in contrast to rodents in which nearly 10% was eliminated by these routes. Coupled with the observation of lower blood levels of ^{14}C in monkeys than in rodents, the results suggest that the skin of monkeys may be less permeable to aqueous formaldehyde than that of rodents.

Formaldehyde is absorbed rapidly and almost completely from the rodent intestinal tract (Buss *et al.*, 1964). In rats, about 40% of an oral dose of [^{14}C]formaldehyde (7 mg/kg) was eliminated as [^{14}C]carbon dioxide within 12 h, while 10% was excreted in the urine and 1% in the faeces. A substantial portion of the radioactivity remained in the carcass as products of metabolic incorporation. In another study in which Sprague-Dawley rats were injected intraperitoneally with 4 or 40 mg/kg bw [^{14}C]formaldehyde, a portion of the injected material (about 3–5% of a dose of 40 mg/kg bw) was excreted unchanged in the urine within 12 h (Mashford & Jones, 1982).

(ii)   In vitro

Since formaldehyde can induce allergic contact dermatitis in humans (see Section 4.2.1), it can be concluded that formaldehyde or its metabolites penetrate human skin (Maibach, 1983). The kinetics of this penetration was determined *in vitro* using an excised full-thickness human skin sample mounted in a diffusion cell at 30 °C (Lodén, 1986). The rate of 'resorption' of [^{14}C]formaldehyde (defined as the uptake of ^{14}C into phosphate-buffered saline, pH 7.4, that flowed unidirectionally beneath the sample) was 16.7 µg/cm^2/h when a 3.7% solution of formaldehyde was used, and increased to 319 µg/cm^2/h when a 37% solution was used. The presence of methanol in both of these solutions (at 1–1.5% and 10–15%, respectively) may have affected the rate of uptake, and it is unclear whether the resorbed ^{14}C was due only to formaldehyde. Skin retention of formaldehyde-derived radioactivity represented a significant fraction of the total amount of formaldehyde absorbed.

(iii)   *Predictive models to analyse the effects of formaldehyde in the respiratory tract*

Computational fluid dynamic models

Anatomically accurate, three-dimensional computational fluid dynamics (CFD) models of formaldehyde in the nasal passages of rat, monkeys and humans have been developed to aid the understanding of absorption and mechanisms of action and risk assessment (Conolly *et al.*, 2000; Kimbell *et al.*, 2001a,b; Georgieva *et al.*, 2003). Conolly *et al.* (2000) sought to increase confidence in predictions of human DNA–protein cross-links (see Fig. 1) by refining earlier models of formaldehyde deposition and DNA–protein cross-links in nasal mucosa. Anatomically accurate CFD models of nasal airways of Fischer 344 rats, rhesus monkeys and humans that were designed to predict the regional flux of formaldehyde were linked to a model of tissue disposition of formaldehyde and kinetics of DNA–protein cross-links. Statistical optimization was used to identify parametric values, and good simulations were obtained. The parametric values obtained for rats and monkeys were used to extrapolate mathematically to the human situation. The results showed that the levels of nasal mucosal DNA–protein cross-links in rats, rhesus monkeys and humans varied with the concentration of formaldehyde inhaled and the predicted DNA–protein cross-link dose–response curves for the three species were similar, in spite of the significant interspecies differences in nasal anatomy and breathing rates.

Kimbell *et al.* (2001a) used anatomically accurate three-dimensional CFD models of nasal air flow and transport of formaldehyde gas in Fischer 344 rats, rhesus monkeys and humans to predict local patterns of wall mass flux ($pmol/(mm^2\ h–ppm)$). The nasal surface of each species was partitioned by flux into smaller regions (flux bins), each of which was characterized by surface area and an average flux value. Flux values higher than half the maximum flux value were predicted for nearly 20% of human, 5% of rat and less than 1% of monkey nasal surfaces at resting inspiratory flow rates. Human nasal flux patterns shifted distally and the percentage of uptake decreased as inspiratory flow rate increased.

Kimbell *et al.* (2001b) used anatomically accurate three-dimensional CFD models of nasal passages in Fischer 344 rats, rhesus monkeys and humans to estimate and compare the regional patterns of uptake of inhaled formaldehyde that were predicted among these species. Maximum flux values, averaged over one breath, in non-squamous epithelium were estimated to be 2620, 4492 and 2082 $pmol/(mm^2\ h–ppm)$ in rats, monkeys and humans, respectively. At sites where cell proliferation rates had been measured and found to be similar in rats and monkeys, predicted flux values were also similar, as were predicted fluxes in a region of high tumour incidence in the rat nose and anterior portion of the human nose.

Thermodynamic model: exposure to particle-adsorbed formaldehyde

The possibility that gaseous formaldehyde may be adsorbed to respirable particles, inhaled and subsequently released into the lung has been examined in a thermodynamic model based on measurable physicochemical properties of particles and volatile pollutants. In this model, analysis of the adsorption of formaldehyde to and its release from respirable carbon black particles showed that only 2 ppb [0.0025 mg/m³] of an airborne formaldehyde concentration of 6 ppm [7.4 mg/m³] would be adsorbed to carbon black (Risby *et al.*, 1990).

4.1.2   *Biomonitoring and metabolism of formaldehyde*

(*a*)   *Humans*

(i)   *Biological monitoring*

A quantitative method that was developed for the determination of formaldehyde in biological tissues used stable-isotope dilution combined with GC–MS. Multilabelled form-aldehyde that contained 90 atom-% ^{13}C and 98 atom-% deuterium (^{2}H) was used as the isotopic diluent, which was added to homogenized tissue. Derivatization was conducted *in situ* with pentafluorophenylhydrazine, followed by extraction and analysis of the penta-fluorophenylhydrazone by selected ion monitoring. With this method, endogenous formal-dehyde could be analysed quantitatively in tissue samples as small as 20 mg wet wt (Heck *et al.*, 1982).

Blood

Concentrations of formaldehyde were determined by the method described above in samples of venous blood that were collected before and after exposure of six human volunteers to 1.9 ppm [2.3 mg/m³] formaldehyde by inhalation for 40 min. Average concentrations of formaldehyde were 2.61 ± 0.14 µg/g blood before and 2.77 ± 0.28 µg/g blood after exposure. These values were not significantly different. However, the subjects exhibited significant inter-individual variation with respect to their blood concentrations of formal-dehyde, and some showed significant differences — either an increase or a decrease — before and after exposure, which suggests that individual blood concentrations of formal-dehyde vary with time. The results are consistent with the assumption that toxicity due to exposure to formaldehyde is unlikely to occur at sites that are distant from the portal of entry (Heck *et al.*, 1985). The absence of an exposure-related increase in blood concentration of formaldehyde in this study can be explained by the fact this chemical is rapidly metabolized by human erythrocytes (Malorny *et al.*, 1965), which contain FDH (Uotila & Koivusalo, 1987) and ALDH (Inoue *et al.*, 1979) (see also Section 4.1.1(*a*)).

DNA–protein cross-links in blood leukocytes were used as a marker for exposure to formaldehyde in a study that involved 12 workers (Anatomy Department and Pathology Institute; duration of exposure, 2–31 years) and eight controls. Protein-bound DNA was separated from protein-free DNA by precipitation with sodium dodecylsulfate (Zhitkovich & Costa, 1992). A significantly higher ($p = 0.03$) level of cross-links was measured among exposed workers (mean ± SD, 28 ± 5%; min., 21%; max., 38%) than among the unexposed controls (mean ± SD, 22 ± 6%; min., 16%; max., 32%). Of the 12 exposed workers, four (33%) showed cross-link values above the upper range of the controls. The level of cross-links was generally higher in workers exposed for longer periods, and was reported not to be influenced by tobacco smoking. The data suggest that

DNA–protein cross-links can be used as a method for the biological monitoring of exposure to formaldehyde (Shaham *et al.*, 1996a).

Urine

Exposure to formaldehyde was monitored in a group of 35 students of veterinary medicine who were enrolled for 3 consecutive weeks in a functional anatomy class, where they worked extensively with animal tissue preserved in formalin. The biological monitoring was based on the known metabolism of formaldehyde to formic acid, which may then be excreted in the urine. Urinary formic acid was converted to methyl formate and measured by GC. The average concentration of formate in the urine of the subjects before the class was 12.5 mg/L, and considerable variation was observed both within and among subjects (range, 2.4–28.4 mg/L). No significant changes in concentration were detected over the 3-week period of exposure to formaldehyde at a concentration in air of < 0.4 ppm [0.5 mg/m^3]. Biological monitoring of exposure to formaldehyde by measurement of urinary formic acid does not appear to be a suitable method at these levels of exposure (Gottschling *et al.*, 1984) (see also Section 4.1.1(*a*)).

Respiratory tract: animal models and extrapolation to humans

The pharmacokinetics of formaldehyde-induced formation of DNA–protein cross-links in the nose was investigated by use of a model in which the rate of formation is proportional to the tissue concentration of this chemical. The model includes both saturable and non-saturable elimination pathways and regional differences in DNA binding are attributed to anatomical rather than biochemical factors. Using this model, the concentration of DNA–protein cross-links formed in corresponding tissues of different species can be predicted by scaling the pharmacokinetic parameter that depends on minute volume and quantity of nasal mucosal DNA. The concentration–response curve for the average rate of formation of cross-links in the turbinates, lateral wall and septum of rhesus monkeys was predicted from that of Fischer 344 rats that were exposed under similar conditions. A significant overlap was observed between predicted and fitted curves, which implies that minute volume and nasal mucosal DNA are major determinants of the rate of formation of DNA–protein cross-links in the nasal mucosa of different species. Concentrations of DNA–protein cross-links that may be produced in the nasal mucosa of adult humans were predicted on the basis of experimental data in rats and monkeys. The authors suggested from their results that formaldehyde would generate lower concentrations of DNA–protein cross-links in the nasal mucosa of humans than that of monkeys, and much lower concentrations in humans than in rats. The rate of formation of DNA–protein cross-links can be regarded as a surrogate for the delivered concentration of formaldehyde (Casanova *et al.*, 1991).

(ii)   *Metabolism of formaldehyde*

Formaldehyde is an endogenous metabolic product of *N*-, *O*- and *S*-demethylation reactions in the cell (Neuberger, 1981). During exogenous exposure, gaseous formaldehyde — which is highly soluble in water — is virtually completely removed by the nose during nasal respiration (Ballenger, 1984). In recent years, the metabolic capacities of nasal cavity tissues have been investigated extensively in mammals, including humans. ALDHs, cytochrome P450 (CYP)-dependent monooxygenases, glutathione (GSH) transferases (GSTs), epoxide hydrolases, flavin-containing monooxygenases and carboxyl esterases have all been reported to occur in substantial quantities in the nasal cavity. The contributions of some of these enzyme activities to the induction of toxic effects from volatile chemicals have been the subject of numerous studies (see reviews by Dahl & Hadley, 1991; Thornton-Manning & Dahl, 1997). The two main enzymes involved in the metabolism of formaldehyde in humans — a dehydrogenase and a hydrolase — are discussed in detail below.

Formaldehyde is detoxified by oxidation to formate by different enzyme systems (Fig. 2; from Hedberg *et al.*, 2002). The primary and generally most important system initially involves GSH-dependent FDH (Uotila & Koivusalo, 1974), which is identical to alcohol dehydrogenase 3 (ADH3; Koivusalo *et al.*, 1989), that oxidizes *S*-hydroxymethyl-glutathione (the thiohemiacetal that is formed spontaneously from formaldehyde and GSH) to *S*-formylglutathione. The systematic name for the enzyme is formaldehyde:NAD+ oxidoreductase (glutathione-formylating) (CAS Registry No. 9028-84-6, IUBMB code EC1.2.1.1). (Other names for this enzyme are formaldehyde dehydrogenase, formaldehyde dehydrogenase (glutathione), NAD-linked formaldehyde dehydrogenase and formic dehydrogenase.) This intermediate is then further metabolized by *S*-formylglutathione

Figure 2. Fate and metabolism of formaldehyde

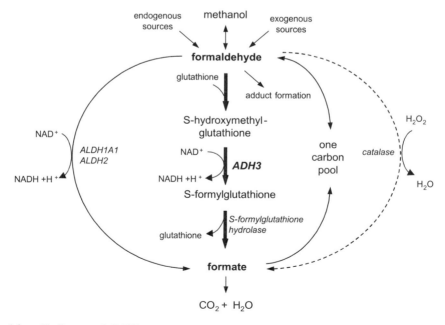

Adapted from Hedberg *et al.* (2002)

hydrolase to yield formate and reduced GSH (Uotila & Koivusalo, 1997). Analyses across species and among various mammalian tissues and cell types imply that ADH3 represents a ubiquitous enzyme, and that it is the ancestral form of ADH from which other types of vertebrate ADH have evolved (Estonius *et al.*, 1996; Hedberg *et al.*, 2000; Jörnvall *et al.*, 2000; Hedberg *et al.*, 2001; Höög *et al.*, 2001, 2003). The activities of ADH3 are two to three orders of magnitude lower than those of *S*-formylglutathione hydrolase and thus the ADH3-catalysed step is rate-limiting (Uotila & Koivusalo, 1997). Formation of *S*-hydroxymethylglutathione efficiently counteracts the existence of free formaldehyde, a reaction that is determined by the fact that cellular GSH is an abundant molecule and is often present in millimolar concentration levels (Meister & Anderson, 1983). The equilibrium constant (K_{eq}) for the formation of this adduct — under conditions of excess GSH — was determined to be 1.77 ± 0.13 mM (Naylor *et al.*, 1988; Sanghani *et al.*, 2000). Furthermore, when formaldehyde is reacted with the thiols, cysteine and cysteinylglycine, it can function as an alternative substrate to *S*-hydroxymethylglutathione for ADH3, but at a far lower turnover (Holmquist & Vallee, 1991). The mechanism for the ADH3-dependent step is identical to any alcohol oxidation by ADH enzymes; it requires catalysis by zinc and uses NAD$^+$/NADH as the electron acceptor and donor, respectively (Höög *et al.*, 2001). The second enzyme system is the ALDHs — class 1 (cytosolic ALDH; ALDH1A1) and class 2 (mitochondrial ALDH; ALDH2) — which have an affinity for free formaldehyde. Because the Michaelis-Menten constant (K_m) is less than micromolar for aldehyde substrates, they are called low-K_m ALDHs (Petersen & Lindahl, 1997), except for free formaldehyde for which the K_m values are high (in the range of 0.6 mM; Mukerjee & Pietruszko, 1992). This value is about 100-fold higher than the K_m displayed by ADH3 for *S*-hydroxymethylglutathione (4 µM) (Holmquist & Vallee, 1991; Uotila & Koivusalo, 1997; Hedberg *et al.*, 1998). Therefore, ADH3 is probably the predominant enzyme responsible for the oxidation of formaldehyde at physiologically relevant concentrations, while low-K_m ALDHs contribute increasingly when the concentrations of formaldehyde increase (Dicker & Cederbaum, 1986). Catalase may also contribute to the oxidation of formaldehyde to formate, but only under circumstances in which hydrogen peroxide is formed (Jones *et al.*, 1978; Uotila & Koivusalo, 1989). Formaldehyde may also be reduced to methanol and then be re-converted to formaldehyde, when ADH1 is involved (Pocker & Li, 1991). Many endogenous and exogenous factors can contribute to the generation of formaldehyde in cells (Grafström, 1990). Both formaldehyde and formate contribute to the 'one-carbon pool', which involves the folic acid metabolic pathway for synthesis of certain nucleic acids and amino acids, and, eventually, cellular macromolecules (Neuberger, 1981). *S*-Hydroxymethylglutathione and *S*-formylglutathione are among the most notable components of this pool, which also includes the tetrahydrofolate adducts, N^5-hydroxymethyl-, N^5,N^{10}-methylene, and N^5- and N^{10}-formyl-tetrahydrofolate, serine, methionine, histamine and methylamine, other reversible amine adducts and hydrated formaldehyde.

ADH3 is the only ADH that can participate in the cellular detoxification of formaldehyde. The nomenclature recommended by Duester *et al.* (1999) defines the protein as

ADH3 and the gene as *ADH3*, whereas previous nomenclature used χ (chi) for the protein and *ADH5* for the gene (Jörnvall & Höög, 1995). The older nomenclature used *ADH3* to define the gene that codes for *ADH1C*, which is important for the oxidation of ethanol, and studies of the latter protein, including the role of polymorphisms in the causation of cancer (Schwartz *et al.*, 2001; Yokoyama *et al.*, 2002), should not be confused with the enzyme that is involved in the oxidation of formaldehyde. *S*-Nitrosoglutathione consti-tutes an excellent substrate for reductive cleavage by ADH3, and, accordingly, ADH3 is also termed *S*-nitrosoglutathione reductase (Jensen *et al.*, 1998; Liu *et al.*, 2001). Com-parative analysis indicates that ADH3 oxidizes GSH-conjugated formaldehyde (i.e. *S*-hydroxymethylglutathione) and reduces *S*-nitrosoglutathione with catalytic efficiencies of 58 000 $min^{-1}.mM^{-1}$ and 90 000 $min^{-1}.mM^{-1}$, respectively (Hedberg *et al.*, 2003). Con-sidering both reactions, exposure to formaldehyde would naturally favour the oxidant activity of ADH3, whereas nitrosative stress leading to the formation of *S*-nitrosogluta-thione would favour reductive activity (Liu *et al.*, 2001; Hedberg *et al.*, 2003). The cellular levels of NAD^+ are normally two orders of magnitude higher than those of NADH and thus, under physiological conditions, the oxidation of *S*-hydroxymethylglutathione would be favoured rather than the reduction of *S*-nitrosoglutathione (Svensson *et al.*, 1999; Molotkov *et al.*, 2002; Höög *et al.*, 2003). Although it has a lower efficiency than other ADH enzymes, ADH3 also mediates oxidation of all-*trans*-retinol to retinal, and may also oxidize ethanol to acetaldehyde at levels of exposure that are reached during alcohol intoxication (Svensson *et al.*, 1999; Molotkov *et al.*, 2003). ADH3 also shows oxidizing activity towards longer-chain primary alcohols, methylglyoxal, ketoxal, hydroxypyruvaldehyde, 20-hydroxy-leukotriene B_4 and ω-hydroxy fatty acids, e.g. 12-hydroxydodecanoic acid (Wagner *et al.*, 1984; Gotoh *et al.*, 1990; Jörnvall *et al.*, 2000).

The physiological relevance of these activities remains unclear, since the catalytic effi-ciencies for these substrates are considerably lower than those of *S*-hydroxymethylgluta-thione and *S*-nitrosoglutathione. However, all of these substrates compete with *S*-hydroxy-methylglutathione and *S*-nitrosoglutathione for the active site of ADH3, and thereby influence the catalytic activity for formaldehyde scavenging. The *ADH3* gene promoter sequence shows several polymorphisms that might influence *ADH3* transcription, but such polymorphisms were not observed in exons that code for the *ADH3* gene (Hedberg *et al.*, 2001). In contrast, polymorphisms in *ALDH*, including *ALDH2*, may reduce the capacity for the oxidation of formaldehyde to less than half of that of the wild-type activity (Wang *et al.*, 2002). Transcription of *ADH3* is coupled to proliferative states in human oral kera-tinocytes where *ADH3* mRNA exhibits a short half-life (7 h); when the protein is formed, it remains highly stable and metabolically active during cellular life expectancy (Hedberg *et al.*, 2000; Nilsson *et al.*, 2004). Formaldehyde and *S*-hydroxymethylglutathione regulate *ADH3* transcription in the bacterium *Rhodobacter sphaeriodes*, and wounding and growth hormones regulate ADH3 in the plant *Arabidopsis*, which provides examples of ADH3 regulation through feed-back control and from both external and internal signals (Barber & Donohue, 1998; Diaz *et al.*, 2003). [The Working Group did not find evidence of such regulation in humans.] The biochemistry that underlies the metabolism of formaldehyde indicates that changes in glutathione levels, NAD^+:NADH ratios, other redox changes and oxidant stress in general, including from nitric oxide and S-nitrosoglutathione, protein S-nitrosothiols and intermediates of the folic acid metabolic pathway should be considered in the assessment of the consequences of exposure to formaldehyde.

(b)   Experimental systems

The distribution of selected metabolizing enzymes in the respiratory tract was compared with that in the liver of beagle dogs. Four beagle dogs (two males, two females; 13–18 kg, 13–130 months of age) were euthanized, the liver and respiratory tract were removed and tissues were prepared for isolation of metabolizing enzymes, including infusion of cold agarose into a lung lobe. The respiratory tract was separated into respiratory nasal epithelium, olfactory nasal epithelium, tracheal epithelium, epithelium from proximal middle and distal bronchus and lung parenchyma. The cytosolic fraction was isolated and the activity of sulfite oxidase, ADH, ALDH, FDH, GST and protein contents were quantified. Sulfite oxidase with sulfite as the substrate had greatest activity in the liver (9.95 nkat/mg protein); in the respiratory tract, the greatest activity was in the lung parenchyma (4.62 nkat/mg protein) and activity in the rest of the respiratory tract was below 4 nkat/mg protein. FDH with formaldehyde as the substrate had greatest activity in the nose (10.5 nkat/mg protein) while the liver (2.28 nkat/mg protein) had less activity than any site in the respiratory tract. ALDH with formaldehyde as the substrate had greatest activity in the trachea (1.28 nkat/mg protein), and the rest of the respiratory tract and liver had levels of activity below 1 nkat/mg protein. ADH with ethanol as the substrate had greatest activity in the liver (4.40 nkat/mg protein), and the respiratory tract had levels below 1 nkat/mg protein. All but one of the 1-chloro-2,4-dinitrobenzene-related GSTs had greatest activity in the liver parenchyma, which ranged from 50 to 300% greater than that in the respiratory tract. The cytosolic fraction of the epoxy-3-(*para*-nitrophenoxy)-propane-related GST had greatest activity in the trachea (3.94 nkat/mg protein); activity in the liver (0.24 nkat/mg protein) was less than 20% of that in any part of the respiratory tract on average. In general, metabolizing enzymes are spread throughout the respiratory tract and can have a metabolic capacity the same as or greater than the liver (Maier *et al.*, 1999).

4.2   Toxic effects

4.2.1   Humans

(a)   Irritation

There is extensive literature on domestic exposures to products that contain formaldehyde, such as plywood, and to urea–formaldehyde foam (see Section 1). Irritative effects have consistently been reported after exposure to formaldehyde; these have also been observed in children and a wide variation in susceptibility has been reported. Because these domestic exposures also involve exposure to other agents, this literature is not reviewed in detail here because the findings do not generally add any information on the specific mode of action of formaldehyde as a potential carcinogen.

(i)   *Experimental studies of acute effects*

Airborne formaldehyde irritates the eyes, nose and throat in healthy humans who had clinical disease. Chamber studies and the symptoms reported therein are summarized in Table 30.

Dose–response irritative effects were investigated (Kulle *et al.*, 1987; Kulle, 1993) in nonsmokers who received 3-h exposures to 0, 0.5, 1, 2 and 3 ppm [0, 0.61, 1.22, 2.44 and 3.66 mg/m^3] formaldehyde. The results are shown in Figure 3. Eye irritation increased linearly at doses of 0.5–3 ppm and was the dominant symptom; no effect was observed with 0.5 ppm; 21% of the volunteers had mild eye irritation with 1 ppm and 35% with 2 ppm. Of the volunteers, 40% could smell formaldehyde at 0.5 ppm (5% when no formaldehyde was present). Nose and/or throat irritation was the least sensitive response with an estimated threshold of 1 ppm.

Adult asthmatics

Green *et al.* (1987) exposed 22 healthy subjects and 16 asthmatics to 3 ppm formaldehyde for 1 h during exercise. In the healthy group, 32% of the subjects reported moderate-to-severe nose and throat irritation and 27% moderate-to-severe eye irritation. In the asthmatics, these percentages were 31% and 19%, respectively.

Unsensitized adult asthmatics

The effects of inhaled formaldehyde on the airways of healthy people and unsensitized asthmatics have been reviewed (Smedley, 1996; Krieger *et al.*, 1998; Suh *et al.*, 2000; Bender, 2002; Liteplo & Meek, 2003).

Bender (2002) reviewed nine controlled chamber studies of exposure to formaldehyde of asthmatic subjects (Reed & Frigas 1984; Sauder *et al.*, 1986; Green *et al.*, 1987; Kulle *et al.*, 1987; Schachter *et al.*, 1987; Witek *et al.*, 1987; Harving *et al.*, 1990; Pazdrak *et al.*, 1993; Krakowiak *et al.*, 1998). Exposure to 2–3 ppm formaldehyde for up to 3 h did not provoke asthma in unsensitized asthmatics. There was no asthmatic response to 0.1–3 ppm formaldehyde in 11 women and two men who reported chest tightness, cough and wheeze attributed to exposure to formaldehyde at home or at work (Reed & Frigas, 1984). Similar conclusions were reached in the review of Liteplo and Meek (2003) who included three further studies (Day *et al.*, 1984; Schachter *et al.*, 1986; Sauder *et al.*, 1987).

Studies on nasal lavage

Two studies have investigated the effect of exposure to formaldehyde on nasal lavage. Krakowiak *et al.* (1998) reported on 10 healthy subjects and 10 asthmatics who reported nasal or respiratory symptoms from formaldehyde at work (nurses, textile and shoe workers), who received a single, blind exposure to clean air or 0.5 mg/m^3 formaldehyde (range, 0.2–0.7 mg/m^3) for 2 h. Nasal washings were performed before and 0, 0.5, 4 and 24 h after exposure. During exposure to formaldehyde, all subjects developed sneezing,

Table 30. Studies of acute exposure to formaldehyde that reported irritant-type symptoms

Subjects (no.)	Exposure to formaldehyde	Effect	Reference
Normal (22) Asthmatics (16)	3 ppm [3.7 mg/m^3] for 60 min	Moderate/severe symptoms Eye, 27%; nose/throat, 32% Eye, 19%; nose/throat, 31%	Green et al. (1987)
Normal with no exposure (10) Asthmatics with allergic symptoms due to exposure to formaldehyde (10)	0.5 mg/m^3 for 2 h	Scored on 0–7 point scale Nasal itching and congestion in all Score 4.3/7 in normal subjects Score 4.6/7 in asthmatics	Krakowiak et al. (1998)
Healthy nonsmokers (19)	3 ppm for 3 h	See Figure 3	Kulle et al. (1987); Kulle (1993)
Healthy (11) Formaldehyde contact dermatitis (9)	0.5 mg/m^3 [0.41 ppm] for 2 h	Scored on 0–7 point scale (sneezes, nasal itching and congestion) Mean nasal score 4/7 at 10 min for allergic and healthy subjects	Pazdrak et al. (1993)
Healthy nonsmokers (9)	3 ppm for 3 h	Mean symptom scores (air/formaldehyde) Throat/nose, 0.22/1.33 Eye irritation, 0/0.78	Sauder et al. (1986)
Asthmatic nonsmokers (9)	3 ppm for 3 h	Eye and nose irritation started after 2 min	Sauder et al. (1987)
Normal formaldehyde-exposed (15)	2 ppm [2.5 mg/m^3] for 40 min	Odour, 12/15 (80%) Sore throat, 0/15 (0%) Nasal irritation, 0/15 (0%) Eye irritation, 7/15 (47%)	Schachter et al. (1987)
Asthmatics (15)	2 ppm for 40 min	Odour, 15/15 (100%) Sore throat, 5/15 (33%) Nasal irritation, 7/15 (47%) Eye irritation, 11/15 (73%)	Witek et al. (1987)
Normal (9), asthmatics with UFFI symptoms (9)	3 ppm for 2 h (1 ppm for 90 min and 2 ppm UFFI for 30 min)	Eye irritation, 15/18 Nasal congestion, 7/18 Throat irritation, 5/18 Same in UFFI symptomatic and normal groups	Day et al. (1984)

UFFI, urea–formaldehyde foam insulation

Figure 3. Symptoms reported by 19 nonsmoking healthy adults exposed to formaldehyde for 3 h

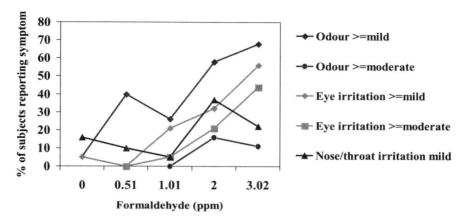

Adapted from Kulle (1993)

itching and congestion, with substantial resolution by 4 h. An increase in total leukocytes and eosinophils was observed immediately after exposure to formaldehyde that was similar in both groups of subjects, with resolution after 4 h. An increase was also observed in the albumin:total protein ratio with a similar time course that was interpreted as an increase in nasal mucosal permeability. No significant increases in tryptase or eosinophil cationic protein were found in either group. An earlier study by the same group (Pazdrak *et al.*, 1993) that used a similar methodology investigated nine workers who had skin hypersensitivity (positive patch test) to formaldehyde and 11 healthy men who had negative formaldehyde patch tests. Nasal lavage was performed at 0, 10 min, 3 (or 4) and 18 h after exposure. Eosinophils increased in the nasal lavage and were maximal immediately after exposure, but were still increased at 4 and 18 h; the percentage of epithelial cells was reduced. Albumin levels were increased in the lavage and albumin:total protein ratios were increased only immediately after exposure. The group that had dermatitis and the normal group had similar responses. The authors concluded that the irritative effects of formaldehyde were confirmed, and also suggested a non-specific, non-allergic pro-inflammatory effect when formaldehyde was inhaled at a low dose (0.5 mg/m^3).

An in-vitro study of human nasal ciliated epithelial cells showed reduced frequency of ciliary beat after exposure to 5000 µg/m^3 formaldehyde for 2 h, but no effect after exposure to 5000 µg/m^3 for 1 h or 500 µg/m^3 for 2 h (Schäfer *et al.*, 1999).

(ii)   *Residential exposure*

Studies have been conducted among residents who were exposed to formaldehyde in the home and school children who were exposed to formaldehyde in classrooms (Broder *et al.*, 1991; Wantke *et al.*, 1996a). These studies are difficult to interpret because they did not control for confounding factors, particularly lack of ventilation and other allergens. It is possible that co-exposures to irritants and allergens increases the risk for allergen sensitization, but this has not been shown reliably for exposures to formaldehyde. Some studies looked for IgG and/or IgE antibodies to formaldehyde/human serum albumin conjugates, but the results were inconsistent (Patterson *et al.*, 1989; Wantke *et al.*, 1996a; Kim *et al.*, 2001; Doi *et al.*, 2003).

(b)   *Pulmonary function: effect of chronic occupational exposure*

Kriebel *et al.* (1993) noted that epidemiological studies of irritants are difficult to perform using standard epidemiological methods because of the reversible nature of the health outcomes, the selection of sensitive individuals from the study population and the wide heterogeneity of normal responses to irritants. Twenty-four physical therapy students, who were exposed to formaldehyde during dissection for 3 h per week over 10 weeks with breathing zone exposures to formaldehyde of 0.49–0.93 ppm, were included in the study. Peak expiratory flow and a symptom questionnaire were completed before and after each exposure, and again before and after 3-h laboratory sessions after several months with no exposure to formaldehyde. Symptoms increased following exposure (eyes, +43%; nose, +21%; throat, +15%; breathing, +20%; and cough, +5%). The intensity of symptoms tended to decrease over time [this might be due to a repeated questionnaire effect with weekly questionnaires]. The peak expiratory flow declined by an average of 4.8 L/min during the morning (pre-dissection to midday) and by 10 L/min before exposure over the 10 weeks of exposure (2% of baseline) with recovery after 12 weeks with no exposure (daily measurements before exposure). The study group included five asthmatics whose peak expiratory flow after exposure fell by 37 L/min (non-asthmatics, 3.9 L/min). [The Working Group noted the lack of controls in this study, to adjust for any seasonal effects over time. The Working Group also noted that this is a difficult study to interpret. The time of day of the dissection sessions is not given, and the peak expiratory flow would be expected to increase for the first 4–10 h after waking, so that the time of day may have affected the outcome of the measurements.]

Akbar-Khanzadeh and Mlynek (1997) compared 50 nonsmoking first-year medical students exposed to breathing zone levels of 1.36–2.58 ppm [1.66–3.2 mg/m^3] formaldehyde with 36 second-year physiotherapy students who had no exposure to formaldehyde. Lung function was measured before exposure, 1 h after exposure and at midday. An increase in lung function was observed in both exposed and unexposed groups during the morning (exposed forced expiry volume in 1 sec (FEV$_1$), +1.2%; control, +2.1% at 1 h; exposed FEV$_1$, + 2.4%; control, +6.2% at 3 h). In the exposed group, 82% reported nose irritation, 76% reported eye irritation (18% wore goggles), 36% reported throat irritation and 14% reported airway irritation. The authors concluded that the reduced increase in lung function during the morning in the exposed group was probably due to the exposure to formaldehyde.

The same group reported a similar study of 34 medical students and instructors who were exposed to 0.07–2.94 ppm (mean, 1.24 ppm) [0.08–3.6 mg/m^3 (mean, 1.22 mg/m^3)]

formaldehyde and 12 control students and instructors who had no exposure to formaldehyde (Akbar-Khanzadeh *et al.*, 1994). Pre- and post-morning sessions showed a 0.03% fall in FEV_1 in the formaldehyde-exposed group compared with a 1% increase in the controls.

(c)   Effect of chronic exposure on nasal mucosa

(i)   Occupational exposure

The possibility that formaldehyde may induce pathological or cytogenetic changes in the nasal mucosa has been examined in subjects exposed either in residential environments or in occupational settings.

Cell smears were collected by a swab that was inserted 6–8 cm into the nose of 42 workers who were employed in two phenol–formaldehyde plants and 38 controls who had no known exposure to formaldehyde. The concentrations of formaldehyde in the plants were 0.02–2.0 ppm [0.02–2.4 mg/m³], with occasional peaks as high as 9 ppm [11.0 mg/m³], and the average length of employment in the plants was about 17 years. Atypical squamous metaplasia was detected as a function of age > 50 years, but no association was found with exposure to formaldehyde (Berke, 1987).

Biopsy samples were taken from the anterior edge of the inferior turbinate of the nose of 37 workers in two particle-board plants, 38 workers in a laminate plant and 25 controls of similar age. The concentrations of formaldehyde in the three plants were 0.1–1.1 mg/m³, with peak concentrations of up to 5 mg/m³. Simultaneous exposure to wood dust occurred in the particle-board plants but not in the laminate plant. The average length of employment was 10.5 years. Exposure to formaldehyde appeared to be associated with squamous metaplasia and mild dysplasia, but no concentration–response relationship was observed, and the histological score was not related to number of years of employment. No difference was detected in the nasal histology of workers exposed to formaldehyde alone or to formaldehyde and wood dust (Edling *et al.*, 1987b, 1988).

Biopsy samples were collected from the medial or inferior aspect of the middle turbinate, 1 cm behind the anterior border, from 62 workers who were engaged in the manufacture of resins for laminate production, 89 workers who were employed in furniture factories and who were exposed to particle-board and glue and 32 controls who were mainly clerks in a local government office. The concentrations of formaldehyde in the resin manufacturing plant were 0.05–0.5 mg/m³, with frequent peaks of over 1 mg/m³, and those in the furniture factories were 0.2–0.3 mg/m³, with rare peaks up to to 0.5 mg/m³; the latter workers were also exposed to wood dust (1–2 mg/m³). The control group was exposed to concentrations of 0.09–0.17 mg/m³ formaldehyde. The average length of employment was about 10 years. The histological scores of workers who were exposed to formaldehyde alone were slightly but significantly higher than those of controls, but the histological scores of workers who were exposed to formaldehyde and wood dust together did not differ from those of controls. No correlation was found between histological score and either duration or concentration of exposure (Holmström *et al.* (1989a). [The possible effect of age on nasal cytology, as noted by Berke (1987), was not determined.]

A nasal biopsy sample was taken from the anterior curvature of the middle turbinate of 37 workers who were exposed at a chemical company where formaldehyde resins were produced and 37 age-matched controls. The concentrations of formaldehyde in the company ranged from 0.5 to > 2 ppm [0.6–> 2.4 mg/m^3], and the average length of employment was 20 years. Hyperplasia and squamous metaplasia were more common among the exposed workers than among the controls, but the difference was not significant. The histological scores increased with age and with concentration and duration of exposure, but the changes were not significant (Boysen *et al.*, 1990).

Histopathological abnormalities of respiratory nasal mucosa cells were determined in 15 nonsmokers (seven women, eight men) who were exposed to formaldehyde that was released from a urea–formaldehyde glue in a plywood factory. Each subject was paired with a control who was matched for age and sex. The mean age of the controls was 30.6 ± 8.7 years and that of exposed workers was 31.0 ± 8.0 years. The mean levels of exposure to formaldehyde (8-h TWA) were about 0.1 mg/m^3 in the sawmill and shearing-press department and 0.39 mg/m^3 in the warehouse area. Peak exposure levels were not given. Concurrent exposure to low levels of wood dust (respirable mass, 0.23 mg/m^3 in the warehouse, 0.73 mg/m^3 during sawing and 0.41 mg/m^3 in shearing-press) occurred. Nasal respiratory cell samples were collected from near the inner turbinate with an endocervical cytology brush. The exposed group had chronic inflammation of the nasal respiratory mucosa and a higher frequency of squamous metaplasia than the controls (mean scores, 2.3 ± 0.5 in the exposed group; 1.6 ± 0.5 in the control group; $p < 0.01$, Mann–Whitney U test) (Ballarin *et al.*, 1992).

(ii)   *Residential exposure*

Samples of cells were collected by a swab that was inserted 2–3 cm into the nostrils of subjects who lived in urea–formaldehyde foam-insulated homes and of subjects who lived in homes without this type of insulation and were examined cytologically. Small but significant increases were observed in the prevalence of squamous metaplastic cells in the samples from the occupants of urea–formaldehyde foam-insulated homes (Broder *et al.*, 1988a,b,c). A follow-up study 1 year later (Broder *et al.*, 1991) showed a decrease in nasal symptoms that was unrelated to any decrease in levels of formaldehyde.

The effects of formaldehyde, other than cancer, on the nasal mucosa are summarized in Table 31.

(d)   *Sensitization to formaldehyde*

Formaldehyde is a well recognized cause of allergic contact dermatitis and an occasional cause of occupational asthma. Provided that suitable control exposures for the affected patient are performed and that similar exposures of unsensitized asthmatics do not provoke asthma, cause and effect can reasonably be implied. The studies on asthma are summarized in Table 32.

Hendrick and Lane (1975) found a late asthmatic reaction following exposure to formaldehyde in a nurse who had no reaction after a control exposure. An asthmatic patho-

Table 31. Findings in the nasal mucosa of people who had occupational exposure to formaldehyde

Industry	Concentration of formaldehyde (mg/m^3)	No. of exposed	No. of controls	Method	Findings	Reference
Formaldehyde (laminate plant)	0.5–1.1	38	25	Nasal biopsy	Histological score: exposed, 2.8; controls, 1.8 ($p < 0.05$). Four exposed men had mild dysplasia.	Edling et al. (1987b)
Formaldehyde Wood dust (laminated particle-board)	0.1–1.1 (peaks to 5) 0.6–1.1	75	25	Nasal biopsy	Histological score: exposed, 2.9; controls, 1.8 ($p < 0.05$). Six men had mild dysplasia.	Edling et al. (1988)
Formaldehyde (phenol?) (laminate)	0.02–2.4 (peaks to 11–18.5)	42	38	Swab smears Clinical examination	No positive correlation between exposure to formaldehyde and abnormal cytology More mucosal abnormalities in non-smoking exposed workers ($p = 0.04$)	Berke (1987)
Formaldehyde (production of formaldehyde and formaldehyde resins)	0.6–> 2.4	37	37	Nasal biopsy	Histological score: exposed, 1.9; controls, 1.4 ($p > 0.05$). Three exposed and no controls had dysplasia.	Boysen et al. (1990)
Formaldehyde (resins for laminate production)	0.05–0.5 (peaks to > 1)	62	32	Nasal biopsy	Histological score: exposed, 2.16; controls, 1.56 ($p < 0.05$). No case of dysplasia	Holmström et al. (1989a)
Formaldehyde Wood dust (plywood factory)	0.1–0.39 0.23–0.73	15	15	Nasal scrapes	Micronuclei in nasal mucosal cells: exposed, 0.90; controls, 0.25 ($p < 0.010$). Cytological score: exposed, 2.3; controls, 1.6 ($p < 0.01$). One exposed had mild dysplasia.	Ballarin et al. (1992)

Table 32. Studies of occupational asthma/dermatitis

Sex	Route	Concentration of formaldehyde	Duration	Effects	Reference
Men (aged 39 years)	Inhalation	0.06 ppm, max. 0.13 ppm 0.01 ppm 0.5 ppm	6 months 20 min 20 min	Asthma None Late asthmatic reaction, IgE negative	Kim et al. (2001)
Men and women	Skin (patch test)	1% in water	Unspecified	Case series of 280 health care workers; 13.9% positive patch test to formaldehyde, little cross reaction with glutaral-dehyde (12.4%) and glyoxal (1.9%)	Kiec-Swierczynska et al. (1998)
Men and women	Inhalation	2.3 mg/m^3 4.8 mg/m^3 31 mg/m^3 4.8 mg/m^3	30 min 30 min 7 min 30 min	Late asthmatic reaction Dual immediate and late asthmatic reaction Irritant asthmatic reaction No reaction in unsensi-tized asthmatics	Burge et al. (1985)
Women	Inhalation	5 ppm 3 ppm	15 min 5 min	Late asthmatic reaction Late asthmatic reaction No reaction in controls	Hendrick & Lane (1975, 1977); Hendrick et al. (1982)
Unspecified	Inhalation			Immediate and late reactions in 2 workers	Popa et al. (1969) [few details]
Men and women	Inhalation	1.2 mg/m^3 2.5 mg/m^3	30 min 30 min	1 worker, early response 11 workers, 6 late response 12/230 exposed sympto-matic workers + specific challenge to formalde-hyde negative in 218, 71 with NSBR	Nordman et al. (1985)
Men	Inhalation (cutting and preparing brain specimens)		2 h	Acute pneumonitis; breath smelled of formaldehyde; resolved	Porter (1975)

NSBR, non-specific bronchial hyper-reactivity

logist had no reaction following a similar 60-min exposure to 5 ppm [6 mg/m³] formaldehyde. A later study (Hendrick *et al.*, 1982) repeated the original exposures, which were reported to be 5 ppm. A second report (Hendrick & Lane, 1977) mentioned a second case who reacted to exposure to 3 ppm [3.6 mg/m³] formaldehyde for 5 min.

Burge *et al.* (1985) reported the results of challenge tests in 15 workers who were exposed to formaldehyde. Three had late asthmatic reactions that suggested sensitization; one reacted following exposure to 2.3 mg/m³ and two after exposure to 4.8 mg/m³. Control asthmatics had no asthma attack provoked by exposures to 4.8 mg/m³; one asthmatic exposed to a sheep dip that contained formaldehyde had an irritant reaction following a 7-min exposure to 31 mg/m³.

Nordman *et al.* (1985) reported the results of inhalation challenges in 230 workers who were investigated at the Finnish Institute of Occupational Medicine. One worker reacted to 1.2 mg/m³ formaldehyde and 11 reacted to 2.5 mg/m³ formaldehyde. No reaction was observed at 2.5 µg/m³ among the remaining 218 workers, 71 of whom had non-specific hyper-responsiveness.

Kim *et al.* (2001) reported on a worker who made crease-resistant trousers and who had a late asthmatic reaction 5 h after exposure to 0.5 ppm [0.6 mg/m³], but not to 0.01 ppm [0.01 mg/m³] formaldehyde (20-min exposures). His IgE to formaldehyde conjugates was negative.

One patient developed anaphylaxis during dialysis with a dialyser that had been sterilized with formaldehyde and contained 5–10 µg/mL residual formaldehyde. She had previously been sensitized to formaldehyde on the skin through contact dermatitis. IgE antibodies to formaldehyde/human serum albumin were strongly positive (Maurice *et al.* (1986).

One case of toxic pneumonitis following a 2-h exposure to a concentration of formaldehyde that was sufficient to be smelled on the breath has been reported (Porter, 1975).

(e)   *Oral poisoning*

Two reports have been made of three patients who were poisoned following ingestion of formaldehyde solution. All three patients died (Eells *et al.*, 1981; Köppel *et al.*, 1990). Two patients had ingested unknown amounts of formalin that had not been contaminated with methanol. Both developed acidosis with raised plasma formic acid levels (6.09 and 4.57 mmol/L) and additional lactic acidosis. Both survived the initial necrosis of the gut mucosa and renal failure, but died from late acute respiratory distress syndrome and cardiac failure at 3 weeks and 8 weeks after ingestion, respectively (Köppel *et al.*, 1990). The third patient had ingested 120 mL (37% w/v) formaldehyde that contained 12.5% v/v methanol. Initial blood levels 30 min after ingestion were 0.48 µg/dL formaldehyde, 44 mg/dL formate and 42 mg/dL methanol. She died after 28 h (Eells *et al.*, 1981).

4.2.2   *Experimental systems*

(*a*)   *In-vitro studies*

(i)   *Cytotoxicity*

The toxicity of formaldehyde was assessed in cultured human bronchial epithelial cells under defined serum- and thiol-free exposure conditions (Grafström *et al.,* 1996). Results obtained from studies of 1-h exposures showed that 0.2 mM and 0.6 mM formaldehyde inhibited cell growth by 50% as measured by loss of clonal growth rate and colony-forming efficiency, respectively. Membrane integrity, i.e. exclusion of trypan blue and cellular uptake of neutral red, an energy-dependent lysosomal accumulation of the dye, was decreased by 50% at concentrations of 2 mM and 6 mM formaldehyde, respectively. Inhibition of growth was also associated with significant decreases in GSH, which occurred without concomitant formation of oxidized GSH and with no alteration of the levels of protein thiols. This result indicated that exposure to formaldehyde was associated with the expected formation of thiohemiacetal, but not with overt oxidative stress as assessed by thiol status, in bronchial cells. Extensive loss of intracellular GSH coincided with loss of membrane integrity, which implies that plasma membrane leakage may have contributed to the effect. Moreover, active re-reduction of oxidized GSH to GSH by GSH reductase could potentially have masked an oxidant effect. Formaldehyde-dependent decreases in thiols provide a mechanism for formaldehyde-induced inhibition of growth, since minor decreases in GSH levels are known to inhibit cell growth efficiently (Atzori *et al.*, 1989, 1994). The steady-state concentration of intracellular Ca^{2+} was increased by 50% within a few minutes after treatment with 0.5 mM formaldehyde, and transient increases were recorded at lower concentrations (Grafström *et al.*, 1996). The toxicity of formaldehyde to keratinocytes is manifested as aberrant induction of terminal differentiation, i.e. increases in involucrin expression and formation of cross-linked envelopes. This cellular response is probably linked to the noted increases in cellular Ca^{2+}, which activates transglutaminase-dependent cross-linking of various proteins, including involucrin, into the cross-linked envelope (Rice & Green, 1979). Various types of genetic damage and mutation are caused by formaldehyde at levels as low as 0.1 mM (see Section 4.4), and may also underlie some of the cytotoxic actions of formaldehyde. Inhibition of DNA repair was shown in bronchial cells following treatment with 0.1–0.3 mM formaldehyde, which implies that inhibition of enzyme function might be an essential aspect of the toxicity of formaldehyde. In this respect, enzymes that carry a thiol moiety in their active site may be particularly sensitive (Grafström *et al.*, 1996).

The toxicity of formaldehyde was evaluated in isolated rat hepatocytes (Teng *et al.*, 2001); exposure to 4 mM for 2 h caused 50% cell lysis. Toxicity was associated with a dose-dependent loss of GSH and mitochondrial membrane potential and, moreover, was associated with inhibition of mitochondrial respiration and the formation of reactive oxygen species. Higher doses were associated with lipid peroxidation. Depletion of GSH and inhibition of ADH and ALDH activities increased the toxicity of formaldehyde, whereas antioxidants such as butylated hydroxytoluene and iron chelators such as desferoxamine protected against toxicity. Prevention of toxicity by cyclosporine or carnitine, agents that prevent the opening of the mitochondrial transition pore, provided evidence that formaldehyde targets mitochondria.

(ii) *Proliferation and apoptosis*

The toxicity of formaldehyde and the influences of exogenous and endogenous thiols were studied in cultured human oral fibroblasts and epithelial cells (Nilsson *et al.*, 1998). The presence of serum and cysteine counteracted the toxicity of formaldehyde, and lower levels of intracellular thiols, including GSH, in fibroblasts (relative to epithelial cells) were associated with greater toxicity. The results emphasize the high thiol-reactivity of formaldehyde and the central role of cellular thiols in the scavenging of formaldehyde. The toxicity of formaldehyde was compared in human dental pulp fibroblasts, buccal epithelial cells and HeLa cervical carcinoma cells (Lovschall *et al.*, 2002). In assessments of proliferation (bromodeoxyuridine incorporation), methylthiazole tetrazolium conversion and neutral red uptake, both of the normal cell types were shown to be more sensitive than the carcinoma cells to the toxicity of formaldehyde. Formaldehyde, applied at concentrations of 0.1–10 mM to HT-29 colon carcinoma and normal endothelial cell cultures, stimulated proliferation at 0.1 mM, inhibited proliferation and induced apoptosis at 1 mM and induced cell lysis at 10 mM (Tyihák *et al.*, 2001). The authors concluded that formaldehyde may either stimulate or inhibit proliferation or induce overt toxicity, depending on the dose. Apoptosis was also induced in rat thymocytes by concentrations of 0.1 mM formaldehyde or more after a 24-h exposure (Nakao *et al.*, 2003). The proliferation-enhancing effects of formaldehyde are supported by studies of gene expression in mouse fibroblast C3H/10T1/2 cells (Parfett, 2003). Formaldehyde at 0.05–0.1 mM, concentrations that are known to induce cell transformation in this system, increased the transcription of proliferin, a response that is also shared by other transformation-promoting agents.

Formaldehyde at doses of 1 ng/mL to 1 µg/mL induced expression of intercellular adhesion molecule-1 and vascular cell adhesion molecule-1 in human microvascular endothelial cells of the nasal mucosa (Kim *et al.*, 2002). Exposures to formaldehyde were also associated with increased adhesiveness of the endothelial cells to eosinophils. The authors concluded that the noted effects and changes in gene expression of intercellular and vascular cell adhesion molecules might underlie the irritant effects of formaldehyde in the nasal mucosa.

(iii) *Effect on the mucociliary apparatus of the respiratory mucosa*

In an ex-vivo study, dose-dependent changes in the mucociliary apparatus of frog respiratory mucosa during exposure to formaldehyde in aqueous solutions were examined. Frog palates (10 per group) were removed and were refridgerated for 2 days to allow the mucous to clear. The palates were then immersed in Ringer solution alone or with 1.25, 2.5 or 5.0 ppm formaldehyde solution. The frequency of ciliary beat, as a measure of the fluctuation of light patterns during the ciliary wave over time, and mucociliary clearance, as a function of the time it took a mucous plug to travel 6 mm of palate, were quantitated. Measurements were taken at time 0, before immersion in formaldehyde solution, and then every 15 min for a total of four measurements over 60 min of exposure at 20 °C and 100% humidity. The later time-points were all compared with their respective 0-time measurement to give a percentage of the baseline measurement. A dose- and time-dependent decrease was observed in both mucociliary clearance and frequency of ciliary beat (Flo-Neyret *et al.*, 2001).

> (*b*)   *In-vivo studies*
>
> (i)   *Acute effects*

Irritation

A quantitative measure of sensory irritation in rodents is provided by the reflex decrease in respiratory rate of mice or rats that is caused by stimulation of trigeminal nerve receptors in the nasal passages. In comparison with other aldehydes (Steinhagen & Barrow, 1984), formaldehyde is a potent respiratory tract irritant, and elicits a 50% decrease in respiratory frequency in B6C3F$_1$ mice at 4.9 ppm [6.0 mg/m^3] and in Fischer 344 rats at 31.7 ppm [38.7 mg/m^3] (Chang *et al.*, 1981). Swiss-Webster mice exposed for 5 days (6 h per day) to formaldehyde at a concentration that elicits a 50% decrease in respiratory frequency (3.1 ppm [3.8 mg/m^3]) developed mild histopathological lesions in the anterior nasal cavity, but no lesions were found in the posterior nasal cavity or in the lung (Buckley *et al.*, 1984).

In addition to decreasing the respiratory rate, formaldehyde may also alter the tidal volume, which results in a decrease in minute ventilation. Exposure to formaldehyde over a 10-min test period induced prompt reductions in both respiratory rates and minute volumes in mice and rats, whether or not they were exposed before testing to 6 ppm [7.4 mg/m^3] formaldehyde for 6 h per day for 4 days (Fig. 4). These effects were observed at lower concentrations of formaldehyde in mice than in rats (Chang *et al.*, 1983). A similar effect has been demonstrated in C57Bl6/F$_1$ mice and CD rats (Jaeger & Gearhart, 1982).

Rats exposed to 28 ppm [34.2 mg/m^3] formaldehyde for 4 days developed tolerance to its sensory irritancy, but those exposed to 15 ppm [18.3 mg/m^3] for 1, 4 or 10 days did not (Chang & Barrow, 1984).

Sensory irritation to formaldehyde, acrolein and acetaldehyde vapours and their mixture was studied in groups of male Wistar rats weighing 240–300 g (four per group) that were exposed to concentrations of the aldehyde vapours up to a level that decreased respiratory frequency by 50%. Formaldehyde vapours were produced by thermal depolymerization of paraformaldehyde in water and evaporation into the in-flow airstream. The maximal decrease in breathing frequency was observed within 3 min of exposure; desensitization occurred within a few minutes after maximal decrease in breathing frequency and only partial recovery was achieved within 10 min after exposure. The authors proposed that the decreased breathing frequency within the first few minutes of exposure is due to trigeminal nerve stimulation from the irritant effect of formaldehyde. The level of exposure to formaldehyde that resulted in a 50% respiratory depression was 10 ppm

Figure 4. Time–response curves for respiratory rate, tidal and minute volume from naive and formaldehyde-pretreated mice and rats (6 ppm, 6 h/day, 4 days) during a 6-h exposure to 6 ppm formaldehyde

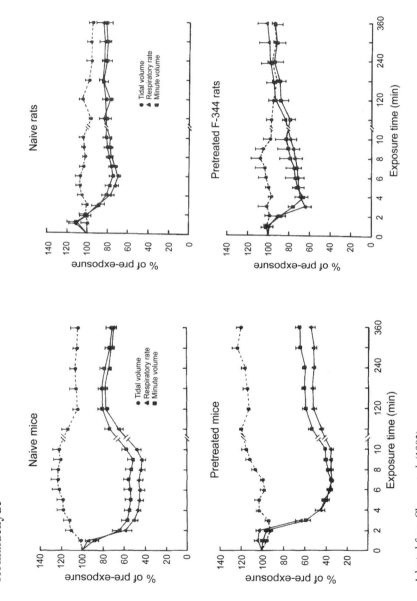

Adapted from Chang *et al.* (1983)

Data shown are $\bar{x} \pm$ SE for each time point; $n = 6$ for each group

[12.3 mg/m³]. Since this was a study of the mixture, the authors also found that the reduction in breathing frequency after exposure to the mixture was always greater than after exposure to the same concentration of any of the components alone (Cassee *et al.*, 1996a).

The retinal toxicity of a single dose of formaldehyde, methanol and formate was investigated in male albino rabbits weighing 2.1–2.3 kg (four per group) by injection into the vitreous cavity of 100 μL of a buffered (pH 7.4) phosphate-saline solution that contained 1% methanol, 0.1% or 1.0% formaldehyde or 1% formate. The final vitreous concentrations were 700 μg/mL methanol, 70 μg/mL formaldehyde, 700 μg/mL formaldehyde and 700 μg/mL formate. The eyeballs were examined with a biomicroscope and ophthalmoscope before treatment and 1, 2, 7, 14 and 30 days after treatment. After 30 days, the rabbits were euthanized and the eyeballs were fixed in formalin for microscopic examination of the retina, choroid, sclera, optic disc and optic nerve. No lesions were observed in the methanol- or formate-treated eyes at any time-point. The eyes treated with formaldehyde had ophthalmoscopic alterations at all time-points and at both doses; the higher dose induced more severe alterations including subcapsular cataract, retinal vessel dilatation and juxtapapillary retinal haemorrhages. Histologically, the eyes treated with 0.1% formaldehyde had disorganization of the ganglion cell and outer nuclear layers of the retina; these symptoms were more severe in eyes treated with 1.0% formaldehyde. The optic nerves had vacuolization after treatment with either dose of formaldehyde (Hayasaka *et al.*, 2001).

Pulmonary hyper-reactivity

Formaldehyde induced pulmonary hyper-reactivity in guinea-pigs: exposure to 0.3 ppm [0.37 mg/m³] for 8 h caused transient bronchoconstriction and hyper-reactivity to infused acetylcholine; exposure to higher concentrations (> 9 ppm [> 11 mg/m³]) for 2 h induced bronchoconstriction. No evidence of tracheal epithelial damage was observed after exposure to 3.4 ppm [4.2 mg/m³] for 8 h. However, the mechanism by which these effects occur is unknown (Swiecichowski *et al.*, 1993).

The effects of formaldehyde (vaporized formalin) on pulmonary flow were determined in cynomolgus monkeys that were tranquilized before exposure and received an endotracheal tube transorally. Pulmonary flow resistance was increased after exposure to formaldehyde at a concentration of 2.5 ppm [3.0 mg/m³] for 2, 5 and 10 min. Narrowing of the airways by formaldehyde was not correlated with methacholine reactivity (Biagini *et al.*, 1989). [The Working Group questioned the relevance of these findings, in view of the method of administration.]

Male Sprague-Dawley rats, 6 weeks of age, were exposed to formaldehyde (10 ppm [12.2 mg/m³]), ozone (0.6 ppm [1 mg/m³]) (with coefficients of variation of less than 12% and 5%, respectively) or a combination of the two during exercise on a treadmill that was modified to deliver a stream of control air or air that contained formaldehyde. The rats were exercised at a moderately fast-walking gait of 15 m/min on a 20% gradient for 3 h, which raised metabolic gas exchange over the resting rate by a factor of at least two. Resting exposure was conducted in a nose-only inhalation tube. Histology, including labelling indices, was examined quantitatively for the nose and lung. Formaldehyde increased labelling in the transitional epithelium in the nose after individual or mixed exposure at rest or after exercise but ozone alone did not. Formaldehyde and ozone after exercice either individually or as a mixture produced injury in the trachea; the mixture caused greater (approximately additive) injury than either of the chemicals alone. The pulmonary parenchyma was unaffected by exposure to formaldehyde. Functional changes included decreased breathing frequency during exposure to formaldehyde; the response to the mixture was lower. Tidal volume decreased after treatment with ozone or formaldehyde but was increased after exposure to the mixture. Formaldehyde produced slow and shallow breathing which resulted in depressed minute ventilation (Mautz, 2003).

Sensitizing effect and inflammatory response

In order to investigate the induction of sensitization to formaldehyde, undiluted formalin was painted on shaven and epilated dorsal sites of guinea-pigs; a second application was administered 2 days later at naive sites, to give a total dose of 74 mg/animal. Other animals received diluted formalin at doses of 0.012–9.3 mg/animal. All animals that received 74 mg formalin developed skin sensitivity when tested 7 days after exposure. A significant dose–response relationship was observed for the degree of sensitization and for the percentage of animals that were sensitized; however, pulmonary sensitization was not induced when formaldehyde was administered dermally, by injection or by inhalation, and no cytophilic antibodies were detected in the blood (Lee *et al.*, 1984).

In the guinea-pig maximization test, 10 guinea-pigs (five per exposure group) received six intradermal injections of saline or 0.25% [2.5 mg/mL] formaldehyde solution followed 6–8 days later by an occlusive dressing of a patch soaked in 10% [100 mg/mL] formaldehyde for 48 h. After an additional 12–14 days, another occlusive dressing was applied for 24 h; 24 h after removal, the size of the area of the erythema was measured. A similar study was conducted in guinea-pigs but only occlusive dressings were used. Both studies resulted in a positive response (Hilton *et al.*, 1996).

The local lymph node assay was conducted in BALB/c mice that received daily applications of 25 µL of 10%, 25% or 50% w/v solutions of formaldehyde on the pinna of both ears for 3 consecutive days. Five days after the initiation of exposure, all mice were injected with tritiated methyl thymidine and were killed 5 h later. The lymph nodes adjacent to the ear were removed and labelled cells were counted to measure the rate of cell proliferation. Formalin induced a strong proliferative response that was considered to be positive for a contact allergen (Hilton *et al.*, 1996).

The mouse IgE test is thought to identify allergens that have the potential to cause sensitivity in the respiratory tract by stimulating a significant increase in serum IgE concentration. This test was conducted in groups of six BALB/c mice that received 50 µL of a 10%, 25% or 50% formalin solution (37% formaldehyde dissolved in dimethylformamide) on an occlusive dressing applied to the shaved flank. Seven days later, 25 µL of the solution of formaldehyde at half the concentration used previously was applied to the dorsum of both ears. Fourteen days after the initial exposure, the mice were exsanguinated and blood was collected for analysis of IgE. There was no significant change in levels of circulating IgE after treatment with formaldehyde (Hilton *et al.*, 1996).

Production of the cytokines interferon-γ (IFN-γ) and interleukin (IL)-10 was measured in draining lymph nodes of the skin of the flanks and the ears of 10 BALB/c mice that had received skin applications of 10%, 25% or 50% formalin solutions (37% formaldehyde in dimethylformamide) on the shaved flank twice a day for 5 days followed by 3 days on the dorsum of the ears. Thirteen days after the initiation of exposure, draining auricular lymph nodes were removed. Lymphocytes were isolated and cultured for up to 120 h, and the supernatant was collected and analysed for IFN-γ and IL-10. The levels of IFN-γ were significantly increased after all concentrations of formaldehyde but not those of IL-10. The authors suggested that formaldehyde causes a contact sensitization reaction in the skin (mediated by Th1-type lymphocytes that secrete IFN-γ) but not sensitization of the respiratory tract (Hilton *et al.*, 1996).

Eighteen 8-week-old male BN/Crj and Fischer 344/DuCrj rats were exposed to an aerosol of 1% formaldehyde solution (equivalent to 15–20 ppm) for 3 h per day for 5 days in a whole-body inhalation exposure system; another nine animals were exposed to an aerosol of ion-exchanged water only. After death by exsanguination, the nose was examined histologically or the nasal epithelium was removed by scraping and used to isolate RNA. Measurements of cDNA were made by reverse-transcriptase polymerase chain reaction (RT-PCR) for quantitative real-time analysis of *IFN-γ*, *IL-2*, *IL-4* and *IL-5* mRNA levels. All samples were examined for levels of glyceraldehyde-3-phosphate dehydrogenase (*GAPDH*) mRNA and quantities of gene were presented as the ratio to *GAPDH*. The histological lesions were consistent with those reported previously and were of greater severity in Fischer 344 than in BN rats (Ohtsuka *et al.*, 1997). Compared with *GAPDH*, *IFN-γ* and *IL-2* (Th1-related cytokines involved in non-allergic inflammation) were expressed at significantly lower levels in BN rats treated with formaldehyde. None of the other mRNA levels were statistically significant, although the expression of *IL-4* and *IL-5* (Th2-related cytokines) in BN rats and that of *IL-2* and *IL-5* in Fischer 344 rats were lower than the levels observed in controls (Ohtsuka *et al.*, 2003).

Cytotoxicity and cell proliferation in the respiratory tract

The acute and subacute effects of formaldehyde in experimental animals are summarized in Table 33. A critical issue for the mechanism of carcinogenesis is whether low concentrations of formaldehyde increase or decrease the rate of cell turnover in the nasal epithelium. Subacute exposure to a low concentration of formaldehyde (1 ppm [1.2 mg/m³]; 6 h per day for 3 days) has been reported to induce a small, transient increase in nasal epithelial cell turnover in Wistar rats (Zwart *et al.*, 1988), but this statistically significant increase was not confirmed in later studies (Reuzel *et al.*, 1990). Other investigators did not detect an increase in cell turnover in the nasal epithelium of Fischer 344 rats exposed to 0.7 or 2 ppm [0.9 or 2.4 mg/m³] (6 h per day for 1, 4 or 9 days) (Monticello *et al.*, 1991) or to 0.5 or 2 ppm [0.6 or 2.4 mg/m³] (6 h per day for 3 days) (Swenberg *et al.*, 1983). Low concentrations of formaldehyde (0.5 or 2 ppm; 6 h per day for 1, 2, 4, 9 or 14 days) also did not

Table 33. Cytotoxicity and cell proliferation induced by acute and subacute exposure to formaldehyde

Strain, species, sex	Exposure	Effects	Reference
Fischer 344 rat, male; B6C3F$_1$ mouse, male	0, 0.6, 2.4, 7.4, 18.5 mg/m^3, 6 h/day, 3 days	0.6, 2.4: no increase in cell replication rate in nasal mucosa; 7.4: increased cell turnover (rats only); 18.5: cell proliferation (rats and mice)	Swenberg et al. (1983)
Fischer 334 rat, male; B6C3F$_1$ mouse, male	0, 18.5 mg/m^3, 6 h/day, 1 or 5 days	18.5: cell proliferation induced in nasal mucosa of both species; rat responses exceeded those of mice.	Chang et al. (1983)
Fischer 344 rat, male	3.7 mg/m^3 × 12 h/day, 7.4 mg/m^3 × 6 h/day, 14.8 mg/m^3 × 3 h/day ($C × t$ = 44 mg/m^3–h/day), 3 or 10 days	Cell proliferation related more closely to concentration than to time; less proliferation after 10 than after 3 days of exposure, indicating adaptation	Swenberg et al. (1983)
Fischer 344 rat, male	0, 0.6, 2.4, 7.4, 18.5 mg/m^3, 6 h/day, 1, 2, 4, 9 or 14 days	0.6: no effects on mucociliary function; 2.4: minimal effects; 7.4: moderate inhibition; 18.5: marked inhibition	Morgan et al. (1986b)
Fischer 344 rat, male	0, 2.4, 18.5 mg/m^3, 10, 20, 45 or 90 min or 6 h	2.4: no effect on mucociliary function; 18.5: inhibition of mucociliary function, marked recovery 1 h after exposure	Morgan et al. (1986c)
Fischer 344 rat, male	0, 0.6, 2.4 mg/m^3, 6 h/day, 1 or 4 days; 7.4 mg/m^3, 6 h/day, 1, 2 or 4 days; 18.5 mg/m^3, 6 h/day, 1 or 2 days	0.6, 2.4: no lesions; 7.4, 18.5: non-cell-specific, dose-related injury, including hypertrophy, non-keratinized squamous cells, nucleolar segregation	Monteiro-Riviere & Popp (1986)
Wistar rat, male	0, 6.2 mg/m^3 × 8 h/day, 12.3 mg/m^3 × 8 h/day ($C × t$ = 49 or 98 mg/m^3–h/day); 12.3 mg/m^3 × 8 × 0.5 h/day, 25 mg/m^3 × 8 × 0.5 h/day ($C × t$ = 49 or 98 mg/m^3–h/day), 5 days/week, 4 weeks	Labelling index increased at all concentrations; cell proliferation more closely related to concentration than to total dose	Wilmer et al. (1987)
Wistar rat, male and female	0, 0.37, 1.2, 3.7 mg/m^3, 6 h/day, 3 days	Significant, transient increase in cell turnover at 1.2 and 3.7 mg/m^3 but not confirmed in later studies at concentration of 1.2 ppm (Reuzel et al., 1990)	Zwart et al. (1988)

Table 33 (contd)

Strain, species, sex	Exposure	Effects	Reference
Rhesus monkey, male	0, 7.4 mg/m³, 6 h/day, 5 days/week, 1 or 6 weeks	Lesions similar to those in rats (Monticello et al., 1991) but more widespread, extending to trachea and major bronchi; increased cell replication in nasal passages, trachea and carina; percentage of nasal surface area affected increased between 1 and 6 weeks.	Monticello et al. (1989)
Wistar rat, male	0, 0.37, 1.2, 3.7 mg/m³, 22 h/day, 3 days Also investigated effect of simultaneous exposure to 0.4, 0.8 or 1.6 mg/m³ ozone	0.37, 1.2: either no increase in or inhibition of cell proliferation; 3.7: increased cell replication; 0.8 mg/m³ ozone + 1.2 or 3.7 mg/m³ formaldehyde: synergistic increase in cell turnover; 1.6 mg/m³ ozone + 1.2 mg/m³ formaldehyde: inhibition of cell turnover	Reuzel et al. (1990)
Fischer 344 rat, male	0, 0.86, 2.4, 7.4, 12.3, 18.5 mg/m³, 6 h/day, 5 days/week, 1, 4, or 9 days or 6 weeks	0.86, 2.4: no effect on cell turnover; 7.4, 12.3, 18.5: concentration- and site-dependent cell proliferation induced at all exposure times	Monticello et al. (1991)
Wistar rat, male	0, 4.43 mg/m³; 8 h followed by 4 h no exposure for 6 consecutive 12-h cycles Also investigated effect of simultaneous exposure to 0.4 ppm ozone.	4.43 mg/m³ resulted in increased GSH peroxidase in nasal respiratory tissue and increased PCNA expression by immunohistochemistry.	Cassee & Feron (1994)
Wistar rat, male	0, 1.23, 3.94, 7.87 mg/m³, 6 h/day, 1 or 3 days Also investigated effect of simultaneous exposure to acetaldehyde (750, 1500 ppm) and acrolein (0.25, 0.67 ppm).	The mixture resulted in more extensive and severe histopathology of the nose than the individual exposure.	Cassee et al. (1996b)
BN/Crj rat, male; Fischer 344/DuCrj rat, male	0 or 18.45–24.6 mg/m³ (estimate), 3 h/day, 5 days	Nasal respiratory degeneration and necrosis more severe in Fischer 344 rats	Ohtsuka et al. (1997)

C, concentration; t, time; PCNA, proliferating cell nuclear antigen inhibit mucociliary function in the nasal passages of Fischer 344 rats (Morgan *et al.*, 1986b,c), and no injury to the nasal epithelium of rats of this strain was detected ultrastructurally after exposure to 0.5 or 2 ppm (6 h per day for 1 or 4 days) (Monteiro-Riviere & Popp, 1986).

Wistar rats exposed to 3 ppm [3.7 mg/m^3] (6 h per day for 3 days (Zwart *et al.*, 1988) or 22 h per day for 3 days (Reuzel *et al.*, 1990)) had a transient increase in cell replication. Higher concentrations of formaldehyde ($\geq$ 6 ppm [7.3 mg/m^3]) induced erosion, epithelial hyperplasia, squamous metaplasia and inflammation in a site-specific manner in the nasal mucosa of Wistar rats (Monticello *et al.*, 1991). Mice are less responsive than rats, probably because they are better able than rats to reduce their minute ventilation when exposed to high concentrations of formaldehyde (Chang *et al.*, 1983; Swenberg *et al.*, 1983). Fischer 344 rats exposed to 6, 10 or 15 ppm [7.3, 12.2 or 18.3 mg/m^3] (6 h per day for 1, 4 or 9 days, or 6 h per day on 5 days per week for 6 weeks) had an enhanced rate of cell turnover (Monticello *et al.*, 1991). The severity of nasal epithelial responses at 15 ppm was much greater than that at 6 ppm (Monteiro-Riviere & Popp, 1986). Rhesus monkeys exposed to 6 ppm (6 h per day for 5 days) developed similar nasal lesions to rats. Mild lesions, characterized as multifocal loss of cilia, were also detected in the larynx, trachea and carina (Monticello *et al.*, 1989).

The relative importance of concentration and total dose on cell proliferation was examined in Fischer 344 and Wistar rats exposed to a range of concentrations for various lengths of time, such that the total inhaled dose was constant. Exposures were for 3 or 10 days (Swenberg *et al.*, 1983) or 4 weeks (Wilmer *et al.*, 1987). All of the investigators concluded that concentration, not total dose, is the primary determinant of the cytotoxicity of formaldehyde. A similar conclusion was reached when rats were exposed for 13 weeks (Wilmer *et al.*, 1989).

Ten 8-week-old male BN/Crj or Fischer 344/DuCrj rats were exposed to 100 L/min (2 mg 1% formaldehyde solution/L air, equivalent to 15–20 ppm) aerosol or water for 3 h per day on 5 days per week for 2 weeks. Clinical signs were monitored and light and scanning electron microscopy were performed. Both strains of rat had abnormal respiration, nasal discharge and sneezing following treatment with formaldehyde; the Fischer 344 rats had a more severe response. Lesions were present only in the nose and trachea from Fischer 344 rats and nose from BN rats; again, Fischer 344 rats were more severely affected. The typical lesions of squamous metaplasia, respiratory hyperplasia and degeneration and necrosis in the nose that were described with Fischer 344 rats affected all sections of the nose examined, whereas BN rats only had squamous metaplasia in the ventral portion of level II. Epithelial hyperplasia was present in the trachea of Fischer 344 rats. By scanning electron microscopy, squamous epithelial-like changes were seen in the anterior nose after treatment with formaldehyde in both rat strains. BN rats were less sensitive to exposure to formaldehyde than Fischer 344 rats (Ohtsuka *et al.*, 1997).

Co-exposure with other agents

Ozone

The effects of simultaneous exposure to formaldehyde and ozone were investigated in Wistar rats exposed to 0.3, 1 or 3 ppm [0.37, 1.2 and 3.7 mg/m³] formaldehyde, 0.2, 0.4 or 0.8 ppm [0.4, 0.8 or 1.6 mg/m³] ozone or mixtures of 0.4 ppm ozone with 0.3, 1 or 3 ppm formaldehyde or 1 ppm formaldehyde with 0.2, 0.4 or 0.8 ppm ozone (22 h per day for 3 days). Both formaldehyde (3 ppm) and ozone (0.4 or 0.8 ppm) induced cell proliferation in the most anterior region of the respiratory epithelium. In a slightly more posterior region, ozone had no effect on cell replication, but formaldehyde either enhanced cell proliferation (3 ppm) or appeared to inhibit it slightly (0.3 or 1 ppm). Combined exposures to low concentrations (0.4 ppm ozone and 0.3 ppm formaldehyde, 0.4 or 0.8 ppm ozone and 1 ppm formaldehyde) induced less cell proliferation than ozone alone; however, more than additive increases in cell proliferation were detected in the anterior nose after exposure to 0.4 ppm ozone in combination with 3 ppm formaldehyde, and in a slightly more posterior region after exposure to 0.4 ppm ozone with 1 or 3 ppm formaldehyde. The results suggested to the authors a complex response of the nasal epithelium to low (non-irritating) concentrations of these irritants but a synergistic increase in cell proliferation at irritating concentrations. To induce a synergistic effect on cell proliferation, at least one of the compounds must be present at a cytotoxic concentration (Reuzel *et al.*, 1990).

The pathophysiology of nasal alterations was investigated in 80 8-week-old male Wistar rats (20 per group) after nose-only exposure to formaldehyde or ozone, or their mixture for 8 h followed by 4 h of no exposure for six consecutive 12-h cycles. The formaldehyde was generated from paraformaldehyde by thermal depolymerization in water and evaporation into the air stream at a concentration of 3.6 ± 0.1 ppm or 3.5 ± 0.1 ppm [4.3 mg/m³] in the individual or ozone mixture exposure groups, respectively (concentration of ozone, 0.4 ppm [0.8 mg/m³]). After euthanasia, the respiratory portion of the nasal epithelium was collected on ice from a subset of the rats and another subset [numbers not specified] was used for microscopic examination of the nose with haematoxylin and eosin, periodic acid Schiff and proliferating cell nuclear antigen immunohistochemistry. The nasal respiratory epithelial samples were pooled (six rats), homogenized and centrifuged for extraction of the supernatant. The enzyme activities of GST, GSH peroxidase, glucose-6-phosphate dehydrogenase, GSH reductase, ADH and FDH were measured. In addition, GSH and protein levels were quantified. All animals lost weight during the exposure period and weight loss was significantly greater in the treated animals compared with controls. Ozone alone resulted in degenerative changes in the respiratory epithelium but formaldehyde alone or in combination with ozone induced necrosis in the respiratory epithelium. Rhinitis was induced by all three treatments but was more severe in rats treated with formaldehyde than in those treated with ozone and was most severe after exposure to the mixture. Cell proliferation was increased after all treatments compared with controls and a uniformly greater increase was observed in rats exposed to formaldehyde combined with ozone compared with those exposed to ozone alone. Rats treated with formaldehyde alone had proliferative rates in most of the measured areas equivalent to those of the ozone–formaldehyde-exposed rats. However, rats that received formaldehyde only had greater proliferation indices in the septum and lateral wall of the posterior section than rats exposed to the mixture. Only GSH peroxidase activity was increased after exposure to formaldehyde and only GST activity was decreased after exposure to the mixture. Ozone alone did not alter any enzyme activities significantly. The authors suggested that there appeared to be no major role for GSH or GSH-dependent enzymes in the pathogenesis of toxicity induced by formaldehyde and/or ozone (Cassee & Feron, 1994).

Other aldehydes

The histological and biochemical effects of exposure to formaldehyde, acetaldehyde and acrolein individually or as mixtures were examined in rats. Groups of male Wistar rats, 8 weeks of age, were exposed to formaldehyde at 0, 1.0, 3.2 or 6.4 ppm [0, 1.23, 3.94 or 7.87 mg/m^3] for 6 h per day for 1 or 3 days in nose-only inhalation chambers. Additional rats were exposed to mixtures of 1.0 ppm formaldehyde and 0.25 ppm acrolein, 1.0 ppm formaldehyde, 0.25 ppm acrolein and 750 ppm acetaldehyde, or 3.2 ppm formaldehyde, 0.67 ppm acrolein and 1500 ppm acetaldehyde. After euthanasia, five or six treated animals per exposure group and a total of 19 control animals from all substudies were used for histology (haematoxylin and eosin and proliferating cell nuclear antigen immunohisto-chemistry) and nine animals from each exposure group were used for biochemical studies. Respiratory and olfactory epithelium were removed separately and homogenized on ice for extraction of the cytosolic fraction and analysis of GSH peroxidase, GST, GSH reductase, ADH, FDH and total amount of protein and non-protein sulfhydryl groups. No histological or biochemical alterations were observed after 1 day of exposure to formaldehyde at any concentration. Only acrolein or the high-dose mixture of all three chemicals induced a biochemical change after 1 day (a decrease in GSH reductase activity). Acetaldyde induced a dose-dependent increase in non-protein sulfhydryls. After 3 days of exposure to 1.0 ppm formaldehyde, no histological alterations were present. Only the group exposed to 3.2 ppm formaldehyde had histopathology that was characterized by degeneration and necrosis of the respiratory epithelium with basal-cell hyperplasia. The lesions were most pronounced along the lateral walls of the naso- and maxilloturbinates. An associated significant increase in cell proliferation was also observed after exposure to 3.2 ppm formaldehyde for 3 days. After 3 days of exposure to 3.2 or 6.4 ppm formaldehyde, only GSH peroxidase activity had increased statistically significantly. Three days of exposure to 1.4 ppm acrolein resulted in a decrease in GST and ADH and an increase in FDH activities while the groups of rats exposed to the mixtures of all three compounds had increased GST and GSH peroxi-dase activities. Histological alterations of the nasal epithelium were more severe after exposure to the mixture than after exposure to any of the components alone at comparable concentrations and duration of exposure. The distribution of the lesions induced by formal-dehyde was different from that produced by acetaldehyde or acrolein, in that lesions pro-duced by formaldehyde were concentrated in the respiratory epithelium (Cassee *et al.*, 1996b).

Enzyme induction

No increase in the activities of FDH or ALDH was seen in the nasal mucosa of Fischer 344 rats exposed to 15 ppm [18.3 mg/m³] formaldehyde (6 h per day on 5 days per week for 2 weeks) (Casanova-Schmitz *et al.*, 1984a). A large increase in the concentration of rat pulmonary CYP was seen, however, after exposure to 0.5, 3 or 15 ppm formaldehyde [0.6, 3.7 or 18.3 mg/m³] (6 h per day for 4 days) (Dallas *et al.*, 1989), although Dinsdale *et al.* (1993) could not confirm these results in the same strain of rat and found no increase in pulmonary concentration of CYP after exposure to 10 ppm [12.3 mg/m³] formaldehyde (6 h per day for 4 days).

The relative contribution of three isoforms of ADH to ethanol, formaldehyde and retinoic acid acute toxicity was examined in knockout mice that had induced deletions of *Adh1*, *Adh3* or *Adh4* genes, which make the enzymes non-functional. The comparison with formaldehyde was based on the LD_{50} after intraperitoneal injection of a 10% formalin solution that resulted in a dose range of 0.09–0.22 g/kg bw formaldehyde. A lethal dose to wild-type mice resulted in death within 90 min. It was assumed in the interpretation of these studies that formaldehyde and not a metabolite was the ultimate toxicant. Mice that had *Adh3* knocked out required significantly lower levels of formaldehyde (0.135 g/kg) than the wild-type control (0.2 g/kg) to achieve an LD_{50} whereas there was no difference between wild-type and mice that had *Adh1* and *Adh4* knocked out. These studies showed that *Adh3* is responsible for the clearance of formaldehyde but does not play a role in the clearance of ethanol or retinoic acid. *Adh1* and *Adh4* demonstrate overlapping functions in the metabolism of ethanol and retinol *in vivo*. *Adh3* is conserved across most levels of biological organization including all mammalian species, invertebrates and plants (Deltour *et al.*, 1999).

Other effects

The nephrotoxicity of formaldehyde after intravascular injection was studied in male Sprague-Dawley rats (eight animals per group) that weighed 200 g. The rats were injected through the tail vein with 7.6 or 38 µM of a saline solution of formaldehyde or normal saline. Blood samples were taken for determination of blood urea and creatinine levels 24 and 48 h after injection of the test solution. Urine was also collected 24 h after injection and analysed for lactate dehydrogenase (LDH) and protein. All rats were killed 48 h after the single injection and the kidneys were removed for histological examination. No histological alterations were present in the kidney. No statistical change in urinary protein or LDH levels nor in blood creatinine was observed. A small but statistically significant increase in blood urea was reported at 24 h (5.23 ± 0.3 versus 4.13 ± 0.5 for control [units not reported]) after treatment which returned to normal levels at 48 h. These data suggested that renal toxicity does not occur after acute intravascular exposure to formaldehyde (Boj *et al.*, 2003).

Twenty-one male (weighing 250–280 g) and 19 female (weighing 180–200 g) 16-week-old Wistar rats were trained over 14 days to find food in a maze and were then tested in the maze after exposure to formaldehyde. The number of mistakes and the length of time to find the food were counted daily for 11 days as a baseline. The animals were exposed to aqueous formaldehyde solutions of either 0.25% (equivalent to 3.06 ± 0.77 mg/m^3; 2.6 ppm) or 0.7% (equivalent to 5.55 ± 1.27 mg/m^3; 4.6 ppm) for 10 min per day on 7 days per week for 90 days. Every 7th day, the animals were tested in the maze prior to exposure. After 90 days of exposure, the animals were then allowed a 30-day recovery and were tested in the maze every 10th day. At the end of the study, the animals were killed and the liver, trachea, lungs, kidneys, heart, spleen, pancreas, testicles, brain and spinal cord were collected and fixed in formalin. Both formaldehyde-exposed groups made more mistakes and took longer to complete the maze than the controls but no difference was observed between the exposed groups. None of the groups differed from one another after the recovery period. There were no treatment-related histological lesions (Pitten *et al.*, 2000). [There is no evidence that the changes seen in this study are due to formaldehyde-induced neurotoxicity, and could have just as easily have been from loss of olfactory capacity and visual difficulties from irritant effects to the cornea which would have improved after the treatment was stopped.]

Lewis rats were exposed to formaldehyde vapours and placed in a water maze to test the effect of formaldehyde on learning. A total of 120 male and female LEW.1K rats, 110–130 days of age, were separated into four groups and exposed to distilled water or 0.1 ± 0.02, 0.5 ± 0.1, or 5.4 ± 0.65 ppm [0.12 mg/m^3, 0.62 mg/m^3 or 6.64 mg/m^3] volatilized formaldehyde for 2 h per day for 10 days. Two hours after exposure, the rats were subjected to the water maze test. The length of time taken to complete the maze and the number of errors while attempting this were measured. At the conclusion of the study, the animals were killed and the lungs, heart, thymus, kidneys, liver, pancreas, skeletal muscle and spleen were examined microscopically. All rats exposed to formaldehyde made more errors in completing the maze, but no difference was observed between exposure groups or sexes. After 10 days, only the 0.5- and 5.4-ppm groups took longer to complete the water maze; no difference was observed between sexes. No histological lesions were found in the tissues examined. The authors suggested that formaldehyde vapours had a central effect on learning and memory. However, none of the tissues sampled were target organs for formaldehyde toxicity in the rat except at very high and prolonged exposure concentrations. [The nose was not examined in this study. Formaldehyde is a surface irritant which would cause degeneration and necrosis of the olfactory epithelium as well as the surface epithelium lining the cornea. The complications of blurry vision and loss of olfactory cues was not controlled for in this study, which suggests that an effect on the central nervous system may not have resulted in the treatment-related response] (Malek *et al.*, 2003).

Forty-two male Wistar rats (weighing approximately 250 g) were divided into six groups (seven rats per group) and exposed by inhalation to 0, 6.1 mg/m^3 or 12.2 mg/m^3 formaldehyde for 8 h per day on 5 days per week for subacute (4 weeks) or subchronic (13 weeks) periods. At the end of the exposure period, the animals were killed and the brains were removed for analysis of zinc, copper and iron levels (mg metal/kg parietal cortex). Both zinc and copper increased in concentration with increasing dose whereas iron decreased in concentration. The increase in copper concentration and decrease in iron concentration were both time-dependent. Exposure to formaldehyde altered the trace element level of copper, zinc and iron in the brain. The greatest change was a 54% increase in levels of zinc after 4 weeks of exposure to the high dose which fell to a 33% increase over controls after 13 weeks (Özen *et al.*, 2003).

Forty male albino Charles Foster rats, weighing 147–171 g, were given daily intraperitoneal injections of 0, 5, 10 or 15 mg/kg bw formaldehyde in saline for 30 days. On day 31, the animals were anaesthetized for blood collection then killed and the thyroid glands were collected, weighed and processed for histology. Thyroid weights were significantly decreased after treatment with 10 and 15 mg/kg per day and histological changes of follicular degeneration, atrophy and epithelial size were observed. Triiodothyronine and thyroxine were significantly decreased and thyroid-stimulating hormone was increased after doses of 10 and 15 mg/kg per day. After treatment with 5 mg/kg per day, triiodothyronine was decreased and thyroid-stimulating hormone was increased but thyroxine was unchanged and the thyroid glands did not differ histologically from those of controls (Patel *et al.*, 2003).

Levels of serum corticosterone were examined in Sprague-Dawley rats (weighing 260–280 g) exposed by inhalation to 0.7 or 2.4 ppm [0.86 or 2.95 mg/m^3] formaldehyde for 20 or 60 min per day on 5 days per week for 2 or 4 weeks. Treatment had no effect after short-term exposure; however, rats exposed to 0.7 ppm for 4 weeks had increased baseline serum corticosterone. Rats treated with 2.4 ppm formaldehyde for 2 or 4 weeks had increased levels of serum corticosterone after a formaldehyde challenge (Sorg *et al.*, 2001).

(ii)   *Chronic effects*

Cytotoxicity and cell proliferation in the respiratory tract

The subchronic and chronic effects of formaldehyde in different animal species exposed by inhalation are summarized in Table 34. No increase in cell turnover or DNA synthesis was found in the nasal mucosa after subchronic or chronic exposure to concentrations of ≤ 2 ppm [≤ 2.4 mg/m^3] formaldehyde (Rusch *et al.*, 1983; Maronpot *et al.*, 1986; Zwart *et al.*, 1988; Monticello *et al.*, 1993; Casanova *et al.*, 1994). Small, site-specific increases in the rate of cell turnover were noted at 3 ppm [3.7 mg/m^3] (6 h per day on 5 days per week for 13 weeks) in Wistar rats (Zwart *et al.*, 1988) and in the rate of DNA synthesis at 6 ppm [7.3 mg/m^3] (6 h per day on 5 days per week for 12 weeks) in Fischer 344 rats (Casanova *et al.*, 1994). At these concentrations, however, an adaptive response occurred in rat nasal epithelium, as cell turnover rates after 6 weeks (Monticello *et al.*, 1991) or 13 weeks (Zwart *et al.*, 1988) were lower than those after 1–3 or 4 days of exposure. Monticello *et al.* (1996) detected no increase in cell turnover in the nasal passages of Fischer 344 rats exposed to 6 ppm [7.3 mg/m^3] formaldehyde for 3 months (6 h per day on 5 days per week). However, as already noted, Casanova *et al.* (1994) detected a small increase in DNA synthesis under these conditions, but after 12 weeks of treatment. Large, sustained increases in cell turnover were observed at 10 and 15 ppm [12.2 and 18.3 mg/m^3] (6 h per day on 5 days per week for 3, 6, 12 or 18 months) (Monticello & Morgan, 1994; Monticello *et al.*, 1996). The effects of subchronic exposure to various concentrations of formaldehyde on DNA synthesis in the rat nose are illustrated in Figure 5.

Table 34. Cytotoxicity and cell proliferation induced by subchronic and chronic exposures to formaldehyde

Strain, species, sex	Exposure	Effects	Reference
Fischer 344 rat, Syrian hamster, male and female; cynomolgus monkey, male	0, 0.25, 1.2, 3.7 mg/m^3, 22 h/day, 7 days/week, 26 weeks	Rat: squamous metaplasia in nasal turbinates at 3.7 mg/m^3 only; hamster: no significant toxic response; monkey: squamous metaplasia in nasal turbinates at 3.7 mg/m^3 only	Rusch et al. (1983)
B6C3F1 mouse, male	0, 2.5, 4.9, 12.3, 24.6, 49.2 mg/m^3, 6 h/day, 5 days/week, 13 weeks	2.5, 4.9: no lesion induced; 12.3, 24.7, 49.2: squamous metaplasia, inflammation of nasal passages, trachea and larynx; 80% mortality at 49.2 mg/m^3	Maronpot et al. (1986)
Wistar rat, male and female	0, 0.37, 1.2, 3.7 mg/m^3, 6 h/day, 5 days/week, 13 weeks	0.37, 1.2: no increase in cell replication; 3.7: increased cell turnover in nasal epithelium but cell proliferation lower than after 3 days of exposure	Zwart et al. (1988)
Wistar rat, male and female	0, 1.2, 12.3, 24.7 mg/m^3, 6 h/day, 5 days/week, 13 weeks	1.2: results inconclusive; 12.3, 24.7: squamous metaplasia, epithelial erosion, cell proliferation in nasal passages and larynx; no hepatotoxicity	Woutersen et al. (1987)
Wistar rat, male	0, 0.12, 1.2, 12.3 mg/m^3, 6 h/day, 5 days/week, 13 or 52 weeks Nasal mucosa of some rats injured by bilateral intranasal electrocoagulation to induce cell proliferation	0: electrocoagulation induced hyperplasia and squamous metaplasia, still visible after 13 weeks but slight after 52 weeks; 0.12, 1.2: focal squamous metaplasia after 13 or 52 weeks; no adverse effects in animals with undamaged nasal mucosa; 12.3: squamous metaplasia in respiratory epithelium (both intact and damaged nose); degeneration with or without hyperplasia of olfactory epithelium (damaged nose only)	Appelman et al. (1988)

Table 34 (contd)

Strain, species, sex	Exposure	Effects	Reference
Wistar rat, male	0, 1.2 mg/m^3 × 8 h/day, 2.4 mg/m^3 × 8 h/day ($C × t$ = 9.8 or 19.7 mg/m^3– h/day), 5 days/week, 13 weeks; 2.4 mg/m^3 × 8 × 0.5 h/day, 4.9 mg/m^3 × 8 × 0.5 h/day ($C × t$ = 9.8 or 19.7 mg/m^3–h/day), 5 days/week, 13 weeks	1.2, 2.5: no observed toxic effect; 4.9: epithelial damage, squamous metaplasia, occasional keratinization; concentration, not total dose, determined severity of toxic effect	Wilmer *et al.* (1989)
Fischer 344 rat, male	0, 0.86, 2.5, 7.4, 12.3, 18.5 mg/m^3, 6 h/day, 5 days/week, 6 weeks	0.86, 2.5: no increase in cell replication detected; 7.4: increase in cell proliferation; 12.3, 18.5: sustained cell proliferation	Monticello *et al.* (1991)
Fischer 334 rat, male	0, 0.86, 2.5, 7.4, 18.5 ppm, 6 h/day, 5 days/week, 12 weeks	0.86, 2.5: DNA synthesis rates in nasal mucosa similar in naive (previously unexposed) and subchronically exposed rats; 7.4, 18.5: DNA synthesis rates higher in subchronically exposed than in naive rats, especially at 18.5 mg/m^3	Casanova *et al.* (1994)
Fischer 344 rat, male	0, 0.86, 2.5, 7.4, 12.3, 18.5 mg/m^3, 6 h/day, 5 days/week, 3 months	0.86, 2.5, 7.4: no increase in cell replication detected; 12.3, 18.5: sustained cell proliferation. Site-specific increase in cell replication corresponded to location of squamous-cell carcinomas.	Monticello *et al.* (1996)

C, concentration; *t*, time

Figure 5. Cell turnover in the lateral meatus (LM) and medial and posterior meatuses (M:PM) of pre-exposed and naive (previously unexposed) Fischer 344 rats, as measured by incorporation of ^{14}C derived from inhaled [^{14}C]formaldehyde (HCHO) into nucleic acid bases (deoxyadenosine, deoxyguanosine and thymidine) and thence into DNA, during a single 3-h exposure to 0.7, 2, 6 or 15 ppm [0.86, 2.5, 7.4 or 18.5 mg/m^3] formaldehyde

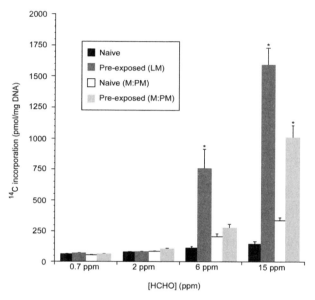

Reproduced, with permission, from Casanova *et al.* (1994)
Pre-exposed rats were exposed subchronically to the same concentrations of unlabelled formaldehyde (6 h per day on 5 days per week for 11 weeks and 4 days), while naive rats were exposed to room air. The exposure to [^{14}C]formaldehyde occurred on the 5th day of the 12th week. The asterisk denotes a significant difference between pre-exposed and naive rats.

Additional studies have shown the importance of increased cell turnover in the induction of rat nasal tumours (Appelman *et al.*, 1988; Woutersen *et al.*, 1989). The nasal mucosa of Wistar rats was damaged by bilateral intranasal electrocoagulation and the susceptibility of the rats to inhalation of formaldehyde at concentrations of 0.1, 1 or 10 ppm [0.1, 1.2 or 12.2 mg/m^3] (for 6 h per day on 5 days per week for 13 or 52 weeks (Appelman *et al.*, 1988), 28 months or 3 months followed by a 25-month observation period (Woutersen *et al.*, 1989)) was evaluated. In rats with undamaged mucosa, the effects of exposure were seen only at 10 ppm; these effects were limited to degenerative, inflammatory and hyperplastic changes, and were increased by electrocoagulation. In the group exposed to 10 ppm for 28 months, nasal tumours were induced in 17/58 rats. No compound-related tumours were induced at 0.1 or 1 ppm. It was concluded that the damaged mucosa was more susceptible to the cyto-toxic effects of formaldehyde and that severe damage contributes to the induction of nasal tumours.

The time-dependent development of formaldehyde-induced lesions was examined in 180 male Fischer 344 rats (six per exposure group), 8–9 weeks of age, that were exposed by inhalation to nominal concentrations of 0, 0.7, 2, 6, 10 or 15 ppm [0, 0.86, 2.46, 7.38, 12.3 or 18.45 mg/m^3, respectively] formaldehyde [thermal depolymerization of para-formaldehyde, purity unspecified] for 6 h per day on 5 days per week for 3, 6, 12, 18 or 24 months. Five days before necropsy, the rats were anaesthetized and received an implant of an osmotic minipump that contained 2mCi [methyl-^{3}H]thymidine for incorporation of the thymidine into DNA during S-phase to allow subsequent quantitation of cell proliferation. A detailed morphological analysis of the nasal cavity of each rat was made in order to collect information on the development and distribution of lesions in seven separate regions of the nose (anterior lateral meatus, posterior lateral meatus, anterior mid-septum, posterior mid-septum, anterior dorsal septum, anterior medial maxilloturbinate and maxillary sinus). The unit length labelling index method was used to establish the proliferation index in each area of the nose. The number of cells in each of the designated areas was also determined through a combination of actual cell counts and estimates of numbers using surface area measurements and a CFD model of the rat nose. A population-weighted unit length labelling index was calculated for direct comparison across time and dose. Survival was not different or greater in controls than in rats treated with 10 ppm formaldehyde or less. Survival was decreased in rats treated with 15 ppm formaldehyde. Formaldehyde-induced lesions were primarily confined to areas lined by respiratory and transitional epithelium and were more prevalent and severe in the anterior portion of the nose. The severity of the lesions was dose-dependent, with only minimal lesions present after exposure to 6 ppm and none after exposure to 2 ppm or 0.7 ppm. The predominant non-neoplastic formaldehyde-induced lesions were epithelial hypertrophy and hyperplasia, squamous metaplasia and inflammatory cell infiltration. The majority of formaldehyde-induced neoplasms were squamous-cell carcinomas with much lower incidences of polypoid adenomas, adenocarcinomas and rhabdomyosarcomas. The 10- and 15-ppm groups had parallel cumulative incidence curves, although the 10-ppm group had a later time to onset of tumours. The squamous-cell carcinomas appeared to arise from regions lined by transitional and respiratory epithelium and were most common in the lateral meatus and mid-septum, the incidence was higher in the more anterior portions (Table 35). Significant increases in the unit length labelling index were only observed in the 10- and 15-ppm groups with the greatest increase in the more anterior portion of the nose where the tumour response was greatest. An elevated unit length labelling index developed in the anterior dorsal septum later in the course of the exposure. This belated elevation in the more posterior nose of animals exposed to the high dose may have been secondary to changes in airflow patterns and resultant local formaldehyde concentrations associated with growth of lesions and distortion of the airspace in the nose. The mapping of cell numbers per area showed significant differences in the total populations of nasal epithelium at risk in the different areas counted for this study. An additional method of examining the association between cells at risk and the labelling index used in this study was the population-weighted unit length labelling index which is the product of the total numbers of cells in the specified

Table 35. Incidences of nasal squamous-cell carcinomas in male Fischer 344 rats exposed by inhalation to formaldehyde

Concentration of formalde-hyde (ppm)	No. of nasal cavities examined	Nasal location							No. of animals with squamous-cell carcinoma[a]
		Anterior lateral meatus	Posterior lateral meatus	Anterior mid-septum	Posterior mid-septum	Anterior dorsal septum	Anterior medial maxillo-turbinate	Maxillary sinus	
0	90	0	0	0	0	0	0	0	0
0.7	90	0	0	0	0	0	0	0	0
2	96	0	0	0	0	0	0	0	0
6	90	1	0	0	0	0	0	0	1
10	90	12	2	0	0	0	0	0	20
15	147	17	9	8	1	3	4	0	69

From Monticello et al. (1996)

[a] Total number of animals with squamous-cell carcinoma, including those too large to allocate and those located in a site not listed in this table

area and the unit length labelling index. This product corresponded very closely with tumour development at all sites in the nose (Figs 6 and 7) (Monticello *et al.*, 1996).

A rat CFD model was used to test whether the distribution of formaldehyde-induced squamous metaplasia was related to the location of high-flux regions posterior to the squamous epithelium. Histological sections of nose corresponding to level 6 (Mery *et al.*, 1994) from male Fischer 344 rats exposed by whole-body inhalation to nominal concentrations of 0, 0.7, 2, 6, 10 and 15 ppm [0, 0.86, 2.46, 7.38, 12.3 and 18.45 mg/m^3] formaldehyde were examined. Distribution of squamous epithelium within 20 subset areas within the section was mapped. Squamous metaplasia was considered to be present when $\geq$ 50% of the epithelium within a subsection was of the squamous type. The regions were then ranked by presence of squamous metaplasia by dose group. Inspiratory airflow and formaldehyde uptake were simulated based on a minute volume of 288 mL/min for a 315-g rat. Steady-state simulations were performed using air concentrations of 6, 10 or 15 ppm formaldehyde. Only these three concentrations were used because no squamous metaplasia was present in sections of nose from rats exposed to 2 ppm or less. Squamous metaplasia was present on the lateral and medial walls of the airway after exposure to 10 or 15 ppm; the highest incidence was on wells of the lateral meatus in all three groups (6, 10 and 15 ppm). The distribution of formaldehyde-induced squamous metaplasia was consistent with the location of high formaldehyde flux in rat noses after exposure to 10 or 15 ppm for 6 months. The data were inconclusive for the 6-ppm group, probably due to the insufficient number of rats examined (Kimbell *et al.*, 1997).

A larger percentage of the nasal mucosal surface area of rhesus monkeys exposed to 6 ppm [7.3 mg/m^3] formaldehyde (6 h per day on 5 days per week) was affected after 6 weeks of exposure than after 5 days. Cell proliferation was detected in the nasal passages, larynx, trachea and carina, but the effects in the lower airways were minimal in comparison with the effects in the nasal passages (Monticello *et al.*, 1989). Other studies showed that Fischer 344 rats exposed to 1 ppm [1.2 mg/m^3] (22 h per day on 7 days per week for 26 weeks) formaldehyde did not develop detectable nasal lesions (Rusch *et al.*, 1983), but that rats exposed to 2 ppm [2.4 mg/m^3] (6 h per day on 5 days per week for 24 months) developed mild squamous metaplasia in the nasal turbinates (Kerns *et al.*, 1983b). Although the total dose received by the former group was 1.5 times higher than that received by the latter group, the incidence and severity of lesions was smaller, which demonstrates the greater importance of concentration than total dose (Rusch *et al.*, 1983).

A computer simulation of the relationship between airflow and the development of formaldehyde-induced lesions was developed for rhesus monkeys. A three-dimensional computer model was developed using video image analysis of serial coronal sections from an 11.9-kg, 7-year-old male rhesus monkey. Coordinates were taken for every 0.1 mm over the 83 mm long nasal passage. Eighty cross sections were used for the final model and spanned 75 mm of airway. Values for airflow simulation were estimated by allometric scaling, using body weight and a calculated minute volume of 2.4 L/min and half maximum nasal airflow calculated to be 3.8 L/min. Simulations were performed using airflow parameters of 0.63–3.8 L/min. The nasal cavity of rhesus monkeys has two air-

Figure 6. Calculated total proliferative population in areas of the nose of rats after exposure to formaldehyde for 3 months and T-site where tumours developed

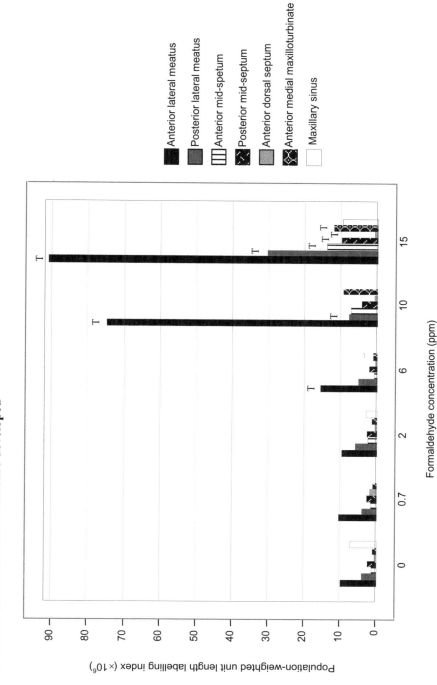

Adapted from Monticello et al. (1996)

Figure 7. Sum of calculated total proliferative population in areas of the nose of rats after exposure to formaldehyde over time and T-site where tumours developed

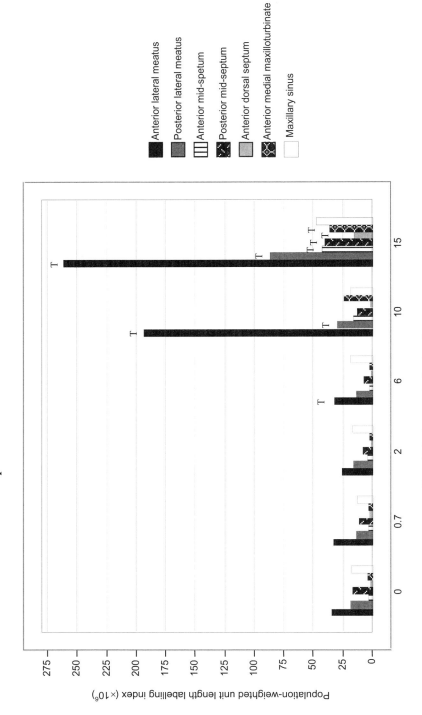

Adapted from Monticello et al. (1996)

ways that are separated by a septum that extends approximately 71.5 mm from the anterior tip of the nares to the nasopharynx. The nose has three distinct regions: the nasal vestibule, the central nasal passage and the nasopharynx. The nasal vestibule extends from the tip of the nostrils to the anterior margin of the middle turbinate. Airflow enters the nasal vestibule in an undeviated pattern and flows along the septal wall to the ventral medial, middle medial and dorsal airways in the central nasal passage. The central nasal passage begins at the anterior margin of the middle turbinate, extends to the middle and ventral turbinates and has a streamlined airflow in the middle portion of the nose which is slower than that of the nasal vestibule. The nasopharynx extends from the posterior nasal passage at the point where the middle turbinate attaches to the nasal wall dorsally to the soft palate and has streamlined airflow in the anterior portion which increases in velocity toward the posterior after the end of the dorsal meatus. The model predicted that 90% of gas uptake would be from the nostrils to the end of the septal wall. In general, the regions where mass flux was predicted to be high (nasal vestibule, mid-septum, floor of the anterior meatus, medial inferior turbinate and the middle turbinate) are also areas where formaldehyde-induced lesions occurred (Monticello *et al.*, 1989). Areas with low mass flux (dorsal meatus and the wall of the ventral lateral meatus) did not develop formaldehyde-induced lesions. An exception was the lateral wall where lesions occurred but mass flux was predicted to be low (Kepler *et al.*, 1998).

Toxicity in the gastrointestinal tract after oral administration

The toxic effects of formaldehyde administered orally have been reviewed (Restani & Galli, 1991).

Formaldehyde was administered orally to rats and dogs at daily doses of 50, 100 or 150 mg/kg bw (rats) or 50, 75 or 100 mg/kg bw (dogs) for 90 consecutive days. Significant changes in body weight were observed at the higher doses, but clinical and pathological studies revealed no specific treatment-related effects on the kidney, liver or lung, which were considered to be possible target organs, or on the gastrointestinal mucosa (Johannsen *et al.*, 1986).

Formaldehyde was administered in the drinking-water to male and female Wistar rats for up to 2 years. In the chronic portion of the study, the mean daily doses of formaldehyde were 1.2, 15 or 82 mg/kg bw (males) and 1.8, 21 or 109 mg/kg bw (females). Controls received drinking-water either *ad libitum* or in an amount equal to that consumed by the highest-dose group, which had a marked decrease in water consumption. Pathological changes after 2 years were essentially restricted to the highest-dose group and consisted of a thickened and raised limiting ridge of the forestomach and gastritis and hyperplasia of the glandular stomach. The no-adverse-effect level was estimated to be 15 mg/kg bw per day (males) or 21 mg/kg bw per day (females) (Til *et al.*, 1989). In a 4-week study, the effects of formaldehyde that were also observed only in the highest-dose group (125 mg/kg bw) were thickening of the limiting ridge and hyperkeratosis in the forestomach and focal gastritis in the glandular stomach (Til *et al.*, 1988).

In another experiment in which formaldehyde was administered in the drinking-water to male and female Wistar rats, fixed concentrations (0, 0.02, 0.1 and 0.5%) were given for up to 2 years. Estimated from the water intake and body weight, these concentrations corresponded, on average, to 0, 10, 50 and 300 mg/kg bw per day. All rats that received the highest dose died during the study. The lesions induced in the stomach were similar to those reported by Til *et al.* (1988, 1989). No treatment-related tumour was found. The no-effect level was estimated to be 0.02% (10 mg/kg bw per day), as forestomach hyper-keratosis was observed in a small number of rats (2/14) that received 0.1% formaldehyde (50 mg/kg bw per day) (Tobe *et al.*, 1989).

(iii)   *Immunotoxicity*

The possibility that formaldehyde may induce changes in the immune response was examined in B6C3F$_1$ mice exposed to 15 ppm [18.3 mg/m^3] formaldehyde (6 h per day on 5 days per week for 3 weeks). A variety of tests of immune function revealed no significant changes, except for an increase in host resistance to challenge with the bacterium, *Listeria monocytogenes*, which implied an increased resistance to infection. Exposure did not alter the number or impair the function of resident peritoneal macrophages, but increased their competence for release of hydrogen peroxide (Dean *et al.*, 1984; Adams *et al.*, 1987). Formaldehyde enhanced the anti-ovalbumin IgE titre after pre-exposure of BALB/c mice to 2 mg/m^3 formaldehyde for 6 h per day for 10 days (Tarkowski & Gorski, 1995) but did not enhance the IgG1 response of ICR mice to a mite allergen in the respiratory tract after exposure to an aerosol of 0.5% formaldehyde saline solution (Sadakane *et al.*, 2002).

Sprague-Dawley rats were exposed to 12.6 ppm [15.5 mg/m^3] formaldehyde (6 h per day on 5 days per week for 22 months), then vaccinated with pneumococcal polysaccharide antigens and tetanus toxoid and were tested 3–4 weeks later for the development of antibodies. An IgG response to pneumococcal polysaccharides and to tetanus toxoid and an IgM response to tetanus toxoid were found in both exposed and control groups. No evidence was obtained that long-term exposure to a high concentration of formaldehyde impairs B-cell function, as measured by antibody production (Holmström *et al.*, 1989c).

4.3   Reproductive and developmental effects

4.3.1   *Humans*

A variety of epidemiological studies are available that have evaluated the reproductive effects of occupational exposures to formaldehyde both directly and indirectly. The outcomes examined in these studies include spontaneous abortions, congenital malformations, birth weight and infertility.

The incidence of spontaneous abortion was studied among hospital staff in Finland who used ethylene oxide (see IARC, 1994b), glutaraldehyde and formaldehyde to sterilize instruments. Potentially exposed women were identified in 1980 with the help of supervising nurses at all of the approximately 80 general hospitals of the country. An equal number of control women were selected by the supervising nurse from among nursing auxiliaries in the same hospitals who had no exposure to sterilizing agents, anaesthetic gases or X-rays. Study subjects were administered a postal questionnaire which requested personal data and information on tobacco smoking habits, intake of alcohol, reproductive history, including the number of pregnancies and their outcome, and occupation at the time of each pregnancy. Information on exposure to chemical sterilizing agents was obtained from the supervising nurses. The crude rates of spontaneous abortion were 16.7% for sterilizing staff who were considered to have been exposed during the first trimester of pregnancy, 6.0% for sterilizing staff who left employment when they learned that they were pregnant (the difference being significant) and 10.6% for controls. When adjusted for age, parity, decade of pregnancy, tobacco smoking habits and alcohol and coffee consumption, the rate associated with exposure to ethylene oxide, with or without other agents, was 12.7%, which was significantly increased ($p < 0.05$), whereas that associated with formaldehyde, with or without other agents, was 8.4%, which was comparable with the reference level of 10.5% and was thus not significantly correlated with spontaneous abortions (Hemminki et al., 1982).

In a nationwide record linkage study in Finland, all nurses who had been pregnant between 1973 and 1979 and who had worked in anaesthesia, surgery, intensive care, operating rooms or internal departments of a general hospital (and in paediatric, gynaecological, cancer and lung departments for the part of the study that was concerned with malformations) were identified. Each of the 217 women treated for spontaneous abortion according to the files of the Finnish hospital discharge register and the 46 women notified to the Register of Congenital Malformations was individually matched on age and hospital with three control women, who were selected at random from the same population of nurses and matched for age and hospital where they were employed. Information was obtained from supervising nurses by postal questionnaires on the exposure of cases and controls to sterilizing agents (ethylene oxide, glutaraldehyde and formaldehyde), anaesthetic gases, disinfectant soaps, cytostatic drugs and X-radiation. Exposure to formaldehyde during pregnancy was reported for 3.7% of the nurses who were later treated for spontaneous abortion and for 5.2% of their controls, yielding a crude odds ratio of 0.7 [95% CI, 0.28–1.7]. Exposure to formaldehyde was also reported for 8.8% of nurses who gave birth to a malformed child and 5.3% of matched controls, to give an odds ratio of 1.74 [95% CI, 0.39–7.7]; the latter analysis was based on eight exposed subjects (Hemminki et al., 1985). [The Working Group noted that these numbers appear to be recalculated from published reports.]

The occurrence of spontaneous abortions among women who worked in laboratories in Finland, and congenital malformations and birth weights of the children were investigated in a matched retrospective case–control study using a case–referent design. The final population in the study of spontaneous abortion was 206 cases and 329 controls; that in the study of congenital malformations was 36 cases and 105 controls. Information on occupational exposure, health status, medication, contraception, tobacco smoking and alcohol consumption during the first trimester of the pregnancy was collected by postal questionnaire. The exposure to individual chemicals was estimated on the basis of a reported frequency of chemical use. An occupational hygienic assessment was conducted and an exposure index was calculated. The odds ratio for spontaneous abortion was increased among women who had been exposed to formalin for at least 3 days per week (odds ratio, 3.5; 95% CI, 1.1–11.2). A greater proportion of the cases (8/10) than the controls (4/7) who had been exposed to formalin had been employed in pathology and histology laboratories. Most of the cases (8/10) and controls (5/7) who were exposed to formalin were also exposed to xylene (see IARC, 1989). The authors stated that the results for individual chemicals should be interpreted with caution because laboratory personnel are often exposed to several solvents and other chemicals simultaneously. No association was observed between exposure to formalin and congenital malformations [data not shown] (Taskinen *et al.*, 1994).

Reduced fertility was investigated in a retrospective study of time to pregnancy that was conducted among female wood workers who were exposed to formaldehyde and who had given birth between 1985 and 1995 (Taskinen *et al.*, 1999). Time to pregnancy was analysed using a discrete proportional hazards regression approach. Study criteria included women who had worked in the wood-processing industry for at least 1 month and for whom employment in wood-related work had started at least 6 months before pregnancy. Exposure assessment was based on responses from a detailed questionnaire that asked women to describe their occupational title and their work tasks. Women estimated the number of hours they spent in various types of factories/enterprises in the industry and the number of hours they were exposed to various chemicals including formaldehyde, organic solvents, wood preservatives, glues or wood-protecting chemicals. The questionnaire also collected information on the use of personal protective equipment, and exposure to welding fumes, exhaust gases, pesticides and tobacco smoke. An occupational hygienist assessed the exposures and calculated a daily exposure index. The authors used workplace exposure measurements to support these exposure estimates. Among the 699 female wood workers, exposure to formaldehyde was significantly associated with delayed conception density, as assessed by an adjusted fecundability density ratio, which was 0.64 (95% CI, 0.43–0.92). When no gloves were used during high levels of exposure, the fecundability density ratio was 0.51 (95% CI, 0.28–0.92). Exposure to phenols, dusts, wood dusts or organic solvents was not related to the time to pregnancy. All women exposed to phenols were also exposed to formaldehyde but the opposite was not true.

Although the study focus was time to pregnancy, other analyses of these workers showed an increased odds ratio for spontaneous abortion (52 pregnancies) of 3.2 (95% CI, 1.2–8.3) in the high-exposure and 2.4 (95% CI, 1.2–4.8) in the low-exposure categories. Exposure to formaldehyde at high levels was also associated with an increased risk (odds ratio, 4.5; 95% CI, 1.0–20.0) for endometriosis (Taskinen *et al.*, 1999).

A meta-risk analysis conducted by Collins *et al.* (2001b) noted that, of the 11 epidemiological studies that they reviewed for their evaluation of reproductive effects among workers exposed to formaldehyde, nine evaluated spontaneous abortions. Four of these studies reported significantly higher rates of spontaneous abortion among women who were occupationally exposed to formaldehyde (Axelsson *et al.*, 1984; John *et al.*, 1994; Taskinen et al., 1994, 1999). Four other studies did not find an increased association (Hemminki et al., 1982, 1985; Stücker et al., 1990; Lindbohm et al., 1991). One study did not report relative risks but showed no increased risk for spontaneous abortion (Shumilina, 1975). Collins et al. (2001b) suggested that there is a reporting bias against negative studies and described some of the difficulties in conducting studies of spontaneous abortions.

Collins et al. (2001b) discussed the four epidemiological studies that used a case–control design to evaluate congenital defects among children of women exposed to form-aldehyde (Axelsson et al., 1984; Ericson et al., 1984; Hemminki et al., 1985; Taskinen et al., 1994).

Three epidemiological studies evaluated birth weights. Neither Taskinen et al. (1994) nor Axelsson et al. (1984) reported associations between exposure to formaldehyde and decreased birth weight among the 500 and 968 births examined, respectively. A study in Russia by Shumilina (1975) reported an elevated number of births of babies that weighed less than 3000 g among 81 newborns of women who were potentially exposed to formal-dehyde; however, if the cut-point of below 2500 g is used (more traditional definition of low birth weight), then these increases disappear.

It is important to note that most of the epidemiological studies reported in this section were not designed to evaluate exposures to formaldehyde specifically. For example, the studies by Taskinen et al. (1994), Hemminki et al. (1982, 1985), Ericson et al. (1984) and Axelsson et al. (1984) were designed to investigate pregnancy outcomes in laboratory workers and that of John et al. (1994) to investigate pregnancy outcomes in cosmeto-logists. All of these studies are confounded by significant co-exposures and, in general, have directed research to examine specific exposures in follow-up studies.

Other studies of reproductive effects in humans have investigated sperm abnormality. Eleven hospital autopsy service workers and 11 matched controls were evaluated for sperm count, abnormal sperm morphology and the frequency of one or two fluorescent F-bodies. Subjects were matched for age and use of alcohol, tobacco and marijuana; additional information was collected on health, medications and other exposure to toxins. Exposed and control subjects were sampled three times at 2–3-month intervals. Ten exposed subjects had been employed for 4.3 months (range, 1–11 months) before the first sample was taken, and one had been employed for several years. Exposure to formaldehyde was intermittent, with a time-weighted average of 0.61–1.32 ppm [0.75–1.6 mg/m^3] (weekly exposure, 3–40 ppm·h [3.7–48.8 mg/m^3·h]). No significant difference was observed between the exposed and control groups with regard to sperm parameters (Ward et al., 1984).

4.3.2   Experimental systems

The reproductive and developmental toxicity of formaldehyde has been reviewed (Feinman, 1988; WHO, 1989; Collins et al., 2001b).

Numerous studies have been performed to examine the potential effects of formal-dehyde on pregnancy and fetal development in rats, mice, hamsters, rabbits and dogs.

Routes of exposure have included inhalation, oral gavage, administration in the drinking-water and dermal application. The inhalation studies (Gofmekler, 1968; Gofmekler *et al.*, 1968; Pushkina *et al.*, 1968; Gofmekler & Bonashevskaya, 1969; Shevelera, 1971; Kilburn & Moro, 1985; Saillenfait *et al.*, 1989; Martin, 1990) and studies of dermal expo-sure (Overman, 1985) use relevant routes of exposure for evaluation. Studies conducted before 1970 (Gofmekler, 1968; Gofmekler *et al.*, 1968; Pushkina *et al.*, 1968; Gofmekler & Bonashevskaya, 1969) reported a prolongation of pregnancy, changes in fetal organ weight and a variety of clinical and biochemical changes in the spleen, liver, kidney, thymus and lymphocytes in rats (Thrasher & Kilburn, 2001; Collins *et al.*, 2001b). Thrasher and Kilburn (2001) reviewed studies of embryotoxicity and teratogenicity (Katakura *et al.*, 1990, 1991, 1993) and reported that [^{14}C]-labelled formaldehyde crossed the placenta and entered fetal tissues at levels greater than those in the dam. Embryotoxic and teratogenic outcomes were a function of the exposure regimen. Rats exposed before mating had increased embryo mortality and those exposed during mating had increased fetal anomalies. [The Working Group agreed with the authors' suggestion that this [C^{14}]-labelling would be consistent with the entry of the [^{14}C]-label from formaldehyde into the one-carbon pool.]

Groups of 25 pregnant Sprague–Dawley rats were exposed by inhalation to formal-dehyde (0, 5, 10, 20 or 40 ppm [0, 6.2, 12.3, 24.6 or 49.2 mg/m^3]) for 6 h per day on days 6–20 of gestation. On day 21, the rats were killed and maternal and fetal parameters were evaluated. The authors concluded that formaldehyde was neither embryolethal nor terato-genic when administered under these conditions. The mean fetal body weight at 20 ppm was 5% less than that of controls ($p < 0.05$) in males but was not reduced in females; at 40 ppm, mean fetal body weight was about 20% less than that in controls ($p < 0.01$) in both males and females. The decrease in fetal weight in the group given the high dose was attributed to maternal toxicity. However, the authors stated that the significant reductions in fetal body weight observed at 20 ppm did not cause overt signs of maternal toxicity (Saillenfait *et al.*, 1989). [The Working Group noted that 20-ppm exposures in other studies would be considered to be 'toxic' doses.]

Groups of 25 mated female Sprague–Dawley rats were exposed by inhalation to form-aldehyde (0, 2, 5 or 10 ppm [2.5, 6.2 or 12.3 mg/m^3]) for 6 h per day on days 6–15 of gestation. At 10 ppm, there was a significant decrease in maternal food consumption and weight gain. None of the parameters of pregnancy, including numbers of corpora lutea, implantation sites, live fetuses, dead fetuses and resorptions or fetal weights, were affected by treatment. An increased incidence of reduced ossification was observed at 5 and 10 ppm in the absence of maternal toxicity (10 ppm) (Martin, 1990). The author of this study noted that the effects at both 5 and 10 ppm were attributed to larger litter sizes which could have reduced fetal body weights (Martin, 1990).

Formaldehyde was applied topically to pregnant Syrian hamsters on day 8, 9, 10 or 11 of gestation by clipping the hair on the dorsal body and applying 0.5 mL formalin (37% formaldehyde) with a syringe directly onto the skin. In order to prevent grooming, the animals were anaesthetized with nembutal (13 mg intraperitoneally) during the 2-h treatment. On day 15, fetuses were removed from four to six hamsters per group and examined. The number of resorptions was increased, but no teratogenic effects or effects on fetal weight or length were detected. The authors suggested that the increase in resorptions may have been caused by stress, as females were anaesthetized during formaldehyde exposures. No effect on maternal weight gain was observed (Overman, 1985).

In a study of post-implantation effects, 27 mature female Wistar rats were exposed by inhalation to 0.5 mg/m³ or 1.5 mg/m³ formaldehyde every day for 4 h for up to 4 months. On day 120, treated females were mated with untreated males. The effect of formaldehyde was evaluated in developing embryos at the 2nd and 3rd day after mating. The authors reported a significant increase in the number of degenerating embryos only from pregnant females who had been exposed to 1.5 mg/m³. The impaired embryonic morphology was reported as structural impairment in blastomers. In a cytogenetic analysis, no increase was found in the number of embryos with chromosomal aberrations in comparison with the controls (Kitaeva et al., 1990).

Reproductive effects were observed in a study of sperm head abnormalities and dominant lethal mutations. Male albino rats (six per group) received five daily intraperitoneal injections of 37% formaldehyde solution to provide 0.125, 0.25 or 0.5 mg/kg bw based on the LD_{50} and a lethal dose of 2 mg/kg bw to examine sperm head abnormalities 3 weeks after the last injection. A separate group of 12 male albino rats was injected intraperitoneally with the same doses, then housed with two untreated virgin female rats that were replaced weekly for 3 weeks to provide 24 females for each treatment group. Mating was detected by the presence of vaginal plugs. All females were killed and necropsied 13 days after the midweek of housing with the males. Total implant scores per female were collected and a dominant lethal mutation index was calculated based on the formula [1–(live implants treated/live implants control)] × 100. Formaldehyde induced sperm head abnormalities at all doses tested, which included pinhead, short hook, long hook, hook at wrong angle, unusual head and wide acrosome; short and long hook were the most common. Only total numbers of abnormalities were compared statistically, and only the incidence of wide acrosome was much greater than that in controls at the lowest dose tested (46 versus 0). In general, there was a decrease in sperm count with increasing dose of formaldehyde. A lower frequency of fertile matings was observed in females within the first 2 weeks after treatment, and the severity of effect was greater when mating took place earlier after treatment. The highest dose with the shortest time between final treatment and mating had the most severe effect and showed a dose- and time-dependent response. By 3 weeks after the last treatment, there was no longer a difference from controls (Odeigah, 1997). Morphological changes in sperm from mice were also identified after five daily intraperitoneal injections of 4, 10 or 30 mg/kg bw formaldehyde. Sperm counts were decreased after 10 and 30 mg/kg bw and deformed sperm were present after all doses (Yi et al., 2000). [The Working Group noted that, because of the reactivity of formaldehyde, the positive results seen after intraperitoneal injection are of questionable biological significance.]

4.4   Genetic and related effects

The genotoxicity of formaldehyde has been reviewed extensively (IARC, 1982, 1987a; Ma & Haris, 1988; WHO, 1989; Feron *et al.*, 1991; Monticello & Morgan, 1994; IARC, 1995; Conaway *et al.*, 1996; Mathison *et al.*, 1997; Monticello & Morgan, 1997; Bolt, 2003; Liteplo & Meek, 2003).

4.4.1   *Humans*

(*a*)   *DNA–protein cross-links*

The induction of DNA–protein cross-links due to exposure to formaldehyde was studied in humans (Shaham *et al.*, 1996a,b, 2003) (see Table 36). The number of DNA–protein cross-links and the amount of p53 protein, both pantropic (wild-type + mutant) and mutant, were measured in peripheral blood lymphocytes and serum, respectively, of 399 workers from 14 hospital pathology departments, 186 of whom were exposed to formaldehyde (59 men and 127 women), and 213 control workers (127 men and 86 women) from the administrative section of the same hospitals. The mean period of exposure to formaldehyde was 15.9 years (range, 1–51 years). The exposed group was divided into two subgroups: (1) low-level exposure (mean, 0.4 ppm [0.5 mg/m³]; range, 0.04–0.7 ppm [0.5–0.62 mg/m³]); and (2) high-level exposure (mean, 2.24 ppm [2.75 mg/m³]; range, 0.72–5.6 ppm [0.88–6.9 mg/m³). Before comparing the results obtained in the exposed and the unexposed group, adjustment was made for age, sex, origin and education. The amount of DNA–protein cross-links was expressed as a ratio to total DNA. The adjusted mean number of DNA–protein cross-links was significantly higher ($p < 0.01$) in all exposed subjects (adjusted mean, 0.21; SE, 0.006) compared with that in all unexposed subjects (adjusted mean, 0.14; SE, 0.006). It was also significantly higher ($p < 0.01$) in the subgroups of exposed men (adjusted mean, 0.21; SE, 0.011) and women (adjusted mean, 0.20; SE, 0.008) compared with that of unexposed men and women (adjusted mean, 0.15 and 0.12; SE, 0.008 and 0.008, respectively). Age, tobacco smoking habits, years of education and origin were not significant confounders. The study population was divided into those who had levels of pantropic p53 protein above or below 150 pg/mL. High levels of p53 (> 150 pg/mL) were more prevalent in the exposed group than in the unexposed (44.1% and 36.3%, respectively). The difference between high and low p53 was significant among exposed men, and exposure to formaldehyde was associated with a higher level of pantropic p53 (> 150 pg/mL). In the exposed group, a significantly ($p < 0.05$) higher proportion of p53 > 150 pg/mL was found among workers with DNA–protein cross-links above the median (0.19). Studies have shown elevated serum levels of p53 protein years before the diagnosis of malignant tumours such as lung cancer (Luo *et al.*, 1994; Hemminki *et al.*, 1996). [The Working Group noted that the reported increases in p53 occurred in the serum and its relationship to the toxicity of formaldehyde is not known.]

Table 36. Genetic effects of formaldehyde in humans

Target tissue	End-point	Response	Comments	Reference
Peripheral blood lymphocytes	Chromosomal aberrations Micronuclei Sister chromatid exchange	+ ($p < 0.01$) + ($p < 0.01$) + ($p < 0.05$)	Exposed, 13; unexposed, 10; chromosomal aberrations included breaks and gaps, which renders interpretation difficult.	He et al. (1988)
Nasal mucosa	Micronuclei	+ ($p < 0.01$)	Exposed, 15; unexposed (control), 15; concurrent exposure to wood dust; no dose–response	Ballarin et al. (1992)
Peripheral blood lymphocytes	Chromosomal aberrations	–	Exposed, 20; unexposed (control), 19; high frequency in controls	Vargova et al. (1992)
Peripheral blood lymphocytes	DNA–protein cross-links	+ ($p = 0.03$)	Exposed, 12; unexposed, 8; pilot study	Shaham et al. (1996a)
Oral mucosa Nasal mucosa	Micronuclei	+ ($p = 0.007$) + (NS)	Exposed, 28; pre- versus post-exposure; no details on tobacco smoking habits	Titenko-Holland et al. (1996)
Peripheral blood lymphocytes	Sister chromatid exchange	+ ($p = 0.05$)	Exposed, 13; unexposed, 20; linear relationship between years of exposure and mean number of sister chromatid exchanges	Shaham et al. (1997)
Nasal mucosa Oral mucosa Peripheral blood lymphocytes	Micronuclei	+ ($p < 0.001$) + ($p < 0.01$) + (NS)	Exposed, 25; pre- versus post-exposure; control for age, sex and tobacco smoking habits questionable	Ying et al. (1997)
Peripheral blood lymphocytes	Sister chromatid exchange	–	Exposed, 23; pre- versus post-exposure	Ying et al. (1999)
Nasal mucosa	Micronuclei	+ ($p < 0.01$)	Exposed, 23; unexposed, 25; no dose–response	Burgaz et al. (2001)

Table 36 (contd)

Target tissue	End-point	Response	Comments	Reference
Oral mucosa	Micronuclei	+ ($p < 0.05$)	Exposed: 22 variable exposures, 28 exposed to formaldehyde; unexposed, 28; unexposed (control), 18; correlation with duration of exposure only in group with variable exposures (not exposed to formaldehyde)	Burgaz et al. (2002)
Peripheral blood lymphocytes	Sister chromatid exchange	+ ($p < 0.01$)	Exposed, 90; unexposed, 52; no dose–response relationship	Shaham et al. (2002)
Peripheral blood lymphocytes	DNA–protein cross-links	+ ($p < 0.01$)	Exposed, 186; unexposed, 213; high levels of p53 protein	Shaham et al. (2003)
Serum	p53 protein	+ ($p < 0.01$)		

NS, not significant

(b)   Chromosomal effects

The effects of formaldehyde on the frequencies of chromosomal aberrations and sister chromatid exchange in peripheral blood lymphocytes and micronuclei in nasal mucosa cells from workers exposed to formaldehyde have been reviewed previously (IARC, 1987a, 1995). Since that time, several further studies have assessed the induction of micronuclei, chromosomal aberrations and sister chromatid exchange in workers exposed to formaldehyde (see Table 36).

In a study of exposure to formaldehyde in a factory that manufactured wood-splinter materials, short-term cultures of peripheral lymphocytes were examined from a group of 20 workers (10 men and 10 women) aged 27–57 years (mean, 42.3 years) who were exposed to 8-h TWA concentrations of 0.55–10.36 mg/m^3 formaldehyde for periods of 5–≥ 16 years. The unexposed group consisted of 19 people [sex and age unspecified] who were employed in the same plant and whose habits and social status were similar to those of the exposed group. No significant difference was observed between control and exposed groups with respect to any chromosomal anomaly (including chromatid and chromosome gaps, breaks, exchanges, breaks per cell, percentage of cells with aberrations) scored in the study (controls: 3.6% aberrant cells, 0.03 breaks per cell; exposed: 3.08% aberrant cells, 0.045 breaks per cell). The authors noted that the frequency of aberrations in the control group was higher than that seen in the general population (1.2–2% aberrant cells) (Vargová et al., 1992). [The Working Group noted that, although the text states that there were 20 people in the exposed group, Table II of the paper gives a figure of 25. The Group also noted the lack of detail on tobacco smoking habits of the subjects.]

In the study of Ballarin et al. (1992), the frequency of micronuclei in respiratory nasal mucosa cells was investigated in 15 nonsmokers who were exposed to formaldehyde in a plywood factory. Mean exposure levels were 0.1–0.39 mg/m^3, with simultaneous exposure to wood dust at a very low level (about one tenth below the threshold limit value). At least 6000 cells from the nasal turbinate area from each individual were scored for micronuclei. A significant increase in the incidence of micronucleated cells was seen in the exposed group (mean percentage of micronucleated cells in the exposed group, 0.90 ± 0.47; range, 0.17–1.83; in controls, 0.25 ± 0.22; range, 0.0–0.66; Mann–Whitney U test, $p < 0.01$). No dose–response relationship between exposure to formaldehyde and the frequency of micronuclei was found. Concurrent exposure to wood dust could have contributed to the increased incidence of micronucleated cells seen in the exposed group.

Burgaz et al. (2001) studied the frequency of micronuclei in cells of the nasal mucosa of 23 individuals (11 women and 12 men) who were exposed to formaldehyde in pathology and anatomy laboratories and 25 healthy men who were not exposed to formaldehyde. The mean age of the exposed group was lower than that of the controls (mean ± SD, 30.56 ± 5.52 and 35.42 ± 9.63 years, respectively). More smokers were included in the control group ($n = 19$) than in the exposed group ($n = 9$). Mean duration of exposure to formaldehyde was 5.06 years (range, 1–13 years). From each individual, 3000 cells were scored for micronuclei. The mean frequency of micronuclei was significantly higher

($p < 0.01$) in the exposed group than in the control group (mean ± SD, $1.01 \pm 0.62\%$ and $0.61 \pm 0.27\%$, respectively). No significant difference in the mean frequency of micronuclei was observed between smokers and nonsmokers in the controls or in the exposed group ($p > 0.05$), but significantly higher ($p < 0.01$) mean frequencies of micronuclei were found in unexposed than in exposed smokers ($1.18 \pm 0.47\%$ and $0.63 \pm 0.29\%$, respectively). No significant difference in the mean frequency of micronuclei was observed between men and women in the exposed group. The air concentration of formaldehyde was 2 ppm [2.4 mg/m³] in the breathing zone of the pathology laboratory workers and 4 ppm [4.9 mg/m³] in that of the anatomy laboratory workers. No dose–response was found between years of exposure and the frequency of micronuclei.

In another study, Burgaz *et al.* (2002) compared the frequency of micronuclei in buccal cells in three groups: group I, 22 workers (all men) from a shoe factory who were exposed to *n*-hexane, toluene and methyl ethyl ketone; group II, 28 workers (15 men and 13 women) who were pathologists or staff in pathology or anatomy laboratories and were exposed to formaldehyde; and group III, 18 unexposed workers (controls), none of whom had been occupationally exposed to potential genotoxic chemicals. The mean duration of exposure to formaldehyde was 4.7 ± 3.33 years (range, 1–13 years). Both exposed and control groups included smokers, most of whom were moderate smokers. There were no significant differences in mean age and smoking habits between the controls and the exposed groups. From each individual, 3000 cells were scored for micronuclei. The concentration of formaldehyde in the breathing zone of the laboratory workers was 2–4 ppm [2.4–4.9 mg/m³]. A significant increase in the frequency of micronucleated cells ($p < 0.05$) was seen in the exposed groups (mean ± SD for workers in group I, group II and controls, $0.62 \pm 0.45\%$, $0.71 \pm 0.56\%$ and $0.33 \pm 0.30\%$, respectively). Analysis of variance indicated that only occupational exposure, but not smoking habits or sex, was associated with an increased frequency of micronuclei in groups I and II ($p < 0.05$). Duration of exposure was significantly associated with the frequency of micronuclei only in group I who were not exposed to formaldehyde ($p < 0.05$).

Titenko-Holland *et al.* (1996) assessed the induction of micronuclei in exfoliated buccal and nasal cells from 28 mortality science students who were exposed to embalming fluid that contained formaldehyde. The original study population included 35 students (seven women and 24 men [specifications of the additional four subjects not given]). Seven were excluded. The students were mainly nonsmokers. Previously unstained and unanalysed slides from the participants in a study by Suruda *et al.* (1993) were used. Each student was sampled before and after the 90-day embalming class. Exposure to formaldehyde was estimated for the 7–10 days before the post-exposure sample in order to correct for the possibility of exposure misclassification. The mean exposure to formaldehyde for the 19 subjects who had data on buccal cell micronuclei was 14.8 ± 7.2 ppm–h [18.2 ± 8.8 mg/m³–h] for the entire 90-day period and 1.2 ± 2.1 ppm–h [1.5 ± 2.6 mg/m³–h] for the 7–10 days before the post-exposure sample. For the 13 subjects who had data on nasal cell micronuclei, the mean exposure to formaldehyde was 16.5 ± 5.8 ppm–h [20.3 ± 7.1 mg/m³–h] for the entire 90-day period and 1.9 ± 2.5 ppm–h [2.3 ± 3 mg/m³–h] during the 7–10 days before the post-exposure sampling. Air samples of glutaraldehyde, phenol, methanol and isopropanol revealed undetectable or very low exposure below the Occupational Safety and Health Administration permissible exposure limits. Quantification of micronuclei was performed by fluorescent in-situ hybridization with a centromeric probe. The mean total frequency of micronuclei was significantly increased in the buccal mucosa (mean ± SD per 1000 epithelial cells, 0.6 ± 0.5 pre-exposure, 2.0 ± 2.0 post-exposure; Wilcoxon rank sum test two-tailed $p = 0.007$), whereas in nasal cells, it was almost the same (2.0 ± 1.3 and 2.5 ± 1.3, respectively; Wilcoxon rank sum test two-tailed $p = 0.2$). Cells with multiple micronuclei were present only in buccal cell samples after exposure to embalming fluid, while in the nasal cell samples, nearly all cells with micronuclei had only one micronucleus per cell in both pre- and post-exposure samples. A weak statistical association (assessed by a Spearman rank order correlation) between cumulative exposure to embalming fluid (90 days) and the change in total micronucleus frequency was observed only in buccal cells ($r = 0.44$; $p = 0.06$). The authors suggested that the main mechanism of micronucleus induction by formaldehyde is due to chromosome breaks.

The frequency of micronuclei in cells of the nasal mucosa, oral mucosa and lymphocytes was evaluated for 25 students (13 men and 12 women; average age, 18.8 ± 1.0 years; all nonsmokers) from anatomy classes. The duration of the anatomy classes was 3 h, three times a week for a period of 8 weeks. The TWA concentrations (mean ± SD) of exposure during the anatomy classes and in the dormitories were 0.508 ± 0.299 mg/m³ (range, 0.071–1.284 mg/m³) and 0.012 ± 0.0025 mg/m³ (range, 0.011–0.016 mg/m³), respectively. Samples of nasal and oral mucosa cells and venous blood were taken before the beginning of the first class and after the end of the last class, so that every student served as his/her own control. A significant difference (paired t-test $p < 0.001$) was found in the mean frequency of micronuclei in the nasal and oral mucosa (mean ± SD per 1000 cells): 1.2 ± 0.67 versus 3.84 ± 1.48 (paired t-test, $p < 0.001$) and 0.568 ± 0.317 versus 0.857 ± 0.558 (paired t-test $p < 0.01$), respectively. The mean frequency of micronuclei in lymphocytes was higher after exposure (1.11 ± 0.543) than before exposure (0.913 ± 0.389), but this difference was not significant (Ying et al., 1997). [The Working Group noted that there were no data related to the possible influence of factors such as age, sex and smoking on the results.]

He et al. (1998) studied the frequency of sister chromatid exchange, chromosomal aberrations and micronuclei in peripheral blood lymphocytes of 13 students from an anatomy class. The duration of the anatomy classes was 10 h per week for 12 weeks. Average exposure to formaldehyde (from breathing-zone air samples) during dissection procedures was 2.37 ppm [3.17 mg/m³]. The unexposed group included 10 students. The sex and age of the two groups were similar and all were nonsmokers. The mean frequency of micronuclei and chromosomal aberrations in the exposed group was significantly higher ($p < 0.01$) than that in the control group (6.38 ± 2.50‰ versus 3.15 ± 1.46‰ and 5.92 ± 2.40% versus 3.40 ± 1.57%, respectively). The main types of chromosomal aberration in the exposed group were chromatid breakages and gaps. A significantly higher ($p < 0.05$) frequency of sister chromatid exchange was observed in the exposed students (5.91 ± 0.71/cell) than in the controls (5.26 ± 0.51/cell). A correlation between micronuclei and chromosomal aberrations was observed. [The Working Group noted that the evaluation of chromosomal aberrations included chromosomal breaks and gaps together, which makes the results difficult to interpret. In addition, the baseline frequencies of sister chromatid exchange and micronuclei in the controls were unusually low.]

Ying *et al.* (1999) studied the frequency of sister chromatid exchange in peripheral blood lymphocytes of 23 students from an anatomy class (11 men and 12 women), all of whom were nonsmokers. The duration of the anatomy classes was 3 h, three times a week for 8 weeks. Peak exposure was during cadaver dissection. TWA (mean ± SD) concentrations of formaldehyde were 0.508 ± 0.299 mg/m^3 (range, 0.071–1.284 mg/m^3) in the laboratory rooms compared with 0.012 ± 0.0025 mg/m^3 (range, 0.011–0.016 mg/m^3) in the dormitories. Blood samples were taken at the beginning of the anatomy classes and again after 8 weeks. No significant difference was found in the mean frequency of sister chromatid exchange before and after exposure, either in the total population (6.383 ± 0.405 versus 6.613 ± 0.786, respectively) or in the subgroups of men and women.

In a pilot study, Shaham *et al.* (1997) studied the frequency of sister chromatid exchange in the peripheral blood lymphocytes of 33 workers, including 13 from a pathology institute who were exposed to formaldehyde and 20 unexposed controls. The mean age of the exposed workers was 42 ± 10 years and that of the control group was 39 ± 14 years. The range of concentrations of formaldehyde was 1.38–1.6 ppm [1.7–2 mg/m^3] in the rooms and 6.9 ppm [8.5 mg/m^3] in the laminar flow. Personal samples showed a range of 2.8–3.1 ppm [3.5–3.7 mg/m^3] formaldehyde at the period when most of the work was in progress and 1.46 ppm [1.8 mg/m^3] at midday, when most of the work had already been carried out. In order to score sister chromatid exchange, cells that had 44–48 clearly visible chromosomes were examined and the sister chromatid exchange count was normalized to the frequency expected for 46 chromosomes. The mean numbers of cells scored per individual were 28 for the exposed group (range, 25–32; SD, 2.36) and 32 for the controls (range, 25–34; SD, 2.0). A significant difference ($p = 0.05$) was found between the mean number of sister chromatid exchanges per chromosome in the exposed workers (mean ± SD, 0.212 ± 0.039) and the controls (mean ± SD, 0.186 ± 0.035). A significant difference ($p < 0.05$) was found between the mean number of sister chromatid exchanges per chromosome of nine exposed and six unexposed nonsmokers and those of three exposed and two unexposed smokers. The group of smokers who were exposed to formaldehyde had the highest mean number of sister chromatid exchanges per chromosome, and a linear relationship was reported between years of exposure and the mean number of sister chromatid exchanges per chromosome.

In a second study, Shaham *et al.* (2002) evaluated the frequency of sister chromatid exchange in peripheral blood lymphocytes of pathology staff exposed to formaldehyde compared with that in unexposed workers. The study population included 90 workers (25 men and 65 women) from 14 hospital pathology departments who were exposed to formaldehyde (mean age, 44.2 ± 8.5 years) and 52 unexposed workers (44 men and eight women) from the administrative section of the same hospitals (mean age, 41.7 ± 11.4 years). Tobacco smoking habits did not differ significantly between the study groups. The exposed group was divided into two subgroups according to levels of exposure to formaldehyde (low-level exposure: mean, 0.4 ppm [0.5 mg/m^3]; range, 0.04–0.7 ppm [0.05–0.86 mg/m^3]; high-level exposure: mean, 2.24 ppm [2.8 mg/m^3]; range, 0.72–5.6 ppm [0.9–6.9 mg/m^3]). The mean duration of exposure to formaldehyde was 15.4 years (range, 1–39 years). The results on the frequency of sister chromatid exchange were expressed in two variables: (a) mean number of sister chromatid exchanges per chromosome; and (b) proportion of high-frequency cells (namely, the proportion of cells with more than eight sister chromatid exchanges). A high correlation between these two variables (rs = 0.94; $p < 0.01$) was found in the study population and in each of the two subgroups (exposed rs = 0.79; $p < 0.01$; unexposed rs = 0.92; $p < 0.01$). Before the results obtained from the exposed and the unexposed groups were compared, adjustment was made for age, sex, origin, education and tobacco smoking. The adjusted mean number of sister chromatid exchanges per chromosome was significantly higher ($p < 0.01$) among the exposed group (0.27; SE, 0.003) than the unexposed group (0.19; SE, 0.004). The adjusted mean of the proportion of high-frequency cells was also significantly higher ($p < 0.01$) among the exposed group (0.88; SE, 0.01) than the controls (0.44; SE, 0.02). After adjustment for potential confounders, the adjusted mean of the two variables of sister chromatid exchange were similar for the two periods of exposure (up to 15 years and more than 15 years). Tobacco smoking was found to be a significant confounder. With regard to levels of exposure, both variables of sister chromatid exchange were similar in the low- and high-level exposure subgroups. However, among smokers, both variables of sister chromatid exchange were higher in the high-exposure subgroup than in the low-exposure subgroup.

(c) DNA repair

Hayes *et al.* (1997) studied the effect of formaldehyde on DNA repair capacity by assessing the activity of O^6-alkylguanine–DNA alkyltransferase (AGT), which was found to be involved in the repair of DNA damage due to exposure to formaldehyde *in vitro*. AGT activity was measured in peripheral blood lymphocytes of 23 mortuary science students (seven women and 16 men), of whom 17 were nonsmokers and six were smokers. Blood samples were taken before the beginning of the course and after 9 weeks of practice. The number of embalmings that the students experienced varied, both before and during the course. The average air concentration of formaldehyde during embalming was about 1.5 ppm and, during some peak exposures, was three to nine times that of the corresponding TWA. Measurements of glutaraldehyde and phenol were below the limit of detection. Total exposure to formaldehyde during the study period, including embalming carried out outside the school, was within the range of 5.7–82.0 ppm–h [7–100 mg/m^3–h] (mean ± SD, 18.4 ± 15.6 ppm [22.5 ± 19.2 mg/m^3]). The total number of embalmings was correlated with the estimated total exposure to formaldehyde (r = 0.59; $p < 0.01$). Students who had had previous experience of embalming had greater estimated exposure to formaldehyde during the study period ($p < 0.05$), and their DNA repair capacity at baseline was reduced ($p = 0.08$). No exposure–response relationship was found between the number of embalmings during the 90 days before the course and the AGT activity ($r = -0.29$; $p = 0.19$). Sex, age and tobacco smoking were not clearly related to pre-exposure DNA repair activity. Post-exposure and pre-exposure AGT activity were correlated ($r = 0.42$; $p < 0.05$). At the end of the course, a reduction in DNA repair capacity was found in 17 students and an increase in DNA repair capacity in six ($p < 0.05$). These findings were confirmed after analysis of variance, including adjustment for age, sex and tobacco smoking status. Among the eight students who had no embalming experience during the 90 days before the study, seven (88%) had decreased and only one had increased AGT activity during the study period ($p < 0.05$). Of the 15 students who had had previous embalming experience, 10 (67%) had decreased and five (33%) had increased AGT activity ($p > 0.05$). No relation was found between the extent of the decrease in AGT activity and the levels of exposure to formaldehyde throughout the 9-week study period or during the last 28 days. As was also noted by the authors, the limitation of the study was the small study population and the fact that many of the students had previous embalming experience.

Schlink *et al.* (1999) studied the activitity of the DNA repair enzyme, O^6-methyl-guanine–DNA methyltransferase (MGMT). The study population included 57 medical students from two universities who were exposed to formaldehyde during anatomy courses. Blood samples of 41 students from the first university were collected before (day 0, control group No. 1), during (day 50) and after (day 111) the course, which lasted 111 days; two 3-h courses were held per week. Additional blood samples from 16 students from the second university were taken at the end of their course, namely 98 days after the start, and an additional 10 blood samples were taken from unexposed students (control group No. 2). The first group of 41 students was exposed to levels of formaldehyde between 0.14 mg/m^3 and 0.3 mg/m^3 (mean ± SD, 0.2 ± 0.05 mg/m^3). The mean MGMT activity (± 95% CI) was 133.2 ± 14.9 fmol MGMT/10^6 cells. No significant difference was observed before and after 50 days of exposure or after 111 days of exposure. Age, sex, cigarette smoking, alcohol consumption and allergic disease had no influence on MGMT activities in either the exposed group or the controls. The exposure level of the second group of 16 students was 0.8 ± 0.6 mg/m^3. No significant difference in MGMT activity was observed between this exposed group and the controls (146.9 ± 22.3 fmol MGMT/10^6 cells and 138.9 ± 22.1 fmol MGMT/10^6 cells, respectively). In addition, the activity of MGMT of students at the second university who were exposed to a higher level of formaldehyde than those at the first university was not statistically significant from that of control group No. 1, and very similar results were obtained in both control groups.

(*d*)	*Urinary mutagenicity*

Hospital autopsy service workers in Galveston, TX (USA) (15 men and four women), aged < 30–> 50 years, and a control group from the local medical school (15 men and five women), who were in the same age range and were matched for consumption of tobacco, marijuana, alcohol and coffee, were studied for urinary mutagenicity (Connor *et al.*, 1985). Individuals were sampled three times at approximately 2-month intervals. The TWA exposures to formaldehyde in the work areas were estimated to be 0.61–1.32 ppm [0.73–1.58 mg/m^3]. Urine (150–200 mL from each subject) was treated with β-glucuronidase and passed through an XAD-2 column, which was then washed with water. The fraction that eluted with acetone was assayed for mutagenicity in *Salmonella typhimurium* TA98 and TA100 in the presence and absence of an exogenous metabolic activation system from the livers of Aroclor-1254-induced rats. No increase in mutagenicity was seen in the autopsy workers compared with the control group.

4.4.2   *Experimental systems*

(a)   *DNA–protein cross-links*

(i)   *In-vitro studies*

Formaldehyde induces DNA–protein cross-links in animal and human cells *in vitro* (see Table 37). The precise nature of these cross-links is unknown.

(ii)   *In-vivo studies in animals*

Groups of four male Fischer 344 rats were exposed for 6 h to 0.3, 0.7, 2, 6 or 10 ppm [0.37, 0.9, 2.4, 7.4 or 12.3 mg/m^3] [^{14}C]formaldehyde in a nose-only inhalation chamber. Individual male rhesus monkeys (*Macaca mulatta)* were exposed for 6 h to 0.7, 2 or 6 ppm [^{14}C]formaldehyde in a head-only inhalation chamber. DNA–protein cross-links induced by exposure to formaldehyde were measured in the nasal mucosa of several regions of the upper respiratory tract of exposed animals. The concentrations of cross-links increased non-linearly with the airborne concentration in both species, but those in the turbinates and anterior nasal mucosa were significantly lower in monkeys than in rats. Cross-links were also formed in the nasopharynx and trachea of monkeys, but were not detected in the sinus, proximal lung or bone marrow. The authors suggested that the differences between the species with respect to DNA–protein cross-link formation may be due to differences in nasal cavity deposition and in the elimination of absorbed formaldehyde (Heck *et al.*, 1989; Casanova *et al.*, 1991).

In order to determine whether the yields of DNA–protein cross-links after chronic and acute exposures are equivalent and to locate the site of DNA–protein cross-links and of DNA replication in the rat nasal respiratory mucosa in relation to tumour incidence, groups of rats were exposed (whole body) to concentrations of 0.7, 2, 6 or 15 ppm [0.8, 2.4, 7.4 or 18.5 mg/m^3] unlabelled formaldehyde for 6 h per day on 5 days per week for 11 weeks and 4 days (pre-exposed rats) while other groups were exposed to room air (naive rats). On day 5 of week 12, the pre-exposed and naive rats were simultaneously exposed (nose only) for 3 h to [^{14}C]-labelled formaldehyde at the same concentrations as those used for pre-exposure to quantitate the acute yield of DNA–protein cross-links and to measure cell proliferation in specific sites of the nose. Alternatively, in order to determine the cumulative yield of DNA–protein cross-links in comparison with unexposed rats, rats that were pre-exposed to 6 or 10 ppm formaldehyde and naive rats that were exposed to room air were simultaneously exposed for 3 h to the same concentration of unlabelled formaldehyde on day 5 or at week 12. The cumulative yield of DNA–protein cross-links was measured immediately after exposure. Nasal mucosal DNA was extracted from proteins, and the percentage of interfacial DNA (an indicator for the concentration of DNA–protein cross-links) was determined. The percentage of interfacial DNA was also determined in a group of unexposed rats. Increases in the percentage of interfacial DNA, namely, decreases in the extractability of DNA from proteins in the exposed rats, was found by the authors to correlate highly with the yield of DNA–protein cross-links (Casanova-Schmitz et al., 1984b). The amount of [^{14}C] incorporation into DNA was an indicator of cell replication. Comparison of cell replication rates in the lateral meatus with those in the medial and posterior meatus showed no significant difference at 0.7 and 2 ppm formaldehyde, but this difference became significant at 6 and 15 ppm formaldehyde in pre-exposed rats ($p \leq 0.02$, Scheffé's test). At 6 and 15 ppm formaldehyde, a significantly ($p \leq 0.01$, Scheffé's test) greater amount of [^{14}C] was incorporated into the DNA in the lateral meatus of pre-exposed rats compared with naive rats and, at 15 ppm, into the DNA in the medial and posterior meatus of pre-exposed rats compared with naive rats. The acute yield of DNA–protein cross-links increased non-linearly with concentrations and, in naive rats, was approximately sixfold greater in the lateral than in the medial and posterior meatus at all concentrations. At 0.7 and 2 ppm, the acute yield was not significantly different between naive and pre-exposed rats. However, at both 6 and 15 ppm formaldehyde, a greater acute yield of DNA–protein cross-links was found in the lateral meatus of naive rats than in that of pre-exposed rats, a difference that was significant at 15 ppm formaldehyde ($p = 0.028$, paired t test). Based on histopathological evidence, this difference can be attributed to an increase in the quantity of DNA due to an increase in the number of cells in the nasal mucosa of the lateral meatus at high concentrations, which results in a dilution of the DNA–protein cross-links. No significant difference was found between naive and pre-exposed rats in relation to acute yield of DNA–protein cross-links in the medial and posterior meatus at any concentration of formaldehyde. Since measurement of the percentage of interfacial DNA does not require the use of [^{14}C]formaldehyde, this parameter was used to investigate whether DNA–protein cross-links accumulated during subchronic, whole-body exposure to formaldehyde. The percentage of interfacial DNA following acute exposure (3-h nose-only exposure) to formaldehyde increased significantly ($p < 0.02$, Scheffé's test) at 6 and 10 ppm. However, at these levels, the percentage of interfacial DNA was lower in pre-exposed rats than in naive rats, a difference that was significant at 10 ppm formaldehyde ($p = 0.01$, Scheffé's test). The authors suggested that the cumulative and acute yields of DNA–protein cross-links in rats exposed to formaldehyde are essentially identical (Casanova et al., 1994). [The Working Group noted that there is doubt about the adequacy of the methods that use interfacial DNA to detect DNA–protein cross-links; the connection between DNA yield needs to be clarified.]

Table 37. Genetic and related effects of formaldehyde in experimental systems and animals

Test system	Result[a] Without exogenous metabolic system	Result[a] With exogenous metabolic system	Dose[b] (LED/HID)	Reference
Misincorporation of DNA bases into synthetic polynucleotides in vitro	+	NT	30	Snyder & Van Houten (1986)
pUC13 plasmid DNA bound to calf-thymus histones, DNA–protein cross-links	+	NT	0.0075	Kuykendall & Bogdanffy (1992)
Escherichia coli PQ37, SOS repair test, DNA strand breaks, cross-links or related damage	+	NT	20	Le Curieux et al. (1993)
Escherichia coli K12 (or E. coli DNA), DNA strand breaks, cross-links or related damage; DNA repair	+	NT	60	Poverenny et al. (1975)
Escherichia coli K12, DNA strand breaks, cross-links or related damage; DNA repair	+	NT	600	Wilkins & MacLeod (1976)
Escherichia coli K12 KS160-KS66 polAI, differential toxicity	+	NT	60	Poverenny et al. (1975)
Escherichia coli polA$^+$/W3110 and polA$^-$ p3478, differential toxicity (spot test)	+	NT	10 μL of pure substance	Leifer et al. (1981)
Salmonella typhimurium TA100, TA1535, TA1537, TA1538, TA98, reverse mutation	−	−	60 μg/plate	Gocke et al. (1981)
Salmonella typhimurium TA100, reverse mutation	−	+	10 μg/plate	Haworth et al. (1983)
Salmonella typhimurium TA100, reverse mutation	(+)	+	30 μg/plate (toxic above 125 μg/plate)[c]	Connor et al. (1983)
Salmonella typhimurium TA100, reverse mutation	+	+[d]	9 μg/plate	Pool et al. (1984)
Salmonella typhimurium TA100, reverse mutation	(+)	NT	51 μg/plate[c]	Marnett et al. (1985)
Salmonella typhimurium TA100, reverse mutation	+	NT	6 μg/plate	Takahashi et al. (1985)
Salmonella typhimurium TA100, reverse mutation	(+)	+	3	Schmid et al. (1986)
Salmonella typhimurium TA100, reverse mutation	+	NT	9.3	O'Donovan & Mee (1993)
Salmonella typhimurium TA100, TA104, reverse mutation	+	+	6.25–50 μg/plate	Dillon et al. (1998)
Salmonella typhimurium TA102, TA104, reverse mutation	+	NT	21 μg/plate[c]	Marnett et al. (1985)

Table 37 (contd)

Test system	Result[a]		Dose[b] (LED/HID)	Reference
	Without exogenous metabolic system	With exogenous metabolic system		
Salmonella typhimurium TA102, reverse mutation	+	NT	10	Le Curieux *et al.* (1993)
Salmonella typhimurium TA102, reverse mutation	+	NT	25 μg/plate	O'Donovan & Mee (1993)
Salmonella typhimurium TA102, reverse mutation	+	NT	0.1–0.25 μg/plate	Chang *et al.* (1997)
Salmonella typhimurium TA102, reverse mutation	+	?	6.25–50 μg/plate	Dillon *et al.* (1998)
Salmonella typhimurium TA1535, TA1537, reverse mutation	–	–[d]	100–200 μg/plate	Haworth *et al.* (1983)
Salmonella typhimurium TA1535, reverse mutation	NT	–[d]	18 μg/plate	Pool *et al.* (1984)
Salmonella typhimurium TA1535, TA1537, TA1538, reverse mutation	–	NT	100 μg/plate	O'Donovan & Mee (1993)
Salmonella typhimurium TA98, reverse mutation	+	NT	12 μg/plate	Marnett *et al.* (1985)
Salmonella typhimurium TA98, reverse mutation	–	(+)	10 μg/plate	Haworth *et al.* (1983)
Salmonella typhimurium TA98, reverse mutation	(+)	(+)	30 μg/plate (toxic above 100 μg/plate)	Connor *et al.* (1983)
Salmonella typhimurium TA98, reverse mutation	NT	(+)[d]	9 μg/plate	Pool *et al.* (1984)
Salmonella typhimurium TA98, reverse mutation	+	NT	12.5 μg/plate	O'Donovan & Mee (1993)
Salmonella typhimurium (other miscellaneous strains), reverse mutation	–	–	100 μg/plate (toxic at 250 μg/plate)	Connor *et al.* (1983)
Salmonella typhimurium TM677, forward mutation to 8-azaguanine	+	+	5; 10[e]	Temcharoen & Thilly (1983)
Salmonella typhimurium TA97, reverse mutation	+	NT	12 μg/plate[c]	Marnett *et al.* (1985)
Salmonella typhimurium TA7005 (*his*[+]), reverse mutation	+	NT	1.5 μg/plate	Ohta *et al.* (2000)
Escherichia coli K12, forward or reverse mutation (*gpt* locus)	+	NT	120	Crosby *et al.* (1988)
Escherichia coli K12, forward or reverse mutation	+	NT	60	Zijlstra (1989)
Escherichia coli K12, forward or reverse mutation	+	NT	18.8	Graves *et al.* (1994)

Table 37 (contd)

Test system	Result[a]		Dose[b] (LED/HID)	Reference
	Without exogenous metabolic system	With exogenous metabolic system		
Escherichia coli WP2 *uvr*A, reverse mutation	+	NT	15	Takahashi *et al.* (1985)
Escherichia coli WP2 *uvr*A (pKM101), reverse mutation	+	NT	12.5 µg/plate	O'Donovan & Mee (1993)
Escherichia coli WP2, reverse mutation	+	NT	1200	Nishioka (1973)
Escherichia coli WP2, reverse mutation	+	NT	60	Takahashi *et al.* (1985)
Escherichia coli WP2 (pKM101), reverse mutation	+	NT	25 µg/plate	O'Donovan & Mee (1993)
Escherichia coli (other miscellaneous strains), reverse mutation	+	NT	100	Demerec *et al.* (1951)
Escherichia coli (other miscellaneous strains), reverse mutation	+	NT	900	Panfilova *et al.* (1966)
Escherichia coli (other miscellaneous strains), reverse mutation	+	NT	30	Takahashi *et al.* (1985)
Escherichia coli WP3104P, reverse mutation	(+)	NT	5 µg/plate	Ohta *et al.* (1999)
Escherichia coli WP3104P, reverse mutation	+	NT	~2 µg/plate	Ohta *et al.* (2000)
Saccharomyces species, DNA strand breaks and DNA repair	+	NT	990	Magaña-Schwencke *et al.* (1978)
Saccharomyces species, DNA strand breaks, DNA–protein cross links or related damage	+	NT	500	Magaña-Schwencke & Ekert (1978); Magaña-Schwencke & Moustacchi (1980)
Saccharomyces cerevisiae, gene conversion	+	NT	540	Chanet *et al.* (1975)
Saccharomyces cerevisiae, homozygosis by mitotic recombination or gene conversion	+	NT	18.5	Zimmermann & Mohr (1992)
Neurospora crassa heterokaryons H-12 strain, forward mutation	(+)	NT	250	de Serres *et al.* (1988); de Serres & Brockman (1999)

Table 37 (contd)

Test system	Result[a]		Dose[b] (LED/HID)	Reference
	Without exogenous metabolic system	With exogenous metabolic system		
Neurospora crassa heterokaryons H-59 strain, forward mutation	+	NT	100	de Serres et al. (1988); de Serres & Brockman (1999)
Neurospora crassa, reverse mutation	−	NT	732	Dickey et al. (1949)
Neurospora crassa, reverse mutation	+	NT	300	Jensen et al. (1951)
Neurospora crassa, reverse mutation	−	NT	300	Kölmark & Westergaard (1953)
Agaricus bisporus, Glycine max, Lycopersicon esculentum, P. americana, Pinus resinosa, Pisum sativum, Populus × eur-americana, Vicia faba, Zea mays, DNA damage	+	NT	3.7% solution, pH 3 and 7, 37 000 µg/mL	Douglas & Rogers (1998)
Plants (other), mutation	+	NT	NG	Auerbach et al. (1977)
Tradescantia pallida, micronucleus formation	+	NT	250 ppm [250 µg/mL], 6 h	Batalha et al. (1999)
Drosophila melanogaster, genetic crossing over or recombination	+		1260	Sobels & van Steenis (1957)
Drosophila melanogaster, genetic crossing over or recombination	+		420	Alderson (1967)
Drosophila melanogaster, genetic crossing over or recombination	+		2500	Ratnayake (1970)
Drosophila melanogaster, sex-linked recessive lethal mutations	+		1000	Kaplan (1948)
Drosophila melanogaster, sex-linked recessive lethal mutations	+		1800	Auerbach & Moser (1953)
Drosophila melanogaster, sex-linked recessive lethal mutations	+		1260	Sobels & van Steenis (1957)
Drosophila melanogaster, sex-linked recessive lethal mutations	+		420	Alderson (1967)
Drosophila melanogaster, sex-linked recessive lethal mutations	+		420	Khan (1967)
Drosophila melanogaster, sex-linked recessive lethal mutations	(+)		2000	Ratnayake (1968)
Drosophila melanogaster, sex-linked recessive lethal mutations	+		250	Stumm-Tegethoff (1969)

Table 37 (contd)

Test system	Result[a]		Dose[b] (LED/HID)	Reference
	Without exogenous metabolic system	With exogenous metabolic system		
Drosophila melanogaster, sex-linked recessive lethal mutations	+		2200	Ratnayake (1970)
Drosophila melanogaster, heritable translocation	+		420	Khan (1967)
Drosophila melanogaster, heritable translocation	+		2500	Ratnayake (1970)
Drosophila melanogaster, dominant lethal mutation	+		1800	Auerbach & Moser (1953)
Drosophila melanogaster, dominant lethal mutation	+		1300	Šrám (1970)
Caenorhabditis elegans, recessive lethal mutations	+		700	Johnsen & Baillie (1988)
DNA strand breaks, DNA–protein cross-links or related damage, mouse leukaemia L1210 cells *in vitro*	+	NT	6	Ross & Shipley (1980)
DNA–protein cross-links, mouse leukaemia L1210 cells *in vitro*	+	NT	3.75	Ross et al. (1981)
DNA single strand breaks, DNA–protein cross-links or related damage, sarcoma rat cell line *in vitro*	+	NT	7.5	O'Connor & Fox (1987)
DNA single strand breaks or related damage, rat hepatocytes *in vitro*	+	NT	22.5	Demkowicz-Dobrzanski & Castonguay (1992)
DNA–protein cross-links, Chinese hamster ovary cells *in vitro*	+	NT	7.5	Olin et al. (1996)
DNA–protein cross-links, male B6C3F₁ mouse hepatocytes *in vitro*	+	NT	15	Casanova et al. (1997)
DNA–protein cross-links, Chinese hamster V79 lung fibroblast cells *in vitro*	+	NT	4	Merk & Speit (1998, 1999)
Unscheduled DNA synthesis, Syrian hamster embryo cells *in vitro*	+	NT	3	Hamaguchi et al. (2000)
Gene mutation, Chinese hamster V79 cells, *Hprt* locus	+	NT	9	Grafström et al. (1993)
Gene mutation, Chinese hamster V79 cells, *Hprt* locus	–	NT	15	Merk & Speit (1998, 1999)
Gene mutation, mouse lymphoma L5178Y cells, $Tk^{+/-}$ locus *in vitro*	NT	+	24	Mackerer et al. (1996)
Gene mutation, mouse lymphoma L5178Y cells *in vitro*	+	NT	> 2	Speit & Merk (2002)
Sister chromatid exchange, Chinese hamster cells *in vitro*	+	NT	1	Obe & Beek (1979)
Sister chromatid exchange, Chinese hamster cells *in vitro*	+	+	3.2	Natarajan et al. (1983)

Table 37 (contd)

Test system	Result[a]		Dose[b] (LED/HID)	Reference
	Without exogenous metabolic system	With exogenous metabolic system		
Sister chromatid exchange, Chinese hamster cells *in vitro*	+	–	2	Basler *et al.* (1985)
Sister chromatid exchange, Chinese hamster V79 cells *in vitro*	+	NT	4	Merk & Speit (1998, 1999)
Micronucleus formation, Chinese hamster V79 cells *in vitro*	+	NT	4	Merk & Speit (1998, 1999)
Chromosomal aberrations, Chinese hamster cells *in vitro*	+	NT	18	Ishidate *et al.* (1981)
Chromosomal aberrations, Chinese hamster cells *in vitro*	+	+	6.3	Natarajan *et al.* (1983)
Cell transformation, C3H10T1/2 mouse cells	+[f]	NT	0.5	Ragan & Boreiko (1981)
DNA single strand breaks, DNA–protein cross-links, human bronchial cells *in vitro*	+	NT	24	Fornace *et al.* (1982)
DNA single strand breaks, DNA–protein cross-links or related damage, human bronchial and skin cells *in vitro*	+	NT	3	Grafström *et al.* (1984)
DNA single strand breaks, DNA–protein cross-links or related damage, human bronchial cells *in vitro*	+	NT	3	Saladino *et al.* (1985)
DNA single strand breaks, DNA–protein cross-links or related damage, human bronchial cells *in vitro*	+	NT	3	Grafström *et al.* (1986)
DNA strand breaks, cross-links or related damage, human fibroblast cells *in vitro*	+	NT	3	Snyder & Van Houten (1986)
DNA strand breaks, DNA–protein cross-links or related damage, human lymphoblast cells *in vitro*	+	NT	1.5	Craft *et al.* (1987)
DNA strand breaks, DNA–protein cross-links or related damage, human bronchial cells *in vitro*	+	NT	12	Grafström (1990)
DNA–protein cross-links, human fibroblasts *in vitro*	+	NT	7.5	Olin *et al.* (1996)
DNA–protein cross-links, human white blood cells *in vitro*	+	NT	3	Shaham *et al.* (1996)
DNA–protein cross-links, EBV-BL human lymphoma cells *in vitro*	+	NT	37 × 18 h	Costa *et al.* (1997)

Table 37 (contd)

Test system	Result[a]		Dose[b] (LED/HID)	Reference
	Without exogenous metabolic system	With exogenous metabolic system		
DNA double-strand breaks, human lung epithelial (A549) cells *in vitro*	+	NT	30 (8, 24, 72 h)	Vock *et al.* (1999)
DNA–protein cross-links, Comet assay, human gastric mucosa cells *in vitro*	+	NT	30	Blasiak *et al.* (2000)
DNA–protein cross-links, human lymphocytes *in vitro*	+	–	3	Andersson *et al.* (2003)
DNA repair exclusive of unscheduled DNA synthesis, human bronchial and skin cells *in vitro*	+	NT	6	Grafström *et al.* (1984)
DNA repair, human MRC5CV1 normal cell line, XP12 ROSV cell line, GMO6914 FA cell line, *in vitro*	+	NT	3.75	Speit *et al.* (2000)
Unscheduled DNA synthesis, human bronchial epithelial cells *in vitro*	-	NT	3 (> 3 was lethal)	Doolittle *et al.* (1985)
Gene mutation, human lymphoblasts TK6 line (*TK* locus) *in vitro*	+	NT	3.9	Goldmacher & Thilly (1983)
Gene mutation, human fibroblasts *in vitro*	+	NT	3	Grafström *et al.* (1985)
Gene mutation, human lymphoblasts TK6 line (*TK* locus) *in vitro*	+	NT	0.9	Craft *et al.* (1987)
Gene mutation, human lymphoblasts TK6 line (*HPRT* locus)	+	NT	4.5, 2 h, × 8 times	Crosby *et al.* (1988)
Gene mutation, human lymphoblasts TK6 line (*HPRT* locus) *in vitro*	+	NT	4.5, 2 h, × 8 times	Liber *et al.* (1989)
Gene mutation, human bronchial fibroblasts (*HPRT* locus) *in vitro*	+	NT	3	Grafström (1990)
Sister chromatid exchange, human lymphocytes *in vitro*	+	NT	5	Obe & Beek (1979)
Sister chromatid exchange, human lymphocytes *in vitro*	+	NT	5	Kreiger & Garry (1983)
Sister chromatid exchange, human lymphocytes *in vitro*	+	+	3.75	Schmid *et al.* (1986)
Micronucleus formation, human MRC5CV1 normal cell line, XP12 ROSV cell line, GMO6914 FA cell line, *in vitro*	+	NT	3.75	Speit *et al.* (2000)
Chromosomal aberrations, human fibroblasts *in vitro*	+	NT	60	Levy *et al.* (1983)

Table 37 (contd)

Test system	Result[a] Without exogenous metabolic system	Result[a] With exogenous metabolic system	Dose[b] (LED/HID)	Reference
Chromosomal aberrations, human lymphocytes *in vitro*	+	NT	10	Miretskaya & Shvartsman (1982)
Chromosomal aberrations, human lymphocytes *in vitro*	+	+	7.5	Schmid *et al.* (1986)
Chromosomal aberrations, premature chromosome condensation technique, human lymphocytes *in vitro*	+	NT	3.75	Dresp & Bauchinger (1988)
DNA–protein cross-links, rat respiratory and olfactory mucosa and bone marrow *in vivo*	+		2 ppm [2.5 mg/m^3], 6 h	Casanova-Schmitz *et al.* (1984b)
DNA–protein cross-links, rat nasal mucosa *in vivo*	+		6 ppm [7.4 mg/m^3], 6 h	Lam *et al.* (1985)
DNA–protein cross-links, rat respiratory mucosa *in vivo*	+		2 ppm [2.5 mg/m^3], 3 h	Heck *et al.* (1986)
DNA–protein cross-links, rat respiratory and olfactory mucosa and bone marrow *in vivo*	+		2 ppm [2.5 mg/m^3], 3 h	Casanova & Heck (1987)
DNA–protein cross-links, rat tracheal implant cells *in vivo*	+		50 ppm [50 µg/mL], instil.	Cosma *et al.* (1988)
DNA–protein cross-links, rat nasal respiratory mucosa *in vivo*	+		0.3 ppm [0.4 mg/m^3], inhal. 6 h	Casanova *et al.* (1989)
DNA–protein cross-links, rhesus monkey nasal turbinate cells *in vivo*	+		0.7 ppm [0.9 mg/m^3], inhal. 6 h	Heck *et al.* (1989)
DNA–protein cross-links, rhesus monkey nasal turbinate cells *in vivo*	+		0.7 ppm [0.9 mg/m^3], inhal. 6 h	Casanova *et al.* (1991)
Gene mutation, rat cells *in vivo* (*p53* point mutations in nasal squamous-cell carcinomas)	+		15 ppm [18.45 mg/m^3], inhal. 6 h/d, 5 d/wk, 2 y	Recio *et al.* (1992)
Mouse spot test	−		15 ppm [18 mg/m^3], inhal. 6 h/d × 3	Jensen & Cohr (1983) [Abstract]

Table 37 (contd)

Test system	Result[a] Without exogenous metabolic system	With exogenous metabolic system	Dose[b] (LED/HID)	Reference
Sister chromatid exchange, rat cells in vivo	−		15 ppm [18.45 mg/m³], inhal. 6 h/d × 5	Kligerman et al. (1984)
Micronucleus formation, mouse bone-marrow cells in vivo	−		30 ip × 1	Gocke et al. (1981)
Micronucleus formation, mouse bone-marrow cells in vivo	−		25 ip × 1	Natarajan et al. (1983)
Micronucleus formation, rat gastrointestinal tract in vivo	+		200 po × 1	Migliore et al. (1989)
Micronucleus formation, newt (Pleurodeles waltl) in vivo	−		5 µg/mL, 8 d	Siboulet et al. (1984)
Chromosomal aberrations, mouse bone-marrow cells in vivo	−		25 ip × 1	Natarajan et al. (1983)
Chromosomal aberrations, rat bone-marrow cells in vivo	+		0.4 ppm [0.5 mg/m³] inhal. 4 h/d, 4 mo	Kitaeva et al. (1990)
Chromosomal aberrations, rat bone-marrow cells in vivo	−		15 ppm [18.45 mg/m³], inhal. 6 h/d × 5, 8 wk	Dallas et al. (1992)
Chromosomal aberrations, rat leukocytes in vivo	−		15 ppm [18.45 mg/m³], inhal. 6 h/d × 5	Kligerman et al. (1984)
Chromosomal aberrations, mouse spermatocytes treated in vivo, spermatocytes observed	−		50 ip × 1	Fontignie-Houbrechts (1981)
Chromosomal aberrations, mouse spleen cells in vivo	−		25 ip × 1	Natarajan et al. (1983)
Chromosomal aberrations, rat pulmonary lavage cells in vivo	+		15 ppm [18.45 mg/m³] inhal. 6 h/d × 5	Dallas et al. (1992)

Table 37 (contd)

Test system	Result[a] Without exogenous metabolic system	With exogenous metabolic system	Dose[b] (LED/HID)	Reference
Dominant lethal mutation, mouse	–		20 ip × 1	Epstein & Shafner (1968)
Dominant lethal mutation, mouse	–		20 ip × 1	Epstein et al. (1972)
Dominant lethal mutation, mouse	(+)		50 ip × 1	Fontignie-Houbrechts (1981)
Dominant lethal mutation, rat	(+)		1.2 ppm [1.5 mg/m^3] inhal. 4 h/d, 4 mo	Kitaeva et al. (1990)

EBV, Epstein–Barr virus; BL, Burkitt lymphoma; XP, xeroderma pigmentosum; FA, Fanconi anaemia

[a] +, positive; (+) weak positive; –, negative; NT, not tested; ?, inconclusive (variable response in several experiments within an adequate study)

[b] In-vitro tests, µg/mL; in-vivo tests, mg/kg bw; d, day; inhal., inhalation; instil., instillation; ip, intraperitoneal; mo, month; NG, not given; po, oral; wk, weeks; y, year

[c] Estimated from the graph in the paper

[d] Tested with exogenous metabolic system without co-factors

[e] LED with exogenous metabolic system is 0.33 mM [10 µg/mL].

[f] Positive only in presence of 12-O-tetradecanoylphorbol 13-acetate

(b)   *Mutation and allied effects* (see also Table 37)

(i)   *In-vitro studies*

Formaldehyde induced mutation and DNA damage in bacteria, mutation, gene conversion, DNA strand breaks and DNA–protein cross-links in fungi and DNA damage in plants. In *Drosophila melanogaster*, administration of formaldehyde in the diet induced sex-linked recessive lethal mutations, dominant lethal effects, heritable translocations and crossing-over in spermatogonia. In a single study, it induced recessive lethal mutations in a nematode. It induced chromosomal aberrations, sister chromatid exchange, DNA strand breaks and DNA–protein cross-links in animal cells and, in single studies, gene mutation, sister chromatid exchange and micronuclei in Chinese hamster V79 cells and transformation of mouse C3H10T1/2 cells *in vitro*. Formaldehyde induced DNA–protein cross-links, chromosomal aberrations, sister chromatid exchange and gene mutation in human cells *in vitro*. Experiments in human and Chinese hamster lung cells indicate that formaldehyde can inhibit repair of DNA lesions caused by the agent itself or by other mutagens, such as *N*-nitroso-*N*-methylurea or ionizing radiation (Grafström, 1990; Grafström *et al.*, 1993).

(ii)   *In-vivo studies in animals*

Formaldehyde induces cytogenetic damage in the cells of tissues of animals exposed either by gavage or by inhalation. Groups of five male Sprague–Dawley rats were given 200 mg/kg bw formaldehyde orally, were killed 16, 24 or 30 h after treatment and were examined for the induction of micronuclei and nuclear anomalies in cells of the gastrointestinal epithelium. The frequency of mitotic figures was used as an index of cell proliferation. Treated rats had significant (greater than fivefold) increases in the frequency of micronucleated cells in the stomach, duodenum, ileum and colon; the stomach was the most sensitive, with a 20-fold increase in the frequency of micronucleated cells 30 h after treatment, and the colon was the least sensitive. The frequency of nuclear anomalies was also significantly increased at these sites. These effects were observed in conjunction with signs of severe local irritation (Migliore *et al.*, 1989).

Male Sprague–Dawley rats were exposed by inhalation to 0, 0.5, 3 or 15 ppm [0, 0.62, 3.7 or 18.5 mg/m^3] formaldehyde for 6 h per day on 5 days per week for 1 and 8 weeks. No significant increase in chromosomal abnormalities in the bone-marrow cells of formaldehyde-exposed rats was observed relative to controls, but the frequency of chromosomal aberrations was significantly increased in pulmonary lavage cells (lung alveolar macrophages) from rats that inhaled 15 ppm formaldehyde. Aberrations, which were predominantly chromatid breaks, were seen in 8.0 and 9.2% of the scored pulmonary lavage cells from treated animals and in 3.5 and 4.4% of cells from controls after 1 and 8 weeks, respectively (Dallas *et al.*, 1992).

In a second in-vivo study on bone-marrow cytogenetics, Wistar rats were exposed by inhalation to formaldehyde (0.5 or 1.5 mg/m^3) every day for 4 h (except for non-working days) for 4 months (Kitaeva *et* al., 1990). The concentration of 1.5 mg/m^3 formaldehyde caused diverse effects on germ cells that the authors correlated with their subsequent studies that showed impairment of early embryonic development (see Section 4.3.2). Both concentrations (0.5 and 1.5 mg/m^3) caused a significantly increased number of chromoso-mal aberrations in the bone marrow that were of the chromatid (at 0.5 mg/m^3) and chromo-somal (at 1.5 mg/m^3) type. The number of hypoploidal and hyperploidal cells was increased. The increase in aneuploidy was due only to chromosomal loss, not to chromo-somal gain. At the higher exposure, chromosomal type aberrations were observed. [The Working Group noted that this was the only study that evaluated bone-marrow cyto-genetics. Since chromosomal loss can frequently occur as an artefact of sample prepa-ration, these studies should be repeated.] The study showed that exposure to formaldehyde at the lower dose was cytotoxic and mutagenic to bone-marrow cells. In an in-vitro part of this study, exposure to 0.5 mg/m^3 formaldehyde caused a decrease in the mitotic index in bone-marrow cells while, at 1.5 mg/m^3, the mitotic index was increased (Kitaeva *et al.*, 1990). [The Working Group noted that this is the only in-vivo study that showed positive cytogenetic effects of formaldehyde in the bone marrow.]

(c)   Mutational spectra

(i)   *In-vitro studies* (see also Table 37 and references therein)

The spectrum of mutations induced by formaldehyde was studied in human lympho-blasts *in vitro*, in *Escherichia coli* and in naked pSV2*gpt* plasmid DNA (Crosby *et al.*, 1988). Thirty mutant TK6 X-linked *HPRT*⁻ human lymphoblast colonies induced by eight repetitive treatments with 150 μmol/L [4.5 μg/mL] formaldehyde were characterized by southern blot analysis. Fourteen (47%) of these mutants had visible deletions of some or all of the X-linked *HPRT* bands, indicating that formaldehyde can induce large losses of DNA in human TK6 lymphoblasts. The remainder of the mutants showed normal restric-tion patterns, which, according to the authors, probably consisted of point mutations or smaller insertions or deletions that were too small to detect by southern blot analysis.

Sixteen of the 30 formaldehyde-induced human lymphoblast TK6 X-linked *HPRT* mutants referred to above that were not attributable to deletion were examined by southern blot, northern blot and DNA sequence analysis (Liber *et al.*, 1989). Of these, nine produced mRNA of normal size and amount, three produced mRNA of normal size but in reduced amounts, one had a smaller size of mRNA and three produced no detectable mRNA. Sequence analyses of cDNA prepared from *HPRT* mRNA were performed on one sponta-neous and seven formaldehyde-induced mutants indicated by normal northern blotting. The spontaneous mutant was caused by an AT→GC transition. Six of the formaldehyde-induced mutants were base substitutions, all of which occurred at AT base-pairs. There was an apparent hot spot, in that four of six independent mutants were AT→CG transversions at a specific site. The remaining mutant had lost exon 8.

In *E. coli*, the mutations induced by formaldehyde were characterized with the use of the xanthine guanine phosphoribosyl transferase gene as the target gene. Exposure of *E. coli* to 4 mmol/L [120 μg/mL] formaldehyde for 1 h induced large insertions (41%), large deletions (18%) and point mutations (41%). DNA sequencing revealed that most of the point mutations were transversions at GC base-pairs. In contrast, exposure of *E. coli* to

40 mmol/L formaldehyde for 1 h produced 92% point mutations, 62% of which were transitions at a single AT base-pair in the gene. Therefore, formaldehyde produced different genetic alterations in *E. coli* at different concentrations. When naked pSV2*gpt* plasmid DNA was exposed to 3.3 or 10 mmol/L [99 or 300 μg/mL] formaldehyde and used to transform *E. coli*, most of the resulting mutations were frameshifts that resulted from the addition or deletion of one base, which again suggests a different mechanism of mutation.

The potential of formaldehyde to induce mutation was determined in mouse lymphoma L5178Y cells treated for 2 h with different concentrations (62.5–500 μM [1.9–15 μg/mL]). The mouse lymphoma assay detects gross alterations as large deletions and rearrangements. Treated cells showed a concentration-related increase in mutation frequency. While the frequency of small colonies was increased, only a marginal increase was observed in the frequency of large colonies. The extent of loss of heterozygosity was studied at five polymorphic markers — D11Agll, D11Mit67, D11Mit29, D11Mit21 and D11Mit63 — all of which are equally distributed along chromosome 11. The analysis showed increased loss of heterozygosity at the marker D11Agll, which is located in the tirosine kinase gene. The authors suggested that the main mechanism involved in the mutagenesis of formaldehyde in the mouse lymphoma assay is the production of small-scale chromosomal deletion or recombination (Speit & Merk, 2002).

Exposure of Chinese hamster V79 cells to formaldehyde did not induce gene mutation at the *Hprt* locus, while DNA–protein cross-links, sister chromatid exchange and micronuclei were induced (Merk & Speit, 1998). Formaldehyde induced G:C→T:A transversion in *E. coli* Lac$^+$ WP3104P and in *S. typhimurium* His$^+$ TA7005 (Ohta *et al.*, 1999, 2000).

Specific locus mutations at two closely linked loci in the *adenine-3* (*ad-3*) region were compared in two strains of *Neurospora crassa* (H-12, a DNA repair-proficient heterokaryon; and H-59, a DNA repair-deficient heterokaryon) exposed to formaldehyde. The majority (93.2%) of formaldehyde-induced *ad-3* mutations in H-12 resulted from gene/point mutations and only 6.8% resulted from multilocus deletion mutations. In contrast, a greater percentage of formaldehyde-induced *ad-3* mutations (62.8%) observed in H-59 resulted from multilocus deletion mutations. The distribution of *ad-3* mutation in this mutational spectra is highly significantly different ($p \ll 0.001$). While formaldehyde induced only a 12.8-fold increase in the frequency of *ad-3* mutations over that which occurs spontaneously in H-12, it induced a 412-fold increase in H-59. Formaldehyde induced a 3.4-fold higher ($p \ll 0.001$) *ad-3B^R*/*ad-3A^R* ratio in H-12 than in H-59. According to the authors, these results indicated that there was a quantitative and qualitative strain difference in formaldehyde-induced mutagenesis (de Serres *et al.*, 1988; de Serres & Brockman, 1999).

(ii)   *In-vivo studies in animals*

DNA sequence analysis of PCR-amplified cDNA fragments that contain the evolutionarily conserved regions II–V of the rat *p53* gene was used to examine *p53* mutations in 11 primary nasal squamous-cell carcinomas induced in rats that had been exposed by inhalation to 15 ppm [18.5 mg/m³] formaldehyde for up to 2 years. Point mutations at GC base-pairs in the *p53* complementary DNA sequence were found in five of the tumours

(Table 38). The authors pointed out that all five human counterparts of the mutated *p53* codons listed in Table 38 have been identified as mutants in a variety of human cancers; the CpG dinucleotide at codon 273 (codon 271 in the rat) is a mutational hot spot that occurs in many human cancers (Recio *et al.*, 1992).

Table 38. DNA sequence analysis of *p53* cDNA (PCR fragment D) from squamous-cell carcinomas of nasal passages induced in rats by formaldehyde

DNA sequence[a]	Mutation (codon)[b]			Equivalent human *p53* codon no.	Location in conserved region
$_{396}$C→A	TTC→TT**A** (132)	phe→leu		134	II
$_{398}$G→T	T**G**C→T**T**C (133)	cys→phe		135	II
$_{638}$G→T	A**G**C→A**T**C (213)	ser→ile		215	
$_{812}$G→A	C**G**T→C**A**T (271)	arg→his		273	V
$_{842}$G→C	C**G**G→C**C**G (281)	arg→pro		283	V

From Recio *et al.* (1992)
[a] The A in the start codon is designated as base position 1.
[b] The start codon ATG is designated as codon 1.

An immunohistochemical technique was used to assess the presence of p53 protein, a marker of cell proliferation (proliferating cell nuclear antigen) and tumour growth factor-α in the histopathological sections of the above tumours. In addition to the positive p53 immunostaining in squamous-cell carcinomas, especially in cells with keratization, p53-positive immunostaining was also observed in preneoplastic hyperkeratotic plaques while normal nasal mucosa immunostained negatively. A correlation was found between both the pattern and the distribution of immunostaining of proliferating cell nuclear antigen and p53 (Wolf *et al.*, 1995).

Cell lines were established from the above set of squamous-cell carcinomas and, when injected into nude mice, two of them that contained the *p53* mutation were tumorigenic while the two cell lines that contained wild-type *p53* were not. The author suggested that these findings indicate that *p53* mutation occurs in the development of certain rodent nasal squamous-cell carcinomas and that it is associated with tumorigenicity (Recio, 1997). All the mutated *p53* codons that were identified in formaldehyde-induced rat squamous-cell carcinomas have also been found to be mutated in a variety of human cancers (for example, rat codon 271, human codon 273). *P53* is mutated in various human squamous-cell carcinomas including those of the respiratory tract, skin and oesophagus. It was suggested that these data indicate that the development of certain human and rat squamous-cell carcinomas share a molecular change. The author proposed a possible mechanistic explanation, which is based on the fact that the induction of nasal squamous-cell carcinomas by formaldehyde is accompanied by cytotoxicity and inflammation followed by cell proliferation that may induce genetic alterations.

Formaldehyde is also known to be genotoxic; a number of lesions have been proposed to explain this genotoxic effect, including DNA–protein cross-links (reviewed in IARC, 1995). Studies on the *HPRT* mutation spectrum in formaldehyde-exposed human cells revealed that 50% of the mutations are deletions, while 50% are due to point mutation at the A:T base-pair (Liber *et al.*, 1989). The finding of deletions as part of the formaldehyde mutation spectrum may explain the homozygous nature of pair mutations observed in *p53* in formaldehyde-induced squamous-cell carcinomas. However, there is an inconsistency with regard to the base-pair that is found to be A:T in *HPRT* in human (Liber *et al.*, 1989) and mammalian cell lines (Graves *et al.*, 1996) and G:C in *p53* in formaldehyde-induced squamous-cell carcinomas. The author suggested that an indirect mechanism of genotoxicity and not a direct effect of formaldehyde on the genome is involved in the carcinogenic process of formaldehyde (Recio, 1997).

In order to evaluate transcriptional changes involved with acute exposure to formaldehyde, two groups of male Fischer 344 rats received either 40 µL distilled water or formaldehyde (400 mM [12 mg/mL]) instilled into each nostril. Twenty-four hours after this treatment, total RNA was extracted from the nasal epithelium to generate cDNA. Adjusted signal intensity was obtained from image analysis of 1185 genes from samples from four controls and three formaldehyde-treated rats. Significance analysis of microarray hybridization data using Clontech™ Rat Atlas 1.2 arrays revealed that 24/1185 genes studied were significantly up-regulated and 22 genes were significantly down-regulated. Ten of the most highly expressed genes for formaldehyde-treated animals included the *N*-methyl-D-aspartate receptor, inducible nitric oxide synthase, macrophage inflammatory protein 1 α and macrophage inflammatory protein 2, Wilms tumour protein homologue 1, tumour necrosis factor ligand, methyl-CpG-binding protein 2, GABA receptor, Fos-responsive gene 1 and presomatotrophin. Of the 24 significantly up-regulated genes, six were receptors, six were involved in extracellular cell signalling and four were oncogene/tumour-suppressor genes, all of which are pathways that could be affected by treatment with formaldehyde. Of the 22 significantly down-regulated genes, five were involved in ion channel regulation and four were involved in protein turnover which suggests that an early response to treatment with formaldehyde may be impaired ion channel function and interruption of protein processing. Many phase I and phase II genes that regulate xenobiotic metabolism and oxidative stress — the CYP and glutathione family, respectively — were altered in treated but not in controls rats. In order to validate the direction of gene expression observed on the microarray, results for 10 of the differentially expressed genes were confirmed by quantitative real-time PCR. Eight of the 10 gene expression values were in positive agreement. No significant difference was found between formaldehyde-treated and control groups in relation to the expression of apoptosis genes. However, in comparison with the control group, the formaldehyde-treated group had a general trend of lower levels of expression of nine apoptic genes that represent three of the major apoptosis regulation pathways, including receptor-mediated, caspase and the mitochondrial-associated *bcl2* family of genes. The authors suggested that their results indicated that exposure to formaldehyde can cause alteration in the levels of expression of genes that are involved in several functional categories including xenobiotic metabolism, cell cycle regulation, DNA synthesis and repair, oncogenes and apoptosis (Hester *et al.*, 2003).

4.5   Mechanistic considerations

4.5.1   *Deposition (airway deposition models)*

Anatomically accurate CFD models have been applied to study the role of nasal airflow and formaldehyde flux in rats, monkeys and humans in order to achieve more accurate risk assessments (Kimbell & Subramaniam, 2001; Kimbell *et al.*, 2002). The use of DNA–protein cross-links as a measure of internal dose, as opposed to the use of air concentration, coupled with the use of monkey-based as opposed to rat-based predictions, resulted in a 50-fold reduction in risk for humans (McClellan, 1995).

Using the Fischer 344 rat CFD model, a sharp anterior to posterior gradient of formaldehyde deposition in the rat nose is predicted, which agrees with observed patterns of formation of DNA–protein cross-links and effects on cell replication (Monticello *et al.*, 1996; Cohen Hubal *et al.*, 1997). In another study, predictions of formaldehyde dosimetry in the non-squamous epithelium in the rat CFD model were used to analyse the role of local flux on the distribution of squamous metaplasia induced by 10 ppm and 15 ppm formaldehyde (Kimbell *et al.*, 1997). Squamous metaplasia is a useful indicator for formaldehyde-induced squamous-cell carcinoma in rodents due to its temporal relevance and consistency (McMillan *et al.*, 1994). Predictions obtained with the model illustrate how, as squamous metaplasia develops, the sites of maximum absorption of formaldehyde move further back in the nose.

In the rhesus monkey, a CFD model of the nasal passages was used to facilitate species-to-species extrapolation of data on the toxicity of formaldehyde (Kepler *et al.*, 1998). As with rats, an anterior to posterior gradient in formaldehyde deposition was predicted and a strong correlation was observed between patterns of airflow and the occurrence of nasal lesions.

In a comparison of Fischer 344 rats, rhesus monkeys and humans, the role of mucous- and non-mucous-coated tissue on formaldehyde uptake was analysed (Kimbell *et al.*, 2001b). Flux values for rats and monkeys were found to be very similar at sites where the effects of formaldehyde on cell proliferation had previously been observed. Similar flux values were predicted in a region of the nasal passage where a high incidence of tumours had been observed in rats and in an anterior region of the human nasal passage. It was suggested that a similar formaldehyde-induced response in rats might be expected in humans when regional fluxes are similar.

CFD models of Fischer 344 rat, rhesus monkey and human nasal passages were also used to predict patterns of wall mass flux in order to reduce the uncertainty in interspecies extrapolation of dose within the nasal passages (Kimbell *et al.*, 2001a). In all cases, steep anterior-to-posterior gradients of formaldehyde deposition were predicted. The surface area and average flux were estimated for the flux bins at different airflow rates. At a minute volume of 15 L/min, approximately 20% of the surface area of the human nasal passages had a predicted flux value greater than the median flux value. Increasing airflow in humans was also associated with a distal shift in flux patterns and a reduced percentage of uptake in the nasal passages. Differences across species in nasal anatomy and associated differences in flux were also suggested to play a potentially large role in the occurrence of local adverse effects due to the non-linear relationships of flux with DNA–protein cross-links and with cell proliferation. The adsorption of formaldehyde on inhaled particles does not appreciably alter the patterns of formaldehyde deposition associated with the inhalation of formaldehyde vapour (Rothenberg *et al.*, 1989; Risby *et al.*, 1990).

4.5.2   *Metabolism*

Formaldehyde is an endogenous metabolite that is formed by demethylation reactions and used in the biosynthesis of macromolecules. Average concentrations, including bound and free forms, in cells and biological fluids are reported to be about 0.1 mM (Heck *et al.*, 1985). Formaldehyde readily combines with GSH to form hydroxymethylglutathione, which is converted to formate in a two-step enzymatic reaction that initially involves ADH3. The K_m for the initial binding of hydroxymethylglutathione with ADH3 is in the order of 4 μM and the level of free formaldehyde is probably even lower (Holmquist & Vallee, 1991; Uotila & Koivusalo, 1997; Hedberg *et al.*, 1998). The half-life of formaldehyde in plasma is very short, and is approximately 1 min in rats exposed intravenously (Rietbrock, 1965).

4.5.3   *Genotoxicity*

Formaldehyde induced DNA–protein cross-links *in vitro* in human bronchial epithelial cells, fibroblasts and lymphocytes, in Chinese hamster ovary cells and in non-transformed human fibroblasts (Grafström *et al.*, 1984; Olin *et al.*, 1996; Shaham *et al.*, 1996a,b). The formation of DNA–protein cross-links showed a consistent dose–effect relationship and was induced at concentrations of formaldehyde that allowed survival of up to 75% of the cells (Merk & Speit, 1998, 1999). A range of half-lives for the removal of DNA–protein cross-links from the cells has been reported (3–66 h), but most of the values are in the vicinity of 24 h (Gräfstrom *et al.*, 1984; Merk & Speit, 1998, 1999; Quievryn & Zhitkovich, 2000).

Several studies that compared the kinetics of the formation and removal of DNA–protein cross-links in a variety of cell types reported no differences among normal and DNA repair-deficient cell types (Grafström *et al.*, 1984; Speit *et al.*, 2000). DNA single-strand breaks and/or alkali-labile sites are generated from the repair of formaldehyde damage in normal cells (Grafström *et al.*, 1984). Formaldehyde is more toxic to Xeroderma Pigmentosum cells, which also show a higher percentage of micronuclei than normal cells. The data suggested that neither defective nucleotide excision repair (Xeroderma Pigmentosum cells) nor defective cross-link repair (Fanconi anaemia cells) seem to delay the removal of formaldehyde-induced DNA–protein cross-links significantly and that more than one repair pathway may be involved in the removal of cross-links (Grafström et al., 1984; Speit et al., 2000). Human peripheral blood lymphocytes lost DNA–protein cross-links at a significantly slower rate than established cell lines (Quievryn & Zhitkovich, 2000). Repair of formaldehyde-induced DNA–protein cross-links was not changed significantly due to loss of GSH. Additional studies have indicated that the active removal of DNA–protein cross-links from cells may involve proteolytic degradation of cross-link proteins (Quievryn & Zhitkovich, 2000). Several studies indicate that formaldehyde may also interfere with the processes of repair of DNA by (a) inhibiting DNA repair enzymes, (b) inhibiting the removal of DNA lesions and (c) altering gene expression (Grafström et al., 1996).

Assessment of DNA–protein cross-links and sister chromatid exchange in peripheral lymphocytes from formaldehyde-exposed workers demonstrated an association with overall exposure (Shaham et al., 1996a,b, 2003). It remains unclear to what extent these endpoints contribute to the mutagenesis and carcinogenicity of formaldehyde (Recio et al., 1992; Merk & Speit, 1998; Speit et al., 2000; Liteplo & Meek, 2003).

Studies in humans have reported both positive and negative results for the incidence of micronuclei in nasal and buccal mucosa in workers exposed to formaldehyde (see Table 36). In one study of both buccal and nasal mucosa, a greater increase was observed in centromere-negative micronuclei than centromere-positive micronuclei, which implicates chromosome breakage as the major mechanism responsible for these effects (Titenko-Holland et al., 1996). Although micronuclei are correlated with risk for cancer in animals, the association between micronuclei and cancer in humans requires clarification because of the high degree of inter-individual variability within the human population (Fenech et al., 1999).

The formation of DNA–protein cross-links in the nasal respiratory mucosa of rats after inhalation exposure to 6 ppm [7.4 mg/m^3] formaldehyde and higher has been demonstrated by a variety of techniques, including decreased extractability of DNA from proteins (Casanova-Schmitz & Heck, 1983), double-labelling studies with [^{3}H]- and [^{14}C]formaldehyde (Casanova-Schmitz et al., 1984b; Casanova & Heck, 1987; Heck & Casanova, 1987) and isolation of DNA from respiratory mucosal tissue and quantification by HPLC of formaldehyde released from cross-links after exposure to [^{14}C]formaldehyde (Casanova et al., 1989, 1994). The formation of DNA–protein cross-links is a non-linear function of concentration (Casanova & Heck, 1987; Casanova et al., 1989, 1994; Heck & Casanova, 1995; see Fig. 8) and correlates with the site-specificity of tumours (Casanova et al., 1994). Cross-links were not detected in the olfactory mucosa or in the bone marrow of rats (Casanova-Schmitz et al., 1984b; Casanova & Heck, 1987).

DNA–protein cross-links were also measured in the respiratory tract of groups of three rhesus monkeys immediately after single 6-h exposures to airborne [^{14}C]formaldehyde (0.7, 2 or 6 ppm [0.9, 2.4 or 7.4 mg/m^3]) (Casanova et al., 1991). The concentrations of cross-linked formaldehyde in the nose of monkeys decreased in the order: middle

Figure 8. Average concentration of DNA–protein cross-links formed per unit time in the turbinates and lateral wall/septum of Fischer 344 rats and rhesus monkeys versus the airborne concentration of formaldehyde (CH₂O)

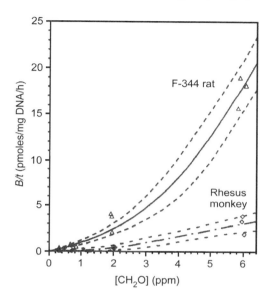

Adapted from Casanova *et al.* (1991)

All animals were exposed to formaldehyde for 6 h. Data in rats are taken from Casanova *et al.* (1989). (Results obtained in rats at 10 ppm are omitted for clarity.) Dashed lines are the 95% confidence limits about the mean for each species.

turbinates > lateral wall–septum > nasopharynx, which is consistent with the location and severity of lesions in monkeys exposed to 6 ppm (Monticello *et al.*, 1989). Very low levels of cross-links were also found in the trachea and carina of some monkeys. The yield of cross-links in the nose of monkeys was an order of magnitude lower than that in the nose of rats, due largely to species differences in minute volume and quantity of exposed tissue (Casanova *et al.*, 1991; Fig. 8). A pharmacokinetic model based on these results indicated that the concentrations of DNA–protein cross-links in the human nose would be lower than those in the noses of monkeys and rats (Casanova *et al.*, 1991).

In order to determine whether DNA–protein cross-links accumulate with repeated exposure, the yield of formaldehyde from cross-links was investigated in rats that were exposed either once or subchronically to unlabelled formaldehyde (6 or 10 ppm [7.4 or 12.3 mg/m³]) for 6 h per day on 5 days per week for 11 weeks and 4 days (Casanova *et al.*, 1994). The yield was not higher in pre-exposed than in naive rats, which suggests that no accumulation had occurred in the former. The results also suggest that DNA–protein cross-links in the rat nasal mucosa are removed rapidly.

Conolly *et al.* (2000) described a model of tissue disposition of formaldehyde, which included CFD and measurements of mucosal epithelial thickness in order to refine previous predictions of the occurrence of DNA–protein cross-links in rats, monkeys and humans. The thickness of the epithelial tissue is approximately 4.5 times greater in humans than in rats, which results in a lesser net dose of formaldehyde in humans at concentrations that saturate the metabolic capacity of rats (Schlosser *et al.*, 2003). Good correlations of model predictions and data of cross-links were obtained in association with the regions of high and low tumour response in the rat nose (Conolly *et al.*, 2000).

Merk and Speit (1998) evaluated the significance of DNA–protein cross-links for mutagenesis in V79 Chinese hamster cells. Formaldehyde was seen to induce DNA–protein cross-links, sister chromatid exchange and micronuclei in conjunction with a reduction in relative cloning efficiency. However, no gene mutations were observed in the *Hprt* test. It was concluded that DNA–protein cross-links were related to chromosomal effects, but not directly to gene mutations.

Shaham *et al.* (2003) reported that the formation of DNA–protein cross-links in peripheral lymphocytes in exposed workers was associated with increased serum p53 protein, including wild-type and mutant forms. Recio *et al.* (1992) found *p53* point mutations in 5/11 squamous-cell carcinomas in formaldehdye-exposed rats. Studies have shown (Luo *et al.*, 1994; Hemminki *et al.*, 1996) that higher levels of p53 protein are found in serum years before the diagnosis of malignant tumours such as lung cancer. [The Working Group felt that there may be an association, although further studies are needed to clarify the association between DNA–protein cross-links and effects on the state of p53.]

4.5.4   *Cytotoxicity and cell proliferation*

Formaldehyde is well established as a toxicant at the site of contact. Following inhalation exposure, cytotoxicity was evident in the nasal passages of rats and mice (Chang *et al.*, 1983). Toxicity was greatest in the respiratory epithelium of rats, and the median septum and nasoturbinates were the sites most affected. At 15 ppm [18.45 mg/m^3], necrosis and sloughing of respiratory epithelium was evident immediately after a single 6-h exposure and early hyperplasia was present 18 h after a single exposure. Mice exhibited lower toxicity in the nasal epithelium associated with reduced exposure due to reduced minute volume. Severe ulcerative rhinitis, inflammation, epithelial hyperplasia and increased cell proliferation were observed in rats exposed to 15 ppm formaldehyde for 5 days (6 h per day). A second study examined cell proliferation and histopathology in rats exposed to 0, 0.7, 2, 6, 10 or 15 ppm [0, 0.86, 2.46, 7.38, 12.3, 18.45 mg/m^3] formaldehyde. Increased cell proliferation was evident at 6 and 15 ppm, but not at 2 ppm or lower following 9 days or 6 weeks of exposure (Monticello *et al.*, 1991).

In a mechanistic 24-month carcinogenesis bioassay with interim sacrifices at 1, 4 and 9 days, 6 weeks, and 3, 6, 12 and 18 months, increased cell proliferation was demonstrated at all time-points in rats exposed to 6, 10 and 15 ppm (Monticello *et al.*, 1991, 1996).

Monticello *et al.* (1996) evaluated the relationship of regional increases in nasal epithelial cell proliferation with nasal cancer in rats. Sublinear increases in both cell proliferation and squamous-cell carcinoma were observed with increasing concentration of formaldehyde. A good correlation was observed between site-specific tumour occurrence and the population-weighted unit length labelling index, which incorporates information on both the rate of cell replication and the numbers of cells at specific sites. It was therefore suggested that not only the rate at which cells divided but also the size of the target cell population that underwent DNA replication were crucial factors in the development of formaldehyde-induced nasal squamous-cell carcinoma. Both the rate of cell division and the number of cells in the proliferative pool are thought to increase the chance for mutation at a given dose of formaldehyde. Monticello *et al.* (1996) stated that, although there is evidence to suggest that concentration is more important than duration of exposure in determining the extent of formaldehyde-induced nasal epithelial damage, the development of formaldehyde-induced nasal squamous-cell carcinoma probably requires repeated and prolonged damage to the nasal epithelium. Sustained cellular proliferation, which was seen at 6, 10 and 15 ppm, is thought to play a crucial role in carcinogenesis through the transformation of cells with damaged DNA to mutated cells and the clonal expansion of the mutated cell population (McClellan, 1995).

Studies of cell cultures provide some support that proliferation is stimulated after exposure to formaldehyde (Tyihák *et al.*, 2001). Transcription of *ADH3* was associated with proliferative states (Nilsson *et al.*, 2004), formaldehyde and formate were shown to serve as donors to the one-carbon pool synthesis of macromolecules and, in one study, exposure to formaldehyde was shown to increase cell proliferation (Tyihák *et al.*, 2001).

4.5.5   *Cancer*

Nasal squamous-cell carcinomas have been observed in toxicological studies of rats exposed to concentrations of at least 6 ppm formaldehyde (Swenberg *et al.*, 1980; Kerns *et al.*, 1983a,b). Epidemiological studies have also suggested increases in risk for sinonasal carcinomas and particularly for nasopharyngeal carcinoma in humans following exposure to formaldehyde. The exact biological mechanism by which exposure to formaldehyde may cause cancer is currently unknown (Conolly, 2002; Liteplo & Meek, 2003); however, formaldehyde causes formation of DNA–protein cross-links and increases cellular proliferation in the upper respiratory tracts of rats and monkeys.

However, most epidemiological studies of sinonasal cancer have not distinguished tumours that arise in the nose from those that develop in the nasal sinuses. Thus, any effect on the risk for nasal cancer specifically would tend to be diluted if there were no corresponding effect on the risk for cancer in the sinuses, and could easily be undetectable through the lack of statistical power.

4.5.6   *Computational dose–response modelling*

A theoretical model for DNA replication in the presence of DNA cross-links was developed by Heck and Casanova (1999). This model assumes that DNA–protein cross-links are formed randomly in the DNA and that replication can advance up to but not past a DNA–protein cross-link. This analysis is consistent with the experimental observation of decreased cell proliferation in the nasal epithelium of rats exposed to concentrations of 0.7 and 2.0 ppm [0.86 and 2.46 mg/m^3] formaldehyde.

A biologically based model of carcinogenesis of formaldehyde was described by Conolly (2002), which included a two-stage clonal growth model and used the incorporation of both DNA–protein cross-links and cell proliferation, together with linked regional dosimetry predictions, into the model to predict tumour incidence. Through inclusion of this information, the author suggested that a smaller degree of uncertainty was associated with the model.

Since both squamous-cell carcinoma and preneoplastic lesions develop in a characteristic site-specific pattern, Conolly *et al.* (2003) used anatomically accurate three-dimensional CFD models to predict the site-specific flux of formaldehyde from inhaled air into the tissues in rats. Flux into tissues was used as a dose metric for two modes of action: direct mutagenicity and cytolethality–regenerative cellular proliferation (CRCP). The two modes were linked to key parameters of a two-stage model of clonal growth. The direct mutagenic mode of action was represented by a low linear dose–response model of DNA–protein cross-link formation. An empirical J-shaped dose–response model and a threshold model fit to experimental data were used to describe CRCP. The J-shaped dose–response for CRCP provided a better description of the data on squamous-cell carcinoma than the threshold model. Sensitivity analysis indicated that the rodent tumour response is primarily due to the CRCP mode of action and the direct mutagenic pathway has little or no influence. The study suggests a J-shaped dose–response for formaldehyde-mediated nasal squamous-cell carcinoma in Fischer 344 rats. [The Working Group felt that uncertainty remains on some components and parameters of this model, which can affect both predictions of risk and qualitative aspects of model behaviour, and warrants further developmental work.]

Gaylor *et al.* (2004) conducted an analysis of the concentration–response relationship for formaldehyde-induced cell proliferation in rats using statistical methods designed to identify J-shaped concentration–response curves. Such J-shaped curves demonstrate an initial decline in response, followed by a return to background response rates at the zero equivalent dose and then an increase above background response at concentrations above the zero equivalent dose. This analysis demonstrated a statistically significant reduction in cytotoxicity at concentrations below the zero equivalent dose. The authors suggested that, at low doses, the increased risk for nasal cancer due to DNA damage may be offset by a reduction in cell proliferation, a postulate that is consistent with the threshold-like behaviour of the concentration–response curve observed for nasal cancer in rats.

Schlosser *et al.* (2003) described a dose–response assessment of formaldehyde that used a combination of benchmark dose and pharmacokinetic methods. Following the identification of points of departure for both tumours and cell proliferation in rats by analysis of the benchmark dose, extrapolation to humans was performed using either a CFD model alone to predict formaldehyde flux or a CFD model in combination with a pharmacokinetic model to predict the tissue dose and the formaldehyde-induced DNA–protein cross-links as a dose metric. Risk predictions obtained with the benchmark dose model are similar to earlier risk predictions obtained with previous benchmark dose models. The benchmark dose risk predictions are substantially higher than those obtained from the clonal growth time-to-tumour model (Liteplo & Meek, 2003).

4.5.7 *Summary of experimental data*

Formaldehyde is an essential metabolic intermediate in all cells, and average concentrations in the blood of unexposed subjects has been reported to be about 0.1 mmol/L. It is a potent nasal irritant, is cytotoxic at high doses and induces nasal cancer in rats exposed to high airborne concentrations. Nasal squamous-cell carcinomas have been observed in toxicological studies of rats exposed to concentrations of at least 6 ppm; the incidence of these tumours increases sharply with further increases in concentration (Monticello *et al.*, 1996). In addition, at concentrations of 2 ppm or less, no histological changes have been observed in rodents, although changes at these concentrations have been seen in humans (IARC, 1995; Liteplo & Meek, 2003).

Early assessments estimated the risk for cancer from exposure to low concentrations of formaldehyde using linear extrapolations from data on high concentrations in animals. However, linear low-dose extrapolation does not account for the sublinearities in the observed concentration–response relationship (Casanova *et al.*, 1994; Monticello *et al.*, 1996; Bolt, 2003). It was suggested that the risk for cancer in humans was probably overestimated by linear low-dose extrapolation from rats at concentrations that do not increase cell proliferation or the size of the cell population at risk (Monticello *et al.*, 1996). Bolt (2003) recommended that predictions of risk at low (≤ 2 ppm) versus high (≥ 6 ppm) concentrations be made separately.

Formaldehyde demonstrates positive effects in a large number of in-vitro tests for genotoxicity, including bacterial mutation, DNA strand breaks, chromosomal aberrations and sister chromatid exchange. Studies in humans showed inconsistent results with regard to cytogenetic changes (micronuclei, chromosomal aberrations and sister chromatid exchange). The frequency of DNA–protein cross-links was found to be significantly higher in peripheral lymphocytes from exposed workers (Shaham *et al.*, 1996, 2003).

In-vitro studies have shown that 0.1 mM [3 µg/mL] formaldehyde increases cell proliferation without detectable cytotoxicity (Tyihák *et al.*, 2001). Formaldehyde also induces genetic damage at concentrations as low as 0.1 mM and inhibits DNA repair in bronchial cells at 0.1–0.3 mM [3–9 µg/mL], although it does not appear to be associated with oxidative stress. Formaldehyde inhibits cell growth at 0.2 mM [6 µg/mL] and 0.6 mM

[18 µg/mL], as expressed by loss of clonal growth rate and colony-forming efficiency, respectively. It alters membrane integrity, which leads to increases in cellular Ca^{2+} and could affect cell death rates by accelerating terminal differentiation (Grafström *et al.*, 1996). Apoptosis has been demonstrated in rat thymocytes at concentrations at or above 0.1 mM (Nakao *et al.*, 2003). HeLa cervical carcinoma cells have been shown to be fairly resistant to the toxic effects of formaldehyde in comparison with untransformed human dental pulp fibroblasts and buccal epithelial cells (Lovschall *et al.*, 2002). In contrast, formaldehyde is only weakly genotoxic in in-vivo tests.

Using a variety of techniques, inhalation of formaldehyde has been shown to induce the formation of DNA–protein cross-links in nasal tissue from rats and monkeys, including decreased extractability of DNA from proteins, labelling studies and isolation of DNA by HPLC. The formation of DNA–protein cross-links is a non-linear function of formaldehyde concentration, described by an initial linear component with a shallow slope and a second linear component with a steeper slope that follows a significant decrease in survival of the cells and depletion of GSH at about 0.1 mM (Merk & Speit, 1998).

Species-specific differences in the rate of formation of DNA–protein cross-links, in the prevalence of squamous metaplasia (McMillan *et al.*, 1994) and in the occurrence of nasal cancer have also been observed at given concentrations of formaldehyde in rats, mice and monkeys (McMillan *et al.*, 1994; McClellan, 1995). Differences in nasal anatomy and regional airflow as well as differences in the absorptive properties of the nasal lining between species have been suggested to influence greatly the dose of formaldehyde that reaches different anatomical regions and subsequent formaldehyde-induced lesions at a given exposure concentration (Kimbell *et al.*, 1997; Kepler *et al.*, 1998; Zito, 1999; Kimbell *et al,*. 2001b; Conolly, 2002).

Anatomically accurate CFD models have been developed to describe the nasal uptake of formaldehyde in rats, monkeys and humans (Conolly, 2000). Interspecies differences in formaldehyde-induced DNA–protein cross-links and nasal lesions appear to be related to species-specific patterns in formaldehyde flux in different regions within the nasal passages (see Fig. 9; Kimbell *et al.*, 2001a). CFD modelling predicts anterior-to-posterior gradients of formaldehyde deposition in the noses of rats, rhesus monkeys and humans (Kimbell *et al.*, 2001a). This might suggest that formaldehyde is more likely to cause cancer of the nose than of the nasopharynx in humans.

Although formaldehyde is mainly deposited in the upper respiratory tract, the distribution of the deposition is expected to vary by species (Conaway *et al.*, 1996; Liteplo & Meek, 2003). The lack of parallel data on the formation of nasal mucosal DNA–protein cross-links and on cell proliferation in humans complicates the extrapolation of the animal data, in particular rodent data, to humans (Conolly *et al.*, 2000; Liteplo & Meek, 2003).

The current data indicate that both genotoxicty and cytoxicity play important roles in the carcinogenesis of formaldehyde in nasal tissues. DNA–protein cross-links provide a potentially useful marker of genotoxicity. The concentration–response curve for the formation of DNA–protein cross-links is bi-phasic, and the slope increases at concentrations of formaldehyde of about 2–3 ppm [2.5–3.7 mg/m³] in Fischer 344 rats. Similar results have been

Figure 9. Allocation of nasal surface area to flux bins in rats, monkeys and humans

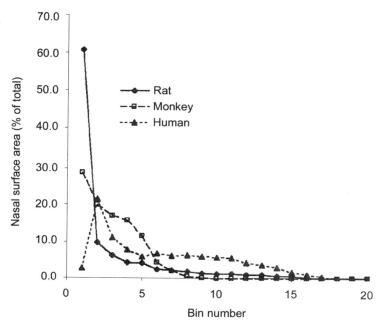

Adapted from Kimbell *et al.* (2001a)
Low bin numbers are associated with low flux values. Inspiratory airflow rates were 0.576 L/min in rats, 4.8 L/min in monkeys and 15 L/min in humans.

observed in rhesus monkeys, although the dose–response curve for DNA–protein cross-links is less well defined in this species. Cellular proliferation, which appears to amplify the genotoxic effects of formaldehyde greatly, increases considerably at concentrations of formaldehyde of about 6 ppm [7.4 mg/m^3], and results in a marked increase in the occurrence of malignant lesions in the nasal passages of rats at concentrations of formaldehyde above this level (Monticello *et al.*, 1996). Recent evidence suggests that cytotoxicity may demonstrate a J-shaped concentration–response curve, with a significant reduction in cellular proliferation rates at concentrations of 0.7–2 ppm [0.86–2.5 mg/m^3] (Conolly & Lutz, 2004; Gaylor *et al.*, 2004).

4.5.8 *Leukaemia*

The epidemiological evidence that formaldehyde may cause acute myelogenous leukaemia raises a number of mechanistic questions, including the processes by which inhaled formaldehyde may reach a myeloid progenitor (Heck & Casanova, 2004). The possibility that formaldehyde causes leukaemia is supported by the detection of cytogenetic abnormalities and an increase in the fraction of DNA–protein cross-links in circulating lymphocytes following occupational exposure to formaldehyde, as well as chromosomal aberrations in bone marrow in a single inhalation study in rats (Kitaeva *et al.*, 1990, 1996; Shaham *et al.*, 1996a,b, 1997, 2003).

It is possible that formaldehyde itself can reach the bone marrow following inhalation, although the evidence is inconsistent (Kitaeva *et al.*, 1990; Dallas *et al.*, 1992; Heck & Casanova, 2004). The relatively rapid rate of metabolism of formaldehyde by circulating red blood cells suggests that little if any inhaled formaldehyde could reach any tissue beyond the respiratory tract. [The Working Group noted that a clastogenic product of formaldehyde could conceivably be formed in the blood and circulate to the bone marrow, although this has not been suggested in the literature. Alternatively, it is possible that circulating myeloid progenitor stem cells could be the source of leukaemia. Such stem cells are known to be present in the blood and plausibly could be exposed to formaldehyde in the respiratory tract vasculature; however, there is currently no known prototype for such a mechanism of leukaemogenesis.]

Another mechanistic issue is the relation of cellular background levels of formaldehyde, as part of the one-carbon pool, to any risk from exogenous formaldehyde. Cellular background concentrations of formaldehyde are about 0.1 mM. In one study in humans, inhalation of 1.9 ppm [2.3 mg/m^3] formaldehyde for 40 min did not alter blood concentrations (Heck *et al.*, 1985). Elevated concentrations of formaldehyde were not observed in the blood of rats and rhesus monkeys exposed to formaldehyde at concentrations of up to 14.4 ppm [17.7 mg/m^3] (Heck *et al.*, 1985; Casanova *et al.*, 1988); nor were protein adducts or DNA–protein cross-links observed in the bone marrow of rats or rhesus monkeys exposed to formaldehyde at concentrations of up to 15 or 6 ppm [18.4 or 7.4 mg/m^3], respectively (Casanova-Schmitz *et al.*, 1984b; Heck *et al.*, 1989).

Known human myeloid leukaemogens include ionizing radiation, benzene and chemotherapeutic agents such as alkylators, DNA topoisomerase inhibitors and DNA-complexing agents. All of these agents produce overt bone marrow toxicity, including pancytopenia and aplastic anaemia in both laboratory animals and humans. Agents known to cause leukaemia in humans and animals are also known to induce chromosomal aberrations in peripheral lymphocytes. The absence of clear evidence of bone-marrow toxicity, even at high doses, indicates that, if formaldehyde is a human myeloid leukaemogen, its mechanism of action differs from those by which the known myeloid leukaemogens noted above operate. This is not inconceivable, because there is epidemiological evidence that butadiene and ethylene oxide are probably human leukaemogens, although neither is a classic bone-marrow toxicant.

Studies of workers exposed to benzene and of individuals who received cancer chemotherapy suggest that the induction period for acute myeloid leukaemia is less than 20 years, and is usually in the range of 2–15 years (Goldstein, 1990). This relatively short lag time for carcinogenesis reflects the intrinsic biology of the myeloid progenitor cell, irrespective of the mechanism that caused the initial cancer mutation. The epidemiological reports that suggest an association of formaldehyde with myeloid leukaemia have not clearly defined an induction period for the effect.

[The Working Group could not identify any rodent model for acute myeloid leukaemia. The lack of evidence of increased risk for leukaemia in long-term studies of formaldehyde in rodents is not informative with respect to myeloid leukaemogenesis in humans. The Working Group felt that, based on the data available at this time, it was not possible to identify a mechanism for the induction of myeloid leukaemia in humans by formaldehyde.]

5. Summary of Data Reported and Evaluation

5.1 Exposure data

Formaldehyde is produced worldwide on a large scale by catalytic, vapour-phase oxidation of methanol. Annual world production is about 21 million tonnes. Formaldehyde is used mainly in the production of phenolic, urea, melamine and polyacetal resins. Phenolic, urea and melamine resins have wide uses as adhesives and binders in wood product, pulp and paper, and synthetic vitreous fibre industries, in the production of plastics and coatings and in textile finishing. Polyacetal resins are widely used in the production of plastics. Formaldehyde is also used extensively as an intermediate in the manufacture of industrial chemicals, such as 1,4-butanediol, 4,4′-methylenediphenyl diisocyanate, pentaerythritol and hexamethylenetetramine. Formaldehyde is used directly in aqueous solution (formalin) as a disinfectant and preservative in many applications.

Occupational exposure to formaldehyde occurs in a wide variety of occupations and industries. The highest continuous exposures (2–5 ppm) [2.5–6.1 mg/m^3] were measured in the past during the varnishing of furniture and wooden floors, in the finishing of textiles, in the garment industry, in the treatment of fur and in certain jobs within manufactured board mills and foundries. Shorter-term exposures to high levels (3 ppm and higher) [3.7 mg/m^3 and higher] have been reported for embalmers, pathologists and paper workers. Lower levels have usually been encountered during the manufacture of man-made vitreous fibres, abrasives and rubber, and in formaldehyde production industries. A very wide range of exposure levels has been observed in the production of resins and plastic products. The development of resins that release less formaldehyde and improved ventilation have resulted in decreased levels of exposure in many industrial settings in recent decades.

Formaldehyde occurs as a natural product in most living systems and in the environment. In addition to these natural sources, common non-occupational sources of exposure include vehicle emissions, particle boards and similar building materials, carpets, paints and varnishes, food and cooking, tobacco smoke and the use of formaldehyde as a disinfectant. Levels of formaldehyde in outdoor air are generally below 0.001 mg/m^3 in remote areas and below 0.02 mg/m^3 in urban settings. The levels of formaldehyde in the indoor air of houses are typically 0.02–0.06 mg/m^3. Average levels of 0.5 mg/m^3 or more have been measured in 'mobile homes', but these have declined since the late 1980s as a result of standards that require that building materials emit lower concentrations of formaldehyde.

5.2   Human data

Nasopharyngeal cancer

Since the last monograph on formaldehyde (in 1995), the follow-up of three major cohort studies has been extended and three new case–control studies have been published.

In the largest and most informative cohort study of industrial workers exposed to formaldehyde, a statistically significant excess of deaths from nasopharyngeal cancer was observed in comparison with the US national population, with statistically significant exposure–response relationships for peak and cumulative exposure. An excess of deaths from nasopharyngeal cancer was also observed in a proportionate mortality analysis of the largest US cohort of embalmers and in a Danish study of proportionate cancer incidence among workers at companies that used or manufactured formaldehyde. In three other cohort studies of US garment manufacturers, British chemical workers and US embalmers, cases of nasopharyngeal cancer were fewer than expected, but the power of these studies to detect an effect on nasopharyngeal cancer was low and the deficits were small.

The relationship between nasopharyngeal cancer and exposure to formaldehyde has also been investigated in seven case–control studies, five of which found elevated risks for overall exposure to formaldehyde or in higher exposure categories, including one in which the increase in risk was statistically significant; three studies (two of which have been published since the last monograph) found higher risks among subjects who had the highest probability, level or duration of exposure.

The most recent meta-analysis, which was published in 1997, included some but not all of the above studies and found an increased overall meta-relative risk for nasopharyngeal cancer.

The Working Group considered it improbable that all of the positive findings for naso-pharyngeal cancer that were reported from the epidemiological studies, and particularly from the large study of industrial workers in the USA, could be explained by bias or un-recognized confounding effects.

Overall, the Working Group concluded that the results of the study of industrial workers in the USA, supported by the largely positive findings from other studies, provided sufficient epidemiological evidence that formaldehyde causes nasopharyngeal cancer in humans.

Leukaemia

Excess mortality from leukaemia has been observed relatively consistently in six of seven studies of professional workers (i.e. embalmers, funeral parlour workers, patho-logists and anatomists). A recently published meta-analysis of exposure to formaldehyde among professionals and the risk for leukaemia reported increased overall summary rela-tive risk estimates for embalmers, and for pathologists and anatomists, which did not vary significantly between studies (i.e. the results were found to be homogeneous). The excess incidence of leukaemia seen in several studies appeared to be predominantly of a myeloid type. There has been speculation in the past that these findings might be explained by exposures to viruses that are experienced by anatomists, pathologists and perhaps funeral workers. However, there is currently little direct evidence that these occupations have a higher incidence of viral infections than that of the general population or that viruses play a causal role in myeloid leukaemia. Professionals may also be exposed to other chemicals, but they have no material exposure to known leukaemogens. Furthermore, the exposure to other chemicals would differ between anatomists, pathologists and funeral workers, which reduces the likelihood that such exposures could explain the observed increases in risk.

Until recently, the findings for leukaemia in studies of professional workers appeared to be contradicted by the lack of such findings among industrial workers. However, some evidence for an excess of deaths from leukaemia has been reported in the recent updates of two of the three major cohort studies of industrial workers. A statistically significant exposure–response relationship was observed between peak exposures to formaldehyde and mortality from leukaemia in the study of industrial workers in the USA. This relationship was found to be particularly strong for myeloid leukaemia, a finding that was also observed in the study of anatomists and in several of the studies of embalmers. However, in the study of industrial workers in the USA, mortality from leukaemia was lower than expected when comparisons were made using the general population as the referent group. This raises concerns about whether these findings are robust with respect to the choice of a comparison group. Leukaemia has been found to be associated with socioeconomic status, and that of industrial workers tends to be low. Thus, the lack of an overall finding of an excess of deaths from leukaemia in the cohort of industrial workers in the USA might be explained by biases in the comparison between the study and referent populations. The study also failed to demonstrate an exposure–response relationship with cumulative exposure, although other metrics may sometimes be more relevant.

Mortality from leukaemia was also found to be in excess in the recent update of the study of garment workers exposed to formaldehyde in the USA. A small and statistically non-significant excess was observed for the entire cohort in comparison with rates among the general population. This excess was somewhat stronger for myeloid leukaemia, which is consistent with the findings from the study of industrial workers in the USA and several of the studies of medical professionals and embalmers. The excess was also stronger among workers who had a long duration of exposure and long follow-up, and who had been employed early in the study period when exposures to formaldehyde were believed to be highest. This pattern of findings is generally consistent with what might be expected if, in fact, exposure to formaldehyde were causally associated with a risk for leukaemia. The positive associations observed in many of the subgroup analyses presented in the study of garment workers in the USA were based on a relatively small number of deaths, and were thus not statistically stable.

The updated study of British industrial workers failed to demonstrate excess mortality among workers exposed to formaldehyde. The lack of positive findings in this study is difficult to reconcile with the findings from the studies of garment workers and industrial workers in the USA and studies of professionals. This was a high-quality study of adequate size and with sufficiently long follow-up to have had a reasonable chance to detect an excess of deaths from leukaemia. The British study did not include an evaluation of peak exposures, but neither did the study of garments workers in the USA nor the studies of professionals. Also, the British study did not examine specifically the risk for myeloid leukaemia, which represented the strongest findings in the studies of garment workers and industrial workers in the USA and in several of the studies of medical professionals and funeral workers.

In summary, there is strong but not sufficient evidence for a causal association between leukaemia and occupational exposure to formaldehyde. Increased risk for leukaemia has consistently been observed in studies of professional workers and in two of three of the most relevant studies of industrial workers. These findings fall slightly short of being fully persuasive because of some limitations in the findings from the cohorts of industrial and garment workers in the USA and because they conflict with the non-positive findings from the British cohort of industrial workers.

Sinonasal cancer

The association between exposure to formaldehyde and the risk for sinonasal cancer has been evaluated in six case–control studies that primarily focused on formaldehyde. Four of these studies also contributed to a pooled analysis that collated occupational data from 12 case–control investigations. After adjustment for known occupational confounders, this analysis showed an increased risk for adenocarcinoma in both men and women and also (although on the basis of only a small number of exposed cases) in the subset of subjects who were thought never to have been occupationally exposed to wood or leather dust. Moreover, a dose–response trend was observed in relation to an index of cumulative exposure. There was little evidence of an association with squamous-cell carcinoma, although in one of the two other case–control studies, a positive association was found particularly for squamous-cell carcinomas. An analysis of proportionate cancer incidence among industrial workers in Denmark also showed an increased risk for squamous-cell carcinomas.

Against these largely positive findings, no excess of mortality from sinonasal cancer was observed in other cohort studies of formaldehyde-exposed workers, including the three recently updated studies of industrial and garment workers in the USA and of chemical workers in the United Kingdom.

Most epidemiological studies of sinonasal cancer have not distinguished between tumours that arise in the nose and those that develop in the nasal sinuses. Thus, any effect on the risk for nasal cancer specifically would tend to be diluted if there were no corresponding effect on the risk for cancer in the sinuses, and would thus mask its detection, particularly in cohort studies that have relatively low statistical power. However, the apparent discrepancy between the results of the case–control as compared with the cohort studies might also reflect residual confounding by wood dust in the former. Almost all of the formaldehyde-exposed cases in the case–control studies were also exposed to wood dust, which resulted in a high relative risk, particularly for adenocarcinomas. Thus, there is only limited epidemiological evidence that formaldehyde causes sinonasal cancer in humans.

Cancer at other sites

A number of studies have found associations between exposure to formaldehyde and cancer at other sites, including the oral cavity, oro- and hypopharynx, pancreas, larynx, lung and brain. However, the Working Group considered that the overall balance of epidemiological evidence did not support a causal role for formaldehyde in relation to these other cancers.

5.3   Animal carcinogenicity data

Several studies in which formaldehyde was administered to rats by inhalation showed evidence of carcinogenicity, particularly the induction of squamous-cell carcinomas of the nasal cavities. A similar study in hamsters showed no evidence of carcinogenicity, and one study in mice showed no effect.

In four studies, formaldehyde was administered in the drinking-water to rats. One study in male rats showed an increased incidence of forestomach papillomas. In a second study in male and female rats, the incidence of gastrointestinal leiomyosarcomas was increased in females and in males and females combined. In a third study in male and female rats, the number of males that developed malignant tumours and the incidences of haemolymphoreticular tumours (lymphomas and leukaemias) and testicular interstitial-cell adenomas in males were increased. A fourth study gave negative results.

Skin application of formaldehyde concomitantly with 7,12-dimethylbenz[*a*]anthracene reduced the latency of skin tumours in mice. In rats, concomitant administration of formaldehyde and *N*-methyl-*N*'-nitro-*N*-nitrosoguanidine in the drinking-water increased the incidence of adenocarcinomas of the glandular stomach. Exposure of hamsters by inhalation to formaldehyde increased the multiplicity of tracheal tumours induced by subcutaneous injections of *N*-nitrosodiethylamine.

5.4   Other relevant data

Toxicokinetics and metabolism

The concentration of endogenous formaldehyde in human blood is about 2–3 mg/L; similar concentrations are found in the blood of monkeys and rats. Exposure of humans, monkeys or rats to formaldehyde by inhalation has not been found to alter these concentrations. The average level of formate in the urine of people who are not occupationally exposed to formaldehyde is 12.5 mg/L and varies considerably both within and between individuals. No significant changes in urinary formate were detected in humans after exposure to 0.5 ppm [0.6 mg/m^3] formaldehyde for up to 3 weeks. More than 90% of inhaled formaldehyde is absorbed in the upper respiratory tract. In rats, it is absorbed almost entirely in the nasal passages; in monkeys, it is also absorbed in the nasopharynx, trachea and proximal regions of the major bronchi. Absorbed formaldehyde can be oxidized to formate and carbon dioxide or may be incorporated into biological macromolecules via tetrahydrofolate-dependent one-carbon biosynthetic pathways. Formaldehyde has a half-life of about 1 min in rat plasma. Rats exposed to [^{14}C]formaldehyde eliminated about 40% of the ^{14}C as exhaled carbon dioxide, 17% in the urine and 5% in the faeces; 35–39% remained in the tissues and carcass. After dermal application of aqueous [^{14}C]formaldehyde, approximately 7% of the dose was excreted in the urine by rodents and 0.2% by monkeys. After oral administration, about 40% of [^{14}C]formaldehyde was excreted as exhaled carbon dioxide, 10% in the urine and 1% in the faeces within 12 h.

Toxic effects in humans

Many studies have evaluated the health effects of inhalation of formaldehyde in humans. Most were carried out in unsensitized subjects and revealed consistent evidence of irritation of the eyes, nose and throat. Symptoms are rare below 0.5 ppm, and become increasingly prevalent in studies in exposure chambers as concentrations increase. Exposures to up to 3 ppm [3.7 mg/m^3] formaldehyde are unlikely to provoke asthma in an unsensitized individual.

Nasal lavage studies show increased numbers of eosinophils and protein exudation following exposures to 0.5 mg/m^3 formaldehyde. Bronchial provocation tests have confirmed the occurrence of occupational asthma due to formaldehyde in small numbers of workers from several centres. The mechanism is probably hypersensitivity, because the reactions are often delayed, there is a latent period of symptomless exposure and unexposed asthmatics do not react to the same concentrations. One case of pneumonitis was reported in a worker who was exposed for 2 h to a level that was sufficient for his breath to smell of formaldehyde. High levels of formaldehyde probably cause asthmatic reactions by an irritant mechanism. Formaldehyde is one of the commoner causes of contact dermatitis and is thought to act as a sensitizer on the skin.

Toxic effects in animals

Formaldehyde is a well documented irritant that causes mild inflammation to severe ulceration. It caused direct toxicity in the upper respiratory system in a concentration- and location-specific manner. There is evidence that formaldehyde can induce irritation to the forestomach after high-dose oral exposure. Formaldehyde is also a sensory irritant that induces a decrease in respiratory rate in rodents; mice are more sensitive than rats, as measured by respiratory depression. This respiratory depression is thought to be secondary to stimulation of the trigeminal nerve by the irritant effect of formaldehyde. Formaldehyde can also result in pulmonary hyperactivity through transient bronchoconstriction.

It can also act as a skin contact sensitizer via a type IV T-cell mediated hypersensitivity reaction. Formaldehyde does not induce haematological effects.

In-vitro toxicity

Formaldehyde exerts dose-dependent toxicity in cell cultures. Cytotoxicity involves loss of glutathione, altered Ca^{2+}-homeostatis and impairment of mitochondrial function. Thiols, including glutathione, and metabolism through alcohol dehydrogenase 3, act in a protective manner.

Reproductive and developmental effects

Eleven epidemiological studies have evaluated directly or indirectly the reproductive effects of occupational exposures to formaldehyde. The outcomes examined in these studies included spontaneous abortions, congenital malformations, birth weights, infertility and endometriosis. Inconsistent reports of higher rates of spontaneous abortion and lowered birth weights were reported among women occupationally exposed to formaldehyde. Studies of inhalation exposure to formaldehyde in animal models have evaluated the effects of formaldehyde on pregnancy and fetal development, which have not been clearly shown to occur at exposures below maternally toxic doses.

Genetic and related effects

There is evidence that formaldehyde is genotoxic in multiple in-vitro models and in exposed humans and laboratory animals. Studies in humans revealed increased DNA–protein cross-links in workers exposed to formaldehyde. This is consistent with laboratory studies, in which inhaled formaldehyde reproducibly caused DNA–protein cross-links in rat and monkey nasal mucosa. A single study reported cytogenetic abnormalities in the bone marrow of rats that inhaled formaldehyde, while other studies did not report effects in bone marrow.

Mechanistic considerations

The current data indicate that both genotoxicty and cytoxicity play important roles in the carcinogenesis of formaldehyde in nasal tissues. DNA–protein cross-links provide a potentially useful marker of genotoxicity. The concentration–response curve for the formation of DNA–protein cross-links is bi-phasic, and the slope increases at formaldehyde concentrations of about 2–3 ppm [2.4–3.7 mg/m^3] in Fischer 344 rats. Similar results are found in rhesus monkeys, although the dose–response curve is less well defined in this species. Cell proliferation, which appears to amplify greatly the genotoxic effects of formaldehyde, is increased considerably at concentrations of formaldehyde of about 6 ppm [7.4 mg/m^3], and results in a marked increase in the occurrence of malignant lesions in the nasal passages of rats at concentrations above this level.

Several possible mechanisms were considered for the induction of human leukaemia, such as clastogenic damage to circulatory stem cells. The Working Group was not aware of any good rodent models that simulate the occurrence of acute myeloid leukaemia in humans. Therefore, on the basis of the data available at this time, it was not possible to identify a mechanism for the induction of myeloid leukaemia in humans.

5.5   Evaluation

There is *sufficient evidence* in humans for the carcinogenicity of formaldehyde.

There is *sufficient evidence* in experimental animals for the carcinogenicity of formaldehyde.

Overall evaluation

Formaldehyde is *carcinogenic to humans (Group 1)*.

6.   References

Abdel Hameed, A.A., Khoder, M.I. & Farag, S.A. (2000) Organic dust and gaseous contaminants at wood working shops. *J. environ. Monit.*, **2**, 73–76

ACGIH® Worldwide (2003) *Documentation of the TLVs® and BEIs® with Other Worldwide Occupational Exposure Values — 2003 CD-ROM*, Cincinnati, OH, American Conference of Government Industrial Hygienists

Acheson, E.D., Barnes, H.R., Gardner, M.J., Osmond, C., Pannett, B. & Taylor, C.P. (1984a) Formaldehyde in the British chemical industry: An occupational cohort study. *Lancet*, **i**, 611–616

Acheson, E.D., Barnes, H.R., Gardner, M.J., Osmond, C., Pannett, B. & Taylor, C.P. (1984b) Formaldehyde process workers and lung cancer. *Lancet*, **i**, 1066–1067

Adams, D.O., Hamilton, T.A., Lauer, L.D. & Dean, J.H. (1987) The effect of formaldehyde exposure upon the mononuclear phagocyte system of mice. *Toxicol. appl. Pharmacol.*, **88**, 165–174

Åhman, M., Alexandersson, R., Ekholm, U., Bergström, B., Dahlqvist, M. & Ulfvarsson, U. (1991) Impeded lung function in moulders and coremakers handling furan resin sand. *Int. Arch. occup. environ. Health*, **63**, 175–180

Akbar-Khanzadeh, F. & Mlynek, J.S. (1997) Changes in respiratory function after one and three hours of exposure to formaldehyde in non-smoking subjects. *Occup. environ. Med.*, **54**, 296–300

Akbar-Khanzadeh, F., Vaquerano, M.U., Akbar-Khanzadeh, M. & Bisesi, M.S. (1994) Formaldehyde exposure, acute pulmonary response, and exposure control options in a gross anatomy laboratory. *Am. J. ind. Med.*, **26**, 61–75

Albert, R.E., Sellakumar, A.R., Laskin, S., Kuschner, M., Nelson, N. & Snyder, C.A. (1982) Gaseous formaldehyde and hydrogen chloride induction of nasal cancer in the rat. *J. natl Cancer Inst.*, **68**, 597–603

Alderson, T. (1967) Induction of genetically recombinant chromosomes in the absence of induced mutation. *Nature*, **215**, 1281–1283

Alexandersson, R. & Hedenstierna, G. (1988) Respiratory hazards associated with exposure to formaldehyde and solvents in acid-curing paints. *Arch. environ. Health*, **43**, 222–227

Altshuller, A.P. (1993) Production of aldehydes as primary emissions and from secondary atmospheric reactions of alkenes and alkanes during the night and early morning hours. *Atmos. Environ.*, **27**, 21–32

Alves Pereira, E., Carrilho, E. & Tavares, M.F.M. (2002) Laser-induced fluorescence and UV detection of derivatized aldehydes in air samples using capillary electrophoresis. *J. Chromatogr.*, **A979**, 409–416

Andersen, S.K., Jensen, O.M. & Oliva, D. (1982) [Exposure to formaldehyde and lung cancer in Danish physicians.] *Ugeskr. Laeg.*, **144**, 1571–1573 (in Danish)

Anderson, L.G., Lanning, J.A., Barrell, R., Miyagishima, J., Jones, R.H. & Wolfe, P. (1996) Sources and sinks of formaldehyde and acetaldehyde: An analysis of Denver's ambient concentration data. *Atmos. Environ.*, **30**, 2113–2123

Andersson, M., Agurell, E., Vaghef, H., Bolcsfoldi, G. & Hellman, B. (2003) Extended-term cultures of human T-lymphocytes and the comet assay: A useful combination when testing for genotoxicity in vitro? *Mutat. Res.*, **540**, 43–55

Andjelkovich, D.A., Mathew, R.M., Richardson, R.B. & Levine, R.J. (1990) Mortality of iron foundry workers. I. Overall findings. *J. occup. Med.*, **32**, 529–540

Andjelkovich, D.A., Shy, C.M., Brown, M.H., Janszen, D.B., Levine, R.J. & Richardson, R.B. (1994) Mortality of iron foundry workers. III. Lung cancer case–control study. *J. occup. Med.*, **36**, 1301–1309

Andjelkovich, D.A., Janszen, D.B., Brown, M.H., Richardson, R.B. & Miller, F.J. (1995) Mortality of iron foundry workers: IV. Analysis of a subcohort exposed to formaldehyde. *J. occup. environ. Med.*, **37**, 826–837

de Andrade, J.B., Andrade, M.V. & Pinheiro, H.L.C. (1998) Atmospheric levels of formaldehyde and acetaldehyde and their relationship with the vehicular fleet composition in Salvador, Bahia, Brazil. *J. Braz. chem. Soc.*, **9**, 219–223

Andreini, B.P., Baroni, R., Galimberti, E. & Sesana, G. (2000) Aldehydes in the atmospheric environment: Evaluation of human exposure in the north-west area of Milan. *Microchem. J.*, **67**, 11–19

AOAC (Association of Official Analytical Chemists) (2003) *Official Methods of Analysis of AOAC International*, 17th Ed., Rev. 2, Gaithersburg, MD [CD-ROM]

Appelman, L.M., Woutersen, R.A., Zwart, A., Falke, H.E. & Feron, V.J. (1988) One-year inhalation toxicity study of formaldehyde in male rats with a damaged or undamaged nasal mucosa. *J. appl. Toxicol.*, **8**, 85–90

Arbejdstilsynet [Danish Working Environment Authority] (2002) *Limit Values for Substances and Material*, Copenhagen, WEA-Guide

Armstrong, R.W., Imrey, P.B., Lye, M.S., Armstrong, M.J., Yu, M.C. & Sani, S. (2000) Nasopharyngeal carcinoma in Malaysian Chinese: Occupational exposures to particles, formaldehyde and heat. *Int. J. Epidemiol.*, **29**, 991–998

ASTM International (1990) *Standard Test Method for Determining Formaldehyde Levels from Wood Products Under Defined Test Conditions Using a Large Chamber* (Method E1333-90), Philadelphia, American Society for Testing and Materials

ASTM International (2000) *Standard Test Method for Determining Formaldehyde Levels from Wood Products using a Desiccator* (ASTM D5582-00), Philadelphia, American Society for Testing and Materials

ASTM International (2002a) *Standard Test Method for Determining Formaldehyde Concentration in Air from Wood Products Using a Small Scale Chamber* (ASTM D6007-02), Philadelphia, American Society for Testing and Materials

ASTM International (2002b) *Standard Test Method for Determining Formaldehyde Concentrations in Air and Emission Rates from Wood Products Using a Large Chamber* (ASTM E1333-96, Reapproved 2002), Philadelphia, American Society for Testing and Materials

ATSDR (Agency for Toxic Substances and Disease Registry) (1999) *Toxicological Profile for Formaldehyde*, Atlanta, GA, US Department of Health and Human Services, Public Health Service [http://atsdr.cdc.gov/toxprofiles/tp111.html]

Atzori, L., Dore, M. & Congiu, L. (1989) Aspects of allyl alcohol toxicity. *Drug Metabol. Drug. Interactions*, **7**, 295–319

Atzori, L., Dypbukt, J.M., Hybbinette, S.S., Moldéus, P. & Grafström, R.C. (1994) Modifications of cellular thiols during growth and squamous differentiation of cultured human bronchial epithelial cells. *Exp. Cell Res.*, **211**, 115–120

Auerbach, C. & Moser, H. (1953) Analysis of the mutagenic action of formaldehyde on food. II. The mutagenic potentialities of the treatment. *Zeitschr. indukt. Abstamm. Verebungs.*, **85**, 547–563

Auerbach, C., Moutschen-Dahmen, M. & Moutschen, J. (1977) Genetic and cytogenetical effects of formaldehyde and related compounds. *Mutat. Res.*, **39**, 317–361

Axelsson, G., Lütz, C. & Rylander, R. (1984) Exposure to solvents and outcome of pregnancy in university laboratory employees. *Br. J. ind. Med.*, **41**, 305–312

Azuma, M., Endo, Y., Miyazaki, T., Hikita, Y., Ikeda, H., Moriya, Y., Hara, I. & Araki, S. (2003) Efficacy of a detector tube method in formaldehyde measurement. *Ind. Health*, **41**, 306-312

Baez, A.P., Belmont, R. & Padilla, H. (1995) Measurements of formaldehyde and acetaldehyde in the atmosphere of Mexico City. *Environ. Pollut.*, **89**, 163–167

Báez, A., Padilla, H., García, R., Torres, M.C., Rosas, I. & Belmont, R. (2003) Carbonyl levels in indoor and outdoor air in Mexico City and Xalapa, Mexico. *Sci. total Environ.*, **302**, 211–226

Ballarin, C., Sarto, F., Giacomelli, L., Bartolucci, G.B. & Clonfero, E. (1992) Micronucleated cells in nasal mucosa of formaldehyde-exposed workers. *Mutat. Res.*, **280**, 1–7

Ballenger, J.J. (1984) Some effects of formaldehyde on the upper respiratory tract. *Laryngoscope*, **94**, 1411–1413

Barber, R.D. & Donohue, T.J. (1998) Pathways for transcriptional activation of a glutathione-dependent formaldehyde dehydrogenase gene. *J. mol. Biol.*, **280**, 775–784

Basler, A., van der Hude, W. & Scheutwinkel-Reich, M. (1985) Formaldehyde-induced sister chromatid exchanges in vitro and the influence of the exogenous metabolizing systems S9 mix and primary hepatocytes. *Arch. Toxicol.*, **58**, 10–13

Batalha, J.R.F., Guimarães, E.T., Lobo, D.J.A., Lichtenfels, A.J.F.C, Deur, T., Carvalho, H.A., Alves, E.S., Domingos, M., Rodrigues, G.S. & Saldiva, P.H.N. (1999) Exploring the clastogenic effects of air pollutants in São Paulo (Brazil) using the *Tradescantia* micronuclei assay. *Mutat. Res.*, **426**, 229–232

Baumann, K. & Angerer, J. (1979) Occupational chronic exposure to organic solvents. VI. Formic acid concentration in blood and urine as an indicator of methanol exposure. *Int. Arch. occup. environ. Health*, **42**, 241–249

Belanger, P.L. & Kilburn, K.H. (1981) *California Society for Histotechnology, Los Angeles, CA, Health Hazard Evaluation Report* (NIOSH Report No. HETA 81-422-1387), Cincinnati, OH, US Department of Health and Human Services, Public Health Service, Centers for Disease Control, National Institute for Occupational Safety and Health

Bender, J. (2002) The use of noncancer endpoints as a basis for establishing a reference concentration for formaldehyde. *Regul. Toxicol. Pharmacol.*, **35**, 23–31

Berke, J.H. (1987) Cytologic examination of the nasal mucosa in formaldehyde-exposed workers. *J. occup. Med.*, **29**, 681–684

Bernardini, P., Carelli, G., Rimatori, V. & Contegiacomo, P. (1983) Health hazard for hospital workers from exposure to formaldehyde. *Med. Lav.*, **74**, 106–110

Berrino, F., Richiardi, L., Boffetta, P., Estève, J., Belletti, I., Raymond, L., Troschel, L., Pisani, P., Zubiri, L., Ascunce, N., Gubéran, E., Tuyns, A., Terracini, B., Merletti, F. & the Milan JEM Working Group (2003) Occupation and larynx and hypopharynx cancer: A job–exposure matrix approach in an international case–control study in France, Italy, Spain and Switzerland. *Cancer Causes Control*, **14**, 213–223

Bertazzi, P.A., Pesatori, A.C., Radice, L., Zocchetti, C. & Vai, T. (1986) Exposure to formaldehyde and cancer mortality in a cohort of workers producing resins. *Scand. J. Work Environ. Health*, **12**, 461–468

Bertazzi, P.A., Pesatori, A.C., Guercilena, S., Consonni, D. & Zocchetti, C. (1989) [Cancer risk among workers producing formaldehyde-based resins: Extension of follow-up.] *Med. Lav.*, **80**, 111–122 (in Italian)

Biagini, R.E., Moorman, W.J., Knecht, E.A., Clark, J.C. & Bernstein, I.L. (1989) Acute airway narrowing in monkeys from challenge with 2.5 ppm formaldehyde generated from formalin. *Arch. environ. Health*, **44**, 12–17

Binding, N. & Witting, U. (1990) Exposure to formaldehyde and glutardialdehyde in operating theatres. *Int. Arch. occup. environ. Health*, **62**, 233–238

Bizzari, S.N. (2000) *CEH Marketing Research Report: Formaldehyde*, Palo Alto, CA, SRI International

Blade, L.M. (1983) Occupational exposure to formaldehyde — Recent NIOSH involvement. In: Clary, J.J., Gibson, J.E. & Waritz, R.S., eds, *Formaldehyde — Toxicology, Epidemiology, Mechanisms*, New York, Marcel Dekker, pp. 1–23

Blair, A. & Stewart, P.A. (1989) Comments on the reanalysis of the National Cancer Institute study of workers exposed to formaldehyde. *J. occup. Med.*, **31**, 881

Blair, A. & Stewart, P.A. (1990) Correlation between different measures of occupational exposure to formaldehyde. *Am. J. Epidemiol.*, **131**, 510–516

Blair, A., Stewart, P.A., O'Berg, M., Gaffey, W., Walrath, J., Ward, J., Bales, R., Kaplan, S. & Cubit, D. (1986) Mortality among industrial workers exposed to formaldehyde. *J. natl Cancer Inst.*, **76**, 1071–1084

Blair, A., Stewart, P.A., Hoover, R.N., Fraumeni, J.F., Jr, Walrath, J., O'Berg, M. & Gaffey, W. (1987) Cancers of the nasopharynx and oropharynx and formaldehyde exposure (Letter to the Editor). *J. natl Cancer Inst.*, **78**, 191–193

Blair, A., Stewart, P.A. & Hoover, R.N. (1990a) Mortality from lung cancer among workers employed in formaldehyde industries. *Am. J. ind. Med.*, **17**, 683–699

Blair, A., Saracci, R., Stewart, P.A., Hayes, R.B. & Shy, C. (1990b) Epidemiologic evidence on the relationship between formaldehyde exposure and cancer. *Scand. J. Work Environ. Health*, **16**, 381–393

Blair, A., Zheng, T., Linos, A., Stewart, P.A., Zhang, Y.W. & Cantor, K.P. (2000) Occupation and leukemia: A population-based case–control study in Iowa and Minnesota. *Am. J. ind. Med.*, **40**, 3–14

Blasiak, J., Trzeciak, A., Malecka-Panas, E., Drzewoski, J. & Wojewódzka, M. (2000) *In vitro* genotoxicity of ethanol and acetaldehyde in human lymphocytes and the gastrointestinal tract mucosa cells. *Toxicol. in Vitro*, **14**, 287–295

Boj, J.R., Marco, I., Cortès, O. & Canalda, C. (2003) The acute nephrotoxicity of systemically administered formaldehyde in rats. *Eur. J. paediat. Dent.*, **4**, 16–20

Bolm-Audorff, U., Vogel, C. & Woitowitz, H. (1990) Occupation and smoking as risk factors of nasal and nasopharyngeal cancer. In: Sakurai, H., ed., *Occupational Epidemiology*, New York, Elsevier Science, pp. 71–74

Bolstad-Johnson, D.M., Burgess, J.L., Crutchfield, C.D., Storment, S., Gerkin, R. & Wilson, J.R. (2000) Characterization of firefighter exposures during fire overhaul. *Am. ind. Hyg. Assoc. J.*, **61**, 636–641

Bolt, H.M. (1987) Experimental toxicology of formaldehyde. *Cancer Res. clin. Oncol.*, **113**, 305–309

Bolt, H.M. (2003) Genotoxicity — Threshold or not? Introduction of cases of industrial chemicals. *Toxicol. Lett.*, **140–141**, 43–51

Bond, G.G., Flores, G.H., Shellenberger, R.J., Cartmill, J.B., Fishbeck, W.A. & Cook, R.R. (1986) Nested case–control study of lung cancer among chemical workers. *Am. J. Epidemiol.*, **124**, 53–66

Boysen, M., Zadig, E., Digernes, V., Abeler, V. & Reith, A. (1990) Nasal mucosa in workers exposed to formaldehyde: A pilot study. *Br. J. ind. Med.*, **47**, 116–121

Brandt-Rauf, P.W., Fallon, L.F., Jr, Tarantini, T., Idema, C. & Andrews, L. (1988) Health hazards of fire fighters: Exposure assessment. *Br. J. ind. Med.*, **45**, 606–612

Brickus, L.S.R., Cardoso, J.N. & Aquino Neto, F.R. (1998) Distributions of indoor and outdoor air pollutants in Rio de Janeiro, Brazil: Implications to indoor air quality in bayside offices. *Environ. Sci. Technol.*, **32**, 3485–3490

Brinton, L.A., Blot, W.J., Becker, J.A., Winn, D.M., Browder, J.P., Farmer, J.C., Jr & Fraumeni, J.F., Jr (1984) A case–control study of cancers of the nasal cavity and paranasal sinuses. *Am. J. Epidemiol.*, **119**, 896–906

Brinton, L.A., Blot, W.J. & Fraumeni, J.F., Jr (1985) Nasal cancer in the textile and clothing industries. *Br. J. ind. Med.*, **42**, 469–474

Broder, I., Corey, P., Cole, P., Lipa, M., Mintz, S. & Nethercott, J.R. (1988a) Comparison of health of occupants and characteristics of houses among control homes and homes insulated with urea formaldehyde foam. I. Methodology. *Environ. Res.*, **45**, 141–155

Broder, I., Corey, P., Cole, P., Lipa, M., Mintz, S. & Nethercott, J.R. (1988b) Comparison of health of occupants and characteristics of houses among control homes and homes insulated with urea formaldehyde foam. II. Initial health and house variables and exposure–response relationships. *Environ. Res.*, **45**, 156–178

Broder, I., Corey, P., Brasher, P., Lipa, M. & Cole, P. (1988c) Comparison of health of occupants and characteristics of houses among control homes and homes insulated with urea formaldehyde foam. III. Health and house variables following remedial work. *Environ. Res.*, **45**, 179–203

Broder, I., Corey, P., Brasher, P., Lipa, M. & Cole, P. (1991) Formaldehyde exposure and health status in households. *Environ. Health Perspect.*, **95**, 101–104

Brownson, R.C., Alavanja, M.C.R. & Chang, J.C. (1993) Occupational risk factors for lung cancer among nonsmoking women: A case–control study in Missouri (United States). *Cancer Causes Control*, **4**, 449–454

Buckley, L.A., Jiang, X.Z., James, R.A., Morgan, K.T. & Barrow, C.S. (1984) Respiratory tract lesions induced by sensory irritants at the RD50 concentration. *Toxicol. appl. Pharmacol.*, **74**, 417–429

Burgaz, S., Cakmak, G., Erdem, O., Yilmaz, M. & Karakaya, A.E. (2001) Micronuclei frequencies in exfoliated nasal mucosa cells from pathology and anatomy laboratory workers exposed to formaldehyde. *Neoplasma*, **48**, 144–147

Burgaz, S., Erdem, O., Çakmak, G., Erdem, N., Karakaya, A. & Karakaya, A.E. (2002) Cytogenetic analysis of buccal cells from shoe-workers and pathology and anatomy laboratory workers exposed to *n*-hexane, toluene, methyl ethyl ketone and formaldehyde. *Biomarkers*, **7**, 151–161

Burge, P.S., Harries, M.G., Lam, W.K., O'Brien, I.M. & Patchett, P. (1985) Occupational asthma due to formaldehyde. *Thorax*, **40**, 255–260

Buss, J., Kuschinsky, K., Kewitz, H. & Koransky, W. (1964) [Enteric resorption of formaldehyde.] *Naunyn-Schmiedeberg's Arch. exp. Pathol. Pharmakol.*, **247**, 380–381 (in German)

California Air Resources Board (2004) *California Ambient Air Quality Data 1990–2002*, Los Angeles, CA, Planning & Technical Support Division

Callas, P.W., Pastides, H. & Hosmer, D.W., Jr (1996) Lung cancer mortality among workers in formaldehyde industries. *J. occup. environ. Med.*, **38**, 747–748

Cantor, K.P., Stewart, P.A., Brinton, L.A. & Dosemeci, M. (1995) Occupational exposures and female breast cancer mortality in the United States. *J. occup. environ. Med.*, **37**, 336–348

CAREX (2003) Available at http://www.ttl.fi/NR/rdonlyres/407B368B-26EF-475D-8F2B-DA0024B853E0/0/5_exposures_by_agent_and_industry.pdf

Carraro, E., Gasparini, S. & Gilli, G. (1999) Identification of a chemical marker of environmental exposure to formaldehyde. *Environ. Res.*, **A80**, 132–137

Casanova, M. & Heck, H.d'A. (1987) Further studies of the metabolic incorporation and covalent binding of inhaled [^{3}H]- and [^{14}C]formaldehyde in Fischer-344 rats: Effects of glutathione depletion. *Toxicol. appl. Pharmacol.*, **89**, 105–121

Casanova, M., Heck, H.d'A., Everitt, J.I., Harrington, W.W., Jr & Popp, J.A. (1988) Formaldehyde concentrations in the blood of rhesus monkeys after inhalation exposure. *Food chem. Toxicol.*, **26**, 715–716

Casanova, M., Deyo, D.F. & Heck, H.d'A. (1989) Covalent binding of inhaled formaldehyde to DNA in the nasal mucosa of Fischer 344 rats: Analysis of formaldehyde and DNA by high-performance liquid chromatography and provisional pharmacokinetic interpretation. *Fundam. appl. Toxicol.*, **12**, 397–417

Casanova, M., Morgan, K.T., Steinhagen, W.H., Everitt, J.I., Popp, J.A. & Heck, H.d'A. (1991) Covalent binding of inhaled formaldehyde to DNA in the respiratory tract of rhesus monkeys: Pharmacokinetics, rat-to-monkey interspecies scaling, and extrapolation to man. *Fundam. appl. Toxicol.*, **17**, 409–428

Casanova, M., Morgan, K.T., Gross, E.A., Moss, O.R. & Heck, H.d'A. (1994) DNA–protein cross-links and cell replication at specific sites in the nose of F344 rats exposed subchronically to formaldehyde. *Fundam. appl. Toxicol.*, **23**, 525–536

Casanova, M., Bell, D.A. & Heck, H.d'A. (1997) Dichloromethane metabolism to formaldehyde and reaction of formaldehyde with nucleic acids in hepatocytes of rodents and humans with and without glutathione S-transferase *T1* and *M1* genes. *Fundam. appl. Toxicol.*, **37**, 168–180

Casanova-Schmitz, M. & Heck, H.d'A. (1983) Effects of formaldehyde exposure on the extractability of DNA from proteins in the rat nasal mucosa. *Toxicol. appl. Pharmacol.*, **70**, 121–132

Casanova-Schmitz, M., David, R.M. & Heck, H.d'A. (1984a) Oxidation of formaldehyde and acetaldehyde by NAD$^+$-dependent dehydrogenases in rat nasal mucosal homogenates. *Biochem. Pharmacol.*, **33**, 1137–1142

Casanova-Schmitz, M., Starr, T.B. & Heck, H.d'A. (1984b) Differentiation between metabolic incorporation and covalent binding in the labeling of macromolecules in the rat nasal mucosa and bone marrow by inhaled [^{14}C]- and [^{3}H]formaldehyde. *Toxicol. appl. Pharmacol.*, **76**, 26–44

Cassee, F.R. & Feron, V.J. (1994) Biochemical and histopathological changes in nasal epithelium of rats after 3-day intermittent exposure to formaldehyde and ozone alone or in combination. *Toxicol. Lett.*, **72**, 257–268

Cassee, F.R., Arts, J.H.E., Groten, J.P. & Feron, V.J. (1996a) Sensory irritation to mixtures of formaldehyde, acrolein and acetaldehyde in rats. *Arch. Toxicol.*, **70**, 329–337

Cassee, F.R., Groten, J.P. & Feron, V.J. (1996b) Changes in the nasal epithelium of rats exposed by inhalation to mixtures of formaldehyde, acetaldehyde, and acrolein. *Fundam. appl. Toxicol.*, **29**, 208–218

Cecinato, A., Yassaa, N., Di Palo, V. & Possanzini, M. (2002) Observation of volatile and semi-volatile carbonyls in an Algerian urban environment using dinitrophenylhydrazine/silica-HPLC and pentafluorophenylhydrazine/silica-GC-MS. *J. environ. Monit.*, **4**, 223–228

Centers for Disease Control (1986) Occupational exposure to formaldehyde in dialysis units. *J. Am. med. Assoc.*, **256**, 698–703

Chan, W.H., Shuang, S. & Choi, M.M.F. (2001) Determination of airborne formaldehyde by active sampling on 3-methyl-2-benzothiazolinone hydrazone hydrochloride-coated glass fibre filters. *Analyst*, **126**, 720–723

Chanet, R., Izard, C. & Moustacchi, E. (1975) Genetic effects of formaldehyde in yeast. I. Influence of the growth stages on killing and recombination. *Mutat. Res.*, **33**, 179–186

Chang, J.C.F. & Barrow, C.S. (1984) Sensory irritation tolerance and cross-tolerance in F-344 rats exposed to chlorine or formaldehyde gas. *Toxicol. appl. Pharmacol.*, **76**, 319–327

Chang, J.-Y. & Lin, J.-M. (1998) Aliphatic aldehydes and allethrin in mosquito-coil smoke. *Chemosphere*, **36**, 617–624

Chang, J.C.F., Steinhagen, W.H. & Barrow, C.S. (1981) Effect of single or repeated formaldehyde exposure on minute volume of B6C3F1 mice and F-344 rats. *Toxicol. appl. Pharmacol.*, **61**, 451–459

Chang, J.C.F., Gross, E.A., Swenberg, J.A. & Barrow, C.S. (1983) Nasal cavity deposition, histopathology and cell proliferation after single or repeated formaldehyde exposures in B6C3F1 mice and F-344 rats. *Toxicol. appl. Pharmacol.*, **68**, 161–176

Chang, H.L., Kuo, M.L. & Lin J.M. (1997) Mutagenic activity of incense smoke in comparison to formaldehyde and acetaldehyde in *Salmonella typhimurium* TA102. *Bull. environ. Contam. Toxicol.*, **58**, 394–401

Chemical Information Services (2004) *Directory of World Chemical Producers*, Dallas, TX [www.chemicalinfo.com]

Chiazze, L., Jr, Watkins, D.K., Fryar, C. & Kozono, J. (1993) A case–control study of malignant and non-malignant respiratory disease among employees of a fiberglass manufacturing facility. II. Exposure assessment. *Br. J. ind. Med.*, **50**, 717–725

Chiazze, L., Watkins, D.K. & Fryar, C. (1997) Historical cohort mortality study of a continuous filament fiberglass manufacturing plant. I. White men. *J. occup. environ. Med.*, **39**, 432–441

Christensen, C.S., Skov, H., Nielsen, T. & Lohse, C. (2000) Temporal variation of carbonyl compound concentrations at a semi-rural site in Denmark. *Atmos. Environ.*, **34**, 287–296

Chung, K.Y.K., Cuthbert, R.J., Revell, G.S., Wassel, S.G. & Summers, N. (2000) A study on dust emission, particle size distribution and formaldehyde concentration during machining of medium density fibreboard. *Ann. occup. Hyg.*, **44**, 455–466

Clarisse, B., Laurent, A.M., Seta, N., Le Moullec, Y., El Hasnaoui, A. & Momas, I. (2003) Indoor aldehydes: Measurement of contamination levels and identification of their determinants in Paris dwellings. *Environ. Res.*, **92**, 245–253

Coggon, D., Pannett, B. & Acheson, E.D. (1984) Use of job–exposure matrix in an occupational analysis of lung and bladder cancers on the basis of death certificates. *J. natl Cancer Inst.*, **72**, 61–65

Coggon, D., Harris, E.C., Poole, J. & Palmer, K.T. (2003) Extended follow-up of a cohort of British chemical workers exposed to formaldehyde. *J. natl Cancer Inst.*, **95**, 1608–1615

Cohen Hubal, E.A., Schlosser, P.M., Conolly, R.B. & Kimbell, J.S. (1997) Comparison of inhaled formaldehyde dosimetry predictions with DNA–protein cross-link measurements in the rat nasal passages. *Toxicol. appl. Pharmacol.*, **143**, 47–55

Coldiron, V.R., Ward, J.B., Jr, Trieff, N.M., Janssen, E., Jr & Smith, J.H. (1983) Occupational exposure to formaldehyde in a medical center autopsy service. *J. occup. Med.*, **25**, 544–548

Collins, J.J. & Lineker, G.A. (2004) A review and meta-analysis of formaldehyde exposure and leukemia. *Regul. Toxicol. Pharmacol.*, **40**, 81–91

Collins, J.J., Acquavella, J.F. & Esmen, N.A. (1997) An updated meta-analysis of formaldehyde exposure and upper respiratory tract cancers. *J. occup. environ. Med.*, **39**, 639–651

Collins, J.J., Esmen, N.A. & Hall, T.A. (2001a) A review and meta-analysis of formaldehyde exposure and pancreatic cancer. *Am. J. ind. Med.*, **39**, 336–345

Collins, J.J., Ness, R., Tyl, R.W., Krivanek, N., Esmen, N.A. & Hall, T.A. (2001b) A review of adverse pregnancy outcomes and formaldehyde exposure in human and animal studies. *Regul. Toxicol. Pharmacol.*, **34**, 17–34

Comba, P., Barbieri, P.G., Battista, G., Belli, S., Ponterio, F., Zanetti, D. & Axelson, O. (1992a) Cancer of the nose and paranasal sinuses in the metal industry: A case–control study. *Br. J. ind. Med.*, **49**, 193–196

Comba, P., Battista, G., Belli, S., de Capua, B., Merler, E., Orsi, D., Rodella, S., Vindigni, C. & Axelson, O. (1992b) A case–control study of cancer of the nose and paranasal sinuses and occupational exposures. *Am. J. ind. Med.*, **22**, 511–520

Composite Panel Association (1999) *American National Standard — Particleboard* (ANSI A208.1-1999), Gaithersburg, MD

Composite Panel Association (2002) *American National Standard — Medium Density Fiberboard (MDF) for Interior Applications* (ANSI A208.2-2002), Gaithersburg, MD

Conaway, C.C., Whysner, J., Verna, L.K. & Williams, G.M. (1996) Formaldehyde mechanistic data and risk assessment: Endogenous protection from DNA adduct formation. *Pharmacol. Ther.*, **71**, 29–55

Connor, T.H., Barrie, M.D., Theiss, J.C., Matney, T.S. & Ward, J.B., Jr (1983) Mutagenicity of formalin in the Ames assay. *Mutat. Res.*, **119**, 145–149

Connor, T.H., Ward, J.B., Jr & Legator, M.S. (1985) Absence of mutagenicity in the urine of autopsy service workers exposed to formaldehyde: Factors influencing mutagenicity testing of urine. *Arch. occup. environ. Health*, **56**, 225–237

Conolly, R.B. (2002) The use of biologically based modeling in risk assessment. *Toxicology*, **181–182**, 275–279

Conolly, R.B. & Lutz, W.K. (2004) Nonmonotonic dose–response relationships: Mechanistic basis, kinetic modeling, and implications for risk assessment. *Toxicol. Sci.*, **77**, 151–157

Conolly, R.B., Lilly, P.D. & Kimbell, J.S. (2000) Simulation modeling of the tissue disposition of formaldehyde to predict nasal DNA–protein cross-links in Fischer 344 rats, rhesus monkeys and humans. *Environ. Health Perspect.*, **108** (Suppl. 5), 919–924

Conolly, R.B., Kimbell, J.S., Janszen, D., Schlosser, P.M., Kalisak, D., Preston, J. & Miller, F.J. (2003) Biologically motivated computational modeling of formaldehyde carcinogenicity in the F344 rat. *Toxicol. Sci.*, **75**, 432–447

Corrêa, S.M., Martins, E.M. & Arbilla, G. (2003) Formaldehyde and acetaldehyde in a high traffic street of Rio de Janeiro, Brazil. *Atmos. Environ.*, **37**, 23–29

Cosma, G.N., Wilhite, A.S. & Marchok, A.C. (1988) The detection of DNA–protein cross-links in rat tracheal implants exposed *in vivo* to benzo[a]pyrene and formaldehyde. *Cancer Lett.*, **42**, 13–21

Cosmetic Ingredient Review Expert Panel (1984) Final report on the safety assessment of formaldehyde. *J. Am. Coll. Toxicol.*, **3**, 157–184

Costa, M., Zhitkovich, A., Harris, M., Paustenbach, D. & Gargas, M. (1997) DNA–protein cross-links produced by various chemicals in cultured human lymphoma cells. *J. Toxicol. environ. Health*, **50**, 433–449

Craft, T.R., Bermudez, E. & Skopek, T.R. (1987) Formaldehyde mutagenesis and formation of DNA–protein crosslinks in human lymphoblasts *in vitro*. *Mutat. Res.*, **176**, 147–155

Crosby, R.M., Richardson, K.K., Craft, T.R., Benforado, K.B., Liber, H.L. & Skopek, T.R. (1988) Molecular analysis of formaldehyde-induced mutations in human lymphoblasts and *E. coli*. *Environ. mol. Mutag.*, **12**, 155–166

Dahl, A.R. & Hadley, W.M. (1991) Nasal cavity enzymes involved in xenobiotic metabolism: Effects on the toxicity of inhalants. *Crit. Rev. Toxicol.*, **21**, 345–372

Dalbey, W.E. (1982) Formaldehyde and tumors in hamster respiratory tract. *Toxicology*, **24**, 9–14

Dallas, C.E., Badeaux, P., Theiss, J.C. & Fairchild, E.J. (1989) The influence of inhaled formaldehyde on rat lung cytochrome P450. *Environ. Res.*, **49**, 50–59

Dallas, C.E., Scott, M.J., Ward, J.B., Jr & Theiss, J.C. (1992) Cytogenetic analysis of pulmonary lavage and bone marrow cells of rats after repeated formaldehyde inhalation. *J. appl. Toxicol.*, **12**, 199–203

Day, J.H., Lees, R.E.M., Clark, R.H. & Pattee, P.L. (1984) Respiratory response to formaldehyde and off-gas of urea formaldehyde foam insulation. *Can. med. Assoc. J.*, **131**, 1061–1065

Dean, J.H., Lauer, L.D., House, R.V., Murray, M.J., Stillman, W.S., Irons, R.D., Steinhagen, W.H., Phelps, M.C. & Adams, D.O. (1984) Studies of immune function and host resistance in B6C3F1 mice exposed to formaldehyde. *Toxicol. appl. Pharmacol.*, **72**, 519–529

Delfino, R.J., Gong, H., Jr, Linn, W.S., Pellizzari, E.D. & Hu, Y. (2003) Asthma symptoms in Hispanic children and daily ambient exposures to toxic and criteria air pollutants. *Environ. Health Perspect.*, **111**, 647–656

Dell, L. & Teta, M.J. (1995) Mortality among workers at a plastics manufacturing and research and development facility: 1946–1988. *Am. J. ind. Med.*, **28**, 373–384

Deltour, L., Foglio, M.H. & Duester, G. (1999) Metabolic deficiencies in alcohol dehydrogenase *Adh1*, *Adh3*, and *Adh4* null mutant mice. Overlapping roles of *Adh1* and *Adh4* in ethanol clearance and metabolism of retinol to retinoic acid. *J. biol. Chem.*, **274**, 16796–16801

Demerec, M., Bertani, G. & Flint, J. (1951) A survey of chemicals for mutagenic action on E. coli. *Am. Naturalist*, **85**, 119–136

Demkowicz-Dobrzanski, K. & Castonguay, A. (1992) Modulation by glutathione of DNA strand breaks induced by 4-(methylnitrosamino)-1-(3-pyridyl)-1-butanone and its aldehyde metabolites in rat hepatocytes. *Carcinogenesis*, **13**, 1447–1454

Department of Housing and Urban Development (2003) Manufactured home construction and safety standards. *US Code fed. Regul.*, **Title 24**, Part 3280.308, pp. 133–134

Deutsche Forschungsgemeinschaft (1993) Aldehydes (formaldehyde, acetaldehyde, propion-aldehyde, butyraldehyde, glutaraldehyde). In: Henschler, D. & Kettrup, A., eds, *Analyses of Hazardous Substances in Air*, Vol. 2, Weinheim, VCH, Commission for the Investigation of Health Hazards of Chemical Compounds in the Work Area, pp. 15–28

Deutsche Forschungsgemeinschaft (2003) *List of MAK and BAT Values 2003 — Commission for the Investigation of Health Hazards of Chemical Compounds in the Work Area* (Report No. 39), Weinheim, Wiley-VCH Verlag GmbH, pp. 64, 132, 157–169

Deutsche Norm (1992) *Wood-based Panels Products. Determination of Formaldehyde Content. Extraction Method (Known as Perforator Method)* (DIN EN 120:1992), Berlin, German Norm Institute

Deutsche Norm (1994) *Wood-based Panel Products. Determination of Formaldehyde Release by the Gas Analysis Method* (DIN EN 717-2:1994), Berlin, German Norm Institute

Deutsche Norm (1996) *Wood-based Panel Products. Determination of Formaldehyde Release by the Flask Method* (DIN EN 717-3:1996), Berlin, German Norm Institute

Diaz, M., Achkor, H., Titarenko, E. & Martinez, M.C. (2003) The gene encoding glutathione-dependent formaldehyde dehydrogenase/GSNO reductase is responsive to wounding, jasmonic acid and salicylic acid. *FEBS Lett.*, **543**, 136–139

Dicker, E. & Cederbaum, A.I. (1986) Inhibition of the low-K_m mitochondrial aldehyde dehydrogenase by diethyl maleate and phorone *in vivo* and *in vitro*. Implications for formaldehyde metabolism. *Biochem. J.*, **240**, 821–827

Dickey, F.H., Cleland, G.H. & Lotz, C. (1949) The role of organic peroxides in the induction of mutations. *Proc. natl Acad. Sci. USA*, **35**, 581–586

Dillon, D., Combes, R. & Zeiger, E. (1998) The effectiveness of *Salmonella* strains TA100, TA102 and TA104 for detecting mutagenicity of some aldehydes and peroxides. *Mutagenesis*, **13**, 19–26

Dingle P., Tapsell, P. & Hu, S. (2000) Reducing formaldehyde exposure in office environments using plants. *Bull. environ. Contam. Toxicol.*, **64**, 302–308

Dinsdale, D., Riley, R.A. & Verschoyle, R.D. (1993) Pulmonary cytochrome P450 in rats exposed to formaldehyde vapor. *Environ. Res.*, **62**, 19–27

Doi, S., Suzuki, S., Morishita, M., Yamada, M., Kanda, Y., Torii, S. & Sakamoto, T. (2003) The prevalence of IgE sensitization in asthmatic children. *Allergy*, **58**, 668–671

Doolittle, D.J., Furlong, J.W. & Butterworth, B.E. (1985) Assessment of chemically induced DNA repair in primary cultures of human bronchial epithelial cells. *Toxicol. appl. Pharmacol.*, **79**, 28–38

Douglas, M.P. & Rogers, S.O. (1998) DNA damage caused by common cytological fixatives. *Mutat. Res.*, **401**, 77–88

Draeger Safety (undated) *Draeger-Tubes® and Accuro® Pump*, Pittsburgh, PA

Dresp, J. & Bauchinger, M. (1988) Direct analysis of the clastogenic effect of formaldehyde in unstimulated human lymphocytes by means of the premature chromosome condensation technique. *Mutat. Res.*, **204**, 349–352

Duester, G., Farrés, J., Felder, M.R., Holmes, R.S., Höög, J.-O., Parés, X., Plapp, B.V., Yin, S.-J. & Jörnvall, H. (1999) Recommended nomenclature for the vertebrate alcohol dehydrogenase gene family. *Biochem. Pharmacol.*, **58**, 389–395

Dufresne, A., Infante-Rivard, C., Malo, J.L. & Gautrin, D. (2002) Exposure to formaldehyde among animal health students. *Am. ind. Hyg. Assoc. J.*, **63**, 647–650

Dumas, S., Parent, M.-E., Siemiatycki, J. & Brisson, J. (2000) Rectal cancer and occupational risk factors: A hypothesis-generating, exposure-based case–control study. *Int. J. Cancer*, **87**, 874–879

Echt, A. & Burr, G.A. (1997) Exposure to formaldehyde during garment manufacturing. *Appl. occup. environ. Hyg.*, **12**, 451–455

Edling, C., Järvholm, B., Andersson, L. & Axelson, O. (1987a) Mortality and cancer incidence among workers in an abrasive manufacturing industry. *Br. J. ind. Med.*, **44**, 57–59

Edling, C., Hellquist, H. & Ödkvist, L. (1987b) Occupational formaldehyde exposure and the nasal mucosa. *Rhinology*, **25**, 181–187

Edling, C., Hellquist, H. & Ödkvist, L. (1988) Occupational exposure to formaldehyde and histopathological changes in the nasal mucosa. *Br. J. ind. Med.*, **45**, 761–765

Eells, J.T., McMartin, K.E., Black, K., Virayotha, V., Tisdell, R.H. & Tephly, T.R. (1981) Formaldehyde poisoning. Rapid metabolism to formic acid. *J. am. Med. Assoc.*, **246**, 1237–1238

Eitzer, B.D., Iannucci-Berger, W.A., Mark, G. & Zito, C. (1997) Fate of toxic compounds during composting. *Bull. environ. Contam. Toxicol.*, **58**, 953–960

Elci, O.C., Akpinar-Elci, M., Blair, A. & Dosemeci, M. (2003) Risk of laryngeal cancer by occupational chemical exposure in Turkey. *J. occup. environ. Med.*, **45**, 1100–1106

Elias, I. (1987) [Evaluation of methods for disinfection of operating theatres in hospitals according to the concentration of formaldehyde in the air.] *Zbl. Arbeitsmed.*, **37**, 389–397 (in German)

Elliott, L.J., Stayner, L.T., Blade, L.M., Halperin, W. & Keenlyside, R. (1987) *Formaldehyde Exposure Characterization in Garment Manufacturing Plants: A Composite Summary of Three In-depth Industrial Hygiene Surveys*, Cincinnati, OH, US Department of Health and Human Services, Public Health Service, Centers for Disease Control, National Institute for Occupational Safety and Health

Enterline, P.E., Marsh, G.M., Henderson, V. & Callahan, C. (1987) Mortality update of a cohort of US man-made mineral fibre workers. *Ann. occup. Hyg.*, **31**, 625–656

Environment Canada (1997) *Results of the CEPA Section 16 Notice to Industry Respecting the Second Priority Substances List and Di(2-ethylhexyl) Phthalate*, Hull, Quebec, Use Patterns Section, Commercial Chemicals Evaluation Branch

Environment Canada (1999) *Canadian Environmental Protection Act — Priority Substances List — Supporting Document for the Environmental Assessment of Formaldehyde*, Hull, Quebec, Commercial Chemicals Evaluation Branch

Environment Canada/Health Canada (2001) *Canadian Environmental Protection Act, 1999. Priority Substances List Assessment Report: Formaldehyde*, Ottawa, Ontario

Environmental Protection Agency (1976) *Investigation of Selected Potential Environmental Contaminants: Formaldehyde* (Report No. EPA-560/2-76-009; PB 256 839), Washington DC, Office of Toxic Substances

Environmental Protection Agency (1988) *Compendium of Methods for the Determination of Toxic Organic Compounds in Ambient Air* (Report No. EPA-600/4-89-017; US NTIS PB90-116989), Research Triangle Park, NC, Office of Research and Development, pp. TO5-1–TO5-22

Environmental Protection Agency (1999a) *Method 318 — Extractive FTIR method for the Measurement of Emissions from the Mineral Wool and Wool Fiberglass Industries*, Washington DC

Environmental Protection Agency (1999b) *Test Method 320 — Measurement of Vapor Phase Organic and Inorganic Emissions by Extractive Fourier Transform Infrared (FTIR) Spectroscopy*, Washington DC

Environmental Protection Agency (1999c) *Compendium of Methods for the Determination of Toxic Organic Compounds in Ambient Air* (Report No. EPA-625/R-96-010b), 2nd Ed., Cincinnati, OH, Office of Research and Development, pp. TO11A-1–TO11A-56

Epstein, S.S. & Shafner, H. (1968) Chemical mutagens in the human environment. *Nature*, **219**, 385–387

Epstein, S.S., Arnold, E., Andrea, J., Bass, W. & Bishop, Y. (1972) Detection of chemical mutagens by the dominant lethal assay in the mouse. *Toxicol. appl. Pharmacol.*, **23**, 288–325

Erdei, E., Bobvos, J., Brózik, M., Páldy, A., Farkas, I., Vaskövi, E. & Rudnai, P. (2003) Indoor air pollutants and immune biomarkers among Hungarian asthmatic children. *Arch. environ. Health*, **58**, 337–347

Ericson, A., Källén, B., Zetterström, R., Eriksson, M. & Westerholm, P. (1984) Delivery outcome of women working in laboratories during pregnancy. *Arch. environ. Health*, **39**, 5–10

Estonius, M., Svensson, S. & Höög, J.-O. (1996) Alcohol dehydrogenase in human tissues: localisation of transcripts coding for five classes of the enzyme. *FEBS Lett.*, **397**, 338–342

European Commission (1989) *Formaldehyde Emission from Wood Based Materials: Guideline for the Determination of Steady State Concentrations in Test Chambers* (EUR 12196 EN; Report No. 2), Luxembourg, European Concerted Action: Indoor Air Quality and Its Impact on Man (COST Project 613)

European Commission (1990) Proposal for a Council Directive on the approximation of the laws of the Member States relating to cosmetic products (90/C322/06). *Off. J. Eur. Commun.*, **C322**, 29–77

European Union (1989) *Council Directive 89/106/EEC of 21 December 1988 on the Approximation of the Laws, Regulations and Administrative Provisions of the Member States Relating to Construction Products, Annex on Legislation on the Release of Dangerous Substances* (89/106/EEC) [Available at: http://europa.eu.int/comm/enterprise/construction/internal/dangsub/dangcount. htm; accessed 01/03/2004]

Fantuzzi, G., Aggazzotti, G., Righi, E., Cavazzuti, L., Predieri, G. & Franceschelli, A. (1996) Indoor air quality in the university libraries of Modena (Italy). *Sci. total Environ.*, **193**, 49–56

Fayerweather, W.E., Pell, S. & Bender, J.R. (1983) Case–control study of cancer deaths in DuPont workers with potential exposure to formaldehyde. In: Clary, J.C., Gibson, J.E. & Waritz, R.S., eds, *Formaldehyde. Toxicology, Epidemiology, and Mechanisms*, New York, Marcel Dekker, pp. 47–121

Feinman, S.E. (1988) Formaldehyde genotoxicity and teratogenicity. In: Feinman, S.E., ed., *Formaldehyde. Sensitivity and Toxicity*, Boca Raton, FL, CRC Press, pp. 167–178

Fenech, M., Holland, N., Chang, W.P., Zeiger, E. & Bonassi, S. (1999) The Human Micronucleus Project — An international collaborative study on the use of the micronucleus technique for measuring DNA damage in humans. *Mutat. Res.*, **428**, 271–283

Feng, Y., Wen, S., Wang, X., Sheng, G., He, Q., Tang, J. & Fu, J. (2004) Indoor and outdoor carbonyl compounds in the hotel ballrooms in Guangzhou, China. *Atmos. Environ.*, **38**, 103–112

Feron, V.J., Bruyntjes, J.P., Woutersen, R.A., Immel, H.R. & Appelman, L.M. (1988) Nasal tumours in rats after short-term exposure to a cytotoxic concentration of formaldehyde. *Cancer Lett.*, **39**, 101–111

Feron, V.J., Til, H.P. & Woutersen, R.A. (1990) Letter to the Editor. *Toxicol. ind. Health*, **6**, 637–639

Feron, V.J., Til, H.P., de Vrijer, F., Woutersen, R.A., Cassee, F.R. & van Bladeren, P.J. (1991) Aldehydes: Occurrence, carcinogenic potential, mechanism of action and risk assessment. *Mutat. Res.*, **259**, 363–385

Ferrari, C.P., Kaluzny, P., Roche, A., Jacob, V. & Foster, P. (1998) Aromatic hydrocarbons and aldehydes in the atmosphere of Grenoble, France. *Chemosphere*, **37**, 1587–1601

Finnish Institute of Occupational Health (1994) *Measurements of Formaldehyde, Industrial Hygiene Data Base*, Helsinki

Fló-Neyret, C., Lorenzi-Filho, G., Macchione, M., Garcia, M.L.B. & Saldiva, P.H.N. (2001) Effects of formaldehyde on the frog's mucociliary epithelium as a surrogate to evaluate air pollution effects on the respiratory epithelium. *Braz. J. med. biol. Res.*, **34**, 639–643

Fontignie-Houbrechts, N. (1981) Genetic effects of formaldehyde in the mouse. *Mutat. Res.*, **88**, 109–114

Food & Drug Administration (2003) Food and drugs. *US Code fed. Regul.*, **Title 21**, Parts 173.340, 175.105, 176.170, 176.180, 176.200, 176.210, 177.2800, 178.3120, 529.1030, 573.460 [www.fda.gov]

Fornace, A.J., Jr, Lechner, J.F., Grafström, R.C. & Harris, C.C. (1982) DNA repair in human bronchial epithelial cells. *Carcinogenesis*, **3**, 1373–1377

Fransman, W., McLean, D., Douwes, J., Demers, P.A., Leung, V. & Pearce, N. (2003) Respiratory symptoms and occupational exposures in New Zealand plywood mill workers. *Ann. occup. Hyg.*, **47**, 287–295

Friedfeld, S., Fraser, M., Lancaster, D., Leleux, D., Rehle, D. & Tittel, F. (2000) Field intercomparison of a novel optical sensor for formaldehyde quantification. *Geophys. Res. Lett.*, **27**, 2093–2096

Friedman, G.D. & Ury, H.K. (1983) Screening for possible drug carcinogenicity: Second report of findings. *J. natl Cancer Inst.*, **71**, 1165–1175

Fritschi, L. & Siemiatycki, J. (1996) Lymphoma, myeloma and occupation: Results of a case–control study. *Int. J. Cancer*, **67**, 498–503

Gaffney, J.S., Marley, N.A., Martin, R.S., Dixon, R.W., Reyes, L.G. & Popp, C.J. (1997) Potential air quality effects of using ethanol–gasoline fuel blends: A field study in Albuquerque, New Mexico. *Environ. Sci. Technol.*, **31**, 3053–3061

Gallagher, R.P., Threlfall, W.J., Band, P.R., Spinelli, J.J. & Coldman, A.J. (1986) *Occupational Mortality in British Columbia 1950–1978*, Ottawa, Statistics Canada, Health and Welfare Canada

Gallagher, R.P., Threlfall, W.J., Band, P.R. & Spinelli, J.J. (1989) *Occupational Mortality in British Columbia 1950–1984*, Vancouver, Canadian Cancer Association of British Columbia

Gammage, R.B. & Gupta, K.C. (1984) Formaldehyde. In: Walsh, P.J., Dudney, C.S. & Copenhaver, E.D., eds, *Indoor Air Quality*, Boca Raton, FL, CRC Press, pp. 109–142

Gammage, R.G. & Travis, C.C. (1989) Formaldehyde exposure and risk in mobile homes. In: Paustenbach, D.J., ed., *The Risk Assessment of Environmental and Human Health Hazards: A Textbook of Case Studies*, New York, John Wiley & Sons, pp. 601–611

García-Alonso, S. & Pérez-Pastor, R.M. (1998) Use of C_{18} and silica-gel coated Sep-Pak cartridges for the determination of carbonyls in air by liquid chromatography. *Anal. chim. Acta*, **367**, 93–99

Gardner, M.J., Pannett, B., Winter, P.D. & Cruddas, A.M. (1993) A cohort study of workers exposed to formaldehyde in the British chemical industry: An update. *Br. J. ind. Med.*, **50**, 827–834

Garrett, M.H., Hooper, M.A. & Hooper, B.M. (1997) Formaldehyde in Australian homes; levels and sources. *Clean Air*, **31**, 28–32

Garrett, M.H., Hooper, M.A.; Hooper, B.M., Rayment, P.R. & Abramson, M.J. (1999) Increased risk of allergy in children due to formaldehyde exposure in homes. *Allergy*, **54**, 330–337

Gaylor, D.W., Lutz, W.K. & Conolly, R.B. (2004) Statistical analysis of nonmonotonic dose–response relationships: Research design and analysis of nasal cell proliferation in rats exposed to formaldehyde. *Toxicol. Sci.*, **77**, 158–164

Georghiou, P.E., Winsor, L., Sliwinski, J.F. & Shirtliffe, C.J. (1993) Method 11. Determination of formaldehyde in indoor air by a liquid sorbent technique. In: Seifert, B., van de Wiel, H., Dodet, B. & O'Neill, I.K., eds, *Environmental Carcinogens: Methods of Analysis and Exposure Measurement. Vol. 12*: *Indoor Air Contaminants* (IARC Scientific Publications No. 109), Lyon, IARC, pp. 245–249

Georgieva, A.V., Kimbell, J.S. & Schlosser, P.M. (2003) A distributed-parameter model for formaldehyde uptake and disposition in the rat nasal lining. *Inhal. Toxicol.*, **15**, 1435–1463

Gerberich, H.R. & Seaman, G.C. (2004) Formaldehyde. In: Kroschwitz, J.I. & Howe-Grant, M., eds, *Kirk–Othmer Encyclopedia of Chemical Technology*, 5th Ed., Vol. 11, New York, John Wiley & Sons, pp. 929–951

Gérin, M., Siemiatycki, J., Nadon, L., Dewar, R. & Krewski, D. (1989) Cancer risks due to occupational exposure to formaldehyde: Results of a multi-site case–control study in Montreal. *Int. J. Cancer*, **44**, 53–58

Gibson, J.E. (1984) Coordinated toxicology: An example study with formaldehyde. *Concepts Toxicol.*, **1**, 276–282

Gocke, E., King, M.-T., Eckhardt, K. & Wild, D. (1981) Mutagenicity of cosmetics ingredients licensed by the European Communities. *Mutat. Res.*, **90**, 91–109

Gofmekler, V.A. (1968) [Embryotropic action of benzol and formaldehyde on experimental introduction by the respiratory route.] *Gig. Sanit.*, **33**, 327–332 (in Russian)

Gofmekler, V.A. & Bonashevskaya, T.I. (1969) [Experimental studies of teratogenic properties of formaldehyde, based on pathological investigations.] *Hyg. Sanit.*, **34**, 266–268 (in Russian)

Gofmekler, V.A., Pushkina, N.N. & Klevtsova. G.N. (1968) [Some biochemical aspects of the embryotropic effect of benzene and formaldehyde.] *Hyg. Sanit.*, **33**, 112–116 (in Russian)

Goldmacher, V.S. & Thilly, W.G. (1983) Formaldehyde is mutagenic for cultured human cells. *Mutat. Res.*, **116**, 417–422

Goldoft, M., Weiss, N., Vaughan, T. & Lee, J. (1993) Nasal melanoma. *Br. J. ind. Med.*, **50**, 767–768

Goldstein, H.B. (1973) Textiles and the chemical industry: A marriage. *J. am. Assoc. Text. Chem. Color.*, **5**, 209–214

Goldstein, B.D. (1990) Is exposure to benzene a cause of human multiple myeloma? *Ann. N.Y. Acad. Sci.*, **609**, 225–234

Gosselin, N.H., Brunet, R.C. & Carrier, G. (2003) Comparative occupational exposures to formaldehyde released from inhaled wood product dusts versus that in vapor form. *Appl. occup. environ. Hyg.*, **18**, 384–393

Gotoh, Y., Sumimoto, H. & Minakami, S. (1990) Formation of 20-oxoleukotriene B_4 by an alcohol dehydrogenase isolated from human neutrophils. *Biochim. biophys. Acta*, **1043**, 52–56

Gottschling, L.M., Beaulieu, H.J. & Melvin, W.W. (1984) Monitoring of formic acid in urine of humans exposed to low levels of formaldehyde. *Am. ind. Hyg. Assoc. J.*, **45**, 19–23

Grafström, R.C (1990) In vitro studies of aldehyde effects related to human respiratory carcinogenesis. *Mutat. Res.*, **238**, 175–184

Grafström, R.C., Fornace, A., Jr & Harris, C.C. (1984) Repair of DNA damage caused by formaldehyde in human cells. *Cancer Res.*, **44**, 4323–4327

Grafström, R.C., Curren, R.D., Yang, L.L. & Harris, C.C. (1985) Genotoxicity of formaldehyde in cultured human bronchial fibroblasts. *Science*, **228**, 89–91

Grafström, R.C., Willey, J.C., Sundqvist, K. & Harris, C.C. (1986) Pathobiological effects of tobacco smoke-related aldehydes in cultured human bronchial epithelial cells. In: Hoffmann, D. & Harris, C.C., eds, *Mechanisms in Tobacco Carcinogenesis* (Banbury Report 23), Cold Spring Harbor, NY, CSH Press, pp. 273–285

Grafström, R.C., Hsu, I.-C. & Harris, C.C. (1993) Mutagenicity of formaldehyde in Chinese hamster lung fibroblasts: Synergy with ionizing radiation and *N*-nitroso-*N*-methylurea. *Chem.-biol. Interactions*, **86**, 41–49

Grafström, R.C., Jernelöv, M.I., Dypbukt, J.M., Sundqvist, K., Atzori, L. & Zheng, X. (1996) Aldehyde toxicity and thiol redox state in cell cultures from human aerodigestive tract. In: Mohr, U., Adler, K.B., Dungworth, D.I., Harris, C.C., Plopper, C.G. & Saracci, R., eds, *Correlations Between In Vitro and In Vivo Investigations in Inhalation Toxicology*, Washington DC, ILSI Press, pp. 319–336

Granby, K., Christensen, C.S. & Lohse, C. (1997) Urban and semi-rural observations of carboxylic acids and carbonyls. *Atmos. Environ.*, **31**, 1403–1415

Graves, R.J., Callander, R.D. & Green, T. (1994) The role of formaldehyde and *S*-chloromethylglutathione in the bacterial mutagenicity of methylene chloride. *Mutat. Res.*, **320**, 235–243

Graves, R.J., Trueman, P., Jones, S. & Green, T. (1996) DNA sequence analysis of methylene chloride-induced HPRT mutations in Chinese hamster ovary cells: Comparison with the mutation spectrum obtained for 1,2-dibromoethane and formaldehyde. *Mutagenesis*, **11**, 229–233

Green, D.J., Sauder, L.R., Kulle, T.J. & Bascom, R. (1987) Acute response to 3.0 ppm formaldehyde in exercising healthy nonsmokers and asthmatics. *Am. Rev. respir. Dis.*, **135**, 1261–1266

Groah, W.J., Bradfield, J., Gramp, G., Rudzinski, R. & Heroux, G. (1991) Comparative response of reconstituted wood products to European and North American test methods for determining formaldehyde emissions. *Environ. Sci. Technol.*, **25**, 117–122

Grosjean, E., Williams, E.L., II & Grosjean, D. (1993) Ambient levels of formaldehyde and acetaldehyde in Atlanta, Georgia. *J. Air Waste Manage. Assoc.*, **43**, 469–474

Grosjean, E., Grosjean, D., Fraser, M.P. & Cass, G.R. (1996) Air quality model evaluation data for organics. 2. C_1-C_{14} carbonyls in Los Angeles air. *Environ. Sci. Technol.*, **30**, 2687–2703

Grosjean, D., Grosjean, E. & Moreira, L.F.R. (2002) Speciated ambient carbonyls in Rio de Janeiro, Brazil. *Environ. Sci. Technol.*, **36**, 1389–1395

Gustavsson, P., Jakobsson, R., Johansson, H., Lewin, F., Norell, S. & Rutkvist, L.-E. (1998) Occupational exposures and squamous cell carcinoma of the oral cavity, pharynx, larynx, and oesophagus: A case–control study in Sweden. *Occup. environ. Med.*, **55**, 393–400

Gylseth, B. & Digernes, V. (1992) The European development of regulations and standards for formaldehyde in air and in wood composite boards. In: *Proceedings of the Pacific Rim Biobased Composites Symposium, 9–13 November 1992, Rotorua, New Zealand*, Rotorua, Forest Products Research Institute, pp. 199–206

Hagberg, M., Kolmodin-Hedman, B., Lindahl, R., Nilsson, C.-A. & Nordström, Å. (1985) Irritative complaints, carboxyhemoglobin increase and minor ventilatory function changes due to exposure to chain-saw exhaust. *Eur. J. respir. Dis.*, **66**, 240–247

Hagen, J.A., Nafstad, P., Skrondal, A., Bjørkly, S. & Magnus, P. (2000) Associations between outdoor air pollutants and hospitalization for respiratory diseases. *Epidemiology*, **11**, 136–140

Hall, A., Harrington, J.M. & Aw, T.-C. (1991) Mortality study of British pathologists. *Am. J. ind. Med.*, **20**, 83–89

Hamaguchi, F. & Tsutsui, T. (2000) Assessment of genotoxicity of dental antiseptics: Ability of phenol, guaiacol, *p*-phenolsulfonic acid, sodium hypochlorite, *p*-chlorophenol, *m*-cresol or formaldehyde to induce unscheduled DNA synthesis in cultured Syrian hamster embryo cells. *Jpn J. Pharmacol.*, **83**, 273–276

Hansch, C., Leo, A. & Hoekman (1995) *Exploring QSAR — Hydrophobic, Electronic, and Steric Constants*, Washington DC, American Chemical Society

Hansen, J. & Olsen, J.H. (1995) Formaldehyde and cancer morbidity among male employees in Denmark. *Cancer Causes Control*, **6**, 354–360

Hansen, J. & Olsen, J.H. (1996) [Occupational exposure to formaldehyde and risk for cancer.] *Ugeskr. Laeger.*, **158**, 4191–4194 (in Danish)

Hardell, L., Johansson, B. & Axelson, O. (1982) Epidemiological study of nasal and nasopharyngeal cancer and their relation to phenoxy acid or chlorophenol exposure. *Am. J. ind. Med.*, **3**, 247–257

Harrington, J.M. & Oakes, D. (1984) Mortality study of British pathologists 1974–80. *Br. J. ind. Med.*, **41**, 188–191

Harrington, J.M. & Shannon, H.S. (1975) Mortality study of pathologists and medical laboratory technicians. *Br. med. J.*, **i**, 329–332

Harving, H., Korsgaard, J., Pedersen, O.F., Mølhave, L. & Dahl, R. (1990) Pulmonary function and bronchial reactivity in asthmatics during low-level formaldehyde exposure. *Lung*, **168**, 15–21

Haszpra, L. Szilágyi, I., Demeter, A., Turányi, T. & Bérces, T. (1991) Non-methane hydrocarbon and aldehyde measurements in Budapest, Hungary. *Atmos. Environ.*, **25**, 2103–2110

Hauptmann, M., Lubin, J.H., Stewart, P.A., Hayes, R.B. & Blair, A. (2003) Mortality from lymphohematopoietic malignancies among workers in formaldehyde industries. *J. natl Cancer Inst.*, **95**, 1615–1623

Hauptmann, M., Lubin, J.H., Stewart, P.A., Hayes, R.B. & Blair, A. (2004) Mortality from solid cancers among workers in formaldehyde industries. *Am. J. Epidemiol.*, **159**, 1117–1130

Haworth, S., Lawlor, T., Mortelmans, K., Speck, W. & Zeiger, E. (1983) Salmonella mutagenicity test results for 250 chemicals. *Environ. Mutag.*, **Suppl. 1**, 3–142

Hayasaka, Y., Yayasaka, S. & Nagaki, Y. (2001) Ocular changes after intravitreal injection of methanol, formaldehyde, or formate in rabbits. *Pharmacol. Toxicol.*, **89**, 74–78

Hayes, R.B., Raatgever, J.W., de Bruyn, A. & Gerin, M. (1986a) Cancer of the nasal cavity and paranasal sinuses, and formaldehyde exposure. *Int. J. Cancer*, **37**, 487–492

Hayes, R.B., Gérin, M., Raatgever, J.W. & de Bruyn, A. (1986b) Wood-related occupations, wood dust exposure, and sinonasal cancer. *Am. J. Epidemiol.*, **124**, 569–577

Hayes, R.B., Blair, A., Stewart, P.A., Herrick, R.F. & Mahar, H. (1990) Mortality of US embalmers and funeral directors. *Am. J. ind. Med.*, **18**, 641–652

Hayes, R.B., Klein, S., Suruda, A., Schulte, P., Boeniger, M., Stewart, P., Livingston, G.K. & Oesch, F. (1997) O⁶-Alkylguanine DNA alkyltansferase activity in student embalmers. *Am. J. ind. Med.*, **31**, 361–365

He, J.-L., Jin, L.-F. & Jin, H.-Y. (1998) Detection of cytogenetic effects in peripheral lymphocytes of students exposed to formaldehyde with cytokinesis-blocked micronucleus assay. *Biomed. environ. Sci.*, **11**, 87–92

Health & Safety Executive (2002) *Occupational Exposure Limits 2002* (EH40/2002), Norwich, Her Majesty' Stationery Office

Health Canada (2000) *Draft Supporting Documentation for PSL2 Assessments. Human Exposure Assessment for Formaldehyde*, Ottawa, Ontario, Priority Substances Section, Health Protection Branch

Heck, H.d'A. & Casanova, M. (1987) Isotope effects and their implications for the covalent binding of inhaled [³H]- and [¹⁴C]formaldehyde in the rat nasal mucosa. *Toxicol. appl. Pharmacol.*, **89**, 122–134

Heck, H.d'A. & Casanova, M. (1995) Nasal dosimetry of formaldehyde: Modelling site specificity and the effects of pre-exposure. In: Miller, F.J., ed., *Nasal Toxicity and Dosimetry of Inhaled Xenobiotics: Implications for Human Health*, Washington DC, Taylor Francis, pp. 159–175

Heck, H.d'A. & Casanova, M. (1999) Pharmacodynamics of formaldehyde: Applications of a model for the arrest of DNA replication by DNA–protein cross-links. *Toxicol. appl. Pharmacol.*, **160**, 86–100

Heck, H.d'A. & Casanova, M. (2004) The implausibility of leukemia induction by formaldehyde: A critical review of the biological evidence on distant-site toxicity. *Regul. Toxicol. Pharmacol.*, **40**, 92–106

Heck, H.d'A., White, E.L. & Casanova-Schmitz, M. (1982) Determination of formaldehyde in biological tissues by gas chromatography/mass spectrometry. *Biomed. mass Spectrom.*, **9**, 347–353

Heck, H.d'A., Chin, T.Y. & Schmitz, M.C. (1983) Distribution of [¹⁴C]formaldehyde in rats after inhalation exposure. In: Gibson, J.E., ed., *Formaldehyde Toxicity*, Washington DC, Hemisphere, pp. 26–37

Heck, H.d'A., Casanova-Schmitz, M., Dodd, P.B., Schachter, E.N., Witek, T.J. & Tosun, T. (1985) Formaldehyde (CH₂O) concentrations in the blood of humans and Fischer-344 rats exposed to CH₂O under controlled conditions. *Am. ind. Hyg. Assoc. J.*, **46**, 1–3

Heck, H.d'A., Casanova, M., Lam, C.-W. & Swenberg, J.A. (1986) The formation of DNA–protein cross-links by aldehydes present in tobacco smoke. In: Hoffmann, D. & Harris, C.C., eds,

Mechanisms in Tobacco Carcinogenesis (Banbury Report 23), Cold Spring Harbor, NY, CSH Press, pp. 215–230

Heck, H.d'A., Casanova, M., Steinhagen, W.H., Everitt, J.I., Morgan, K.T. & Popp, J.A. (1989) Formaldehyde toxicity: DNA–protein cross-linking studies in rats and nonhuman primates. In: Feron, V.J. & Bosland, M.C., eds, *Nasal Carcinogenesis in Rodents: Relevance to Human Risk*, Wageningen, Pudoc, pp. 159–164

Hedberg, J.J., Strömberg, P. & Höög, J.-O. (1998) An attempt to transform class characteristics within the alcohol dehydrogenase family. *FEBS Lett.*, **436**, 67–70

Hedberg, J.J., Höög, J.-O., Nilsson, J.A., Zheng, X., Elfwing, A. & Grafström, R.C. (2000) Expression of alcohol dehydrogenase 3 in tissue and cultured cells from human oral mucosa. *Am. J. Pathol.*, **157**, 1745–1755

Hedberg, J.J., Backlund, M., Strömberg, P., Lönn, S., Dahl, M.-L., Ingelman-Sundberg, M. & Höög, J.-O. (2001) Functional polymorphism in the alcohol dehydrogenase 3 (*ADH3*) promoter. *Pharmacogenetics*, **11**, 815–824

Hedberg, J.J., Höög, J.-O. & Grafström R.C. (2002) Assessment of formaldehyde metabolizing enzymes in human oral mucosa and cultured oral keratinocytes indicate high capacity for detoxification of formaldehyde. In: Heinrich, U. & Mohr, U., eds, *Crucial Issues in Inhalation Research — Mechanistic, Clinical and Epidemiologic* (INIS Monographs), Stuttgart, Fraunhofer IRB Verlag, pp. 103–115

Hedberg, J.J., Griffiths, W.J., Nilsson, S.J.F. & Höög, J.-O. (2003) Reduction of *S*-nitrosoglutathione by human alcohol dehydrogenase 3 is an irreversible reaction as analysed by electrospray mass spectrometry. *Eur. J. Biochem.*, **270**, 1249–1256

Heikkilä, P., Priha, E. & Savela, A. (1991) [Formaldehyde (Exposures at Work No. 14)], Helsinki, Finnish Institute of Occupational Health and Finnish Work Environment Fund (in Finnish)

Hemminki, K., Mutanen, P., Saloniemi, I., Niemi, M.-L. & Vainio, H. (1982) Spontaneous abortions in hospital staff engaged in sterilising instruments with chemical agents. *Br. med. J.*, **285**, 1461–1463

Hemminki, K., Kyyrönen, P. & Lindbohm, M.-L. (1985) Spontaneous abortions and malformations in the offspring of nurses exposed to anaesthetic gases, cytostatic drugs, and other potential hazards in hospitals, based on registered information of outcome. *J. Epidemiol. Community Health*, **39**, 141–147

Hemminki, K., Partanen, R., Koskinen, H., Smith, S., Carney, W. & Brandt-Rauf, P.W. (1996) The molecular epidemiology of oncogens. Serum p53 protein in patients with asbestosis. *Chest*, **109**, 22S–26S

Hendrick, D.J. & Lane, D.J. (1975) Formalin asthma in hospital staff. *Br. med. J.*, **i**, 607–608

Hendrick, D.J. & Lane, D.J. (1977) Occupational formalin asthma. *Br. J. ind. Med.*, **34**, 11–18

Hendrick, D.J., Rando, R.J., Lane, D.J. & Morris, M.J. (1982) Formaldehyde asthma: Challenge exposure levels and fate after five years. *J. occup. Med.*, **24**, 893–897

Herbert, F.A., Hessel, P.A., Melenka, L.S., Yoshida, K. & Nakaza, M. (1995) Pulmonary effects of simultaneous exposures to MDI formaldehyde and wood dust on workers in an oriented strand board plant. *J. occup. environ. Med.*, **37**, 461–465

Hernberg, S., Westerholm, P., Schultz-Larsen, K., Degerth, R., Kuosma, E., Englund, A., Engzell, U., Sand Hansen, H. & Mutanen, P. (1983a) Nasal and sinonasal cancer. Connection with occupational exposures in Denmark, Finland and Sweden. *Scand. J. Work Environ. Health*, **9**, 315–326

Hernberg, S., Collan, Y., Degerth, R., Englund, A., Engzell, U., Kuosma, E., Mutanen, P., Nordlinder, H., Sand Hansen, H., Schultz-Larsen, K., Søgaard, H. & Westerholm, P. (1983b) Nasal cancer and occupational exposures. Preliminary report of a joint Nordic case–referent study. *Scand. J. Work Environ. Health*, **9**, 208–213

Hester, S.D., Benavides, G.B., Yoon, L., Morgan, K.T., Zou, F., Barry, W. & Wolf, D.C. (2003) Formaldehyde-induced gene expression in F344 rat nasal respiratory epithelium. *Toxicology*, **187**, 13–24

Hildesheim, A., West, S., DeVeyra, E., De Guzman, M.F., Jurado, A., Jones, C., Imai, J. & Hinuma, Y. (1992) Herbal medicine use, Epstein–Barr virus, and risk of nasopharyngeal carcinoma. *Cancer Res.*, **52**, 3048–3051

Hildesheim, A., Dosemeci, M., Chan, C.-C., Chen, C.-J., Cheng, Y.-J., Hsu, M.-M., Chen, I.-H., Mittl, B.F., Sun, B., Levine, P.H., Chen, J.-Y., Brinton, L.A. & Yang, C.-S. (2001) Occupational exposure to wood, formaldehyde, and solvents and risk of nasopharyngeal carcinoma. *Cancer Epidemiol. Biomarkers Prev.*, **10**, 1145–1153

Hilton, J., Dearman, R.J., Basketter, D.A., Scholes, E.W. & Kimber, I. (1996) Experimental assessment of the sensitizing properties of formaldehyde. *Food chem. Toxicol.*, **34**, 571–578

Ho, K.F., Lee, S.C., Louie, P.K.K. & Zou, S.C. (2002) Seasonal variation of carbonyl compound concentrations in urban area of Hong Kong. *Atmos. Environ.*, **36**, 1259–1265

Hodgson, A.T., Wooley, J.D. & Daisey, J.M. (1993) Emissions of volatile organic compounds from new carpets measured in a large-scale environmental chamber. *J. Air Waste Manage. Assoc.*, **43**, 316–324

Hodgson, A.T., Rudd, A.F., Beal, D. & Chandra, S. (2000) Volatile organic compound concentrations and emission rates in new manufactured and site-built houses. *Indoor Air*, **10**, 178–192

Hodgson, A.T., Beal, D. & McIlvane, J.E.R. (2002) Sources of formaldehyde, other aldehydes and terpenes in a new manufactured house. *Indoor Air*, **12**, 235–242

Holly, E.A., Aston, D.A., Ahn, D.K. & Smith, A.H. (1996) Intraocular melanoma linked to occupations and chemical exposures. *Epidemiology*, **7**, 55–61

Holmquist, B. & Vallee, B.L. (1991) Human liver class III alcohol and glutathione dependent formaldehyde dehydrogenase are the same enzyme. *Biochem. biophys. Res. Commun.*, **178**, 1371–1377

Holmström, M., Wilhelmsson, B., Hellquist, H. & Rosén, G. (1989a) Histological changes in the nasal mucosa in persons occupationally exposed to formaldehyde alone and in combination with wood dust. *Acta otolaryngol.*, **107**, 120–129

Holmström, M., Wilhelmsson, B. & Hellquist, H. (1989b) Histological changes in the nasal mucosa in rats after long-term exposure to formaldehyde and wood dust. *Acta otolaryngol.*, **108**, 274–283

Holmström, M., Rynnel-Dagöö, B. & Wilhelmsson, B. (1989c) Antibody production in rats after long-term exposure to formaldehyde. *Toxicol. appl. Pharmacol.*, **100**, 328–333

Höög, J.-O., Hedberg, J.J., Strömberg, P. & Svensson, S. (2001) Mammalian alcohol dehydrogenase — Functional and structural implications. *J. biomed. Sci.*, **8**, 71–76

Höög, J.-O., Strömberg, P., Hedberg, J.J. & Griffiths, W.J. (2003) The mammalian alcohol dehydrogenases interact in several metabolic pathways. *Chem.-biol. Interactions*, **143–144**, 175–181

Horton, A.W., Tye, R. & Stemmer, K.L. (1963) Experimental carcinogenesis of the lung. Inhalation of gaseous formaldehyde or an aerosol of coal tar by C3H mice. *J. natl Cancer Inst.*, **30**, 31–43

IARC (1979) *IARC Monographs on the Evaluation of the Carcinogenic Risk of Chemicals to Humans*, Vol. 19, *Some Monomers, Plastics and Synthetic Elastomers, and Acrolein*, Lyon, pp. 314–340

IARC (1982) *IARC Monographs on the Evaluation of the Carcinogenic Risk of Chemicals to Humans*, Vol. 29, *Some Industrial Chemicals and Dyestuffs*, Lyon, pp. 345–389

IARC (1983) *IARC Monographs on the Evaluation of the Carcinogenic Risk of Chemicals to Humans*, Vol. 32, *Polynuclear Aromatic Compounds, Part 1, Chemical, Environmental and Experimental Data*, Lyon

IARC (1984) *IARC Monographs on the Evaluation of the Carcinogenic Risk of Chemicals to Humans*, Vol. 34, *Polynuclear Aromatic Compounds, Part 3, Industrial Exposures in Aluminium Production, Coal Gasification, Coke Production, and Iron and Steel Founding*, Lyon

IARC (1986) *IARC Monographs on the Evaluation of the Carcinogenic Risk of Chemicals to Humans*, Vol. 39, *Some Chemicals Used in Plastics and Elastomers*, Lyon, pp. 287–323

IARC (1987a) *IARC Monographs on the Evaluation of Carcinogenic Risks to Humans*, Suppl. 7, *Overall Evaluations of Carcinogenicity: An Updating of* IARC Monographs *Volumes 1–42*, Lyon, pp. 211–216

IARC (1987b) *IARC Monographs on the Evaluation of Carcinogenic Risks to Humans*, Suppl. 7, *Overall Evaluations of Carcinogenicity: An Updating of* IARC Monographs *Volumes 1–42*, Lyon, pp. 131–134

IARC (1987c) *IARC Monographs on the Evaluation of Carcinogenic Risks to Humans*, Suppl. 7, *Overall Evaluations of Carcinogenicity: An Updating of* IARC Monographs *Volumes 1–42*, Lyon, pp. 152–154

IARC (1987d) *IARC Monographs on the Evaluation of the Carcinogenic Risk of Chemicals to Humans*, Vol. 42, *Silica and Some Silicates*, Lyon, pp. 39–143

IARC (1987e) *IARC Monographs on the Evaluation of Carcinogenic Risks to Humans*, Suppl. 7, *Overall Evaluations of Carcinogenicity: An Updating of* IARC Monographs *Volumes 1–42*, Lyon, pp. 106–116

IARC (1989a) *IARC Monographs on the Evaluation of Carcinogenic Risks to Humans*, Vol. 47, *Some Organic Solvents, Resin Monomers and Related Compounds, Pigments and Occupational Exposures in Paint Manufacture and Painting*, Lyon, pp. 125–156

IARC (1989b) *IARC Monographs on the Evaluation of Carcinogenic Risks to Humans*, Vol. 47, *Some Organic Solvents, Resin Monomers and Related Compounds, Pigments and Occupational Exposures in Paint Manufacture and Painting*, Lyon, pp. 79–123

IARC (1989c) *IARC Monographs on the Evaluation of Carcinogenic Risks to Humans*, Vol. 47, *Some Organic Solvents, Resin Monomers and Related Compounds, Pigments and Occupational Exposures in Paint Manufacture and Painting*, Lyon, pp. 263–287

IARC (1990a) *IARC Monographs on the Evaluation of Carcinogenic Risks to Humans*, Vol. 48, *Some Flame Retardants and Textile Chemicals, and Exposures in the Textile Manufacturing Industry*, Lyon, pp. 181–212

IARC (1990b) *IARC Monographs on the Evaluation of Carcinogenic Risks to Humans*, Vol. 48, *Some Flame Retardants and Textile Chemicals, and Exposures in the Textile Manufacturing Industry*, Lyon, pp. 215–280

IARC (1994a) *IARC Monographs on the Evaluation of Carcinogenic Risks to Humans*, Vol. 60, *Some Industrial Chemicals*, pp. 445–474

IARC (1994b) *IARC Monographs on the Evaluation of Carcinogenic Risks to Humans*, Vol. 60, *Some Industrial Chemicals*, pp. 73–159

IARC (1995) *IARC Monographs on the Evaluation of Carcinogenic Risks to Humans*, Vol. 62, *Wood Dust and Formaldehyde*, Lyon, pp. 217–362

IARC (1999) *IARC Monographs on the Evaluation of Carcinogenic Risks to Humans*, Vol. 71, *Re-evaluation of Some Organic Chemicals, Hydrazine and Hydrogen Peroxide*, Lyon

IARC (2002) *IARC Monographs on the Evaluation of Carcinogenic Risks to Humans*, Vol. 81, *Man-made Vitreous Fibres*, Lyon

IARC (2004) *IARC Monographs on the Evaluation of Carcinogenic Risks to Humans*, Vol. 83, *Tobacco Smoke and Involuntary Smoking*, Lyon

Inoue, K., Nishimukai, H. & Yamasawa, K. (1979) Purification and partial characterization of aldehyde dehydrogenase from human erythrocytes. *Biochim. biophys. Acta*, **569**, 117–123

INRS (Institut national de Recherche et de Sécurité) (2005) [Threshold Limit Values for Occupational Exposure to Chemicals in France] (Notes documentaires 2098), Paris, Hygiène et Sécurité du Travail (in French)

International Labour Office (2001) *Safety in the Use of Synthetic Vitreous Fibre Insulation Wool (Glass Wool, Rockwool, Slag Wool)*, Geneva, International Labour Organization, p. 20

Interscan Corporation (undated) *Portable Analyzer (4000 Series) with Digital Display — Formaldehyde*, Chatsworth, CA

Ishidate, M., Jr, Sofuni, T. & Yoshikawa, K. (1981) Chromosomal aberration tests *in vitro* as a primary screening tool for environmental mutagens and/or carcinogens. *Gann Monogr. Cancer Res.*, **27**, 95–108

Iversen, O.H. (1986) Formaldehyde and skin carcinogenesis. *Environ. int.*, **12**, 541–544

Jaeger, R.J. & Gearhart, J.M. (1982) Respiratory and metabolic response of rats and mice to formalin vapor. *Toxicology*, **25**, 299–309

James, J.T. (1997) Carcinogens in spacecraft air. *Radiat. Res.*, **148**, S11–S16

Jankovic, J., Jones, W., Burkhart, J. & Noonan, G. (1991) Environmental study of firefighters. *Ann. occup. Hyg.*, **35**, 581–602

Jann, O. (1991) Present state and developments in formaldehyde regulations and testing methods in Germany. In: *Proceedings of the 25th International Particleboard/Composite Materials Symposium*, Pullman, WA, Washington State University

Japanese Standards Association (2001) *Japanese Industrial Standard: Building Boards. Determination of Formaldehdye Emission — Dessicator Method* (JIS A-1460:2001), Tokyo

Jeffcoat, A.R., Chasalow, F., Feldman, D.B. & Marr, H. (1983) Disposition of [^{14}C]formaldehyde after topical exposure to rats, guinea pigs, and monkeys. In: Gibson, J.E., ed., *Formaldehyde Toxicity*, Washington DC, Hemisphere, pp. 38–50

Jensen, O.M. & Andersen, S.K. (1982) Lung cancer risk from formaldehyde. *Lancet*, **i**, 913

Jensen, N.J. & Cohr, K.-H. (1983) Testing of formaldehyde in the mammalian spot test by inhalation (Abstract No. 73). *Mutat. Res.*, **113**, 266

Jensen, K.A., Kirk, I., Kølmark, G. & Westergaard, M. (1951) Chemically induced mutations in Neurospora. *Cold Spring Harbor Symp. quant. Biol.*, **16**, 245–261

Jensen, D.E., Belka, G.K. & Du Bois, G.C. (1998) S-Nitrosoglutathione is a substrate for rat alcohol dehydrogenase class III isoenzyme. *Biochem. J.*, **331**, 659–668

Johannsen, F.R., Levinskas, G.J. & Tegeris, A.S. (1986) Effects of formaldehyde in the rat and dog following oral exposure. *Toxicol. Lett.*, **30**, 1–6

John, E.M., Savitz, D.A. & Shy, C.M. (1994) Spontaneous abortions among cosmetologists. *Epidemiology*, **5**, 147–155

Johnsen, R.C. & Baillie, D.L. (1988) Formaldehyde mutagenesis of the eT1 balanced region in *Caenorhabditis elegans*: Dose–response curve and the analysis of mutation events. *Mutat. Res.*, **201**, 137–147

Jones, D.P., Thor, H., Andersson, B. & Orrenius, S. (1978) Detoxification reactions in isolated hepatocytes. Role of glutathione peroxidase, catalase, and formaldehyde dehydrogenase in reactions relating to *N*-demethylation by the cytochrome P-450 system. *J. biol. Chem.*, **253**, 6031–6037

Jörnvall, H. & Höög, J.-O. (1995) Nomenclature of alcohol dehydrogenases. *Alcohol Alcohol.*, **30**, 153–161

Jörnvall, H., Höög, J.-O., Persson, B. & Parés, X. (2000) Pharmacogenetics of the alcohol dehydrogenase system. *Pharmacology*, **61**, 184–191

Jurvelin, J., Vartiainen, M., Jantunen, M. & Pasanen, P. (2001) Personal exposure levels and micro-environmental concentrations of formaldehyde and acetaldehyde in the Helsinki metropolitan area, Finland. *J. Air Waste Manage. Assoc.*, **51**, 17–24

Jurvelin, J.A., Edwards, R.D., Vartiainen, M., Pasanen, P. & Jantunen, M.J. (2003) Residential indoor, outdoor, and workplace concentrations of carbonyl compounds: Relationships with personal exposure concentrations and correlation with sources. *J. Air Waste Manage. Assoc.*, **53**, 560–573

Kalabokas, P., Carlier, P., Fresnet, P., Mouvier, G. & Toupance, G. (1988) Field studies of aldehyde chemistry in the Paris area. *Atmos. Environ.*, **22**, 147–155

Kalász, H. (2003) Biological role of formaldehyde, and cycles related to methylation, demethylation, and formaldehyde production. *Mini Rev. med. Chem.*, **3**, 175–192

Kamata, E., Nakadate, M., Uchida, O., Ogawa, Y., Suzuki, S., Kaneko, T., Saito, M. & Kurokawa, Y. (1997) Results of a 28-month chronic inhalation toxicity study of formaldehyde in male Fisher-344 rats. *J. toxicol. Sci.*, **22**, 239–254

Kaplan, W.D. (1948) Formaldehyde as a mutagen in *Drosophila*. *Science*, **108**, 43

Karlberg, A.-T., Skare, L., Lindberg, I. & Nyhammar, E. (1998) A method for quantification of formaldehyde in the presence of formaldehyde donors in skin-care products. *Contact Derm.*, **38**, 20–28

Katakura, Y., Kishi, R., Ikeda, T. & Miyake, H. (1990) [Distributions of [^{14}C]-formaldehyde and their metabolites in pregnant mice.] *Sangyo Igaku*, **32**, 42–43 (in Japanese)

Katakura, Y., Okui, T., Kishi, R., Ikeda, T. & Miyake, H. (1991) [Distribution of ^{14}C-formaldehyde in pregnant mice: A study by liquid scintillation counter and binding to DNA.] *Sangyo Igaku*, **33**, 264–265 (in Japanese)

Katakura, Y., Kishi, R., Okui, T., Ikeda, T. & Miyake, H. (1993) Distribution of radioactivity from ^{14}C-formaldehyde in pregnant mice and their fetuses. *Br. J. ind. Med.*, **50**, 176–182

Kato, S., Burke, P.J., Koch, T.H. & Bierbaum, V.M. (2001) Formaldehyde in human cancer cells: Detection by preconcentration-chemical ionization mass spectrometry. *Anal. Chem.*, **73**, 2992–2997

Kauppinen, T. (1986) Occupational exposure to chemical agents in the plywood industry. *Ann. occup. Hyg.*, **30**, 19–29

Kauppinen, T. & Niemelä, R. (1985) Occupational exposure to chemical agents in the particleboard industry. *Scand. J. Work Environ. Health*, **11**, 357–363

Kauppinen, T. & Partanen, T. (1988) Use of plant- and period-specific job–exposure matrices in studies on occupational cancer. *Scand. J. Work Environ. Health*, **14**, 161–167

Kauppinen, T., Toikkanen, J., Pedersen, D., Young, R., Ahrens, W., Boffetta, P., Hansen, J., Kromhout, H., Maqueda Blasco J., Mirabelli, D., de la Orden-Rivera, V., Pannett, B., Plato, N., Savela, A., Vincent, R. & Kogevinas, M. (2000) Occupational exposure to carcinogens in the European Union. *Occup. environ. Med.*, **57**, 10–18

Keil, C.B., Akbar-Khanzadeh, F. & Konecny, K.A. (2001) Characterizing formaldehyde emission rates in a gross anatomy laboratory. *Appl. occup. environ. Hyg.*, **16**, 967–972

Kelly, T.J., Smith, D.L. & Satola, J. (1999) Emission rates of formaldehyde from materials and consumer products found in California homes. *Environ. Sci. Technol.*, **33**, 81–88

Kennedy, E.R., Gagnon, Y.T., Teass, A.W. & Seitz, T. (1992) Development and evaluation of a method to estimate potential formaldehyde dose from inhalable dust/fibers. *Appl. occup. environ. Hyg.*, **7**, 231–240

Kepler, G.M., Richardson, R.B., Morgan, K.T. & Kimbell, J.S. (1998) Computer simulation of inspiratory nasal airflow and inhaled gas uptake in a rhesus monkey. *Toxicol. appl. Pharmacol.*, **150**, 1–11

Kerfoot, E.J. & Mooney, T.F., Jr (1975) Formaldehyde and paraformaldehyde study in funeral homes. *Am. ind. Hyg. Assoc. J.*, **36**, 533–537

Kernan, G.J., Ji, B.-T., Dosemeci, M., Silverman, D.T., Balbus, J. & Zahm, S.H. (1999) Occupational risk factors for pancreatic cancer: A case–control study based on death certificates from 24 US states. *Am. J. ind. Med.*, **36**, 260–270

Kerns, W.D., Pavkov, K.L., Donofrio, D.J., Gralla, E.J. & Swenberg, J.A. (1983a) Carcinogenicity of formaldehyde in rats and mice after long-term inhalation exposure. *Cancer Res.*, **43**, 4382–4392

Kerns, W.D., Donofrio, D.J. & Pavkov, K.L. (1983b) The chronic effects of formaldehyde inhalation in rats and mice: A preliminary report. In: Gibson, J.E., ed., *Formaldehyde Toxicity*, Washington DC, Hemisphere, pp. 111–131

Khan, A.H. (1967) The induction of crossing over in the absence of mutation. *Sind Univ. Sci. Res. J.*, **3**, 103–106

Khoder, M.I., Shakour, A.A., Farag, S.A. & Abdel Hameed, A.A. (2000) Indoor and outdoor formaldehyde concentrations in homes in residential areas in Greater Cairo. *J. environ. Monit.*, **2**, 123–126

Khwaja, H.A. (1995) Atmospheric concentrations of carboxylic acids and related compounds at a semiurban site. *Atmos. Environ.*, **29**, 127–139

Kiec-Swierczynska, M., Krecisz, B., Krysiak, B., Kuchowicz, E. & Rydzynski, K. (1998) Occupational allergy to aldehydes in health care workers. Clinical observations. Experiments. *Int. J. occup. Med. environ. Health*, **11**, 349–358

Kilburn, K.H. & Moro, A. (1985) Reproductive and maternal effects of formaldehyde (HCHO) in rats (Abstract). *Fed. Proc.*, **44**, 535

Kilburn, K.H., Seidman, B.C. & Warshaw, R. (1985) Neurobehavioral and respiratory symptoms of formaldehyde and xylene exposure in histology technicians. *Arch. environ Health*, **40**, 229–233

Kim, H., Kim, Y.-D. & Cho, S.-H. (1999) Formaldehyde exposure levels and serum antibodies to formaldehyde–human serum albumin of Korean medical students. *Arch. environ. Health*, **54**, 115–118

Kim, C.-W., Song, J.-S., Ahn, Y.-S., Park, S.-H., Park, J.-W., Noh, J.-H. & Hong, C.-S. (2001) Occupational asthma due to formaldehyde. *Yonsei med. J.*, **42**, 440–445

Kim, W.J., Terada, N., Nomura, T., Takahashi, R., Lee, S.D., Park, J.H. & Konno, A. (2002) Effect of formaldehyde on the expression of adhesion molecules in nasal microvascular endothelial cells: The role of formaldehyde in the pathogenesis of sick building syndrome. *Clin. exp. Allergy*, **32**, 287–295

Kimbell, J.S. & Subramaniam, R.P. (2001) Use of computational fluid dynamics models for dosimetry of inhaled gases in the nasal passages. *Inhal. Toxicol.*, **13**, 325–334

Kimbell, J.S., Gross, E.A., Richardson, R.B., Conolly, R.B. & Morgan, K.T. (1997) Correlation of regional formaldehyde flux predictions with the distribution of formaldehyde-induced squamous metaplasia in F344 rat nasal passages. *Mutat. Res.*, **380**, 143–154

Kimbell, J.S., Overton, J.H., Subramaniam, R.P., Schlosser, P.M., Morgan, K.T., Conolly, R.B. & Miller, F.J. (2001a) Dosimetry modeling of inhaled formaldehyde: Binning nasal flux predictions for quantitative risk assessment. *Toxicol. Sci.*, **64**, 111–121

Kimbell, J.S., Subramaniam, R.P., Gross, E.A., Schlosser, P.M. & Morgan, K.T. (2001b) Dosimetry modeling of inhaled formaldehyde: Comparisons of local flux predictions in the rat, monkey, and human nasal passages. *Toxicol. Sci.*, **64**, 100–110

Kimbell, J.S., Schlosser, P.M., Conolly, R.B. & Miller, F.J. (2002) Dosimetry modelling of inhaled formaldehyde. *CIIT Activities*, **22**, 1–8

Kinney, P.L., Chillrud, S.N., Ramstrom, S., Ross, J. & Spengler, J.D. (2002) Exposures to multiple air toxics in New York City. *Environ. Health Perspect.*, **110** (Suppl. 4), 539–546

Kirchstetter, T.W., Singer, B.C., Harley, R.A., Kendall, G.R. & Chan, W. (1996) Impact of oxygenated gasoline use on California light-duty vehicle emissions. *Environ. Sci. Technol.*, **30**, 661–670

Kitaeva, L.V., Kitaev, E.M. & Pimenova, M.N. (1990) [The cytopathic and cytogenetic effects of chronic inhalation of formaldehyde on germ and marrow cells of the female rat.] *Tsitologiia*, **32**, 1212–1216 (in Russian)

Kitaeva, L.V., Mikheeva, E.A., Shelomova, L.F. & Shvartsman, P.Y. (1996) [Genotoxic effect of formaldehyde in somatic human cells in vivo.] *Genetika*, **32**, 1298–1290 (in Russian)

Kligerman, A.D., Phelps, M.C. & Erexson, G.L. (1984) Cytogenetic analysis of lymphocytes from rats following formaldehyde inhalation. *Toxicol. Lett.*, **21**, 241–246

Koeck, M., Pichler-Semmelrock, F.P. & Schlacher, R. (1997) Formaldehyde — Study of indoor air pollution in Austria. *Centr. Eur. J. public Health*, **5**, 127–130

Koivusalo, M., Baumann, M. & Uotila, L. (1989) Evidence for the identity of glutathione-dependent formaldehyde dehydrogenase and class III alcohol dehydrogenase. *FEBS Lett.*, **257**, 105–109

Kölmark, G. & Westergaard, M. (1953) Further studies on chemically induced reversions at the adenine locus of *Neurospora*. *Hereditas*, **39**, 209–224

Köppel, C., Baudisch, H., Schneider, V. & Ibe, K. (1990) Suicidal ingestion of formalin with fatal complications. *Intensive Care Med.*, **16**, 212–214

Korczynski, R.E. (1994) Formaldehyde exposure in the funeral industry. *Appl. occup. environ. Hyg.*, **9**, 575–579

Korczynski, R.E. (1996) Effectiveness of downdraft ventilation in morgues. *Appl. occup. environ. Hyg.*, **11**, 5–8

Korhonen, K., Liukkonen,T., Ahrens, W., Astrakianakis, G., Boffetta, P., Burdorf, A., Heederik, D., Kauppinen, T., Kogevinas, M., Osvoll, P., Rix, B.A., Saalo, A., Sunyer, J., Szadkowska-

Stanczyk, I., Teschke, K., Westberg, H. & Widerkiewicz, K. (2004) Occupational exposure to chemical agents in the paper industry. *Int. Arch. occup. environ. Health*, **77**, 451–460

Korky, J.K., Schwarz, S.R. & Lustigman, B.K. (1987) Formaldehyde concentrations in biology department teaching facilities. *Bull. environ. Contam. Toxicol.*, **38**, 907–910

Krakowiak, A., Górski, P., Pazdrak, K. & Ruta, U. (1998) Airway response to formaldehyde inhalation in asthmatic subjects with suspected respiratory formaldehyde sensitization. *Am. J. ind. Med.*, **33**, 274–281

Kreiger, R.A. & Garry, V.F. (1983) Formaldehyde-induced cytotoxicity and sister-chromatid exchanges in human lymphocyte cultures. *Mutat. Res.*, **120**, 51–55

Kriebel, D., Sama, S.R. & Cocanour, B. (1993) Reversible pulmonary responses to formaldehyde. A study of clinical anatomy students. *Am. Rev. respir. Dis.*, **148**, 1509–1515

Krieger, P., De Blay, F., Pauli, G. & Kopferschmitt, M.-C. (1998) [Asthma and domestic chemical pollutants (except for tobacco).] *Rev. Mal. respir.*, **15**, 11–24 (in French)

Kulle, T.J. (1993) Acute odor and irritation response in healthy nonsmokers with formaldehyde exposure. *Inhal. Toxicol.*, **5**, 323–332

Kulle, T.J., Sauder, L.R., Hebel, J.R., Green, D.J. & Chatham, M.D. (1987) Formaldehyde dose–response in healthy nonsmokers. *J. Air Pollut. Control Assoc.*, **37**, 919–924

Kuykendall, J.R. & Bogdanffy, M.S. (1992) Efficiency of DNA–histone crosslinking induced by saturated and unsaturated aldehydes *in vitro*. *Mutat. Res.*, **283**, 131–136

Laforest, L., Luce, D., Goldberg, P., Bégin, D., Gérin, M., Demers, P.A., Brugère, J. & Leclerc, A. (2000) Laryngeal and hypopharyngeal cancers and occupational exposure to formaldehyde and various dusts: A case–control study in France. *Occup. environ. Med.*, **57**, 767–773

Lam, C.-W., Casanova, M. & Heck, H.d'A. (1985) Depletion of nasal mucosal glutathione by acrolein and enhancement of formaldehyde-induced DNA–protein cross-linking by simultaneous exposure to acrolein. *Arch. Toxicol.*, **58**, 67–71

Lamont Moore, L. & Ogrodnik, E.C. (1986) Occupational exposure to formaldehyde in mortuaries. *J. environ. Health*, **49**, 32–35

Lancaster, D.G., Fried, A., Wert, B., Henry, B. & Tittel, F.K. (2000) Difference-frequency-based tunable absorption spectrometer for detection of atmospheric formaldehyde. *Appl. Optics*, **39**, 4436–4443

Leclerc, A., Martinez Cortes, M., Gérin, M., Luce, D. & Brugère, J. (1994) Sinonasal cancer and wood dust exposure: Results from a case–control study. *Am. J. Epidemiol.*, **140**, 340–349

Le Curieux, F., Marzin, D. & Erb, F. (1993) Comparison of three short-term assays: Results on seven chemicals. Potential contribution to the control of water genotoxicity. *Mutat. Res.*, **319**, 223–236

Lee, S. & Radtke, T. (1998) Exposure to formaldehyde among fish hatchery workers. *Appl. occup. environ. Hyg.*, **13**, 3–6

Lee, H.K., Alarie, Y. & Karol, M.H. (1984) Induction of formaldehyde sensitivity in guinea pigs. *Toxicol. appl. Pharmacol.*, **75**, 147–155

Lehmann, W.F. & Roffael, E. (1992) International guidelines and regulations for formaldehyde emissions. In: *Proceedings of the 26th Washington State University International Particleboard/Composite Materials Symposium*, Pullman, WA, Washington State University, pp. 124–150

Leifer, Z., Hyman, J. & Rosenkranz, H.S. (1981) Determination of genotoxic activity using DNA polymerase-deficient and -proficient *E. coli*. In: Stich, H.F. & San, R.H.C., eds, *Short-term Tests for Chemical Carcinogenesis*, New York, Springer, pp. 127–139

Lemus, R., Abdelghani, A.A., Akers, T.G. & Horner, W.E. (1998) Potential health risks from exposure to indoor formaldehyde. *Rev. environ. Health*, **13**, 91–98

Lévesque, B., Allaire, S., Gauvin, D., Koutrakis, P., Gingras, S., Rhainds, M., Prud'Homme, H. & Duchesne, J.-F. (2001) Wood-burning appliances and indoor air quality. *Sci. total Environ.*, **281**, 47–62

Levine, R.J., Andjelkovich, D.A., & Shaw, L.K. (1984) The mortality of Ontario undertakers and a review of formaldehyde-related mortality studies. *J. occup. Med.*, **26**, 740–746

Levy, S., Nocentini, S. & Billardon, C. (1983) Induction of cytogenetic effects in human fibroblast cultures after exposure to formaldehyde or X-rays. *Mutat. Res.*, **119**, 309–317

Lewis, B. (1998) Formaldehyde in dentistry: A review for the millennium. *J. clin. pediatr. Dent.*, **22**, 167–177

Lewis, K.J., Ward, M.K. & Kerr, D.N.S. (1981) Residual formaldehyde in dialyzers: Quantity, location, and the effect of different methods of rinsing. *Artif. Organs*, **5**, 269–277

Liber, H.L., Benforado, K., Crosby, R.M., Simpson, D. & Skopek, T.R. (1989) Formaldehyde-induced and spontaneous alterations in human *hprt* DNA sequence and mRNA expression. *Mutat. Res.*, **226**, 31–37

Lide, D.R., ed. (2003) *CRC Handbook of Chemistry and Physics*, 84th Ed., Boca Raton, FL, CRC Press, p. 3-288

Liebling, T., Rosenman, K.D., Pastides, H., Griffith, R.G., & Lemeshow, S. (1984) Cancer mortality among workers exposed to formaldehyde. *Am. J. ind. Med.*, **5**, 423–428

Lindbohm, M.-L., Hemminki, K., Bonhomme, M.G., Anttila, A., Rantala, K., Heikkilä, P. & Rosenberg, M.J. (1991) Effects of paternal occupational exposure on spontaneous abortions. *Am. J. public Health*, **81**, 1029–1033

Lindstrom, A.B., Proffitt, D. & Fortune, C.R. (1995) Effects of modified residential construction on indoor air quality. *Indoor Air*, **5**, 258–269

Linos, A., Blair, A., Cantor, K.P., Burmeister, L., VanLier, S., Gibson, R.W., Schuman, L. & Everett, G. (1990) Leukemia and non-Hodgkin's lymphoma among embalmers and funeral directors (Letter to the Editor). *J. natl Cancer Inst.*, **82**, 66

Liteplo, R.G. & Meek, M.E. (2003) Inhaled formaldehyde: Exposure estimation, hazard characterization, and exposure–response analysis. *J. Toxicol. environ. Health*, **B6**, 85–114

Liu, L., Hausladen, A., Zeng, M., Que, L., Heitman, J. & Stamler, J.S. (2001) A metabolic enzyme for *S*-nitrosothiol conserved from bacteria to humans. *Nature*, **410**, 490–494

Lodén, M. (1986) The *in vitro* permeability of human skin to benzene, ethylene glycol, formaldehyde, and n-hexane. *Acta pharmacol. toxicol.*, **58**, 382–389

Logue, J.N., Barrick, M.K. & Jessup, G.L., Jr (1986) Mortality of radiologists and pathologists in the radiation registry of physicians. *J. occup. Med.*, **28**, 91–99

Lovschall, H., Eiskjaer, M. & Arenholt-Bindslev, D. (2002) Formaldehyde cytotoxicity in three human cell types assessed in three different assays. *Toxicol. in Vitro*, **16**, 63–69

Luce, D., Leclerc, A., Morcet, J.F., Casal-Lareo, A., Gérin, M., Brugère, J., Haguenoer, J.M. & Goldberg, M. (1992) Occupational risk factors for sinonasal cancer: A case–control study in France. *Am. J. ind. Med.*, **21**, 163–175

Luce, D., Gérin, M., Leclerc, A., Morcet, J.-F., Brugère, J. & Goldberg, M. (1993) Sinonasal cancer and occupational exposure to formaldehyde and other substances. *Int. J. Cancer*, **53**, 224–231

Luce, D., Leclerc, A., Bégin, D., Demers, P.A., Gérin, M., Orlowski, E., Kogevinas, M., Belli, S., Bugel, I., Bolm-Audorff, U., Brinton, L.A., Comba, P., Hardell, L., Hayes, R.B., Magnani, C., Merler, E., Preston-Martin, S., Vaughan, T.L., Zheng, W. & Boffetta, P. (2002) Sinonasal cancer and occupational exposures: A pooled analysis of 12 case–control studies. *Cancer Causes Control*, **13**, 147–157

Luker, M.A. & Van Houten, R.W. (1990) Control of formaldehyde in a garment sewing plant. *Am. ind. Hyg. Assoc. J.*, **51**, 541–544

Luo, J.-C., Zehab, R., Anttila, S., Ridanpaa, M., Husgafvel-Pursiainen, K., Vainio, H., Carney, W., DeVivo, I., Milling, C. & Brandt-Rauf, P.W. (1994) Detection of serum p53 protein in lung cancer patients. *J. occup. Med.*, **36**, 155–160

Luo, W., Li, H., Zhang, Y. & Ang, C.Y.W. (2001) Determination of formaldehyde in blood plasma by high-performance liquid chromatography with fluorescence detection. *J. Chromatogr.*, **B753**, 253–257

Ma, T.-H. & Harris, M.M. (1988) Review of the genotoxicity of formaldehyde. *Mutat. Res.*, **196**, 37–59

Mackerer, C.R., Angelosanto, F.A., Blackburn, G.R. & Schreiner, C.A. (1996) Identification of formaldehyde as the metabolite responsible for the mutagenicity of methyl *tertiary*-butyl ether in the activiated mouse lymphoma assay. *Proc. Soc. exp. Biol. Med.*, **212**, 338–341

Magaña-Schwencke, N. & Ekert, B. (1978) Biochemical analysis of damage induced in yeast by formaldehyde. II. Induction of cross-links between DNA and protein. *Mutat. Res.*, **51**, 11–19

Magaña-Schwencke, N. & Moustacchi, E. (1980) Biochemical analysis of damage induced in yeast by formaldehyde. III. Repair of induced cross-links between DNA and proteins in the wild-type and in excision-deficient strains. *Mutat. Res.*, **70**, 29–35

Magaña-Schwencke, N., Ekert, B. & Moustacchi, E. (1978) Biochemical analysis of damage induced in yeast by formaldehyde. I. Induction of single-strand breaks in DNA and their repair. *Mutat. Res.*, **50**, 181–193

Magnani, C., Comba, P., Ferraris, F., Ivaldi, C., Meneghin, M. & Terracini, B. (1993) A case–control study of carcinomas of the nose and paranasal sinuses in the woolen textile manufacturing industry. *Arch. environ. Health*, **48**, 94–97

Maibach, H. (1983) Formaldehyde: Effects on animal and human skin. In: Gibson, J.E., ed., *Formaldehyde Toxicity*, Washington DC, Hemisphere, pp. 166–174

Maier, K.L., Wippermann, U., Leuschel, L., Josten, M., Pflugmacher, S., Schröder, P., Sandermann, H., Jr, Takenaka, S., Ziesenis, A. & Heyder, J. (1999) Xenobiotic-metabolizing enzymes in the canine respiratory tract. *Inhal. Toxicol.*, **11**, 19–35

Maître, A., Soulat, J.-M., Masclet, P., Stoklov, M., Marquès, M. & de Gaudemaris, R. (2002) Exposure to carcinogenic air pollutants among policemen working close to traffic in an urban area. *Scand. J. Work Environ. Health*, **28**, 402–410

Mäkinen, M., Kalliokoski, P. & Kangas, J. (1999) Assessment of total exposure to phenol–formaldehyde resin glue in plywood manufacturing. *Int. Arch. occup. environ. Health*, **72**, 309–314

Malaka, T. & Kodama, A.M. (1990) Respiratory health of plywood workers occupationally exposed to formaldehyde. *Arch. environ. Health*, **45**, 288–294

Malek, F.A., Möritz, K.-U. & Fanghänel, J. (2003) A study on the effect of inhalative formaldehyde exposure on water labyrinth test performance in rats. *Ann. Anat.*, **185**, 277–285

Malker, H.R. & Weiner, J. (1984) [Cancer–Environment Registry: Examples of the Use of Register Epidemiology in Studies of the Work Environment] (Arbete och Hälsa 1984;9), Stockholm, Arbetarskyddsverket (in Swedish)

Malorny, G., Rietbrock, N. & Schneider, M. (1965) [Oxidation of formaldehyde to formic acid in blood, a contribution to the metabolism of formaldehyde.] *Naunyn–Schmiedeberg's Arch. exp. Pathol. Pharmakol.*, **250**, 419–436 (in German)

't Mannetje, A., Kogevinas, M., Luce, D., Demers, P.A., Bégin, D., Bolm-Audorff, U., Comba, P., Gérin, M., Hardell, L., Hayes, R.B., Leclerc, A., Magnani, C., Merler, E., Tobías, A. & Boffetta, P. (1999) Sinonasal cancer, occupation, and tobacco smoking in European women and men. *Am. J. ind. Med.*, **36**, 101–107

Marnett, L.J., Hurd, H.K., Hollstein, M.C., Levin, D.E., Esterbauer, H. & Ames, B.N. (1985) Naturally occurring carbonyl compounds are mutagens in Salmonella tester strain TA104. *Mutat. Res.*, **148**, 25–34

Maronpot, R.A., Miller, R.A., Clarke, W.J., Westerberg, R.B., Decker, J.R. & Moss, O.R. (1986) Toxicity of formaldehyde vapor in B6C3F1 mice exposed for 13 weeks. *Toxicology*, **41**, 253–266

Maroziene, L. & Grazuleviciene, R. (2002) Maternal exposure to low-level air pollution and pregnancy outcomes: A population-based study. *Environ. Health*, **1**, 6–12

Marsh, G.M. (1982) Proportional mortality patterns among chemical plant workers exposed to formaldehyde. *Br. J. ind. Med.*, **39**, 313–322

Marsh, G.M. (1983) Proportional mortality among chemical workers exposed to formaldehyde. In: Gibson, J.E., ed., *Formaldehyde Toxicity*, Washington DC, Hemisphere, pp. 237–255

Marsh, G.M. & Youk, A.O. (2004) Reevaluation of mortality risks from leukemia in the formaldehyde cohort study of the National Cancer Institute. *Regul. Toxicol. Pharmacol.*, **40**, 113–124

Marsh, G.M., Stone, R.A. & Henderson, V.L. (1992a) A reanalysis of the National Cancer Institute study on lung cancer mortality among industrial workers exposed to formaldehyde. *J. occup. Med.*, **34**, 42–44

Marsh, G.M., Stone, R.A. & Henderson, V.L. (1992b) Lung cancer mortality among industrial workers exposed to formaldehyde: A Poisson regression analysis of the National Cancer Institute study. *Am. ind. Hyg. Assoc. J.*, **53**, 681–691

Marsh, G.M., Stone, R.A., Esmen, N.A. & Henderson, V.L. (1994) Mortality patterns among chemical plant workers exposed to formaldehyde and other substances (Brief communication). *J. natl Cancer Inst.*, **86**, 384–386

Marsh, G.M., Stone, R.A., Esmen, N.A., Henderson, V.L. & Lee, K.Y. (1996) Mortality among chemical workers in a factory where formaldehyde was used. *Occup. environ. Med.*, **53**, 613–627

Marsh, G.M., Youk, A.O., Stone, R.A., Buchanich, J.M., Gula, M.J., Smith, T.J. & Quinn, M.M. (2001) Historical cohort study of US man-made vitreous fiber production workers: I. 1992 fiberglass cohort follow-up: Initial findings. *J. occup. environ. Med.*, **43**, 741–756

Marsh, G.M., Youk, A.O., Buchanich, J.M., Cassidy, L.D., Lucas, L.J., Esmen, N.A. & Gathuru, I.M. (2002) Pharyngeal cancer mortality among chemical plant workers exposed to formaldehyde. *Toxicol. ind. Health*, **18**, 257–268

Martin, W.J. (1990) A teratology study of inhaled formaldehyde in rat. *Reprod. Toxicol.*, **4**, 237–239

Mašek, V. (1972) [Aldehydes in the air of workplaces in coal coking and pitch coking plants.] *Staub-Reinhalt Luft*, **32**, 335–336 (in German)

Mashford, P.M. & Jones, A.R. (1982) Formaldehyde metabolism by the rat: A re-appraisal. *Xeno-biotica*, **12**, 119–124

Matanoski, G.M. (1991) *Risk of Pathologists Exposed to Formaldehyde* (NTIS/PB91-173682), Springfield, VA, National Technical Information Service

Materna, B.L., Jones, J.R., Sutton, P.M., Rothman, N. & Harrison, R.J. (1992) Occupational exposures in California wildland fire fighting. *Am. ind. Hyg. Assoc. J.*, **53**, 69–76

Matheson Tri-Gas® (2004) *Detector Tube Listing for Matheson-Kitagawa Toxic Gas Detector System* (Technical Bulletin 102-1, Issue 3), Irving, TX

Mathew, L., Tai, W.R. & Lo, J.-G. (2001) Measurements of sulfur dioxide and formaldehyde in Taipei using a differential optical absorption spetrometer. *J. Air Waste Manage. Assoc.*, **51**, 94–101

Mathison, B.H., Harman, A.E. & Bogdanffy, M.S. (1997) DNA damage in the nasal passageway: A literature review. *Mutat. Res.*, **380**, 77–96

Maurice, F., Rivory, J.-P., Larsson, P.H., Johansson, S.G.O. & Bousquet, J. (1986) Anaphylactic shock caused by formaldehyde in a patient undergoing long-term hemodialysis. *J. Allergy clin. Immunol.*, **77**, 594–597

Mautz, W.J. (2003) Exercising animal models in inhalation toxicology: Interactions with ozone and formaldehyde. *Environ. Res.*, **92**, 14–26

McClellan, R.O. (1995) Risk assessment and biological mechanisms: Lessons learned, future opportunities. *Toxicology*, **102**, 239–258

McGuire, M.T., Casserly, D.M. & Greff, R.M. (1992) Formaldehyde concentrations in fabric stores. *Appl. occup. environ. Hyg.*, **7**, 112–119

McMillan, A., Whittemore, A.S., Silvers, A. & DiCiccio, Y. (1994) Use of biological markers in risk assessment. *Risk Anal.*, **14**, 807–813

Meister, A. & Anderson, M.E. (1983) Glutathione. *Annu. Rev. Biochem.*, **52**, 711–760

Merk, O. & Speit, G. (1998) Significance of formaldehyde-induced DNA–protein crosslinks for mutagenesis. *Environ. mol. Mutag.*, **32**, 260–268

Merk, O. & Speit, G. (1999) Detection of crosslinks with the comet assay in relationship to geno-toxicity and cytotoxicity. *Environ. mol. Mutag.*, **33**, 167–172

Merler, E., Baldasseroni, A., Laria, R., Faravelli, P., Agostini, R., Pisa, R. & Berrino, F. (1986) On the causal association between exposure to leather dust and nasal cancer: Further evidence from a case–control study. *Br. J. ind. Med.*, **43**, 91–95

Merletti, F., Boffetta, P., Ferro, G., Pisani, P. & Terracini, B. (1991) Occupation and cancer of the oral cavity or oropharynx in Turin, Italy. *Scand. J. Work Environ. Health*, **17**, 248–254

Mery, S., Gross, E.A., Joyner, D.R., Godo, M. & Morgan, K.T. (1994) Nasal diagrams: A tool for recording the distribution of nasal lesions in rats and mice. *Toxicol. Pathol.*, **22**, 353–372

Migliore, L., Ventura, L., Barale, R., Loprieno, N., Castellino, S. & Pulci, R. (1989) Micronuclei and nuclear anomalies induced in the gastro-intestinal epithelium of rats treated with formal-dehyde. *Mutagenesis*, **4**, 327–334

Miguel, A.H., De Aquino Neto, F.R., Cardoso, J.N., Vasconcellos, P.C., Pereira, A.S. & Marquez, K.S.G. (1995) Characterization of indoor air quality in the cities of São Paulo and Rio de Janeiro, Brazil. *Environ. Sci. Technol.*, **29**, 338–345

Milham, S. (1983) *Occupational Mortality in Washington State 1950–1979* (DHHS (NIOSH) Publication No. 83-116), Cincinatti, OH, National Institute for Occupational Safety and Health

Milton, D.K., Walters, M.D., Hammond, K. & Evans, J.S. (1996) Worker exposure to endotoxin, phenolic compounds, and formaldehyde in a fiberglass insulation manufacturing plant. *Am. ind. Hyg. Assoc. J.*, **57**, 889–896

Miretskaya, L.M. & Shvartsman, P.Y. (1982) [Studies of chromosome aberrations in human lymphocytes under the influence of formaldehyde. 1. Formaldehyde treatment of lymphocytes *in vitro*.] *Tsitologiia*, **24**, 1056–1060 (in Russian)

MKS Instruments (2004a) *Application Note: Formaldehyde Emissions Monitoring with Multi-Gas™ 2030* (App. Note #06/03), Wilmington, MA

MKS Instruments (2004b) *MultiGas™ 2030 On-line Gas Analysis*, Wilmington, MA

Molotkov, A., Fan, X., Deltour, L., Foglio, M.H., Martras, S., Farrés, J., Parés, X. & Duester, G. (2002) Stimulation of retinoic acid production and growth by ubiquitously expressed alcohol dehydrogenase *Adh3*. *Proc. natl Acad. Sci. USA*, **99**, 5337–5342

Monteiro-Riviere, N.A. & Popp, J.A. (1986) Ultrastructural evaluation of acute nasal toxicity in the rat respiratory epithelium in response to formaldehyde gas. *Fundam. appl. Toxicol.*, **6**, 251–262

Montero, L., Vasconcellos, P.C., Souza, S.R., Pires, M.A.F., Sanchez-Ccoyllo, O.R., Andrade, M.F. & Carvalho, L.R.F. (2001) Measurements of atmospheric carboxylic acids and carbonyl compounds in São Paulo City, Brazil. *Environ. Sci. Technol.*, **35**, 3071–3081

Monticello, T.M. & Morgan, K.T. (1994) Cell proliferation and formaldehyde-induced respiratory carcinogenesis. *Risk Anal.*, **14**, 313–319

Monticello, T.M. & Morgan, K.T. (1997) Chemically-induced nasal carcinogenesis and epithelial cell proliferation: A brief review. *Mutat. Res.*, **380**, 33–41

Monticello, T.M., Morgan, K.T., Everitt, J.I. & Popp, J.A. (1989) Effects of formaldehyde gas on the respiratory tract of rhesus monkeys. Pathology and cell proliferation. *Am. J. Pathol.*, **134**, 515–527

Monticello, T.M., Miller, F.J. & Morgan, K.T. (1991) Regional increases in rat nasal epithelial cell proliferation following acute and subchronic inhalation of formaldehyde. *Toxicol. appl. Pharmacol.*, **111**, 409–421

Monticello, T.M., Gross, E.A. & Morgan, K.T. (1993) Cell proliferation and nasal carcinogenesis. *Environ. Health Perspect.*, **101** (Suppl. 5), 121–124

Monticello, T.M., Swenberg, J.A., Gross, E.A., Leininger, J.R., Kimbell, J.S., Seilkop, S., Starr, T.B., Gibson, J.E. & Morgan, K.T. (1996) Correlation of regional and nonlinear formaldehyde-induced nasal cancer with proliferating populations of cells. *Cancer Res.*, **56**, 1012–1022

Morgan, K.T., Jiang, X.-Z., Starr, T.B. & Kerns, W.D. (1986a) More precise localization of nasal tumors associated with chronic exposure of F-344 rats to formaldehyde gas. *Toxicol. appl. Pharmacol.*, **82**, 264–271

Morgan, K.T., Patterson, D.L. & Gross, E.A. (1986b) Responses of the nasal mucociliary apparatus of F-344 rats to formaldehyde gas. *Toxicol. appl. Pharmacol.*, **82**, 1–13

Morgan, K.T., Gross, E.A. & Patterson, D.L. (1986c) Distribution, progression, and recovery of acute formaldehyde-induced inhibition of nasal mucociliary function in F-344 rats. *Toxicol. appl. Pharmacol.*, **86**, 448–456

Morgan, K.T., Kimbell, J.S., Monticello, T.M., Patra, A.L. & Fleishman, A. (1991) Studies of inspiratory airflow patterns in the nasal passages of the F344 rat and rhesus monkey using nasal molds: Relevance to formaldehyde toxicity. *Toxicol. appl. Pharmacol.*, **110**, 223–240

MSA (1998) *Detector Tubes and Pumps* (Bulletin 08-00-02-MC), Pittsburgh, PA

Mukerjee, N. & Pietruszko, R. (1992) Human mitochondrial aldehyde dehydrogenase substrate specificity: Comparison of esterase with dehydrogenase reaction. *Arch. Biochem. Biophys.*, **299**, 23–29

Nakao, H., Umebayashi, C., Nakata, M., Nishizaki, Y., Noda, K., Okano, Y. & Oyama, Y. (2003) Formaldehyde-induced shrinkage of rat thymocytes. *J. pharmacol. Sci.*, **91**, 83–86

Natarajan, A.T., Darroudi, F., Bussman, C.J.M. & van Kesteren-van Leeuwen, A.C. (1983) Evaluation of the mutagenicity of formaldehyde in mammalian cytogenetic assays in vivo and in vitro. *Mutat. Res.*, **122**, 355–360

National Library of Medicine (NLM) (2004) *TRI2001 — Toxics Release Inventory*, Bethesda, MD

Naylor, S., Mason, R.P., Sanders, J.K.M., Williams, D.H. & Moneti, G. (1988) Formaldehyde adducts of glutathione. Structure elucidation by two-dimensional n.m.r. spectroscopy and fast-atom-bombardment tandem mass spectrometry. *Biochem. J.*, **249**, 573–579

Neitzert, V. & Seiler, W. (1981) Measurement of formaldehyde in clean air. *Geophys. Res. Lett.*, **8**, 79–82

Neuberger, A. (1981) The metabolism of glycine and serine. In: Neuberger, A. & van Deenen, L.L.M., eds, *Comprehensive Biochemistry*, Vol. 19A, *Amino Acid Metabolism and Sulphur Metabolism*, Amsterdam, Elsevier, pp. 257–303

Nguyen, H.T.-H., Takenaka, N., Bandow, H., Maeda, Y., de Oliva, S.T., Botelho, M.M. & Tavares, T.M. (2001) Atmospheric alcohols and aldehydes concentrations measured in Osaka, Japan and in Sao Paulo, Brazil. *Atmos. Environ.*, **35**, 3075–3083

Nielsen, J. (2002) [Introduction to research in frozen fish and fishing.] In: [Proceedings of a Workshop on 'High Quality Frozen Fish', March 7, 2002], Copenhagen (in Danish)

Niemelä, R. & Vainio, H. (1981) Formaldehyde exposure in work and the general environment. Occurrence and possibilities for prevention. *Scand. J. Work Environ. Health*, **7**, 95–100

Nilsson, J.A., Zheng, X., Sundqvist, K., Liu, Y., Atzori, L., Elfwing, Å., Arvidson, K. & Grafström, R.C. (1998) Toxicity of formaldehyde to human oral fibroblasts and epithelial cells: Influences of culture conditions and role of thiol status. *J. dent. Res.*, **77**, 1896–1903

Nilsson, J.A., Hedberg, J.J., Vondracek, M., Staab, C.A., Hansson, A., Höög, J.-O. & Grafström, R.C. (2004) Alcohol dehydrogenase 3 transcription associates with proliferation of human oral keratinocytes. *Cell. mol. Life Sci.*, **61**, 610–617

NIOSH (National Institute for Occupational Safety and Health) (1994a) *NIOSH Manual of Analytical Methods (NMAM®)* (DHHS (NIOSH) Publ. No. 94-113), 4th Ed., Cincinnati, OH, pp. 3500-1–3500-5 [http://www.cdc.gov/niosh/nmam/]

NIOSH (National Institute for Occupational Safety and Health) (1994b) *NIOSH Manual of Analytical Methods (NMAM®)* (DHHS (NIOSH) Publ. No. 94-113), 4th Ed., Cincinnati, OH, pp. 2539-1–2539-10 [http://www.cdc.gov/niosh/nmam/]

NIOSH (National Institute for Occupational Safety and Health) (1994c) *NIOSH Manual of Analytical Methods (NMAM®)* (DHHS (NIOSH) Publ. No. 94-113), 4th Ed., Cincinnati, OH, pp. 2541-1–2541-5 [http://www.cdc.gov/niosh/nmam/]

NIOSH (National Institute for Occupational Safety and Health) (1994d) *NIOSH Manual of Analytical Methods (NMAM®)* (DHHS (NIOSH) Publ. No. 94-113), 4th Ed., Cincinnati, OH, pp. 5700-1–5700-5 [http://www.cdc.gov/niosh/nmam/]

NIOSH (National Institute for Occupational Safety and Health) (2003a) *NIOSH Manual of Analytical Methods (NMAM®)* (DHHS (NIOSH) Publ. 2003-154), 4th Ed., Supplement 3, Cincinnati, OH, pp. 2016-1–2016-7 [http://www.cdc.gov/niosh/nmam/]

NIOSH (National Institute for Occupational Safety and Health) (2003b) *NIOSH Manual of Analytical Methods (NMAM®)* (DHHS (NIOSH) Publ. 2003-154), 4th Ed., Supplement 3, Cincinnati, OH, pp. 3800-1–3800-47 [http://www.cdc.gov/niosh/nmam/]

Nishioka, H. (1973) Lethal and mutagenic action of formaldehyde in Hcr+ and Hcr– strains of *Escherichia coli*. *Mutat. Res.*, **17**, 261–265

Nisse, C., Haguenoer, J.M., Grandbastien, B., Preudhomme, C., Fontaine, B., Brillet, J.M., Lejeune, R. & Fenaux, P. (2001) Occupational and environmental risk factors of the myelodysplastic syndromes in the North of France. *Br. J. Haematol.*, **112**, 927–935

Norbäck, D., Björnsson, E., Janson, C., Widström, J. & Boman, G. (1995) Asthmatic symptoms and volatile organic compounds, formaldehyde, and carbon dioxide in dwellings. *Occup. environ. Med.*, **52**, 388–395

Norbäck, D., Wålinder, R., Wieslander, G., Smedje, G., Erwall, C. & Venge, P. (2000) Indoor air pollutants in schools: Nasal patency and biomarkers in nasal lavage. *Allergy*, **55**, 163–170

Nordman, H., Keskinen, H. & Tuppurainen, M. (1985) Formaldehyde asthma — Rare or overlooked. *J. Allergy clin. Immunol.*, **75**, 91–99

Nousiainen, P. & Lindqvist, J. (1979) [Chemical Hazards in the Textile Industry. Air Contaminants] (Tiedonanto 16), Tampere, Valtion teknillinen tutkimuskeskus (in Finnish)

Obe, G. & Beek, B. (1979) Mutagenic activity of aldehydes. *Drug Alcohol Dependence*, **4**, 91–94

Occupational Safety & Health Administration (1990a) *OSHA Analytical Methods Manual*, 2nd Ed., Part 1, Vol. 2 (Methods 29–54), Salt Lake City, UT, Method 52 [www.osha.gov]

Occupational Safety & Health Administration (1990b) *OSHA Analytical Methods Manual*, 2nd Ed., Part 2, Vol. 2 (Methods ID-160 to ID-210), Salt Lake City, UT, Method ID-205 [www.osha.gov]

O'Connor, P.M. & Fox, B.W. (1987) Comparative studies of DNA cross-linking reactions following methylene dimethanesulphonate and its hydrolytic product, formaldehyde. *Cancer Chemother. Pharmacol.*, **19**, 11–15

Odeigah, P.G.C. (1997) Sperm head abnormalities and dominant lethal effects of formaldehyde in albino rats. *Mutat. Res.*, **389**, 141–148

O'Donovan, M.R. & Mee, C.D. (1993) Formaldehyde is a bacterial mutagen in a range of Salmonella and Escherichia indicator strains. *Mutagenesis*, **8**, 577–581

Oftedal, B., Nafstad, P., Magnus, P., Bjørkly, S. & Skrondal, A. (2003) Traffic related air pollution and acute hospital admission for respiratory diseases in Drammen, Norway 1995–2000. *Eur. J. Epidemiol.*, **18**, 671–675

Ohta, T., Watanabe-Akanuma, M., Tokishita, S.-I. & Yamagata, H. (1999) Mutation spectra of chemical mutagens determined by Lac+ reversion assay with *Escherichia coli* WP3101P–WP3106P tester strains. *Mutat. Res.*, **440**, 59–74

Ohta, T., Watanabe-Akanuma, M. & Yamagata, H. (2000) A comparison of mutation spectra detected by the *Escherichia coli* Lac+ reversion assay and the *Salmonella typhimurium* His+ reversion assay. *Mutagenesis*, **15**, 317–323

Ohtsuka, R., Shuto, Y., Fujie, H., Takeda, M., Harada, T. & Itagaki, S.-J. (1997) Response of respiratory epithelium of BN and F344 rats to formaldehyde inhalation. *Exp. Anim.*, **46**, 279–286

Ohtsuka, R., Shutoh, Y., Fujie, H., Yamaguchi, S., Takeda, M., Harada, T. & Doi, K. (2003) Rat strain difference in histology and expression of Th1- and Th2-related cytokines in nasal mucosa after short-term formaldehyde inhalation. *Exp. Toxicol. Pathol.*, **54**, 287–291

Ojajärvi, I.A., Partanen, T.J., Ahlbom, A., Boffetta, P., Hakulinen, T., Jourenkova, N., Kauppinen, T.P., Kogevinas, M., Porta, M., Vainio, H.U., Weiderpass, E. & Wesseling, C.H. (2000) Occupational exposures and pancreatic cancer: A meta-analysis. *Occup. environ. Med.*, **57**, 316–324

Olin, K.L., Cherr, G.N., Rifkin, E. & Keen, C.L. (1996) The effects of some redox-active metals and reactive aldehydes on DNA–protein cross-links in vitro. *Toxicology*, **110**, 1–8

Olsen, J.H. & Asnaes, S. (1986) Formaldehyde and the risk of squamous cell carcinoma of the sinonasal cavities. *Br. J. ind. Med.*, **43**, 769–774

Olsen, J.H., Plough Jensen, S., Hink, M., Faurbo, K., Breum, N.O. & Møller Jensen, O. (1984) Occupational formaldehyde exposure and increased nasal cancer risk in man. *Int. J. Cancer*, **34**, 639–644

Ott, M.G., Teta, M.J. & Greenberg, H.L. (1989) Lymphatic and hematopoietic tissue cancer in a chemical manufacturing environment. *Am. J. ind. Med.*, **16**, 631–643

Overman, D.O. (1985) Absence of embryotoxic effects of formaldehyde after percutaneous exposure in hamsters. *Toxicol. Lett.*, **24**, 107–110

Overton, J.H., Kimbell, J.S. & Miller, F.J. (2001) Dosimetry modeling of inhaled formaldehyde: The human respiratory tract. *Toxicol. Sci.*, **64**, 122–134

Özen, O.A., Songur, A., Sarsilmaz, M., Yaman, M. & Kus, I. (2003) Zinc, copper and iron concentrations in cerebral cortex of male rats exposed to formaldehyde inhalation. *J. trace Elem. Med. Biol.*, **17**, 207–209

Panfilova, Z.I., Voronina, E.N., Poslovina, A.S., Goryukhova, N.M. & Salganik, R.I. (1966) Study of the joint action of chemical mutagens and ultra-violet rays upon the appearance of back mutations in *Escherichia coli*. *Sov. Genet.*, **2**, 35–40

Parfett, C.L. (2003) Combined effects of tumor promoters and serum on proliferin mRNA induction: A biomarker sensitive to saccharin, 2,3,7,8-TCDD, and other compounds at minimal concentrations promoting C3H/10T1/2 cell transformation. *J. Toxicol. environ. Health*, **A66**, 1943–1966

Park, J.S. & Ikeda, K. (2003) Database system, AFoDAS/AVODAS, on indoor air organic compounds in Japan. *Indoor Air*, **13** (Suppl. 6), 35–41

Partanen, T. (1993) Formaldehyde exposure and respiratory cancer — A meta-analysis of the epidemiologic evidence. *Scand. J. Work Environ. Health*, **19**, 8–15

Partanen, T., Kauppinen, T., Nurminen, M., Nickels, J., Hernberg, S., Hakulinen, T., Pukkala, E. & Savonen, E. (1985) Formaldehyde exposure and respiratory and related cancers: A case–referent study among Finnish woodworkers. *Scand. J. Work Environ. Health*, **11**, 409–415

Partanen, T., Kauppinen, T., Hernberg, S., Nickels, J., Luukkonen, R., Hakulinen, T. & Pukkala, E. (1990) Formaldehyde exposure and respiratory cancer among woodworkers — An update. *Scand. J. Work Environ. Health*, **16**, 394–400

Partanen, T., Kauppinen, T., Luukkonen, R., Hakulinen, T. & Pukkala, E. (1993) Malignant lymphomas and leukemias, and exposures in the wood industry: An industry-based case–referent study. *Int. Arch. occup. environ. Health*, **64**, 593–596

Patel, K.G., Bhatt, H.V. & Choudhury, A.R. (2003) Alteration in thyroid after formaldehyde (HCHO) treatment in rats. *Ind. Health*, **41**, 295–297

Patterson, R., Dykewicz, M.S., Evans, R.III, Grammer, L.C., Greenberger, P.A., Harris, K.E., Lawrence, I.D., Pruzansky, J.J., Roberts, M., Shaughnessy, M.A. & Zeiss, C.R. (1989) IgG antibody against formaldehyde human serum proteins: A comparison with other IgG antibodies against inhalant proteins and reactive chemicals. *J. Allergy clin. Immunol.*, **84**, 359–366

Paustenbach, D., Alarie, Y., Kulle, T., Schachter, N., Smith, R., Swenberg, J., Witschi, H. & Horowitz, S.B. (1997) A recommended occupational exposure limit for formaldehyde based on irritation. *J. Toxicol. environ. Health*, **50**, 217–263

Pazdrak, K., Górski, P., Krakowiak, A. & Ruta, U. (1993) Changes in nasal lavage fluid due to formaldehyde inhalation. *Int. Arch. occup. environ. Health*, **64**, 515–519

Petersen, D. & Lindahl, R. (1997) Aldehyde dehydrogenases. In: Guengerich, F.P., ed., *Comprehensive Toxicology*, New York, Pergamon, pp. 97–118

Petersen, G.R. & Milham, S. (1980) *Occupational Mortality in the State of California 1959–1961* (DHEW (NIOSH) Publication No. 80-104), Cincinatti, OH, National Institute for Occupational Safety and Health

Pickrell, J.A., Mokler, B.V., Griffis, L.C., Hobbs, C.H. & Bathija, A. (1983) Formaldehyde release rate coefficients from selected consumer products. *Environ. Sci. Technol.*, **17**, 753–757

Pickrell, J.A., Griffis, L.C., Mokler, B.V., Kanapilly, G.M. & Hobbs, C.H. (1984) Formaldehyde release from selected consumer products: Influence of chamber loading, multiple products, relative humidity, and temperature. *Environ. Sci. Technol.*, **18**, 682–686

Pinkerton, L.E., Hein, M.J. & Stayner, L.T. (2004) Mortality among a cohort of garment workers exposed to formaldehyde: An update. *Occup. environ. Med.*, **61**, 193–200

Pitten, F.-A., Kramer, A., Herrmann, K., Bremer, J. & Koch, S. (2000) Formaldehyde neurotoxicity in animal experiments. *Pathol. Res. Pract.*, **196**, 193–198

Pocker, Y. & Li, H. (1991) Kinetics and mechanism of methanol and formaldehyde interconversion and formaldehyde oxidation catalyzed by liver alcohol dehydrogenase. *Adv. exp. Med. Biol.*, **284**, 315–325

Pohanish, R.P. (2002) *Sittig's Handbook of Toxic and Hazardous Chemicals and Carcinogens*, 4th Ed., Norwich, NY, Noyes Publications/William Andrew Publishing, pp. 1179–1182

Pool, B.L., Frei, E., Plesch, W.J., Romruen, K. & Wiessler, M. (1984) Formaldehyde as a possible mutagenic metabolite of *N*-nitrodimethylamine and of other agents which are suggested to yield non-alkylating species *in vitro*. *Carcinogenesis*, **5**, 809–814

Popa, V., Teculescu, D., Stanescu, D. & Gavrilescu, N. (1969) Bronchial asthma and asthmatic bronchitis determined by simple chemicals. *Dis. Chest*, **56**, 395–404

Porter, J.A.H. (1975) Acute respiratory disease following formalin inhalation. *Lancet*, **ii**, 603–604

Possanzini, M., Di Palo, V., Petricca, M., Fratarcangeli, R. & Brocco, D. (1996) Measurements of lower carbonyls in Rome ambient air. *Atmos. Environ.*, **30**, 3757–3764

Poverenny, A.M., Siomin, Y.A., Saenko, A.S. & Sinzinis, B.I. (1975) Possible mechanisms of lethal and mutagenic action of formaldehyde. *Mutat. Res.*, **27**, 123–126

Pratt, G.C., Palmer, K., Wu, C.Y., Oliaei, F., Hollerbach, C. & Fenske, M.J. (2000) An assessment of air toxics in Minnesota. *Environ. Health Perspect.*, **108**, 815–825

Preuss, P.W., Dailey, R.L. & Lehman, E.S. (1985) Exposure to formaldehyde. In: Turoski, V., ed., *Formaldehyde. Analytical Chemistry and Toxicology* (Advances in Chemistry Series, Vol. 210), Washington DC, American Chemical Society, pp. 247–259

Priha, E., Riipinen, H. & Korhonen, K. (1986) Exposure to formaldehyde and solvents in Finnish furniture factories in 1975–1984. *Ann. occup. Hyg.*, **30**, 289–294

Priha, E., Vuorinen, R. & Schimberg, R. (1988) [Textile Finishing Agents] (Työolot 65), Helsinki, Finnish Institute of Occupational Health (in Finnish)

Pushkina, N.N., Gofmekler, V.A. & Klevtsova, T.N. (1968) [Changes in the ascorbic acid titer and in the nucleinic acids following action of benzol and formaldehyde.] *Bjull. eksp. Biol. Med.*, **66**, 51–53 (in Russian)

Puxbaum, H., Rosenberg, C., Gregori, M., Lanzerstorfer, C., Ober, E. & Winiwarter, W. (1988) Atmospheric concentrations of formic and acetic acid and related compounds in eastern and northern Austria. *Atmos. Environ.*, **22**, 2841–2850

Quievryn, G. & Zhitkovich, A. (2000) Loss of DNA–protein crosslinks from formaldehyde-exposed cells occurs through spontaneous hydrolysis and an active repair process linked to proteosome function. *Carcinogenesis*, **21**, 1573–1580

Ragan, D.L. & Boreiko, C.J. (1981) Initiation of C3H/10T1/2 cell transformation by formaldehyde. *Cancer Lett.*, **13**, 325–331

Ratnayake, W.E. (1968) Tests for an effect of the Y-chromosome on the mutagenic action of formaldehyde and X-rays in *Drosophila melanogaster*. *Genet. Res. Camb.*, **12**, 65–69

Ratnayake, W.E. (1970) Studies on the relationship between induced crossing-over and mutation in *Drosophila melanogaster*. *Mutat. Res.*, **9**, 71–83

Recio, L. (1997) Oncogene and tumor suppressor gene alterations in nasal tumors. *Mutat. Res.*, **380**, 27–31

Recio, L., Sisk, S., Pluta, L., Bermudez, E., Gross, E.A., Chen, Z., Morgan, K. & Walker, C. (1992) *p53* Mutations in formaldehyde-induced nasal squamous cell carcinomas in rats. *Cancer Res.*, **52**, 6113–6116

Reed, C.E. & Frigas, E. (1984) Does formaldehyde cause allergic respiratory disease? In: Gammage, R.B. & Kay, S.V., eds, *Indoor Air and Human Health*, Boca Raton, FL, Lewis, pp. 379–386

Reh, C.M., Letts, D. & Deitchman, S. (1994) *National Park Service, Yosemite National Park, CA* (Health Hazard Evaluation Report, HETA 90-0365-2415), Cincinnati, OH, National Institute of Occupational Safety and Health, Centers for Disease Control and Prevention

Reinhardt, T.E., Ottmar, R.D. & Castilla, C. (2001) Smoke impacts from agricultural burning in a rural Brazilian town. *J. Air Waste Manage. Assoc.*, **51**, 443–450

Reiss, R., Ryan, P.B., Tibbetts, S.J. & Koutrakis, P. (1995) Measurement of organic acids, aldehydes, and ketones in residential environments and their relation to ozone. *J. Air Waste Manage. Assoc.*, **45**, 811–822

Restani, P. & Galli, C.L. (1991) Oral toxicity of formaldehyde and its derivatives. *Crit. Rev. Toxicol.*, **21**, 315–328

Restani, P., Restelli, A.R. & Galli, C.L. (1992) Formaldehyde and hexamethylenetetramine as food additives: Chemical interactions and toxicology. *Food Addit. Contam.*, **9**, 597–605

Reuss, G., Disteldorf, W., Gamer, A.O. & Hilt, A. (2003) Formaldehyde. In: *Ullmann's Encyclopedia of Industrial Chemistry*, 6th rev. Ed., Vol. 15, Weinheim, Wiley-VCH Verlag GmbH & Co., pp. 1–34

Reuzel, P.G.J., Wilmer, J.W.G.M., Woutersen, R.A. & Zwart, A. (1990) Interactive effects of ozone and formaldehyde on the nasal respiratory lining epithelium in rats. *J. Toxicol. environ. Health*, **29**, 279–292

Reynolds, S.J., Black, D.W., Borin, S.S., Breuer, G., Burmeister, L.F., Fuortes, L.J., Smith, T.F., Stein, M.A., Subramanian, P., Thorne, P.S. & Whitten, P. (2001) Indoor environmental quality in six commercial office buildings in the Midwest United States. *Appl. occup. environ. Hyg.*, **16**, 1065–1077

Riala, R.E. & Riihimäki, H.A. (1991) Solvent and formaldehyde exposure in parquet and carpet work. *Appl. occup. environ. Hyg.*, **6**, 301–308

Rice, R.H. & Green, H. (1979) Presence in human epidermal cells of a soluble protein precursor of the cross-linked envelope: Activation of the cross-linking by calcium ions. *Cell*, **18**, 681–694

Rietbrock, N. (1965) [Formaldehyde oxidation in the rat.] *Naunyn-Schmiedeberg's Arch. exp. Pathol. Pharmakol.*, **251**, 189–190 (in German)

Risby, T.H., Sehnert, S.S., Jakab, G.J. & Hemenway, D.R. (1990) Model to estimate effective doses of adsorbed pollutants on respirable particles and their subsequent release into alveolar surfactant. I. Validation of the model for the adsorption and release of formaldehyde on a respirable carbon black. *Inhal. Toxicol.*, **2**, 223–239

Robins, J.M., Pambrun, M., Chute, C. & Blevins, D. (1988) Estimating the effect of formaldehyde exposure on lung cancer and non-malignant respiratory disease (NMRD) mortality using a new method to control for the healthy worker survivor effect. In: Hogstedt, C. & Reuterwall, C., eds, *Progress in Occupational Epidemiology*, Amsterdam, Elsevier Science, pp. 75–78

Rosén, G., Bergström, B. & Ekholm, U. (1984) [Occupational exposure to formaldehyde in Sweden.] *Arbete Hälsa*, **50**, 16–21 (in Swedish)

Ross, W.E. & Shipley, N. (1980) Relationship between DNA damage and survival in formaldehyde-treated mouse cells. *Mutat. Res.*, **79**, 277–283

Ross, W.E., McMillan, D.R. & Ross, C.F. (1981) Comparison of DNA damage by methylmelamines and formaldehyde. *J. natl Cancer Inst.*, **67**, 217–221

Rothenberg, S.J., Nagy, P.A., Pickrell, J.A. & Hobbs, C.H. (1989) Surface area, adsorption, and desorption studies on indoor dust samples. *Am. ind. hyg. Assoc. J.*, **50**, 15–23

Roush, G.C., Walrath, J., Stayner, L.T., Kaplan, S.A., Flannery, J.T. & Blair, A. (1987) Nasopharyngeal cancer, sinonasal cancer, and occupations related to formaldehyde: A case–control study. *J natl Cancer Inst.*, **79**, 1221–1224

Rusch, G.M., Clary, J.J., Rinehart, W.E. & Bolte, H.F. (1983) A 26-week inhalation toxicity study with formaldehyde in the monkey, rat, and hamster. *Toxicol. appl. Pharmacol.*, **68**, 329–343

Sadakane, K., Takano, H., Ichinose, T., Yanagisawa, R. & Shibamoto, T. (2002) Formaldehyde enhances mite allergen-induced eosinophilic inflammation in the murine airway. *J. environ. Pathol. Toxicol. Oncol.*, **21**, 267–276

Sadtler Research Laboratories (1991) *Sadtler Standard Spectra. 1981–1991 Supplementary Index*, Philadelphia, PA

Saillenfait, A.M., Bonnet, P. & de Ceaurriz, J. (1989) The effects of maternally inhaled formaldehyde on embryonal and foetal development in rats. *Food chem. Toxicol.*, **27**, 545–548

Sakaguchi, J. & Akabayashi, S. (2003) Field survey of indoor air quality in detached houses in Niigata Prefecture. *Indoor Air*, **13** (Suppl. 6), 42–49

Sakai, K., Norbäck, D., Mi, Y., Shibata, E., Kamijima, M., Yamada, T. & Takeuchi, Y. (2004) A comparison of indoor air pollutants in Japan and Sweden: Formaldehyde, nitrogen dioxide, and chlorinated volatile organic compounds. *Environ. Res.*, **94**, 75–85

Saladino, A.J., Willey, J.C., Lechner, J.F., Grafström, R.C., LaVeck, M. & Harris, C.C. (1985) Effects of formaldehyde, acetaldehyde, benzoyl peroxide, and hydrogen peroxide on cultured normal human bronchial epithelial cells. *Cancer Res.*, **45**, 2522–2526

Salisbury, S. (1983) *Dialysis Clinic Inc., Atlanta, GA, Health Hazard Evaluation Report* (NIOSH Report No. HETA 83-284-1536), Cincinnati, OH, US Department of Health and Human Services, Public Health Service, Centers for Disease Control, National Institute for Occupational Safety and Health

Sandner, F., Dott, W. & Hollender, J. (2001) Sensitive indoor air monitoring of formaldehyde and other carbonyl compounds using the 2,4-dinitrophenylhydrazine method. *Int. J. Hyg. environ. Health*, **203**, 275–279

Sanghani, P.C., Stone, C.L., Ray, B.D., Pindel, E.V., Hurley, T.D. & Bosron, W.F. (2000) Kinetic mechanism of human glutathione-dependent formaldehyde dehydrogenase. *Biochemistry*, **39**, 10720–10729

Sass-Kortsak, A.M., Holness, D.L., Pilger, C.W. & Nethercott, J.R. (1986) Wood dust and formaldehyde exposures in the cabinet-making industry. *Am. ind. Hyg. Assoc. J.*, **47**, 747–753

Satsumabayashi, H., Kurita, H., Chang, Y.-S., Carmichael, G.R. & Ueda, H. (1995) Photochemical formations of lower aldehydes and lower fatty acids under long-range transport in central Japan. *Atmos. Environ.*, **29**, 255–266

Sauder, L.R., Chatham, M.D., Green, D.J. & Kulle, T.J. (1986) Acute pulmonary response to formaldehyde exposure in healthy nonsmokers. *J. occup. Med.*, **28**, 420–424

Sauder, L.R., Green, D.J., Chatham, M.D. & Kulle, T.J. (1987) Acute pulmonary response of asthmatics to 3.0 ppm formaldehyde. *Toxicol. ind. Health*, **3**, 569–578

Schachter, E.N., Witek, T.J., Jr, Tosun, T. & Beck, G.J. (1986) A study of respiratory effects from exposure to 2 ppm formaldehyde in healthy subjects. *Arch. environ. Health*, **41**, 229–239

Schachter, E.N., Witek, T.J., Jr, Brody, D.J., Tosun, T., Beck, G.J. & Leaderer, B.P. (1987) A study of respiratory effects from exposure to 2 ppm formaldehyde in occupationally exposed workers. *Environ. Res.*, **44**, 188–205

Schäfer, D., Brommer, C., Riechelmann, H. & Mann, J.W. (1999) In vivo and in vitro effect of ozone and formaldehyde on human mucociliary transport system. *Rhinology*, **37**, 56–60

Schifter, I., Vera, M., Díaz, L., Guzmán, E., Ramos, F. & López-Salinas, E. (2001) Environmental implications on the oxygenation of gasoline with ethanol in the metropolitan area of Mexico City. *Environ. Sci. Technol.*, **35**, 1893–1901

Schlink, K., Janssen, K., Nitzsche, S., Gebhard, S., Hengstler, J.G., Klein, S. & Oesch, F. (1999) Activity of O^6-methylguanine DNA methyltransferase in mononuclear blood cells of formaldehyde-exposed medical students. *Arch. Toxicol.*, **73**, 15–21

Schlosser, P.M. (1999) Relative roles of convection and chemical reaction for the disposition of formaldehyde and ozone in nasal mucus. *Inhal. Toxicol.*, **11**, 967–980

Schlosser, P.M., Lilly, P.D., Conolly, R.B., Janszen, D.B. & Kimbell, J.S. (2003) Benchmark dose risk assessment for formaldehyde using airflow modeling and a single-compartment, DNA–protein cross-link dosimetry model to estimate human equivalent doses. *Risk Anal.*, **23**, 473–487

Schmid, E., Göggelmann, W. & Bauchinger, M. (1986) Formaldehyde-induced cytotoxic, genotoxic and mutagenic response in human lymphocytes and *Salmonella typhimurium*. *Mutagenesis*, **1**, 427–431

Schreider, J.P. (1986) Comparative anatomy and function of the nasal passages. In: Barrow, C.S., ed., *Toxicology of the Nasal Passages*, Washington DC, Hemisphere, pp. 1–25

Schwartz, S.M., Doody, D.R., Fitzgibbons, E.D., Ricks, S., Porter, P.L. & Chen, C. (2001) Oral squamous cell cancer risk in relation to alcohol consumption and alcohol dehydrogenase-3 genotypes. *Cancer Epidemiol. Biomarkers Prev.*, **10**, 1137–1144

Seila, R.L., Main, H.H., Arriaga, J.L., Martínez, G.V. & Ramadan, A.B. (2001) Atmospheric volatile organic compound measurements during the 1996 Paso del Norte Ozone Study. *Sci. total Environ.*, **276**, 153–169

Sellakumar, A.R., Snyder, C.A., Solomon, J.J. & Albert, R.E. (1985) Carcinogenicity of formaldehyde and hydrogen chloride in rats. *Toxicol. appl. Pharmacol.*, **81**, 401–406

Sensidyne (2004) *Sensidyne Detector Tube Selection Guide*, Clearwater, FL

Sensidyne (undated) *Sensidyne Gas Detector Tube Handbook*, Clearwater, FL, pp. 129–131

de Serres, F.J. & Brockman, H.E. (1999) Comparison of the spectra of genetic damage in formaldehyde-induced *ad-3* mutations between DNA repair-proficient and deficient heterokaryons of *neurospora crassa*. *Mutat. Res.*, **437**, 151–163

de Serres, F.J., Brockman, H.E. & Hung, C.Y. (1988) Effect of the homokaryotic state of the *uvs*-2 allele in *Neurospora crassa* on formaldehyde-induced killing and *ad*-3 mutation. *Mutat. Res.*, **199**, 235–242

de Serves, C. (1994) Gas phase formaldehyde and peroxide measurements in the Arctic atmosphere. *J. geophys. Res.*, **99**, 25391–25398

Sexton, K., Liu, K.-S. & Petreas, M.X. (1986) Formaldehyde concentrations inside private residences: A mail-out approach to indoor air monitoring. *J. Air Pollut. Control Assoc.*, **36**, 698–704

Sexton, K., Petreas, M.X. & Liu, K.-S. (1989) Formaldehyde exposures inside mobile homes. *Environ. Sci. Technol.*, **23**, 985–988

Shah, J.J. & Singh, H.B. (1988) Distribution of volatile organic chemicals in outdoor and indoor air. A national VOCs data base. *Environ. Sci. Technol.*, **22**, 1381–1388

Shaham, J., Bomstein, Y., Meltzer, A., Kaufman, Z., Palma, E. & Ribak, J. (1996a) DNA–protein crosslinks, a biomarker of exposure to formaldehyde — *In vitro* and *in vivo* studies. *Carcinogenesis*, **17**, 121–125

Shaham, J., Bomstein, Y., Meltzer, A. & Ribak, J. (1996b) Response. *Carcinogenesis*, **17**, 2098–2101

Shaham, J., Bomstein, Y., Melzer, A. & Ribak, J. (1997) DNA–protein crosslinks and sister chromatid exchanges as biomarkers of exposure to formaldehyde. *Int. J. occup. environ. Health*, **3**, 95–104

Shaham, J., Gurvich, R. & Kaufman, Z. (2002) Sister chromatid exchange in pathology staff occupationally exposed to formaldehyde. *Mutat. Res.*, **514**, 115–123

Shaham, J., Bomstein, Y., Gurvich, R., Rashkovsky, M. & Kaufman, Z. (2003) DNA–protein crosslinks and p53 protein expression in relation to occupational exposure to formaldehyde. *Occup. environ. Med.*, **60**, 403–409

Shepson, P.B., Hastie, D.R., Schiff, H.I., Polizzi, M., Bottenheim, J.W., Anlauf, K., Mackay, G.I. & Karecki, D.R. (1991) Atmospheric concentrations and temporal variations of C_1–C_3 carbonyl compounds at two rural sites in central Ontario. *Atmos. Environ.*, **25A**, 2001–2015

Shields, P.G., Xu, G.X., Blot, W.J., Fraumeni, J.F., Jr, Trivers, G.E., Pellizzari, E.D., Qu, Y.H., Gao, Y.T. & Harris, C.C. (1995) Mutagens from heated Chinese and US cooking oils. *J. natl Cancer Inst.*, **87**, 836–841

Shumilina, A.V. (1975) [Menstrual and child-bearing functions of female workers occupationally exposed to the effects of formaldehyde.] *Gig. Tr. prof. Zabol.*, **12**, 18–21 (in Russian)

Siboulet, R., Grinfeld, S., Deparis, P. & Jaylet, A. (1984) Micronuclei in red blood cells of the newt *Pleurodeles waltl* Michah: Induction with X-rays and chemicals. *Mutat. Res.*, **125**, 275–281

Siemiatycki, J., Day, N.E., Fabry, J. & Cooper, J.A. (1981) Discovering carcinogens in the occupational environment: A novel epidemiological approach. *J. natl Cancer Inst.*, **66**, 217–225

Siemiatycki, J., Dewar, R., Nadon, L. & Gérin, M. (1994) Occupational risk factors for bladder cancer: Results from a case–control study in Montreal, Quebec, Canada. *Am. J. Epidemiol.*, **140**, 1061–1080

Sin, D.W.M., Wong, Y.-C. & Louie, P.K.K. (2001) Trends of ambient carbonyl compounds in the urban environment of Hong Kong. *Atmos. Environ.*, **35**, 5961–5969

SKC® (2005) *Gastec® Color Detector Tubes Price List*, Eighty Four, PA

Skisak, C.M. (1983) Formaldehyde vapor exposures in anatomy laboratories. *Am. ind. Hyg. Assoc. J.*, **44**, 948–950

Slemr, J. (1992) Development of techniques for the determination of major carbonyl compounds in clean air. In: *EUROTRAC Annual Report for 1991*, Part 9, Mainz, Max Planck Institute for Chemistry, pp. 110–113

Slemr, J., Junkermann, W. & Volz-Thomas, A. (1996) Temporal variations in formaldehyde, acetaldehyde and acetone and budget of formaldehyde at a rural site in southern Germany. *Atmos. Environ.*, **30**, 3667–3676

Smedley, J. (1996) Is formaldehyde an important cause of allergic respiratory disease? *Clin. exp. Allergy*, **26**, 247–249

Smith, E.L., Hill, R.L., Lehman, I.R., Lefkowitz, R.J., Handler, P. & White, A. (1983) *Principles of Biochemistry: Mammalian Biochemistry*, New York, McGraw-Hill, pp. 3–4, 142

Snyder, R.D. & Van Houten, B. (1986) Genotoxicity of formaldehyde and an evaluation of its effects on the DNA repair process in human diploid fibroblasts. *Mutat. Res.*, **165**, 21–30

Sobels, F.H. & van Steenis, H. (1957) Chemical induction of crossing-over in *Drosophila* males. *Nature*, **179**, 29–31

Soffritti, M., Maltoni, C., Maffei, F. & Biagi, R. (1989) Formaldehyde: An experimental multi-potential carcinogen. *Toxicol. ind. Health*, **5**, 699–730

Soffritti, M., Belpoggi, F., Lambertini, L., Lauriola, M., Padovani, M. & Maltoni, C. (2002) Results of long-term experimental studies on the carcinogenicity of formaldehyde and acetaldehyde in rats. *Ann. N.Y. Acad. Sci.*, **982**, 87–105

Sorg, B.A., Bailie, T.M., Tschirgi, M.L., Li, N. & Wu, W.-R. (2001) Exposure to repeated low-level formaldehyde in rats increases basal corticosterone levels and enhances the corticosterone response to subsequent formaldehyde. *Brain Res.*, **898**, 314–320

Spanel, P., Smith, D., Holland, T.A., Al Singary, W. & Elder, J.B. (1999) Analysis of formaldehyde in the headspace of urine from bladder and prostate cancer patients using selected ion flow tube mass spectrometry. *Rapid Commun. mass Spectrom.*, **13**, 1354–1359

Speit, G. & Merk, O. (2002) Evaluation of mutagenic effects of formaldehyde *in vitro*: Detection of crosslinks and mutations in mouse lymphoma cells. *Mutagenesis*, **17**, 183–187

Speit, G., Schütz, P. & Merk, O. (2000) Induction and repair of formaldehyde-induced DNA–protein crosslinks in repair-deficient human cell lines. *Mutagenesis*, **15**, 85–90

Spitzer, H.L. (1997) An analysis of the health benefits associated with the use of MTBE reformulated gasoline and oxygenated fuels in reducing atmospheric concentrations of selected volatile organic compounds. *Risk Anal.*, **17**, 683–691

Šrám, R.J. (1970) The effect of storage on the frequency of dominant lethals in *Drosophila melanogaster*. *Mol. gen. Genet.*, **106**, 286–288

Standardiseringen i Sverige (1996) [Plywood — Formaldehyde Release Classes Determined by the Gas Analysis Method] (SS EN 1084:1995), Stockholm, Swedish Standards Institute (in Swedish)

Stayner, L., Smith, A.B., Reeve, G., Blade, L., Elliott, L., Keenlyside, R. & Halperin, W. (1985) Proportionate mortality study of workers in the garment industry exposed to formaldehyde. *Am. J. ind. Med.*, **7**, 229–240

Stayner, L.T., Elliott, L., Blade, L., Keenlyside, R. & Halperin, W. (1988) A retrospective cohort mortality study of workers exposed to formaldehyde in the garment industry. *Am. J. ind. Med.*, **13**, 667–681

Steenland, K., Nowlin, S., Ryan, B. & Adams, S. (1992) Use of multiple-cause mortality data in epidemiologic analyses: US rate and proportion files developed by the National Institute for Occupational Safety and Health and the National Cancer Institute. *Am. J. Epidemiol.*, **136**, 855–862

Steinhagen, W.H. & Barrow, C.S. (1984) Sensory irritation structure–activity study of inhaled aldehydes in B6C3F1 and Swiss-Webster mice. *Toxicol. appl. Pharmacol.*, **72**, 495–503

Stellman, S.D., Demers, P.A., Colin, D. & Boffetta, P. (1998) Cancer mortality and wood dust exposure among participants in the American Cancer Society Cancer Prevention Study-II (CPS-II). *Am. J. ind. Med.*, **34**, 229–237

Sterling, T.D. & Weinkam, J.J. (1976) Smoking characteristics by type of employment. *J. occup. Med.*, **18**, 743–754

Sterling, T.D. & Weinkam, J.J. (1988) Reanalysis of lung cancer mortality in a National Cancer Institute study on mortality among industrial workers exposed to formaldehyde. *J. occup. Med.*, **30**, 895–901

Sterling, T.D. & Weinkam, J.J. (1989a) Reanalysis of lung cancer mortality in a National Cancer Institute study on 'Mortality among industrial workers exposed to formaldehyde'. *Exp. Pathol.*, **37**, 128–132

Sterling, T.D. & Weinkam, J.J. (1989b) Reanalysis of lung cancer mortality in a National Cancer Institute study of 'Mortality among industrial workers exposed to formaldehyde': Additional discussion. *J. occup. Med.*, **31**, 881–884

Sterling, T.D. & Weinkam, J.J. (1994) Mortality from respiratory cancers (including lung cancer) among workers employed in formaldehyde industries. *Am. J. ind. Med.*, **25**, 593–602

Sterling, T.D. & Weinkam, J.J. (1995) Comments on the Blair and Stewart comments on the Sterling and Weinkam analysis of data from the National Cancer Institute Formaldehyde Study. *Am. J. ind. Med.*, **27**, 301–305

Stewart, P.A., Blair, A., Cubit, D.A., Bales, R.E., Kaplan, S.A., Ward, J., Gaffey, W., O'Berg, M.T. & Walrath, J. (1986) Estimating historical exposures to formaldehyde in a retrospective mortality study. *Appl. ind. Hyg.*, **1**, 34–41

Stewart, P.A., Cubit, D.A. & Blair, A. (1987) Formaldehyde levels in seven industries. *Appl. ind. Hyg.*, **2**, 231–236

Stewart, P.A., Herrick, R.F., Feigley, C.E., Utterback, D.F., Hornung, R., Mahar, H., Hayes, R., Douthit, D.E. & Blair, A. (1992) Study design for assessing exposures of embalmers for a case–control study. Part I. Monitoring results. *Appl. occup. environ. Hyg.*, **7**, 532–540

Stone, R.A., Youk, A.O., Marsh, G.M., Buchanich, J.M., McHenry, M.B. & Smith, T.J. (2001) Historical cohort study of US man-made vitreous fiber production workers: IV. Quantitative exposure–response analysis of the nested case–control study of respiratory system cancer. *J. occup. environ. Med.*, **43**, 779–792

Stragier, A, Wenderickx, D. & Jadoul, M. (1995) Rinsing time and disinfectant release of reused dialyzers: Comparison of formaldehyde, hypochlorite, Warexin, and Renalin. *Am. J. Kidney Dis.*, **26**, 549–553

Stroup, N.E., Blair, A. & Erikson, G.E. (1986) Brain cancer and other causes of death in anatomists. *J. natl Cancer Inst.*, **77**, 1217–1224

Stücker, I., Caillard, J.-F., Collin, R., Gout, M., Poyen, D. & Hémon, D. (1990) Risk of spontaneous abortion among nurses handling antineoplastic drugs. *Scand. J. Work Environ. Health*, **16**, 102–107

Stumm-Tegethoff, B.F.A. (1969) Formaldehyde-induced mutations in *Drosophila melanogaster* in dependence of the presence of acids. *Theoret. appl. Genet.*, **39**, 330–334

Suh, H.H., Bahadori,T., Vallarino, J. & Spengler, J.D. (2000) Criteria air pollutants and toxic air pollutants. *Environ. Health Perspect.*, **108** (Suppl. 4), 625–633

Suruda, A., Schulte, P., Boeniger, M., Hayes, R.B., Livingston, G.K., Steenland, K., Stewart, P., Herrick, R., Douthit, D. & Fingerhut, M.A. (1993) Cytogenetic effects of formaldehyde exposure in students of mortuary science. *Cancer Epidemiol. Biomarkers Prev.*, **2**, 453–460

Suva (2003) *Grenzwerte am Arbeitsplatz 2003*, Luzern, Swiss Accident Insurance [Swiss OELs]

Svensson, S., Some, M., Lundsjö, A., Helander, A., Cronholm, T. & Höög, J.-O. (1999) Activities of human alcohol dehydrogenases in the metabolic pathways of ethanol and serotonin. *Eur. J. Biochem.*, **262**, 324–329

Swenberg, J.A., Kerns, W.D., Mitchell, R.I., Gralla, E.J. & Pavkov, K.L. (1980) Induction of squamous cell carcinomas of the rat nasal cavity by inhalation exposure to formaldehyde vapor. *Cancer Res.*, **40**, 3398–3402

Swenberg, J.A., Gross, E.A., Randall, H.W. & Barrow, C.S. (1983) The effect of formaldehyde exposure on cytotoxicity and cell proliferation. In: Clary, J.J., Gibson, J.E. & Waritz, R.S., eds, *Formaldehyde: Toxicology, Epidemiology, Mechanisms*, New York, Marcel Dekker, pp. 225–236

Swiecichowski, A.L., Long, K.J., Miller, M.L. & Leikauf, G.D. (1993) Formaldehyde-induced airway hyperreactivity *in vivo* and *ex vivo* in guinea pigs. *Environ. Res.*, **61**, 185–199

Takahashi, K., Morita, T. & Kawazoe, Y. (1985) Mutagenic characteristics of formaldehyde on bacterial systems. *Mutat. Res.*, **156**, 153–161

Takahashi, M., Hasegawa, R., Furukawa, F., Toyoda, K., Sato, H. & Hayashi, Y. (1986) Effects of ethanol, potassium metabisulfite, formaldehyde and hydrogen peroxide on gastric carcinogenesis in rats after initiation with *N*-methyl-*N*'-nitro-*N*-nitrosoguanidine. *Jpn. J. Cancer Res.*, **77**, 118–124

Tan, Y.-M., DiBerardinis, L. & Smith, T. (1999) Exposure assessment of laboratory students. *Appl. occup. environ. Hyg.*, **14**, 530–538

Tanaka, K., Nishiyama, K., Yaginuma, H., Sasaki, A., Maeda, T., Kaneko, S.-y., Onami, T. & Tanaka, M. (2003) [Formaldehyde exposure levels and exposure control measure during an anatomy dissecting course.] *Kaibogaku Zasshi*, **78**, 43–51 (in Japanese)

Tanner, R.L., Zielinska, B., Uberna, E., Harshfield, G. & McNichol, A.P. (1996) Concentrations of carbonyl compounds and the carbon isotopy of formaldehyde at a coastal site in Nova Scotia during the NARE summer intensive. *J. geophys. Res.*, **101**, 28961–28970

Tarkowski, M. & Gorski, P. (1995) Increased IgE antiovalbumin level in mice exposed to formaldehyde. *Int. Arch. Allergy Immunol.*, **106**, 422–424

Taskinen, H., Kyyrönen, P., Hemminki, K., Hoikkala, M., Lajunen, K. & Lindbohm, M.-L. (1994) Laboratory work and pregnancy outcome. *J. occup. Med.*, **36**, 311–319

Taskinen, H.K., Kyyrönen, P., Sallmén, M., Virtanen, S.V., Liukkonen, T.A., Huida, O., Lindbohm, M.-L. & Anttila, A. (1999) Reduced fertility among female wood workers exposed to formaldehyde. *Am. J. ind. Med.*, **36**, 206–212

Tatham, L., Tolbert, P. & Kjeldsberg, C. (1997) Occupational risk factors for subgroups of non-Hodgkin's lymphoma. *Epidemiology*, **8**, 551–558

Temcharoen, P. & Thilly, W.G. (1983) Toxic and mutagenic effects of formaldehyde in *Salmonella typhimurium. Mutat. Res.*, **119**, 89–93

Teng, S., Beard, K., Pourahmad, J., Moridani, M., Easson, E., Poon, R. & O'Brien, P.J. (2001) The formaldehyde metabolic detoxification enzyme systems and molecular cytotoxic mechanism in isolated rat hepatocytes. *Chem.-biol. Interactions*, **130–132**, 285–296

Thermo Electron Corporation (2005) *Product Specifications: MIRAN SapphIRe ML Portable Infrared Ambient Analyzer for the Medical Industry*, Franklin, MA

Thornton-Manning, J.R. & Dahl, A.R. (1997) Metabolic capacity of nasal tissue interspecies comparisons of xenobiotic-metabolizing enzymes. *Mutat. Res.*, **380**, 43–59

Thrasher, J.D. & Kilburn, K.H. (2001) Embryo toxicity and teratogenicity of formaldehyde. *Arch. environ. Health*, **56**, 300–311

Tikuisis, T., Phibbs, M.R. & Sonnenberg, K.L. (1995) Quantitation of employee exposure to emission products generated by commercial-scale processing of polyethylene. *Am. ind. Hyg. Assoc. J.*, **56**, 809–814

Til, H.P., Woutersen, R.A., Feron, V.J. & Clary, J.J. (1988) Evaluation of the oral toxicity of acetaldehyde and formaldehyde in a 4-week drinking-water study in rats. *Food chem. Toxicol.*, **26**, 447–452

Til, H.P., Woutersen, R.A., Feron, V.J., Hollanders, V.H.M. & Falke, H.E. (1989) Two-year drinking-water study of formaldehyde in rats. *Food. chem. Toxicol.*, **27**, 77–87

Titenko-Holland, N., Levine, A.J., Smith, M.T., Quintana, P.J.E., Boeniger, M., Hayes, R., Suruda, A. & Schulte, P. (1996) Quantification of epithelial cell micronuclei by fluorescence in situ hybridization (FISH) in mortuary science students exposed to formaldehyde. *Mutat. Res.*, **371**, 237–248

Tobe, M., Naito, K. & Kurokawa, Y. (1989) Chronic toxicity study on formaldehyde administered orally to rats. *Toxicology*, **56**, 79–86

Tokars, J.I., Miller, E.R., Alter, M.J. & Arduino, M.J. (2000) *National Surveillance of Dialysis-associated Diseases in the United States, 1997*, Atlanta, GA, National Center for Infectious Diseases, Centers for Disease Control and Prevention

Triebig, G., Schaller, K.-H., Berger, B., Müller, J. & Valentin, H. (1989) Formaldehyde exposure at various workplaces. *Sci. total Environ.*, **79**, 191–195

Tuomi, T., Engström, B., Niemelä, R., Svinhufvud, J. & Reijula, K. (2000) Emission of ozone and organic volatiles from a selection of laser printers and photocopiers. *Appl. occup. environ. Hyg.*, **15**, 629–634

Tyihák, E., Bocsi, J., Timár, F., Rácz, G. & Szende, B. (2001) Formaldehyde promotes and inhibits proliferation of cultured tumour and endothelial cells. *Cell Prolif.*, **34**, 135–141

Työsuojelusäädöksiä (2002) *HTP arvot 2002*, Helsinki, Sosiaali-ja terveysministeriön [Finnish OELs]

Uotila, L. & Koivusalo, M. (1974) Formaldehyde dehydrogenase from human liver. Purification, properties, and evidence for the formation of glutathione thiol esters by the enzyme. *J. biol. Chem.*, **249**, 7653–7663

Uotila, L. & Koivusalo, M. (1987) Multiple forms of formaldehyde dehydrogenase from human red blood cells. *Hum. Hered.*, **37**, 102–106

Uotila, L. & Koivusalo, M. (1989) Glutathione-dependent oxidoreductases: Formaldehyde dehydrogenase. In: Dolphin, D., Poulson, R. & Avramovic, O., eds, *Coenzymes and Cofactors*, Vol. III, *Glutathione. Chemical, Biochemical and Medical Aspects*, Part A, New York, John Wiley & Sons, pp. 517–551

Uotila, L. & Koivusalo, M. (1997) Expression of formaldehyde dehydrogenase and *S*-formyl-glutathione hydrolase activities in different rat tissues. *Adv. exp. Med. Biol.*, **414**, 365–371

Vargová, M., Janota, S., Karelová, J., Barancokova, M. & Šulcová, M. (1992) Analysis of the health risk of occupational exposure to formaldehyde using biological markers. *Analysis*, **20**, 451–454

Vaughan, T.L. (1989) Occupation and squamous cell cancers of the pharynx and sinonasal cavity. *Am. J. ind. Med.*, **16**, 493–510

Vaughan, T.L. & Davis, S. (1991) Wood dust exposure and squamous cell cancers of the upper respiratory tract. *Am. J. Epidemiol.*, **133**, 560–564

Vaughan, T.L., Strader, C., Davis, S. & Daling, J.R. (1986a) Formaldehyde and cancers of the pharynx, sinus and nasal cavity: I. Occupational exposures. *Int. J. Cancer*, **38**, 677–683

Vaughan, T.L., Strader, C., Davis, S. & Daling, J.R. (1986b) Formaldehyde and cancers of the pharynx, sinus and nasal cavity: II. Residential exposures. *Int. J. Cancer*, **38**, 685–688

Vaughan, T.L., Stewart, P.A., Teschke, K., Lynch, C.F., Swanson, G.M., Lyon, J.L. & Berwick, M. (2000) Occupational exposure to formaldehyde and wood dust and nasopharyngeal carcinoma. *Occup. environ. Med.*, **57**, 376–384

Vaught, C. (1991) *Locating and Estimating Air Emissions From Sources of Formaldehyde (Revised)* (Report No. EPA-450/4-91-012; US NTIS PB91-181842), Research Triangle Park, NC, Environmental Protection Agency

Vinzents, P. & Laursen, B. (1993) A national cross-sectional study of the working environment in the Danish wood and furniture industry — Air pollution and noise. *Ann. occup. Hyg.*, **37**, 25–34

Viskari, E.-L., Vartiainen, M. & Pasanen, P. (2000) Seasonal and diurnal variation in formaldehyde and acetaldehyde concentrations along a highway in Eastern Finland. *Atmos. Environ.*, **34**, 917–923

Vock, E.H., Lutz, W. K., Ilinskaya, O. & Vamvakas, S. (1999) Discrimination between genotoxicity and cytotoxicity for the induction of DNA double-strand breaks in cells treated with aldehydes and diepoxides. *Mutat. Res.*, **441**, 85–93

Wagner, F.W., Parés, X., Holmquist, B. & Vallee, B.L. (1984) Physical and enzymatic properties of a class III isozyme of human liver alcohol dehydrogenase: χ-ADH. *Biochemistry*, **23**, 2193–2199

Walrath, J. & Fraumeni, J.F., Jr (1983) Mortality patterns among embalmers. *Int. J. Cancer*, **31**, 407–411

Walrath, J. & Fraumeni, J.F., Jr (1984) Cancer and other causes of death among embalmers. *Cancer Res.*, **44**, 4638–4641

Walrath, J., Rogot, E., Murray, J. & Blair, A. (1985) *Mortality Patterns among US Veterans by Occupation and Smoking Status* (NIH Publ. No. 85-2756), Bethesda, MD, Department of Health and Human Services

Wang, R.-S., Nakajima, T., Kawamoto, T. & Honma, T. (2002) Effects of aldehyde dehydrogenase-2 genetic polymorphisms on metabolism of structurally different aldehydes in human liver. *Drug Metab. Dispos.*, **30**, 69–73

Wantke, F., Demmer, C.M., Tappler, P., Götz, M. & Jarisch, R. (1996a) Exposure to gaseous formaldehyde induces IgE-mediated sensitization to formaldehyde in school-children. *Clin. exp. Allergy*, **26**, 276–280

Wantke, F., Focke, M., Hemmer, W., Tschabitscher, M., Gann, M., Tappler, P., Götz, M. & Jarisch, R. (1996b) Formaldehyde and phenol exposure during an anatomy dissection course: A possible source of IgE-mediated sensitization? *Allergy*, **51**, 837–841

Wantke, F., Focke, M., Hemmer, W., Bracun, R., Wolf-Abdolvahab, S., Götz, M., Jarisch, R., Tschabitscher, M., Gann, M. & Tappler, P. (2000) Exposure to formaldehyde and phenol during an anatomy dissecting course: Sensitizing potency of formaldehyde in medical students. *Allergy*, **55**, 84–87

Ward, J.B., Jr, Hokanson, J.A., Smith, E.R., Chang, L.W., Pereira, M.A., Whorton, E.B., Jr & Legator, M.S. (1984) Sperm count, morphology and fluorescent body frequency in autopsy service workers exposed to formaldehyde. *Mutat. Res.*, **130**, 417–424

Weast, R.C. & Astle, M.J., eds (1985) *CRC Handbook of Data on Organic Compounds*, Vol. I, Boca Raton, FL, CRC Press, p. 641

Werle, P., Maurer, K., Kormann, R., Mücke, R., D'Amato, F., Lancia, T. & Popov, A. (2002) Spectroscopic gas analyzers based on indium-phosphide, antimonide and lead-salt diode-lasers. *Spectrochim. Acta*, **A58**, 2361–2372

Weschler, C.J. & Shields, H.C. (1996) Production of the hydroxyl radical in indoor air. *Environ. Sci. Technol.*, **30**, 3250–3258

West, S., Hildesheim, A. & Dosemeci, M. (1993) Non-viral risk factors for nasopharyngeal carcinoma in the Philippines: Results from a case–control study. *Int. J. Cancer*, **55**, 722–727

West, R.R., Stafford, D.A., Farrow, A. & Jacobs, A. (1995) Occupational and environmental exposures and myelodysplasia: A case–control study. *Leuk. Res.*, **19**, 127–139

WHO (1989) *Formaldehyde* (Environmental Health Criteria 89), Geneva, International Programme on Chemical Safety

WHO (1991) *Formaldehyde Health and Safety Guide* (Health and Safety Guide No. 57), Geneva, International Programme on Chemical Safety

Wieslander, G., Norbäck, D., Björnsson, E., Janson, C. & Boman, G. (1997) Asthma and the indoor environment: The significance of emission of formaldehyde and volatile organic compounds from newly painted indoor surfaces. *Int. Arch. occup. environ. Health*, **69**, 115–124

Wieslander, G., Norbäck, D., Wålinder, R., Erwall, C. & Venge, P. (1999a) Inflammation markers in nasal lavage, and nasal symptoms in relation to relocation to a newly painted building: A longitudinal study. *Int. Arch. occup. environ. Health*, **72**, 507–515

Wieslander, G., Norbäck, D., Nordström, K., Wålinder, R. & Venge, P. (1999b) Nasal and ocular symptoms, tear film stability and biomarkers in nasal lavage, in relation to building-dampness and building design in hospitals. *Int. Arch. occup. environ. Health*, **72**, 451–461

Wilkins, R.J., & MacLeod, H.D. (1976) Formaldehyde induced DNA–protein crosslinks in *Escherichia coli*. *Mutat. Res.*, **36**, 11–16

Williams, T.M., Levine, R.J. & Blunden, P.B. (1984) Exposure of embalmers to formaldehyde and other chemicals. *Am. ind. Hyg. Assoc. J.*, **45**, 172–176

Williams, I.D., Revitt, D.M. & Hamilton, R.S. (1996) A comparison of carbonyl compound concentrations at urban roadside and indoor sites. *Sci. total Environ.*, **189/190**, 475–483

Wilmer, J.W.G.M., Woutersen, R.A., Appelman, L.M., Leeman, W.R. & Feron, V.J. (1987) Subacute (4-week) inhalation toxicity study of formaldehyde in male rats: 8-hour intermittent *versus* 8-hour continuous exposures. *J. appl. Toxicol.*, **7**, 15–16

Wilmer, J.W.G.M., Woutersen, R.A., Appelman, L.M., Leeman, W.R. & Feron, V.J. (1989) Subchronic (13-week) inhalation toxicity study of formaldehyde in male rats: 8-hour intermittent versus 8-hour continuous exposures. *Toxicol. Lett.*, **47**, 287–293

Wilson, R.T., Moore, L.E. & Dosemeci, M. (2004) Occupational exposures and salivary gland cancer mortality among African American and white workers in the United States. *J. occup. environ. Med.*, **46**, 287–297

Witek, T.J., Jr, Schachter, E.N., Tosun, T., Beck, G.J. & Leaderer, B.P. (1987) An evaluation of respiratory effects following exposure to 2.0 ppm formaldehyde in asthmatics: Lung function, symptoms, and airway reactivity. *Arch. environ. Health*, **42**, 231–237

Wolf, D.C., Gross, E.A., Lyght O., Bermudez, E., Recio, L. & Morgan, K. T. (1995) Immunohistochemical localization of p53, PCNA, and TGF-α proteins in formaldehyde-induced rat nasal squamous cell carcinomas. *Toxicol. appl. Pharmacol.*, **132**, 27–35

Wolkoff, P., Johnsen, C.R., Franck, C., Wilhardt, P. & Albrechtsen, O. (1992) A study of human reactions to office machines in a climatic chamber. *J. Expo. Anal. environ. Epidemiol.*, **Suppl. 1**, 71–96

Wong, O. (1983) An epidemiologic mortality study of a cohort of chemical workers potentially exposed to formaldehyde, with a discussion on SMR and PMR. In: Gibson, J.E., ed., *Formaldehyde Toxicity*, Washington DC, Hemisphere, pp. 256–272

Wortley, P., Vaughan, T.L., Davis, S., Morgan, M.S. & Thomas, D.B. (1992) A case–control study of occupational risk factors for laryngeal cancer. *Br. J. ind. Med.*, **49**, 837–844

Woutersen, R.A., Appelman, L.M., Wilmer, J.W.G.M., Falke, H.E. & Feron, V.J. (1987) Subchronic (13-week) inhalation toxicity study of formaldehyde in rats. *J. appl. Toxicol.*, **7**, 43–49

Woutersen, R.A., van Garderen-Hoetmer, A., Bruijntjes, J.P., Zwart, A. & Feron, V.J. (1989) Nasal tumours in rats after severe injury to the nasal mucosa and prolonged exposure to 10 ppm formaldehyde. *J. appl. Toxicol.*, **9**, 39–46

Wu, P.-C., Li, Y.-Y., Lee, C.-C., Chiang, C.-M. & Su, H.-J.J. (2003) Risk assessment of formaldehyde in typical office buildings in Taiwan. *Indoor Air*, **13**, 359–363

Yanysheva, N.A., Balenko, N.V., Chernichenko, I.A., Litvichenko, O.N., Sovertkova, L.S. & Babij, V.F. (1998) [Characteristics of modifying effects of formaldehyde on carcinogenesis.] *Gig. Sanit.*, **8**, 51–54 (in Russian)

Yasuhara, A. & Shibamoto, T. (1995) Quantitative analysis of volatile aldehydes formed from various kinds of fish flesh during heat treatment. *J. agric. Food Chem.*, **43**, 94–97

Yi, J., Zhang, J. & Gao, Y. (2000) [Experiment on effect of formaldehyde on sperm toxicity of mice] (Abstract). *Gongye Weisheng Yu Zhiyebing*, **26**, 263–264 (in Chinese)

Ying, C.-J., Yan, W.-S., Zhao, M.-Y., Ye, X.-L., Xie, H., Yin, S.-Y. & Zhu, X.-S. (1997) Micronuclei in nasal mucosa, oral mucosa and lymphocytes in students exposed to formaldehyde vapor in anatomy class. *Biomed. environ. Sci.*, **10**, 451–455

Ying, C.-J., Ye, X.-L., Xie, H., Yan, W.-S., Zhao, M.-Y., Xia, T. & Yin, S.-Y. (1999) Lymphocyte subsets and sister-chromatid exchanges in the students exposed to formaldehyde vapor. *Biomed. environ. Sci.*, **12**, 88–94

Yokoyama, A., Kato, H., Yokoyama, T., Tsujinaka, T., Muto, M., Omori, T., Haneda, T., Kumagai, Y., Igaki, H., Yokoyama, M., Watanabe, H., Fukuda, H. & Yoshimizu, H. (2002) Genetic polymorphisms of alcohol and aldehyde dehydrogenases and glutathione *S*-transferase M1 and drinking, smoking, and diet in Japanese men with esophageal squamous cell carcinoma. *Carcinogenesis*, **23**, 1851–1859

Youk, A.O., Marsh, G.M., Stone, R.A., Buchanich, J.M. & Smith, T.J. (2001) Historical cohort study of US man-made vitreous fiber production workers: III. Analysis of exposure-weighted measures of respirable fibers and formaldehyde in the nested case–control study of respiratory system cancer. *J. occup. environ. Med.*, **43**, 767–778

Zhang, J., Wilson, W.E. & Lloy, P.J. (1994) Indoor air chemistry: Formation of organic acids and aldehydes. *Environ. Sci. Technol.*, **28**, 1975–1982

Zhang, L., Chung, F.-L., Boccia, L., Colosimo, S., Liu, W. & Zhang, J. (2003) Effects of garage employment and tobacco smoking on breathing-zone concentrations of carbonyl compounds. *Am. ind. Hyg. Assoc. J.*, **64**, 388–393

Zheng, W., Blot, W.J., Shu, X.O., Diamond, E.L., Gao, Y.T., Ji, B.T. & Fraumeni, J.F., Jr (1992) A population-based case–control study of cancers of the nasal cavity and paranasal sinuses in Shanghai. *Int. J. Cancer*, **52**, 557–561

Zhitkovich, A. & Costa, M. (1992) A simple, sensitive assay to detect DNA–protein crosslinks in intact cells and *in vivo*. *Carcinogenesis*, **13**, 1485–1489

Zijlstra, J.A. (1989) Liquid holding increases mutation induction by formaldehyde and some other cross-linking agents in *Escherichia coli* K12. *Mutat. Res.*, **210**, 255–261

Zimmermann, F.K. & Mohr, A. (1992) Formaldehyde, glyoxal, urethane, methyl carbamate, 2,3-butanedione, 2,3-hexanedione, ethyl acrylate, dibromoacetonitrile and 2-hydroxypropionitrile induce chromosome loss in *Saccharomyces cerevisiae*. *Mutat. Res.*, **270**, 151–166

Zito, R. (1999) Cancer risk assessment of direct acting carcinogens. *J. exp. clin. Cancer Res.*, **18**, 273–278

Zwart, A., Woutersen, R.A., Wilmer, J.W.G.M., Spit, B.J. & Feron, V.J. (1988) Cytotoxic and adaptive effects in rat nasal epithelium after 3-day and 13-week exposure to low concentrations of formaldehyde vapour. *Toxicology*, **51**, 87–99

Zweidinger, R.B., Sigsby, J.E., Jr, Tejada, S.B., Stump, F.D., Dropkin, D.L., Ray, W.D. & Duncan, J.W. (1988) Detailed hydrocarbon and aldehyde mobile source emissions from roadway studies. *Environ. Sci. Technol.*, **22**, 956–962

GLYCOL ETHERS

2-BUTOXYETHANOL

1.   Exposure Data

1.1   Chemical and physical data

1.1.1   *Nomenclature*

Chem. Abstr. Serv. Reg. No.: 111-76-2
Chem. Abstr. Name: 2-Butoxyethanol
IUPAC Systematic Name: 2-Butoxyethanol
Synonyms: Butoxyethanol; β-butoxyethanol; *n*-butoxyethanol; 2-*n*-butoxyethanol; 2-butoxy-1-ethanol; 2-*n*-butoxy-1-ethanol; O-butyl ethylene glycol; butylglycol; butyl monoether glycol; EGBE; ethylene glycol butyl ether; ethylene glycol *n*-butyl ether; ethylene glycol monobutyl ether; ethylene glycol mono-*n*-butyl ether; glycol butyl ether; glycol monobutyl ether; monobutyl ether of ethylene glycol; monobutyl glycol ether; 3-oxa-1-heptanol

1.1.2   *Structural and molecular formulae and relative molecular mass*

$$H_3C—CH_2—CH_2—CH_2—O—CH_2—CH_2—OH$$

$C_6H_{14}O_2$ Relative molecular mass: 118.17

1.1.3   *Chemical and physical properties of the pure substance*

From Lide (2004) unless otherwise specified
(*a*)   *Description*: Liquid
(*b*)   *Boiling-point*: 168.4 °C
(*c*)   *Melting-point*: –74.8 °C
(*d*)   *Density*: 0.9015 g/mL at 20 °C
(*e*)   *Spectroscopy data*: Infrared and nuclear magnetic resonance (proton) spectral data have been reported (National Toxicology Program, 2000)

(*f*)   *Solubility*: Miscible with water, ethanol and diethyl ether; slightly soluble in carbon tetrachloride; soluble in mineral oil and most organic solvents (National Toxicology Program, 2000)

(*g*)   *Volatility*: Vapour pressure, 100 Pa or 0.6 mm Hg at 20 °C; relative vapour density (air = 1), 4.07 (Verschueren, 2001)

(*h*)   *Octanol/water partition coefficient (P)*: log P, 0.83 (Hansch *et al.*, 1995)

(*i*)   *Conversion factor*: mg/m^3 = 4.873 × ppm[1]

1.1.4   *Technical products and impurities*

2-Butoxyethanol is commercially available with the following specifications: purity, 99% min.; acidity (as acetic acid, % wt), 0.005–0.01 max.; water (% wt), 0.1 max.; peroxides (as oxygen), 10 mg/kg max.; ethylene glycol (% wt), 0.2–0.3 max.; n-butyl alcohol (% wt), 0.1 max.; diethylene glycol monobutyl ether (% wt), 0.1 max.; stabilizer (butylated hydroxytoluene), 376 ppm target or 0.1% max. (Eastman Chemical Co., 2000a,b; Dow Chemical Co., 2001; Shell Chemicals, 2002; Eastman Chemical Co., 2003; Shell Chemicals, 2004).

Trade names for 2-butoxyethanol include: Butyl Cellosolve®; n-Butyl Cellosolve®; Butyl Cellosolve® Solvent; Butyl Cellu-Sol; O-Butyl Ethylene Glycol; Butyl Glysolv; Butyl Oxitol®; Butyl Oxital® EB; C4E1; Chimec NR; Dowanol® EB; Eastman® EB; Eastman® EB Solvent; Ektasolve EB; Ektasolve EB Solvent; Gafcol EB; Glycol EB; Glycol Ether EB; Jeffersol EB; Minex BDH; Poly-Solv EB.

1.1.5   *Analysis*

Analytical methods suitable for the determination of 2-butoxyethanol in environmental matrices have been reviewed (ATSDR, 1998). These methods rely principally on adsorption onto charcoal or other suitable material, followed by gas chromatographic (GC) analysis with flame ionization (FID) or mass spectrometric (MS) detection. Lower limits of detection generally range from 0.1 to 2 ppm, depending on the specific analytical method employed and on the sampling procedure used (Boatman & Knaak, 2001). Typical methods include those from the Deutsche Forschungsgemeinschaft (1991), the National Institute for Occupational Safety and Health (2003), the Occupational Safety and Health Administration (1990) and the Institut national de Recherche et de Sécurité (INRS, 2002). Yoshikawa and Tani (2003) reported a reversed-phase high-performance liquid chromatography (HPLC) method with fluorescence detection after derivatization by treatment with 1-anthroylnitrile; the method detects 2-butoxyethanol in workplace air in the low parts per billion range (1–3 pg).

---

[1] Calculated from: mg/m^3 = (relative molecular mass/24.45) × ppm, assuming normal temperature (25 °C) and pressure (103.5 kPa)

Preparation methods for water samples are based on purge-and-trap (Michael *et al.*, 1988, 1991), solvent extractions (Jungclaus *et al.*, 1976; Yasuhara *et al.*, 1981; Nguyen *et al.*, 1994) or direct injection (Beihoffer & Ferguson, 1994). Eckel *et al.* (1996) noted the inefficiency of the common purge-and-trap and solvent extraction methods for the isolation of low-molecular-weight glycol ethers, and recommended instead the use of direct aqueous injection, extractive alkylation or salting-out extraction with derivatization with penta-fluorobenzoyl chloride.

Analytical methods for the determination of 2-butoxyethanol and its metabolites (2-butoxyacetic acid and conjugates) in biological matrices (blood and urine) have also been reviewed (Johanson, 1988; ATSDR, 1998). The methods generally involve extraction, derivatization and analysis by GC with FID, MS or electron capture detection (ECD), or HPLC with ultraviolet (UV) detection (Johanson *et al.*, 1986a; Begerow *et al.*, 1988; Johanson, 1989; Groeseneken *et al.*, 1989; Rettenmeier *et al.*, 1993; Sakai *et al.*, 1993, 1994; Bormett *et al.*, 1995). A more recent method (Shih *et al.*, 1999; Brown *et al.*, 2003) reported improved analysis of butoxyacetic acid in urine without derivatization.

Jones and Cocker (2003) reported that about half of the total 2-butoxyacetic acid in human urine is in the conjugated form, although the percentage is highly variable between and within individuals. The authors recommended total 2-butoxyacetic acid (after acid hydrolysis) in urine as the biomarker of choice to monitor exposure to 2-butoxyethanol.

1.2 Production and use

Glycol ethers began to be used in the 1930s and some have been in general use for nearly 50 years. They form a varied family of more than 30 solvents that commonly dissolve in both water and oil. Traditionally, a distinction is made between two main groups of glycol ethers: the E series and the P series, which derive from the name of the chemical substance that serves as a starting point for their production (ethylene and propylene, respectively). In each series, different derivatives have been developed to provide the properties of solubility, volatility, compatibility and inflammability that are required for different uses (Oxygenated Solvents Producers Association, 2004).

1.2.1 *Production*

Ethylene glycol ethers are manufactured in a closed, continuous process by reacting ethylene oxide with an anhydrous alcohol in the presence of a suitable catalyst. Depending on the molar ratios of the reactants and other process parameters, the mixtures obtained contain varying amounts of the monoethylene, diethylene, triethylene and higher glycol ethers. Typically, the products of these mixtures are separated and purified by fractional distillation (Boatman & Knaak, 2001).

Available information indicates that 2-butoxyethanol was produced by nine companies in China, seven companies in Germany, six companies in India, four companies in Japan, three companies in the USA, two companies each in Argentina, Mexico, Taiwan

(China) and the United Kingdom and one company each in Australia, Brazil, Poland, Russia, Slovakia and Spain (Chemical Information Services, 2004).

Since the early 1980s, 2-butoxyethanol has been the most widely produced and consumed glycol ether in the USA. Production estimates for 2-butoxyethanol in the USA from 1970 to 1999 are presented in Table 1.

Table 1. Production of 2-butoxyethanol in the USA from 1970 to 1999 (thousand tonnes)

1970	1975	1980	1985	1990	1995	1999
48.5	59.2	90.9	125.6	187.5	187.2	226.8

From Chinn *et al.* (2000)

1.2.2   Use

Because of their miscibility with water and with a large number of organic solvents, most ethylene glycol ethers are especially useful as solvents in oil–water compositions. This property, among others, leads to their use in numerous industrial (paints, pharmaceutical products, inks) and consumer (cosmetics, detergents) applications. Their relatively slow rate of evaporation also makes them useful as solvents and coalescing agents in paints. Other uses include inks, cleaning products, chemical intermediates, process solvents, brake fluids and de-icers (Boatman & Knaak, 2001).

Time trends in consumption of 2-butoxyethanol in the USA and western Europe are shown in Tables 2 and 3, respectively. In 1999, consumption in Japan was estimated at 27 600 tonnes (Chinn *et al.*, 2000). Some data on typical uses in Canada, the European Union and the USA are shown in Table 4.

Table 2. Trends in consumption for 2-butoxyethanol in the USA — 1980–99 (thousand tonnes)

	1980	1985	1990	1995	1999
Paints, coatings and inks	36.3	42.6	63.1	68.5	76.7
Metal and liquid household cleaners	11.8	14.5	19.0	21.3	20.4
Other uses	16.8	18.1	25.4	26.8	29.9
Production of 2-butoxyethanol acetate	4.5	6.4	6.4	5.9	6.8
Other production	0.9	4.5	5.9	6.8	7.7
Total	70.3	86.1	119.8	129.3	141.5

From Chinn *et al.* (2000)

Table 3. Trend in consumption of 2-butoxyethanol in selected western European countries[a] from 1987 to 1999 (thousand tonnes)

Year	1987	1991	1993	1995	1997	1999
Consumption	72	90	92	98	104	114

From Chinn et al. (2000)
[a] Countries include, in order of relevance: Austria, Switzerland, Sweden, Norway, Portugal, Finland, Denmark, Ireland and Greece.

Table 4. Typical uses of 2-butoxyethanol in selected regions and countries

Region/country Year	European Union [2001]	Canada 2002	USA [1997]
Industrial use	**87.3%**	**78%**	**61%**
Paints and coatings	75.8%	85%	
Cleaners	3.8%	8%	
Inks	6.4%	5%	
Other[a]	14.0%	2%	
Consumer use	**12.7%**	**22%**	**39%**
Cleaners	8.8%	47%	46%
Paints and coatings	91.2%	32%	32%
Solvents			21.5%
Polishes			0.5%
Other[b]		21%	

From OECD (1997); Boatman & Knaak (2001); ToxEcology Environmental Consulting Ltd (2003)
[a] Includes chemicals used in synthesis and the electronic, rubber and oil industries, agricultural products, adhesives, oil spill dispersants, leather finishing, fire foams, pharmaceuticals and construction materials.
[b] Includes consumer solvents, pesticides and personal care products.

The largest use for 2-butoxyethanol is as a solvent in surface coatings, especially water-based paints and varnishes. Other coatings include spray lacquers, quick-dry lacquers, enamels, varnishes and latex paint. Approximately 80% of 2-butoxyethanol consumed in surface coatings is used for industrial and specialty coatings; the remainder is used in architectural coatings (Chinn et al., 2000).

2-Butoxyethanol also is used as a mutual solvent and coupling agent to stabilize and solubilize immiscible ingredients in emulsion metal and liquid household cleaners. Other solvent applications include printing inks, industrial cleaning fluids, nitrocellulose resins, dry-cleaning compounds, rust-removing liquids, varnish removers, textile and mineral oils, as a formulation solvent for insecticides and herbicides, as a co-solvent in diesel fuel, and use in cosmetic products such as hair dyes, nail polishes, nail polish removers and skin cleansers (Chinn *et al.*, 2000; Boatman & Knaak, 2001; Environment Canada/Health Canada, 2002).

2-Butoxyethanol has a number of important applications as a chemical intermediate, notably to form esters of acetic acid, phthalic anhydride, phosphoric acid, adipic acid and several specialty herbicide products (e.g. the glycol ether esters of 2,4-D and 2,4,5-T) (Chinn *et al.*, 2000; Boatman & Knaak, 2001). It is also used as a component in phthalate and stearate plasticizers.

In the 1980s, 2-butoxyethanol was used in certain automotive brake fluids, but it has mostly been replaced by higher-boiling glycol ethers (Chinn *et al.*, 2000).

2-Butoxyethanol has been replaced in some of its applications by the P-series of glycol ethers, such as propylene glycol mono-*n*-butyl ether, dipropylene glycol mono-*n*-butyl ether and propylene glycol mono-*tert*-butyl ether. Relative consumption of E- and P-series glycol ethers differs by geographical region, ranging in 1999 from 55% E/45% P in western Europe to about 75% E/25% P in the USA and Japan and 94% E/6% P in Mexico (Chinn *et al.*, 2000).

1.3   Occurrence

1.3.1   *Natural occurrence*

2-Butoxyethanol is not known to occur as a natural product.

1.3.2   *Occupational exposure*

Occupational exposure to 2-butoxyethanol may occur during its manufacture and use as an intermediate in the chemical industry, and during the formulation and use of its products. The major routes of exposure are inhalation and skin absorption. Because 2-butoxyethanol is readily absorbed through the skin and has a relatively low vapour pressure, the dermal route may be predominant or may contribute significantly to overall exposure.

Exposure to 2-butoxyethanol by inhalation is well documented; recent high-quality reports prepared by national or international bodies are available (NICNAS, 1996; OECD, 1997; ATSDR, 1998).

Environmental monitoring of air concentrations in the breathing zone or in the work area has been found to be inadequate to assess overall exposures; measurements of total exposure to 2-butoxyethanol should take into account the respiratory uptake of vapours and aerosols and the dermal absorption of 2-butoxyethanol in liquid, vapour and aerosol form (NICNAS, 1996). Biological monitoring of the common urinary metabolite, 2-butoxyacetic acid, is recommended for a complete assessment of exposure (Angerer *et al.*, 1990; Johanson & Johnsson, 1991; Söhnlein *et al.*, 1993; Vincent *et al.*, 1993; Jones

& Cocker, 2003). For workers in high-exposure occupations who do not wear protective gloves, environmental sampling probably underestimates the exposure, and biomonitoring of urinary butoxyacetic acid appears to be the best method for estimating overall exposure.

Data from the National Occupational Exposure Survey (NOES) conducted in the USA by the National Institute for Occupational Safety and Health from 1980 to 1983 indicate that an estimated 2 139 000 workers in 2260 industrial/occupational categories were potentially exposed to 2-butoxyethanol (National Institute for Occupational Safety and Health, 1989; ATSDR, 1998). The NOES database does not contain information on the frequency, level or duration of exposure of workers to any chemical listed therein and does not reflect recent changes in US production. The numbers also do not include workers who were potentially exposed to trade-name compounds (observed in the NOES survey) that contain 2-butoxyethanol.

In Australia, 82 companies were identified that formulate 2-butoxyethanol into cleaning products, some of which produced cleaning products at more than one site; at least 200 workers were involved in the formulation in each company (NICNAS, 1996).

(a) Manufacture and use as an intermediate

2-Butoxyethanol is manufactured continuously, either full-time during the year or within specific periods of several weeks or months. Workers may be exposed for approximately 8 h per day on 5 days per week during specific periods, but, typically, no personnel works constantly at the plant, and fitters, engineers and other technical staff visit the plant occasionally only. The process is enclosed as extensive precautions are taken to prevent and minimize exposure of workers to the toxicity of the ethylene oxide feedstock (ECETOC, 1994; NICNAS, 1996; OECD, 1996).

Exposure during transfer to tankers or drums is generally minimized by the use of automated filling, where the operator is outside of the area during transfer, and the use of local exhaust ventilation. Accidental exposure may occur when the process is breached or when spills occur. Exposure may also occur during maintenance and cleaning activities; however, the prior purging of equipment is generally standard practice (OECD, 1996).

Measurements of airborne concentrations of 2-butoxyethanol provided by manufacturers and collected for the OECD assessment are reported in Table 5.

Measurements in a manufacturing plant in the USA during drum filling operations, the most probable source of exposure, showed levels of 1.7 ppm during area monitoring. The highest personal monitoring reading was 0.1 ppm (Clapp et al., 1984).

Eight-hour time-weighted average (TWA) personal exposures of 2-butoxyethanol in manufacturing plants in Europe were in the range of 0.01–0.4 ppm (production), 0.03–0.3 ppm (drum filling), 0.5–2.7 ppm (blending) and < 1.6 ppm (roadcar filling) (ECETOC, 1985).

Personal exposure measurements of 2-butoxyethanol at a number of production sites during 1988–93 showed concentrations in the range of 0.1–1.6 ppm and a mean of 0.13 ppm (ECETOC, 1994).

Table 5. Airborne concentrations[a] measured during the manufacture of 2-butoxyethanol

Plant location	Activity	No. of readings	Mean (ppm)	Maximum (ppm)
Australia	All (STEL and TWA, personal)		0.1	
	Maintenance (TWA, area)			1.8
European Union	Production	97	0.09	1.2
	Filling	66	1.3	5.3
	Technical unit	9	0.25	1.2
	Laboratory	14	1.3	11
	Various	8	0.5	2.7
European Union	All	311	< 0.1	1.6
European Union	Production	30	< 0.14	< 0.31
	Filling	10	< 0.14	0.22
	Laboratory sampling	20	< 0.38	1.1
USA	Production	16		< 0.04
	Tanker loading	11	< 0.25	1.8

From NICNAS (1996); OECD (1997)
STEL, short-term exposure limit; TWA, time-weighted average
[a] No indications were available as to whether they represent task measurements or 8-h time-weighted averages, except for the plant in Australia.

(b)   Formulation of products containing 2-butoxyethanol

Exposure during formulation strongly depends on the mixing process, which may be enclosed or relatively open. Information obtained from the national assessment of exposure to 2-butoxyethanol in Australia indicated that approximately 50% of formulators of cleaning products that contain 2-butoxyethanol carry out mixing in open-top tanks that provide greater potential for exposure (NICNAS, 1996). Workers are potentially exposed to 2-butoxyethanol for an average of 3 h per week (56% for ≤ 1 h per week; range, 0.1–20 h). For most formulators, 2-butoxyethanol is an ingredient of only some of their products, and therefore exposure is not continuous on a daily or weekly basis.

Personal exposures of 2-butoxyethanol during the formulation of products are presented in Table 6.

(c)   Painting, printing and use of inks and varnishes

Airborne concentrations of 2-butoxyethanol that were measured during painting and printing activities are summarized in Tables 7 and 8, respectively.

In a study performed from 1988 to 1993 (Vincent *et al.*, 1996), exposure measurements were made in 55 companies that covered 18 sectors of activity, including the principal use category of products that contain glycol ethers: paints, inks, diluents and varnishes (Table 9). Exposure of workers was measured by 8-h individual atmospheric sampling and

Table 6. Eight-hour time-weighted average personal exposures to butoxy-ethanol during formulation of products

Product	No. of samples	Mean (ppm)	Range (ppm)	Reference
Printing ink	9	< 1	NR	Winchester (1985)
Varnish	12[a]	1.1	< 0.1–8.1	Angerer *et al.* (1990)
Varnish	12[a] pre-shift	0.5	< 0.1–1.4	Söhnlein *et al.* (1993)
	12[a] post-shift	0.6	< 0.1–1	
Paints	4	1.3	0.41–3.13	Foo *et al.* (1994)
Paints	328	0.4	< 0.1–44.7	Vincent *et al.* (1996)
Paints	179	0.1	0.0–1.4	Wesolowski & Gromiec (1997)

NR, not reported
[a] No. of workers [no. of samples not stated]

biological monitoring of urine at the beginning and at the end of the shift. The people most heavily exposed to 2-butoxyethanol were workers in the area of cataphoresis, where the mean atmospheric exposure was 0.8 ppm, whose concentration of urinary butoxyacetic acid reached 210 mg/g creatinine.

In a survey of industrial solvents conducted in 1994–96 in Japan in 95 different plants (196 unit work areas; 1176 samples), 2-butoxyethanol was detected in 59 samples (eight samples taken in printing areas and 51 samples taken in painting areas) with a median atmospheric concentration of 0.5 ppm and a maximum concentration of 1.3 ppm (Yasugi *et al.*, 1998).

Exposure measurements (sampling period, 60–480 min) registered between 1987 and 1998 in the COLCHIC database in France were analysed by Vincent (1999). Results related to painting and coating are presented in Table 10, and those for the printing industry are given in Table 11.

Referring to the same COLCHIC database, 45 atmospheric personal samples were taken between 1987 and 1998 in the printing industry and resulted in an arithmetic mean concentration of 0.6 ppm (range, 0.02–5.3 ppm; median, 0.04 ppm; 95th percentile, 2.7 ppm) (Vincent, 1999). It should be noted that exposure to 2-butoxyethanol in the printing industry in France has significantly decreased from 1987–92 to 1993–98; the arithmetic mean for personal samples in 1987–92 was 1.4 ppm (median, 1.3 ppm; range, 0.02–6.6 ppm; 68 samples) and that in 1993–98 was 0.3 ppm (median, 0.1 ppm; range, 0.02–2.6 ppm; 79 samples) ($p < 0.01$) (Vincent & Jeandel, 1999).

In another study in France (Delest & Desjeux, 1995), exposures of 54 house painters were assessed by biological monitoring. Only three painters had urinary concentrations of butoxyacetic acid higher than the limit of detection (2 mg/g creatinine) and the maximum concentration was 13.2 mg/g. The main reasons for the low figures observed were the application technique (brush or roller) and the low content of 2-butoxyethanol in the products used (< 5%).

Table 7. Time-weighted average[a] personal exposures to 2-butoxyethanol during painting

Activity	No. of samples (no. of workers)	Mean (ppm)	Max. or range (ppm)	Reference
Furniture production/finishing	64	1.5	0.07–9.9	Zaebst (1984, cited in ATSDR, 1998)
Staining/varnishing of parquet	9[b]	5	71.8	Denkhaus et al. (1986)
Car repair	1[b]	1.2	NA	Veulemans et al. (1987)
General painting	10[b]	3.9	0.7–19.2	Veulemans et al. (1987)
House painting (water-based paints < 1.4% 2-butoxyethanol)	15	NR	0.4–12	Hansen et al. (1987)
Wood cabinet finishing	6 (3)	NR	ND–0.4	Newman & Klein (1990)
Automobile spray painting	8 (8)	0.4	0.2–0.6	Winder & Turner (1992)
Painting (water-based paints < 5 % 2-butoxyethanol)	(54)[b]	< 0.1	< 0.1–0.2	Delest & Desjeux (1995)
Indoor house painting (water-based paints)	20[c]	0.02	< 0.01–0.15	Norbäck et al. (1996)
Painting of plastic material (two plants)	79 (19)	< 0.1	< 0.1–0.8	Vincent et al. (1996)
Cataphoresis (two plants)[d]	66 (12)	0.8	< 0.1–6.2	
Varnishing metallic containers (three plants)	168 (79)	0.2	< 0.1–2.4	
Painting new vehicles (one plant)	39 (20)	< 0.1	< 0.1–0.5	
Can coating (three plants)	261 (143)	0.1	< 0.1–1.0	
Painting of metal frame (two plants)	50 (23)	< 0.1	< 0.1–0.3	
Painting of buildings (11 plants)	63 (63)	< 0.1	< 0.1–0.2	
Printed circuit boards varnishing (two plants)	57 (13)	< 0.2	< 0.1–2.8	
Can coating				Haufroid et al. (1997)
External decoration	20	0.7	0.4–1.3	
Inner protection	11	0.5	0.2–0.7	

NA, not applicable; ND, not detected [limit of detection not reported]; NR, not reported

[a] Unless stated otherwise

[b] Type of sampling not stated

[c] 2-Butoxyethanol found in two samples

[d] Electro-deposition of water-based anticorrosive agent

Table 8. Personal exposures to 2-butoxyethanol during printing

Activity	No. of samples (no. of workers)	Mean (ppm)	Range (ppm)	Content of 2-butoxyethanol (%); comments	Reference
Printing press operators	3	< 0.2	< 0.04–0.49	2% in cleaning printing press rollers	Lewis & Thoburn (1981); ATSDR (1998)
Label printing/plate makers and pressmen	7	[2]	1–2		Apol (1981)
Silkscreen printing and cleaning	6	3.4	1.1–5.2		Boiano (1983)
Silkscreen printing					Baker et al. (1985)
Silk screeners	16	6.8			
Spray printer	5	2.6			
Controls	6	0.3			
Silkscreen printing	3	4	3–5		Apol (1986)
Printing (various)	25[a]	0.8	0.3–3.6		Veulemans et al. (1987)
Printing press operators	1	NA	8		Lee (1988)
Silkscreen clean-up and maintenance	5	5.2	1.7–9.8	10–50% in hydrocarbon-based cleaning solvent	Salisbury et al. (1987)
Printing press operators	2	< 0.33	ND–0.53	2% in cleaning printing press rollers	Kaiser & McManus (1990); ATSDR (1998)
General printing	9	0.64	0.4–0.8		Sakai et al. (1993)
Tampography (three workshops)	84 (29)	0.2	< 0.1–0.7		Vincent et al. (1996)
Silkscreen (six workshops)	295 (110)	0.2	< 0.1–1.6		
Screen printing					Auffarth et al. (1998)
Semi automatic	5	0.5	0.3–0.9		
75% automatic	14	0.6	0.3–1.0		
Fully automatic	3	0.5	0.3–0.9		
Screen cleaning	5	0.6	0.2–0.7		

NA, not applicable; ND, not detected
[a] Type of sampling not stated

Table 9. Biological monitoring during the use of paints, inks and varnishes

Activity	No. of samples		Arithmetic mean urinary excretion (mg/g creatinine) of butoxyacetic acid (range)	
	Pre-shift	Post-shift	Pre-shift	Post-shift
Cataphoresis	51	51	6.3 (< 2–88.3)	17.9 (< 2–210)
Painting new vehicles	40	40	ND	ND
Automobile repainting	8	8	ND	ND
Aircraft repainting	28	28	ND	ND
Silk-screen painting	116	154	ND	ND
Tampography	48	48	< 2[a] (< 2–4.1)	2.2 (< 2–7.1)
Offset printing	9	11	3.2 (< 2–11.0)	2.2 (< 2–3.8)
Can coating	85	213	< 2[a] (< 2–13.6)	2.3 (< 2–28.4)
Varnishing metallic containers for foods	79	79	3.0 (< 2–38.2)	5.0 (< 2–33.9)
Manufacture of paints	112	300	2.2 (< 2–5.2)	3.9 (< 2–59.6)
Painting metal frames	47	46	4.3 (< 2–30.7)	9.4 (< 2–63.0)
Painting buildings	63	63	< 2 (< 2–9.1)	< 2 (< 2–13.2)
Manufacture of printed circuit boards	56	56	< 2 (< 2–15.7)	4.6 (< 2–30.4)
Staining and varnishing furniture	50	50	ND	2.9 (< 2–31.2)
Painting plastic materials	19	19	ND	ND

From Vincent *et al.* (1996)

ND, not detected (< 2 mg/L)

[a] The arithmetic mean was < 2 when calculated by replacing data below the limit of detection by half of the limit of detection.

Table 10. Personal exposures (60–480 min) to 2-butoxyethanol during painting and coating activities in 1987–98

Type of work	No. of positive samples	Mean (ppm)	Median (ppm)	Range (ppm)
Pneumatic coating with paint or varnish	58	0.47	0.2	0.04–4.3
Varnishing (curtain)	19	0.14	0.1	0.02–0.6
Brush or roll coating with paint or varnish	21	0.18	0.1	0.04–0.6
Electrodeposition	3	0.21	NR	0–0.6

From Vincent (1999)

NR, not reported

Table 11. Personal exposures (60–480 min) to 2-butoxyethanol during printing activities in 1987–98

Activity	No. of results	Mean (ppm)	Range (ppm)	Median (ppm)
Manual or automated screen printing	92	1.1	0.02–6.6	0.4
Screen cleaning	9	0.4	0.04–1.6	NR
Offset printing	13	0.3	0.02–1.2	0.04
General cleaning with solvents	2	2.6	1.2–3.9	NR
Flexography	20	0.08	0.04–0.1	0.1
'Rotogravure'	7	0.04	0.02–0.1	NR

From Vincent (1999)
NR, not reported

Twelve workers in a varnish production facility in Germany were found to be exposed to an average concentration of 1.1 ppm 2-butoxyethanol, and individual TWA exposures ranged from < 0.1 to 8.1 ppm. Biological monitoring of 2-butoxyethanol in the blood and butoxyacetic acid in the urine showed average post-shift concentrations of 121.3 µg/L and 10.5 mg/L, respectively. A markedly lower pre-shift concentration of butoxyacetic acid in the urine (3.3 mg/L) was reported. Most of the exposure was attributed to dermal absorption (Angerer *et al.*, 1990).

In another study in Germany, the occupational exposure to glycol ethers of 12 workers in the varnish production industry was evaluated. Urine samples of the workers were collected on the morning of the first day (pre-shift) and at the end of the second day (post-shift). Mean concentrations of 2-butoxyethanol from personal air samples were 0.5 ppm (range, < 0.1–1.4 ppm) on the first day and 0.6 ppm (range, < 0.1–1.0 ppm) on the second day. The mean urinary concentration of butoxyacetic acid was 0.2 mg/L (range, < 0.02–1.3 mg/L) on Monday pre-shift and 16.4 mg/L (range, 0.8–60.6 mg/L) on Tuesday post-shift (Söhnlein *et al.*, 1993).

(d)   Cleaning

Exposure during cleaning is extremely variable, due to differences in the frequency and duration of use of cleaning products, the strength of the solutions used, the method of application of the products and the precautions taken during their use. Monitoring data reported for cleaning activities are summarized in Table 12.

A study was conducted in France to evaluate the occupational exposure to 2-butoxyethanol of 16 office cleaners and 13 automobile cleaners who used window-cleaning agents (Vincent *et al.*, 1993). Table 13 shows the atmospheric concentrations of 2-butoxyethanol and the urinary concentrations of butoxyacetic acid in pre-shift and end-shift samples by occupation. Average urinary concentrations of butoxyacetic acid correlated well with work practices, i.e. with duration of use and daily quantity of window-cleaning agent used.

Table 12. Personal exposures to 2-butoxyethanol during cleaning activities

Activity	No. of samples (no. of workers)	Mean (ppm)	Range (ppm)	% 2-Butoxyethanol; comments	Reference
Window cleaning in hospitals	(4)	< 0.2	< 0.2	Cleaner applied in spray	Apol & Cone (1983)
Cleaning in food plant	(1)		1.6	0.3%; mechanical floor scrubbing, 95-min sampling	Apol & Johnson (1979)
School cleaning	(4)[a]		< 0.7	0.25%; cleaner applied in liquid and	Rhyder (1992), cited in NICNAS (1996)
			< 0.2	spray form	Vincent et al. (1993)
Window cleaning					
Cleaning cars					
Garage A	10 (2)	[0.5]	< 0.1–1.2	14.4%; 0.8–5-h exposure	
Garage B	10 (6)	[0.83]	< 0.1–2.8	21.2%; 0.3–4-h exposure	
Garage C	6 (3)	< 0.1	NR	5.7%; 0.7–2-h exposure	
Garage D	4 (2)	4.9	2.9–7.3	21.2%; 5.3-h exposure	
Office cleaners[b]					
Group A	32 (8)	0.32	< 0.3–0.73	9.8%; 15-min exposure	
Group B	8 (2)	< 0.3	NR	0.9%; 15-min exposure	

Adapted from NICNAS (1996)
NR, not reported
[a] Area monitoring
[b] Half-day shift air samples

Table 13. Results of air and biological sampling for 2-butoxyethanol during cleaning activities

| Job category | Air concentration of 2-butoxyethanol (ppm) | | | Urinary concentration of butoxyacetic acid (mg/g creatinine) | | | | | |
| | | | | Pre-shift | | | End of shift | | |
	No. of samples	AM	Range	No. of samples	AM	Range	No. of samples	AM	Range
Cleaner of new cars	15	2.33	<0.10–7.33	14	17.9	<2–98.6	12	111.3	12.7–371.0
Cleaner of used cars	15	0.36	<0.10–1.52	12	4.8	<2–33	11	6.3	<2–24.4
Office cleaner	32	0.32	<0.30–0.73	32	2.1	<2–4.6	32	2.1	2–3.3

From Vincent et al. (1993)
AM, arithmetic mean

Among workers with the highest exposures, the average TWA concentration of 2-butoxy-ethanol was 2.33 ppm and the maximum urinary concentration of butoxyacetic acid reached 371 mg/g creatinine. Butoxyacetic acid was detected in only three of the 32 post-shift urine samples of the office cleaners. Pre-shift concentrations were generally < 10 mg/g creatinine; however, an isolated reading of 99 mg/g and a few readings of approximately 30 mg/g were obtained for car cleaners (Vincent *et al.*, 1993).

(*e*) Offices

2-Butoxyethanol was measured in indoor air samples at 70 office buildings across the USA in 1991. 2-Butoxyethanol was detected in 24% of the samples from 50 telecommunications offices at concentrations up to 33 μg/m^3 [6.7 ppb] (geometric mean [GM], 0.1 μg/m^3 [0.02 ppb]), in 44% of the samples from nine data centres at concentrations up to 16 μg/m^3 (GM, 0.2 μg/m^3 [0.04 ppb]) and in 73% of the samples from 11 administrative offices at concentrations up to 32 μg/m^3 [6.6 ppb] (GM, 1.0 μg/m^3 [0.2 ppb]). In contrast, 70 samples of outdoor air collected in the immediate vicinities of these office buildings were below the limit of detection of 0.05 μg/m^3 [0.01 ppb] (Shields *et al.*, 1996).

Indoor air was sampled in 1990 in 12 office buildings in the San Francisco Bay area (USA). Concentrations of 2-butoxyethanol ranged from below the limit of detection (1.9 μg/m^3 [0.39 ppb]) to 130 μg/m^3 [26.6 ppb]. The GM concentration was 7.7 μg/m^3 [1.6 ppb] in indoor air compared with < 1.9 μg/m^3 [0.39 ppb] in the air outside these buildings (Daisey *et al.*, 1994).

(*f*) Miscellaneous data

From 1987 to 1998, the French COLCHIC database collected the results of 10 593 samplings of glycol ethers from 620 facilities. 2-Butoxyethanol was detected in 1195 samples; the arithmetic mean (AM) concentration of the 60–480-min personal samplings (347 results) was 0.64 ppm (median, 0.10 ppm; range, 0.02–22.6 ppm) (Vincent, 1999). It should be noted that, globally, personal exposure concentrations have significantly decreased from 1987–92 (147 samples; AM, 1.1 ppm; median, 0.6 ppm; range, 0.02–11.0 ppm) to 1993–98 (178 samples; AM, 0.3 ppm; median, 0.1 ppm; range, 0.02–3.9 ppm) (Vincent & Jeandel, 1999).

Exposure to 2-butoxyethanol was monitored in a 1983 survey of 336 industries and workshops in Belgium (Veulemans *et al.*, 1987). 2-Butoxyethanol was found in 25 of 94 air samples from sites that used printing pastes, in 10 of 81 samples where painting was carried out, in one of 20 samples from automobile repair shops and in 17 of 67 samples from various other industries (production and distribution of chemicals, production and sterilization of medical equipment and cleaning agents). The GM atmospheric concentrations and ranges of 2-butoxyethanol at various sites were: printing shops, 0.8 ppm (range, 0.3–3.6 ppm); painting areas, 3.9 ppm (range, 0.7–19.2 ppm); automobile repair shops, 1.2 ppm (one sample); various other industries, 1.7 ppm (range, < 0.1–367 ppm) (the data that relate to painting and printing activities are also presented in Tables 7 and 8, respectively).

Exposure of 53 hairdressers who worked in 10 workshops was evaluated. The composition of 43 products was analysed; 2-butoxyethanol was detected in eight products at concentrations of 0.5–5% by volume. No solvent was detected in the air samples (Vincent *et al.*, 1996).

Six personal exposure measurements made during the removal of mastic that contained asbestos showed 2-butoxyethanol concentrations in the range of 8–107 mg/m^3 [2–22 ppm] with a mean of 56.5 mg/m^3 [12 ppm] (Kelly, 1993).

Exposure levels of workers who used soluble cutting oils that contained 2-butoxy-ethanol were relatively low; the range of butoxyacetic acid concentrations in post-shift urine samples was in the order of < 2–8.3 mg/g creatinine (Vincent *et al.*, 1996).

1.3.3   *Environmental occurrence*

(*a*)   *Air*

According to data reported under the CEPA Section 16 survey, 319 tonnes of 2-butoxyethanol were released into the air in Canada in 1996, while 63 tonnes were released as waste, 6.5 tonnes were released into landfills and 2 tonnes were released into water (Environment Canada, 1997, cited in Environment Canada/Health Canada, 2002).

Reported levels of 2-butoxyethanol in three samples of ambient air taken from a remote site in Nepal ranged from 0.1 to 1.6 µg/m^3; in forested areas in Germany (one sample) and Italy (one sample), concentrations were 1.3 µg/m^3 and 0.4 µg/m^3, respectively (Ciccioli *et al.*, 1993). In a later study (Ciccioli *et al.*, 1996), levels of 2-butoxyethanol in samples from six sites near the Italian base on Terra Nova Bay, Antartica, ranged from 1.3 to 14.9 µg/m^3. [The source of these unexpectedly high levels is unknown.]

The US Environmental Protection Agency's national volatile organic compounds database, which includes data on indoor air in non-industrial offices (residential and commercial), showed an average level of 0.214 ppb (median, 0.075 ppb) in 14 samples that contained 2-butoxyethanol (Shah & Singh, 1988).

Concentrations of 2-butoxyethanol were measured in the indoor air of flats in France (CSHPF, 2002; Gourdeau *et al.*, 2002; Kirchner, 2002; European Union, 2004). Preliminary results indicate that the 90th percentiles were 3 µg/m^3 in the bedroom of a flat that had a maximum value of 14 µg/m^3, and 3.5 µg/m^3 in the kitchen of a flat that had a maximum value of 23 µg/m^3. Releases from building materials were also evaluated. Simulations were made by installing new carpets or new floor coverings or by applying paints to the walls of reference rooms. After 24 h, the concentrations of 2-butoxyethanol in air ranged from below the limit of detection to 3.8 µg/m^3 (mean, 1.7 µg/m^3; standard deviation [SD], 1.5 µg/m^3) when release from carpets was tested. After 28 days, they ranged from undetectable to 23.3 µg/m^3 (mean, 6.1 µg/m^3; SD, 9.0 µg/m^3). With other categories of floor coverings, concentrations ranged from undetectable to 5.6 µg/m^3 (mean, 2.5 µg/m^3; SD, 2.7 µg/m^3) after 24 h and from undetectable to 59.6 µg/m^3 (mean, 27.5 µg/m^3; SD, 30.9 µg/m^3) after 28 days. Release by paint applied to the wall was at undetectable values after 24 h and reached 24 and 298 μg/m³, respectively, for the two paints tested 28 days after application.

(b)   Drinking-water, groundwater and surface water

2-Butoxyethanol was listed as a contaminant in drinking-water samples analysed between September 1974 and January 1980 in a survey of cities in the USA (Lucas, 1984, cited in ATSDR, 1998).

2-Butoxyethanol was detected in 68% of 50 drinking-water samples (limit of detection, 0.02 μg/L) collected from Ontario, Nova Scotia and Alberta, Canada, in 1997. Concentrations ranged from below the limit of detection to 0.94 μg/L, with a mean concentration of 0.21 μg/L. The authors mentioned that, due to limitations of the analytical methods involved, confidence in the results of this study is low (Environment Canada/Health Canada, 2002).

Leachate from municipal landfills and hazardous waste sites can release 2-butoxyethanol into groundwater (Brown & Donnelly, 1988). Concentrations of 2-butoxyethanol in aqueous samples from a municipal and an industrial landfill in the USA ranged from < 0.4 to 84 mg/L (Beihoffer & Ferguson, 1994). 2-Butoxyethanol was detected at a concentration of 23 μg/L in one of seven groundwater samples collected near the Valley of Drums, KY, USA, in February 1974 (Stonebreaker & Smith, 1980, cited in ATSDR, 1998).

Water samples taken from a polluted river in Japan (Hayashida River, where effluent enters the river from the leather industry) in 1980 contained 2-butoxyethanol at a concentration of 1310–5680 μg/L (Yasuhara et al., 1981).

Environment Canada/Health Canada (2002) have estimated that the average daily intake of 2-butoxyethanol from air and drinking-water for the general Canadian population ranges from 5 to 15 μg/kg bw for various age groups, and that the major contributor is indoor air.

(c)   Occurrence in consumer products

Typical percentage concentrations (ranges) of 2-butoxyethanol in various consumer products are summarized in Table 14.

Emissions of 2-butoxyethanol from 13 consumer products purchased in the Ottawa, Ontario, area were recently investigated by Health Canada (Cao, 1999; Zhu et al., 2001). Products were selected on the basis of their likelihood to contain 2-butoxyethanol. 2-Butoxyethanol was detected in emissions from seven products, including cleaners, nail polish remover and hair colourant, at rates of up to 876 mg/m²/h. Analyses of the products indicated that the cleaners contained 0.5–3.7% 2-butoxyethanol, while the nail polish remover and hair colourant contained 3.8% and 25%, respectively (Environment Canada/Health Canada, 2002).

In the Swedish product register (KEMI, 2002, cited in European Union, 2004), 882 products that contain 2-butoxyethanol have been identified, of which 58% are paints or inks, 16% are cleaning agents, 8% are antirust agents and 8% are polishing agents.

Table 14. Typical levels of 2-butoxyethanol in consumer products (%)

Paints and coatings	2–25
Surface cleaners	0.1–71
Polishes	5–10
Floor strippers	< 1–30.5
Glass and window cleaners	< 1–40
Degreasers	5–15
Carpet cleaners	< 1–30
Laundry detergent	< 1.5–30
Rust removers	< 10–60
Oven cleaners	< 1–30
Ink and resin removers	1–93
Other (including solvents, pesticides and personal care products)	0.1–94

From NICNAS (1996); Boatman & Knaak (2001); ToxEcology Environmental Consulting Ltd (2003)

In the Danish product register (Arbejdstilsynet, 2001), 1204 products that contain 2-butoxyethanol have been identified, of which 76 were private household products. The most common products were paints and varnishes (37%), cleaning/washing agents (20%), surface treatments (8%), corrosion inhibitors (6%), surface active agents (3%), adhesives/binding agents (3%) and solvents (2%).

Data extracted from the French product register SEPIA (INRS, 2003, cited in European Union, 2004) showed that 368 of the 10 345 products registered between 1997 and 2003 contained 2-butoxyethanol. The main use categories were paints, varnishes and inks (39%), cleaning agents (37%) and products for metallurgical and mechanical sectors, e.g. grease cleaners (14%).

Twenty-seven water-based paints and formulations used in the French automotive industry have been analysed (Jargot et al., 1999). 2-Butoxyethanol was found in 18 samples at concentrations ranging from traces to 40%; in thinners, the concentration ranged from 0 to 24.7%.

Concentrations of 2-butoxyethanol in window-cleaning preparations used by car and office cleaners ranged from 0.9 to 21.2% by volume (Vincent et al., 1993).

(d)   Miscellaneous

Potential exposure has been linked to the stoppers of bottles used for perfusion in medicine that are made with natural or artificial rubber. Chemicals used in rubber formulations can leach from rubber stoppers during sterilization and enter the bloodstream of patients when the perfusion is administered. Results indicated a release of 70 and 65 μg/150 mL 2-butoxyethanol from two dextrose solutions and a release of 13 μg/500 mL 2-butoxyethanol from a sodium bicarbonate solution (Danielson, 1992).

1.4   Regulations and guidelines

Occupational exposure limits and guidelines for 2-butoxyethanol in workplace air are presented in Table 15.

Germany recommends a biological tolerance value for occupational exposure to 2-butoxyethanol of 100 mg/L butoxyacetic acid in urine, and recommends that butoxy-acetic acid in urine collected for long-term exposures after several shifts be monitored as an indicator of exposure to 2-butoxyethanol (Deutsche Forschungsgemeinschaft, 2003).

The Health and Safety Executive (2002) in the United Kingdom recommends a biological monitoring guidance value for occupational exposure to 2-butoxyethanol of 240 mmol butoxyacetic acid/mol creatinine in urine [roughly equivalent to 200 mg/L butoxyacetic acid] measured after a shift.

In the European Union, 2-butoxyethanol is environmentally regulated as part of the Volatile Compounds Directive (European Union, 1999).

2.   Studies of Cancer in Humans

In a case–control study at eight haematology departments in France, Hours *et al.* (1996) identified all locally resident patients aged 25–75 years who had acute myeloid leukaemia or myelodysplasia with an excess of blastoids that was newly diagnosed during January 1991–April 1993. The controls were patients from the same hospitals, matched for age (± 3 years), department of residence and nationality (French or other), who had never been hospitalized for cancer or an occupational disease. All subjects were interviewed in hospital by a trained investigator and were asked about their occupational history, including details of tasks and products handled. An occupational hygieniest who was blinded to the case/control status reviewed the information and classified the subject for exposure to each of four categories of glycol ethers, as well as to various potentially confounding substances. Analysis was by conditional logistic regression, and was based on 198 case–control pairs. After adjustment for level of education, exposure to the group of glycol ethers that included 2-butoxyethanol was associated with an odds ratio of 0.64 (95% confidence interval [CI], 0.31–1.29), based on 20 exposed cases and 27 exposed controls. [The Working Group noted that the exposure category analysed included propyl and butyl glycol ethers. Furthermore, the high prevalence of exposure among controls (27/191) suggests that the index of exposure used was relatively non-specific.]

Table 15. Occupational exposure limits and guidelines for 2-butoxyethanol

Country or region	Concentration (ppm) [mg/m³]	Interpretation	Carcinogen classification
Australia	25	TWA	Sk[a]
Austria	20 [100]	TWA	
	40 [200]	STEL	
Belgium	20	TWA	Sk
	50	STEL	
Canada			
(Alberta)	20	TWA	Sk
	75	STEL	Sk
(British Columbia)	25	TWA	Sk
(Ontario)	20	TWA	Sk
(Quebec)	25	TWA	Sk
Brazil	39	TWA	
Czech Republic	[100]	TWA	Sk
	[200]	STEL	
Denmark	20	TWA	Sk
European Commission	20	TWA	Sk
	50	STEL	
Finland	20 [98]	TWA	Sk
	50 [250]	STEL	
France	2 [9.8]	TWA	Sk
	30 [147.6]	STEL	
Germany (MAK)	20 [98]	TWA	Sk
	80	Ceiling	
Hong Kong	25	TWA	Sk
Ireland	20	TWA	Sk
	50	STEL	
Italy	20 [97]	TWA	
Malaysia	20	TWA	Sk
Mexico	26	TWA	Sk
	75	STEL	
Netherlands	20	TWA	Sk
	40	STEL	
New Zealand	25	TWA	Sk
Norway	10	TWA	Sk
Poland	[98]	TWA	Sk
	[200]	STEL	
South Africa	25	TWA	Sk
Spain	20	TWA	Sk
	50	STEL	
Sweden	10	TWA	Sk
	20	STEL	
Switzerland	20 [100]	TWA	Sk
	80 [400]	STEL	

Table 15 (contd)

Country or region	Concentration (ppm) [mg/m³]	Interpretation	Carcinogen classification
United Kingdom (OES)	25	TWA	Sk
	50	STEL	Sk
USA			
ACGIH (TLV)	20	TWA	A3[b]
NIOSH (REL)	5	TWA	Sk
OSHA (PEL)	50	TWA	Sk

From Arbejdstilsynet (2002); Health & Safety Executive (2002); Työsuojelusää-döksiä (2002); Deutsche Forschungsgemeinschaft (2003); Suva (2003); ACGIH Worldwide (2004); European Union (2004); INRS (2005)
MAC/MAK, maximum allowable concentration; OES, occupational exposure standard; PEL, permissible exposure limit; REL, recommended exposure limit; STEL, short-term exposure limit; TLV, threshold limit value; TWA, full-shift time-weighted average
[a] Sk, skin notation
[b] A3, confirmed animal carcinogen with unknown relevance to humans

3.   Studies of Cancer in Experimental Animals

3.1   Inhalation

3.1.1   *Mouse*

Groups of 50 male and 50 female B6C3 F_1 mice, 7–8 weeks of age, were exposed to 2-butoxyethanol (> 99% pure) vapour by whole-body exposure at concentrations of 0, 62.5, 125 or 250 ppm [0, 302, 604 or 1208 mg/m³] for 6 h per day on 5 days per week for 104 weeks. Complete necropsies were performed on all mice, at which time all organs and tissues were examined for macroscopic lesions and all major tissues were examined microscopically. Survival of male mice exposed to 125 or 250 ppm was significantly lower (by pair-wise comparison) than that of the control group (39/50 controls, 39/50 low-dose, 27/50 mid-dose ($p = 0.021$) and 26/50 high-dose ($p = 0.015$)). In females, survival was not affected (29/50 controls, 31/50 low-dose, 33/50 mid-dose and 36/50 high-dose). The body weights in control and treated animals were comparable except in high-dose female mice in which a 17% decrease in body weight was observed. In males, the incidences of haeman-giosarcoma of the liver were: 0/50 (control), 1/50 (low-dose), 2/49 (mid-dose) and 4/49 (high-dose). The incidence in high-dose males (250 ppm) was significantly increased ($p = 0.046$, Poly-3 test) relative to controls and the trend test was positive ($p = 0.014$, Poly-3 test); this incidence exceeded the range in the historical control values (0–4%). Two of the four mice treated with 250 ppm that had liver haemangiosarcomas also had haemangiosarcomas in either the bone marrow and heart or bone marrow and spleen; it was not possible to determine whether these were primary or metastatic tumours. One liver haemangiosarcoma developed in a low-dose female mouse. In female mice, dose-related increases in the incidence of forestomach squamous-cell papilloma were observed (0/50 control, 1/50 low-dose, 2/50 mid-dose and 5/50 high-dose). There was a single fore-stomach squamous-cell carcinoma in the high-dose group only. The combined incidence of forestomach squamous-cell papillomas and carcinoma was significantly increased ($p = 0.034$, Poly-3 test) in the high-dose group (250 ppm) and the trend was positive ($p = 0.002$; Poly-3 test); the incidence exceeded the range (0–3%) in historical controls. In males, the incidences of forestomach squamous-cell papillomas were 1/50 control, 1/50 low-dose, 2/49 mid-dose and 2/49 high-dose animals. One squamous-cell carcinoma deve-loped in the mid-dose group. The incidence in treated males was not significantly different from that in controls. Accompanying these neoplasms in females and, to a lesser extent, in males were exposure-related increases in the incidences of ulcer and epithelial hyperplasia of the forestomach. In addition, there was a possible exposure-related increase in the inci-dence of hepatocellular carcinoma in high-dose males (control, 10/50; low-dose, 11/50; mid-dose, 16/49; and high-dose, 21/49; $p \leq 0.01$, Poly-3 test) (National Toxicology Program, 2000).

3.1.2 *Rat*

Groups of 50 male and 50 female Fischer 344/N rats, 7–8 weeks of age, were exposed to 2-butoxyethanol (> 99% pure) vapour by whole-body exposure at concentrations of 0, 31.2, 62.5 or 125 ppm [0, 151, 302 or 604 mg/m^3] for 6 h per day on 5 days per week for 104 weeks. Complete necropsies were performed on all rats, at which time all organs and tissues were examined for macroscopic lesions and all major tissues were examined micros-copically. No exposure-related adverse effects on survival were observed. The survival rates in males were 19/50 (control), 11/50 (low-dose), 21/50 (mid-dose) and 24/50 (high-dose), and those in females were 29/50 (control), 27/50 (low-dose), 23/50 (mid-dose) and 21/50 (high-dose). No exposure-related increases in the incidence of tumours was found in males. In females, the incidences of benign pheochromocytomas in the adrenal medulla were 3/50 (control), 4/50 (low-dose), 1/49 (mid-dose) and 7/49 (high-dose). In addition, one malignant pheochromocytoma developed in the high-dose (125-ppm) group. The combined incidence of benign and malignant tumours in females had a positive trend ($p = 0.044$, Poly-3 test); however, the incidence in females exposed to 125-ppm was not significantly increased relative to that in concurrent controls, but slightly exceeded the range for historical controls (2–13%) from 2-year inhalation studies. Overall, the slight increase in incidences of pheo-chromocytomas was considered to be an equivocal finding and could not be attributed with certainty to exposure to 2-butoxyethanol (National Toxicology Program, 2000).

4.   Other Data Relevant to an Evaluation of Carcinogenicity and its Mechanisms

4.1   Absorption, distribution, metabolism and excretion

4.1.1   *Toxicokinetics*

(*a*)   *Humans*

2-Butoxyethanol is well absorbed by ingestion, inhalation and through the skin.

Several cases of ingestion of 2-butoxyethanol from suicide attempts have been reported (see Table 16). Rambourg-Schepens *et al.* (1988) described a case report of a suicide attempt by ingestion of 250–500 mL of a window cleaner that contained 12% 2-butoxyethanol. The subject survived but had moderate haemoglobinuria on the 3rd day and peak urinary levels of butoxyacetic acid of approximately 40 g/g creatinine [estimated from a graph]. In another report that involved the ingestion of 8 oz (8×28.4 cm^3 = 227.2 mL) of a cleaner that contained 10–30% 2-butoxyethanol and 10–40% isopropanol, the peak blood concentration of butoxyacetic acid was 900 µg/L (6.8 µM) and declined with a half-life of 12.7 h in samples collected 100 min after ingestion and at different times over 3 days (McKinney *et al.*, 2000). [This is longer than other reported half-lives and may be due to simultaneous treatment of the patient with ethanol to inhibit metabolism.] The subject survived with no reported haemolysis. A third case also involved ingestion of 360–480 mL of a window cleaner that contained 22% 2-butoxyethanol. The highest measured blood concentration of butoxyacetic acid was 4.86 mM in samples collected approximately 16 h after ingestion and at different times over 3 days (Gualtieri *et al.*, 2003).

The blood-to-air partition coefficient of 2-butoxyethanol was reported to be 7965 (Johanson & Dynésius, 1988) and, as a consequence, it is well absorbed by inhalation. Kumagai *et al.* (1999) measured the concentration of 2-butoxyethanol in inspired and expired air of four volunteers exposed to 25 ppm [120.5 mg/m^3] for 10 min at rest and found that 80% of the 2-butoxyethanol was absorbed. Johanson *et al.* (1986a) exposed seven male volunteers by inhalation to 20 ppm [96.4 mg/m^3; 0.85 mmol/m^3] 2-butoxyethanol for 2 h during physical exercise. Respiratory uptake averaged 10.1 µmol/min or 57% of the amount inspired. The concentration of 2-butoxyethanol in blood reached a plateau of 7.4 µmol/L after 1–2 h and the apparent elimination half-life was 40 min. Jones and Cocker (2003) reported a similar apparent elimination half-life of 2-butoxyethanol from blood of 56 min (range, 41–84 min) after exposure of four volunteers to 50 ppm [241 mg/m^3] 2-butoxy-ethanol for 2 h at rest. Peak levels of the metabolite butoxyacetic acid were seen in blood 20 min after the 2-h exposure with a mean concentration of 35 µM (range, 28–43 µM) that declined with a half-life of 13 min (range, 2–42 min). Johanson *et al.* (1986a) reported that

Table 16. Toxic effects of 2-butoxyethanol after its ingestion by humans

Reference	Subject	Glass cleaner (% of 2-butoxyethanol)	Syndrome
Rambourg-Schepens et al. (1988)	50-year-old woman	250–500 mL (12%, ~30–60 g)	Deep coma, poor ventilation, metabolic acidosis, hypokalaemia, haemoglobinuria, oxoluria
Gijsenbergh et al. (1989)	23-year-old woman	~500 mL; estimated absorbed samples, 200–250 mL (12.7%, ~25–30 g)	Coma, hypotension, metabolic acidosis, anaemia, haematuria
Litovitz et al. (1991)	87-year-old woman	Unknown amount (6.5%)	Coma, hypotension, metabolic acidosis, hepatic and renal failure
Bauer et al. (1992)	53-year-old man	500 mL (9.1%, 45.5 g)	Coma, metabolic acidosis, non-cardiogenic pulmonary oedema
Nisse et al. (1998)	52-year-old woman	150 mL (9.1%, 13.65 g)	Poor ventilation, metabolic acidosis, renal injury
Burkhart & Donovan (1998)	19-year-old man	568–852 mL (25–35%, 113–255 g)	Neurotoxicity, lethargy, deep coma, hypotension, metabolic acidosis, aspiration pneumonitis
McKinney et al. (2000)	51-year-old woman	227 mL (10–30%, ~22.7–68 g)	Vomiting, lethargy, metabolic acidosis, hypotension
Osterhoudt (2002)	16-month-old girl	Unknown quantity (10–30%)	Mental state depression, metabolic acidosis
Gualtieri et al. (2003)	18-year-old man	360–480 mL (22%, ~80–105.6 g)	Central nervous system depression, metabolic acidosis

total blood clearance of 2-butoxyethanol was 1.2 L/min and that the steady-state volume of distribution was 54 L.

In-vivo studies have investigated the dermal absorption of 2-butoxyethanol liquid (Johanson et al., 1988; Jakasa et al., 2004) and vapours (Johanson & Bowman, 1991; Corely et al., 1997; Jones et al., 2003). Johanson et al. (1988) conducted experiments of dermal exposure among five male volunteers; two or four of their fingers were exposed to neat 2-butoxyethanol for 2 h. Capillary blood samples were collected from the other arm and were analysed for 2-butoxyethanol. Urine was collected for 24 h and analysed for butoxyacetic acid. The percutaneous uptake rates of 2-butoxyethanol ranged from 7 to 96 nmol/min/cm^2. The authors estimated that, on average, 17% of the absorbed dose was excreted as butoxyacetic acid within 24 h. However, their method for determining butoxyacetic acid did not include hydrolysis of the glutamine conjugate and may therefore underestimate the total amount of butoxyacetic acid excreted. The percutaneous uptake rate ranged from 1 to 16 μmol/min when four fingers were exposed while the respiratory rate ranged from 8 to 14 (average, 10) μmol/min when the same volunteers were exposed to 20 ppm [96.4 mg/m³; 0.85 mmol/m³] butoxyethanol vapour during light work (Johanson *et al.*, 1986a).

In a more recent study, six male volunteers were exposed by dermal application twice to 50%, once to 90% or once to undiluted (neat) 2-butoxyethanol for 4 h on a 40-cm² area of skin. Inhalation exposure with a known input rate and duration was used as a reference dose. Dermal absorption parameters were calculated from 24-h excretion of total (free plus conjugated) butoxyacetic acid in urine and 2-butoxyethanol in blood, measured after both inhalation and dermal exposures. These exposures correlated to pulmonary uptake and dermal uptake. The dermal absorption of 2-butoxyethanol was higher from the aqueous solutions than from neat 2-butoxyethanol. The dermal fluxes obtained from 24-h cumulative excretion of butoxyacetic acid were 1.34 ± 0.49, 0.92 ± 0.6 and 0.26 ± 0.17 mg/cm²/h for 50%, 90% and neat 2-butoxyethanol, respectively. The permeation rates into the blood reached a plateau between 60 and 120 min after the start of exposure, which indicated the achievement of steady-state permeation. The apparent permeability coefficient was $1.75 \pm 0.53 \times 10^{-3}$ and $0.88 \pm 0.42 \times 10^{-3}$ cm/h for 50% and 90% 2-butoxyethanol, respectively. These results show that percutaneous absorption of 2-butoxyethanol increases markedly in aqueous solutions and that a water content as low as 10% can increase permeation rates fourfold. The uptake after dermal exposure to aqueous solutions substantially exceeds pulmonary uptake (Jakasa *et al.*, 2004).

In-vitro studies with human epidermal membranes in glass diffusion cells with water as a receptor fluid show steady-state absorption rates of 0.198 ($\pm$ 0.7) mg/cm²/h for neat 2-butoxyethanol applied as an infinite dose. The permeability constant was 2.14×10^4 cm/h and the lag time was less than 1 h (Dugard *et al.*, 1984). Lower rates of absorption were seen with full thickness human skin and a tissue culture medium that contained 2% bovine serum albumin (used as receptor fluid), in which the steady-state flux was 544 ± 64 nmol/cm²/h (0.046 mg/cm²/h) (Wilkinson & Williams, 2002).

2-Butoxyethanol vapour is also well absorbed through the skin and can contribute significantly to the systemic dose. Corley *et al.* (1997) exposed one arm of each of six volunteers to 50 ppm [24.1 mg/m³] 2-butoxyethanol vapour for 2 h. Blood was collected from both the exposed and unexposed arms and was analysed for 2-butoxyethanol and butoxyacetic acid. Urine was collected and analysed for butoxyacetic acid and its conjugates, ethylene glycol and glycolic acid. The concentration of 2-butoxyethanol was 1500 times greater in fingerprick blood from the exposed arm than that in venous blood from the unexposed arm. This confirmed that the previous estimates of 75% dermal absorption of 2-butoxyethanol calculated by Johanson and Bowman (1991) were probably overestimates due to contamination of the blood sample with 2-butoxyethanol during collection. Estimates of dermal absorption based on butoxyacetic acid and a physiologically based pharmacokinetic model showed that dermal absorption of 2-butoxyethanol probably contributed 15–27% of the total systemic dose. After dermal exposure of one arm to 50 ppm for 2 h, the peak 2-butoxyethanol concentration was 0.07 μM [8.26 μg/L] and occurred at the end of exposure. The half-life for 2-butoxyethanol in blood was 0.66 h. The peak blood concentration of butoxyacetic acid was 0.59 μM [70 μg/L] and occurred 3.7 h after the end of exposure. The half-life of butoxyacetic acid in blood was 3.3 h.

The significance of dermal absorption of 2-butoxyethanol vapour was confirmed by Jones *et al*. (2003) who exposed four volunteers on nine occasions by either 'whole body' (inhalation and dermal absorption) or 'skin only' (breathing clean air) exposure to 50 ppm 2-butoxyethanol for 2 h at different temperatures and humidities. At 25 °C and 40% relative humidity, dermal absorption of vapour accounted for an average of 11% of the total absorbed dose. Dermal absorption increased slightly with increased temperature or humidity; when both were combined (30 °C and 60% relative humidity), dermal absorption contributed 39% of the 'total' absorbed dose.

In humans, the elimination of 2-butoxyethanol is mostly by excretion of butoxyacetic acid in the urine. Johanson *et al*. (1986a) showed that less than 0.03% of the dose was excreted as unchanged 2-butoxyethanol in urine and that butoxyacetic acid (without hydrolysis) accounted for 15–55% of the dose. This value probably underestimates the percentage of 2-butoxyethanol that is excreted as butoxyacetic acid since this metabolite is also excreted as a glutamine conjugate. Sakai *et al*. (1994) showed that the percentage of conjugation of butoxyacetic acid in the urine of workers exposed to 2-butoxyethanol varied from 44 to 92% with a mean value of 71%, a value supported by Corely *et al*. (1997) who estimated butoxyacetic acid–glutamine conjugation to be around 67% and found no ethylene glycol or glycolic acid in the urine. Jones and Cocker (2003) showed that conjugation of butoxyacetic acid was variable both between and within workers and, based on urine samples from 48 workers, that the average level of conjugation was 57% (95% CI, 44–70%).

Studies of volunteers showed that peak urinary excretion of butoxyacetic acid occurs 3–6 h after the end of a 2-h exposure to 2-butoxyethanol by inhalation and then declines with a half-life of approximately 6 h (Johanson *et al*., 1986a; Jones & Cocker, 2003).

The low renal clearance of butoxyacetic acid (23–39 mL/min) indicates extensive binding to protein and absence or low efficiency of tubular secretion of butoxyacetic acid. The low apparent volume of distribution (15 L) is an additional indication of binding of butoxyacetic acid to blood proteins (Johanson & Johnsson, 1991).

(b) Animals

(i) In-vivo studies

2-Butoxyethanol is well absorbed from the stomach in experimental animals.

Poet *et al*. (2003) administered 250 mg/kg bw 2-butoxyethanol by gavage and by intraperitoneal injection and 400 mg/kg bw by subcutaneous injection to $B6C3F_1$ mice and found no significant differences at the end of exposure in blood concentrations of 2-butoxyethanol or butoxyacetic acid between the routes of administration. 2-Butoxyethanol was rapidly eliminated and was no longer detectable 1 h after treatment. The highest measured concentrations of butoxyacetic acid in blood (approx. 1 mM) were found in the samples obtained 0.5 h after administration.

Medinsky *et al.* (1990) administered [^{14}C]2-butoxyethanol in the drinking-water (at concentrations of 290, 860 or 2590 ppm equivalent to 237, 401 or 1190 µmol/kg bw, respectively) for 24 h to Fischer 344N rats and showed that 50–60% of the dose was eliminated in the urine as butoxyacetic acid, 10% as ethylene glycol, 8–10% as carbon dioxide and less than 5% as unmetabolized 2-butoxyethanol.

Sabourin *et al.* (1992a) exposed Fischer 344 rats by inhalation for 6 h to [^{14}C]2-butoxyethanol at concentrations up to 438 ppm [2111 mg/m^3] (at which level 50% died). Uptake and metabolism were linear up to 438 ppm and the major metabolite was butoxyacetic acid with lesser amounts of ethylene glycol and its glucuronide. Over 80% of the [^{14}C]2-butoxyethanol-derived material in blood was in the plasma and the data indicated that formation of the haemolytic metabolite butoxyacetic acid was linearly related to the exposure concentration up to levels that were toxic. Elimination of inhaled 2-butoxyethanol is rapid with half-lives of < 10 min in Fischer 344 rats and < 5 min in B6C3F$_1$ mice after 1 day of exposure (Dill *et al.*, 1998).

Johanson (1994) exposed Sprague-Dawley rats by inhalation continuously for up to 12 days to 20 or 100 ppm [96.4 or 482 mg/m^3] 2-butoxyethanol and showed that it was efficiently metabolized with an average blood clearance of 2.6 L/h/kg. The major (64%) metabolite was butoxyacetic acid and its renal clearance averaged 0.53 L/h/kg. The kinetics of the elimination of 2-butoxyethanol and butoxyacetic acid were linear up to 100 ppm. The average blood concentration of butoxyacetic acid during exposure to 20 and 100 ppm was 41 and 179 µM, respectively.

After topical application of 200 mg/kg bw [^{14}C]2-butoxyethanol to an area of 12 cm^2 of the shaved backs of Wistar rats under non-occlusive conditions, 25–29% was absorbed within 48 h. Peak blood levels of 2-butoxyethanol occurred 2 h after application and butoxyacetic acid was the major metabolite. Haemolysis was noted in rats that received a single dermal application of 260–500 mg/kg bw. In-vitro studies of percutaneous penetration of 2-butoxyethanol showed that, in fresh dorsal skin of hairless rats under non-occlusive conditions, 6% of the dose was absorbed within 1 h (2-butoxyethanol was absorbed or evaporated after 1 h) and that a greater percentage (10%) was absorbed from a 10% aqueous solution of 2-butoxyethanol (Bartnik *et al.*, 1987).

The absorption of 2-butoxyethanol through the skin of anaesthetized guinea-pigs was studied using one or two sealed glass rings (3.14 cm^2 each) that contained 1 mL diluted or undiluted 2-butoxyethanol on the clipped back of the animals. During the latter half of a 2-h exposure to undiluted 2-butoxyethanol of an area of 6.28 cm^2 of skin, the concentration of 2-butoxyethanol in blood appeared to level off with an average concentration of 21 µmol/L (SD, 45%) and the absorption rate through the skin was estimated to be 0.25 (range, 0.05–0.46) µmol/min/cm^2 (SD, 49%) (Johanson & Fernström, 1986). In a later experiment, the relative rates of absorption of aqueous solutions were investigated; 5, 10 and 20% 2-butoxyethanol had rates of absorption similar to undiluted 2-butoxyethanol but 40% and 80% solutions had double the rate. The permeability coefficient of guinea-pig skin for undiluted 2-butoxyethanol was 0.4×10^{-3} cm/h and that for 5% aqueous 2-butoxyethanol was 12×10^{-3} cm/h (Johanson & Fernström, 1988).

Three different amounts (520–2530 µmol/kg bw [30–61.4 mg/kg bw]) of [^{14}C]2-butoxyethanol were applied to three circular areas, 2 cm in diameter, of the clipped backs of Fischer 344N rats (non-occluded); within the dose range studied, absorption and metabolism were linear with dose and 20–25% of the dose was absorbed. The majority (83%) of the absorbed dose was excreted in the urine as butoxyacetic acid; only small amounts of ethylene glycol were formed. Eighty per cent of [^{14}C]2-butoxyethanol was associated with plasma and less than 20% was associated with red cells. Peak levels of [^{14}C]2-butoxyethanol (223 nmol/mL [^{14}C]2-butoxyethanol equivalents) in plasma were reached at about 1 h after dermal administration of 1530 µmol/kg bw [18.5 mg/kg bw] [^{14}C]2-butoxyethanol, after which the concentration decreased with a half-life of about 4 h. The major metabolite (53–75% of [^{14}C]2-butoxyethanol equivalents) in plasma was butoxyacetic acid (Sabourin *et al.*, 1992b). Compared with other studies (Medinsky *et al.*, 1990), the metabolic profile was slightly different after dermal application compared with administration in the drinking-water, which was speculated to be due to different rates of administration and/or local tissue metabolism (Sabourin *et al.*, 1992b).

Johanson and Fernström (1986) gave an intravenous bolus dose of 42 or 92 µmol/kg bw (5 or 11 mg/kg bw) 2-butoxyethanol to pentobarbital-anaesthetized guinea-pigs. The apparent total clearance and mean residence time of 2-butoxyethanol were 128 mL/min/kg bw (± 30%, SD) (which corresponds to 2.7 mL/min/g liver (± 30%, SD)) and 4.7 min (± 30%, SD), respectively.

Ghanayem *et al.* (1990) injected [^{14}C]2-butoxyethanol intravenously into rats of different ages (controls aged 3–4 months and old rats aged 12–13 months). In addition, some rats were also pretreated with pyrazole or cyanamide, which are inhibitors of alcohol dehydrogenase (ADH) or aldehyde dehydrogenase (ALDH), respectively, or probenecid, which is an inhibitor of renal transport of organic acids. The area-under-the-curve (AUC), maximum blood concentration (C_{max}) and systemic clearance of 2-butoxyethanol were dose-dependent. There was no effect of dose on half-life or volume of distribution of 2-butoxyethanol. Age did not effect the half-life, volume of distribution or clearance of 2-butoxyethanol but C_{max} and the AUC of 2-butoxyethanol increased in older rats. Inhibition of ADH and ALDH, the enzymes that metabolize 2-butoxyethanol, increased the half-life and AUC of this substrate and decreased its clearance. For butoxyacetic acid, the half-life, AUC and C_{max} increased in older rats and with dose. Inhibition of ADH and ALDH decreased the C_{max}, AUC and half-life of butoxyacetic acid. Treatments that protect against 2-butoxyethanol-induced haemolytic anaemia in rats were associated with a significant decrease in the concentrations of butoxyacetic acid in blood. When renal transport of organic acids was inhibited, no effect on the AUC, C_{max} or clearance of 2-butoxyethanol but an increase in the half-life and AUC of butoxyacetic acid were observed. The data suggest that a decreased elimination of butoxyacetic acid in older rats may contribute to their increased sensitivity to 2-butoxyethanol-induced haematotoxicity.

Bartnik *et al.* (1987) injected Wistar rats subcutaneously with 118 mg/kg [^{14}C]2-butoxyethanol; 79% of the radioactivity was excreted in the urine, 10% in expired air (as carbon dioxide) and 0.5% in the faeces within 72 h. Thymus and spleen had higher levels of radioactivity than liver, fat, kidney, testes, sternum, carcass and blood [other tissues not examined].

In female B6C3F$_1$ mice, 2-Butoxyethanol and butoxyacetic acid were eliminated more slowly from forestomach tissue than from the blood or other tissues. The half-lives of 2-butoxyethanol after an intraperitoneal dose of 261 mg/kg bw were 2.6 h and 0.6 h for the forestomach and liver, respectively. The same dose of 2-butoxyethanol resulted in half-lives of butoxyacetic acid of 4.6, 1.1 and 1.05 h for the forestomach, liver and blood, respectively. The forestomach was the only tissue that had detectable levels of 2-butoxy-ethanol at 24 h. 2-Butoxyethanol and butoxyacetic acid were excreted in the saliva and were present in the stomach contents for a prolonged period following intraperitoneal and oral administration (Poet *et al.*, 2003).

Ghanayem *et al.* (1987a) administered 125 or 500 mg/kg bw [^{14}C]2-butoxyethanol to Fischer 344 rats by oral gavage and showed that 2-butoxyethanol was distributed at highest concentrations (at 48 h) in the forestomach followed by liver, kidney, spleen and glandular stomach. The tissue concentrations did not increase linearly from low to high doses. The major route of elimination was the urine followed by exhalation of [^{14}C]carbon dioxide. The proportion of the dose excreted as [^{14}C]carbon dioxide was significantly higher in rats treated with 125 mg/kg bw compared with those given 500 mg/kg bw, which may indicate saturation of metabolism. A small proportion of the dose was excreted in the bile (8% of 500 mg/kg bw). The major urinary metabolite was butoxyacetic acid which accounted for more than 75% of ^{14}C in the urine, and the second major metabolite was the glucuronide conjugate of 2-butoxyethanol. Conversely, the major metabolite in bile was the glucuronide conjugate followed by butoxyacetic acid. A small quantity of radioactivity was excreted in the urine as the sulfate conjugate of butoxyethanol at the lower (but not the higher) dose.

Species and sex differences in elimination exist and, overall, mice eliminated 2-butoxy-ethanol and butoxyacetic acid faster than rats. Sex-related differences were most significant in rats and females were less efficient at clearing butoxyacetic acid from blood than males. It was speculated that this might be explained by differences in renal excretion (Dill *et al.*, 1998). As the animals aged, the rates of elimination of butoxyethanol and butoxyacetic acid decreased in both species. Old mice eliminated butoxyacetic acid from blood up to 10 times more slowly than young mice after a single exposure but this difference was reduced after repeated exposure of the old mice to 2-butoxyethanol.

Further evidence of the influence of ethanol on the elimination of 2-butoxyethanol was reported in an earlier study (Romer *et al.*, 1985). Ethanol (20 mmol/kg bw [920 mg/kg bw]) and 2-butoxyethanol (2.5 mmol/kg bw [295 mg/kg bw]) were co-administered intraperito-neally to female Sprague-Dawley rats; blood levels of 2-butoxyethanol were nearly constant as long as blood ethanol levels were above 3 mM [138 µg/mL]. This level of ethanol inhi-bited the metabolism of 2-butoxyethanol by ADH, the enzyme that is common to ethanol and 2-butoxyethanol.

(ii)   *In-vitro studies*

In-vitro studies with isolated perfused rat liver showed dose-dependent Michaelis-Menten kinetics in the elimination of 2-butoxyethanol at doses up to 3 mM [354 µg/mL] (Johanson *et al.*, 1986b). The apparent Michaelis-Menten constant (K_m) ranged from 0.32 to 0.7 mM [38 to 82.6 µg/mL] and the maximum elimination (V_{max}) rate ranged from 0.63 to 1.4 µmol/min/g liver [74.5–165 µg/min/g liver]. The maximum intrinsic clearance was 1.7–2 mL/min/g liver. This in-vitro study also investigated the influence of ethanol on the elimination of 2-butoxyethanol and found that, in the presence of 17 mM [782 µg/mL] ethanol, the extraction ratio of 2-butoxyethanol decreased from 0.44 to 0.11, which supports the hypothesis that 2-butoxyethanol is metabolized by ADH.

(iii)   *Pharmacokinetic models*

Several pharmacologically based pharmacokinetic models have been developed to describe the absorption and elimination of 2-butoxyethanol in humans (Johanson & Näslund, 1988; Corley *et al.*, 1997), rats (Shyr *et al.*, 1993; Lee *et al.*, 1998) or both (Johanson, 1986; Corley *et al.*, 1994). The first model by Johanson (1986) was based on elimination data (K_m and V_{max}) that were extrapolated from perfused rat liver and used blood flows and tissue volumes from the literature. Simulation of arterial blood concentrations of 2-butoxyethanol in a pharmacologically based pharmacokinetic model developed for a man after inhalation exposure to 20 ppm [0.8 mmol/m^3] and physical exercise ('light work'; 50 W) agreed well with data from a study of experimental exposure of human volunteers. In further simulations, the effects of exercise and co-exposure to ethanol were also studied and both predicted increased blood concentrations of 2-butoxyethanol due to increased ventilation (e.g. increased pulmonary uptake of 2-butoxyethanol) and inhibition of its metabolism, respectively. The relatively rapid decay of 2-butoxyethanol in all compartments indicates that it is unlikely to accumulate. The model also predicted that linear kinetics can be expected following occupational inhalation exposures to 2-butoxyethanol of < 100 ppm.

Corley *et al.* (1994) developed a more sophisticated model to include additional routes of exposure, physiological parameters and competing metabolic pathways for 2-butoxyethanol. Model simulations were compared with data from rats following either intravenous infusion or oral or inhalation exposure and from humans following either inhalation or dermal exposure to 2-butoxyethanol. The model accurately simulated observed data and was used to show that the species differences in kinetics resulted in higher blood concentrations of butoxyacetic acid in rats than in humans. This, coupled with the fact that human blood is less susceptible to haemolysis by butoxyacetic acid, predicts less risk for haemolysis in humans as a consequence of exposure to 2-butoxyethanol. In a later model, Corley *et al.* (1997) added parameters to describe the dermal absorption of 2-butoxyethanol vapours and showed that, after exposure to 25 ppm (0.8 mmol/m^3) for 8 h, the concentrations of butoxyacetic acid in human blood would be unlikely to reach levels associated with haemolysis *in vitro*.

4.1.2   *Metabolism*

The general metabolism of 2-butoxyethanol is described in Figure 1 (ATSDR, 1998). In the primary pathway, which occurs in the liver, 2-butoxyethanol is first oxidized via ADH to the intermediate, 2-butoxyacetaldehyde, which is subsequently further oxidized via ALDH to 2-butoxyacetic acid (the principal active metabolite). 2-Butoxyacetic acid may be conjugated with glycine or glutamine to form *N*-butoxyacetylglycine and *N*-butoxyacetylglutamine, respectively, or be metabolized to carbon dioxide. 2-Butoxyethanol can also be *O*-dealkylated via cytochrome P450 (CYP) 2E1 to form ethylene glycol and butyraldehyde. Ethylene glycol is subsequently metabolized to oxalic acid and further to carbon dioxide, while butyraldehyde is oxidized to butyric acid. 2-Butoxyethanol can also be conjugated directly with glucuronide or sulfate via glucuronyl or sulfotransferases, respectively. In addition, conjugation with fatty acids in the liver has been observed in one in-vivo study in rats exposed to 2-butoxyethanol (Kaphalia *et al.*, 1996).

The route of administration appears to influence the relative importance of each metabolic pathway in rats, based on the profile of urinary metabolites (Medinsky *et al.*, 1990; Sabourin *et al.*, 1992a,b). Although 2-butoxyacetic acid is the major metabolite following exposure to 2-butoxyethanol via any route, the formation of ethylene glycol is favoured after inhalation exposure or administration in the drinking-water compared with conjugation with glucuronide. However, at low concentrations in the drinking-water or high concentrations in air, no significant difference in the proportion of these metabolites was observed. Production of the glucuronide conjugate is favoured following dermal exposure.

(*a*)   *Oxidation of 2-butoxyethanol to 2-butoxyacetaldehyde and 2-butoxyacetic acid*

Although it was considered for a long time to be an intermediate step in the conversion of 2-butoxyethanol to butoxyacetic acid, the actual formation of the aldehyde metabolite has only very recently been demonstrated in experimental animals. Deisinger and Boatman (2004) administered a single oral dose of 600 mg/kg bw 2-butoxyethanol to male and female B6C3F₁ mice and detected low but measurable levels of 2-butoxyacetaldehyde in the blood, liver and forestomach at all time-points (5, 15 and 45 min) up to 90 min after exposure. Concentrations were highest in all tissues 5 min after administration and declined thereafter. Initial levels were approximately 10-fold higher in the forestomach than in the blood and liver. Levels of the aldehyde intermediate were significantly higher in tissues of female mice than in those of male mice, and were one to three orders of magnitude less than those of the acid metabolite.

An extensive database of studies in exposed humans and experimental animals shows that the formation of 2-butoxyacetic acid is a principal metabolic end-point for 2-butoxyethanol. Although it mainly occurs in the liver, there is potential for the formation of 2-butoxyacetic acid in tissues at or near the site of contact that contain ALDH and ADH, e.g. the skin, forestomach or glandular stomach (Sabourin *et al.*, 1992a). Aasmoe *et al.* (1998) demonstrated that ADH3 was the only ADH isoenzyme that effectively oxidized

Figure 1. Metabolism of 2-butoxyethanol

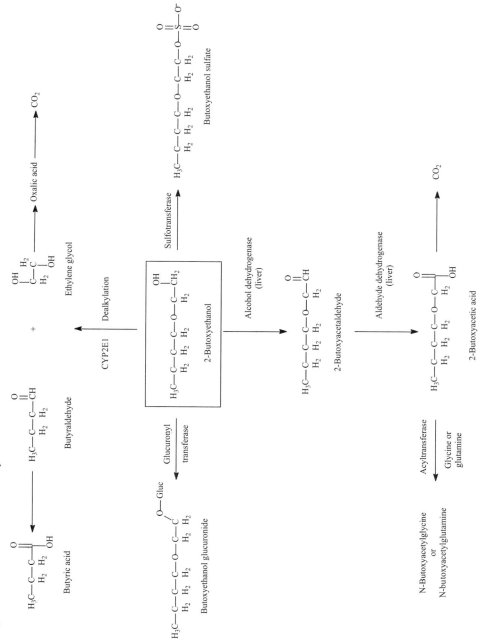

Modified from ATSDR (1998)

2-butoxyethanol in the liver of rats. No information was found on the isoenzyme(s) of ADH that is involved in the metabolism of 2-butoxyethanol to 2-butoxyacetic acid in humans. There are several classes of ADH, for some of which interindividual variation occurs in humans (i.e. polymorphism); thus, there may be substantial variability in the extent to which 2-butoxyethanol is metabolized to 2-butoxyacetic acid in the human population, but this has not been investigated extensively.

Green *et al.* (2002) compared the distribution of ADHs in the forestomach and glandular stomach of rodents with that in the stomach of humans. The authors noted that the enzymes are largely concentrated in the stratified squamous epithelium of the forestomach of rats and mice but are more diffuse in the glandular stomach, and have greater activity in these tissues in mice than in rats. This greater activity corresponds to the greater sensitivity of mice to 2-butoxyethanol-induced effects in the forestomach. In the human stomach, ADH and ALDH are evenly distributed throughout the gastric epithelial cells of the mucosa.

2-Butoxyacetic acid appeared in the urine or was measured in the blood of humans following incidental ingestion or occupational or controlled exposure via inhalation or dermal contact (Johanson *et al.*, 1986a, 1988; Rambourg-Schepens *et al.*, 1988; Angerer *et al.*, 1990; Rettenmeier *et al.*, 1993; Sakai *et al.*, 1993; Söhnlein *et al.*, 1993; Sakai *et al.*, 1994; Corley *et al.*, 1997; Haufroid *et al.*, 1997; Laitinen, 1998; McKinney *et al.*, 2000; Jakasa *et al.*, 2004). In these studies, 2-butoxyacetic acid was the major metabolite identified and was found to correspond to up to 70% of the amount of 2-butoxyethanol absorbed (Jakasa *et al.*, 2004). Some of the 2-butoxyacetic acid is eliminated as the free acid, while a portion is conjugated before elimination (Jakasa *et al.*, 2004). Concentrations of free 2-butoxyacetic acid in the blood of five men exposed to 20 ppm [97 mg/m^3] 2-butoxyethanol by inhalation for 2 h ranged from 18.5 to 56.5 µM [2 to 7 mg/L] (Johanson & Johnsson, 1991). Levels of 2-butoxyacetic acid at the end of a shift in the urine of workers who used glass cleaners that contained 2-butoxyethanol increased linearly with ambient concentration of 2-butoxyethanol (exposure range, < 0.1–7.33 ppm [< 0.5–35 mg/m^3]) (Vincent *et al.*, 1993), which suggests that saturation of this metabolic pathway does not occur at these exposure concentrations. However, in an experimental study, Johanson *et al.* (1986a, 1988) observed substantial variation in the urinary levels of 2-butoxyacetic acid between volunteers exposed to 2-butoxyethanol by dermal application (2.5–39%; five subjects) or by inhalation (15–55%; six subjects). Similarly, Jakasa *et al.* (2004) observed interindividual variations of 42–70% in urinary levels of total 2-butoxyacetic acid (i.e. free and conjugated) of six volunteers exposed by inhalation to approximately 93 mg/m^3 2-butoxyethanol.

2-Butoxyacetic acid is also the major metabolite of 2-butoxyethanol in experimental animals. In rats administered up to 2590 ppm [2.6 mg/L] 2-butoxyethanol in the drinking-water (1.2 mmol/kg bw), 2-butoxyacetic acid eliminated in the urine accounted for up to 60% of the administered dose (Medinsky *et al.*, 1990). 2-Butoxyacetic acid also comprised more than 75% of the radioactivity in the urine of rats administered a single dose of up to 500 mg/kg bw [^{14}C]2-butoxyethanol by gavage (Ghanayem *et al.*, 1987a). Inhibition of

ADH or ALDH by pyrazole or cyanamide, respectively, significantly reduced the extent of conversion of 2-butoxyethanol to 2-butoxyacetic acid in rats administered a single oral dose of 500 mg/kg bw (i.e. from 75–90% of total radioactivity in the urine to 5–13%); the reduction in levels of 2-butoxyacetic acid corresponded with a reduction in toxicity (Ghanayem *et al.*, 1987b) (see also Section 4.1.1). Similarly, competitive inhibition of ADH by ethanol, *n*-propanol or *n*-butanol reduced the production of 2-butoxyacetic acid from 2-butoxyethanol by 43, 33 and 31%, respectively (consistent with the greater affinity of the enzyme for alcohols than for glycol ether), which was accompanied by a corresponding reduction in the toxicity of 2-butoxyethanol (Morel *et al.*, 1996). Exposure of rats to airborne concentrations of up to 483 ppm [2333 mg/m^3] 2-butoxyethanol did not appear to exceed the saturation level of its conversion to 2-butoxyacetic acid, based on the increase in concentrations of this metabolite measured in the urine (Sabourin *et al.*, 1992a; Johanson, 1994).

In an investigation of the metabolism of 2-butoxyethanol to 2-butoxyacetic acid during long-term inhalation exposure of rats and mice (Dill *et al.*, 1998; National Toxicology Program, 2000), the rate of elimination of 2-butoxyethanol from blood followed linear kinetics, which suggests that the production of 2-butoxyacetic acid in both species was also linear. However, the rate of disappearance of 2-butoxyethanol from blood was greater in mice than in rats. Similarly, mice were more efficient at eliminating 2-butoxyacetic acid from the blood, although elimination followed non-linear kinetics in both species (see also Section 4.1.1(*b*)). In addition, the rate of elimination of both 2-butoxyethanol and 2-butoxyacetic acid from blood decreased with increasing duration of exposure, particularly in rats. Thus, although mice may metabolize 2-butoxyethanol to 2-butoxyacetic acid at a greater rate than rats, the metabolite is subsequently cleared much more rapidly in mice, which is consistent with the apparently greater sensitivity to 2-butoxyethanol-induced haematological effects of rats than mice in both short- and long-term studies. Similarly, the greater sensitivity of female rats than male rats is probably related to slower clearance of the active acid metabolite than to sex-related differences in its production, although the activity of the hepatic ADH isoenzyme involved (ADH3) was reported to be greater in female rats than in male rats (Aasmoe *et al.*, 1998; Aasmoe & Aarbakke, 1999). The activities of gastric ADH are greater in male than in female rats [however, the sex difference was only significant when octanol was the substrate; 2-butoxyethanol was not tested in this study] (Aasmoe & Aarbakke, 1999). Consistent with the less pronounced sex-specific sensitivities to 2-butoxyethanol-induced toxicity in mice, little sex difference in the formation or elimination of 2-butoxyacetic acid was observed in this species.

Ghanayem *et al.* (1987c) observed that older rats metabolized 2-butoxyethanol to 2-butoxyacetic acid to a greater extent than younger rats following oral administration of 500 mg/kg bw, based on a comparison of the levels of 2-butoxyacetic acid in the urine. Similar results were obtained in rats that were administered a single intravenous dose of up to 125 mg/kg bw 2-butoxyethanol, based on greater values of the AUC and C_{max} of 2-butoxyethanol and in C_{max} and half-life of 2-butoxyacetic acid in older rats compared with younger rats (Ghanayem *et al.*, 1990). In mice, although no significant difference in the rate of clearance of 2-butoxyethanol (and presumably the formation of 2-butoxyacetic acid) was observed between older and younger animals exposed to up to 125 ppm [603 mg/m³] by inhalation for 1 day, younger mice cleared 2-butoxyacetic acid at a 10-fold greater rate than older mice after 1 day. However, this difference was less obvious after 3 weeks of exposure (Dill *et al.*, 1998) (see also Section 4.1.1(*b*)).

In an in-vitro investigation of the comparative metabolism of 2-butoxyethanol in hepatocytes from humans and rats, Green *et al.* (1996) observed that cells from rats were more efficient at converting 2-butoxyethanol to 2-butoxyacetic acid than those from humans (four men and three women). Saturation of this pathway appeared to occur at much lower doses in hepatocytes from humans than in those from rats, since the percentage of total radioactivity identified as 2-butoxyacetic acid was only 1.5-fold greater in rat hepatocytes than in human hepatocytes at 0.02 mM, while the difference was 6.1-fold at 10 mM. The percentage that was converted to 2-butoxyacetic acid increased with up to 10 mM glycol ether in rat hepatocytes but decreased in human hepatocytes between 0.02 and 0.2 mM.

(*b*)   *Conjugation of 2-butoxyacetic acid with glutamine or glycine*

Conjugation of 2-butoxyacetic acid with glutamine via acyltransferase has been demonstrated in humans. Rettenmeier *et al.* (1993) reported that *N*-butoxyacetylglutamine accounted for a mean of 48% (range, 16–64%) of the 2-butoxyacetic acid that was detected in urine collected at the end of the work week from six lacquerers who were exposed to 2-butoxyethanol (the remainder was free 2-butoxyacetic acid). Hence, conjugation with glutamine may represent an important route of removal of 2-butoxyacetic acid. Sakai *et al.* (1994) reported that a larger proportion (mean, 71%; range, 44–92%) of total 2-butoxyacetic acid was present as conjugates [not further identified] in the urine of six workers who were exposed to 2-butoxyethanol. They also determined that the fraction of 2-butoxyacetic acid eliminated as conjugates decreased throughout the work week, which may reflect a decline in the capacity for conjugation with continued exposure. These data are consistent with the lower proportions of conjugated 2-butoxyacetic acid observed by Rettenmeier *et al.* (1993) in the urine of workers after several days of exposure. More recently, Jones and Cocker (2003) determined that the mean extent of conjugation of 2-butoxyacetic acid [not further identified] was 57% (95% CI, 44–70%) in a group of 48 exposed workers, in six of whom there was no evidence of conjugation. These authors also observed substantial intra-individual variability in volunteers who were exposed repeatedly to 50 ppm [242 mg/m³] 2-butoxyethanol for 2 h (i.e. nearly 0–100%) and hypothesized that this large variability was not related to polymorphisms but to other factors such as levels of glutamine. Corley *et al.* (1997) observed that about two-thirds (67%) of the 2-butoxyacetic acid excreted in the urine of male volunteers exposed dermally (one arm) to airborne concentrations of 50 ppm [242 mg/m³] 2-butoxyethanol was present as *N*-butoxyacetylglutamine.

Little information was available on the conjugation of 2-butoxyacetic acid with glycine. No evidence of conjugation with this amino acid was found in rats that were administered up to 2590 ppm [2590 µg/mL] 2-butoxyethanol in the drinking-water for 1 day and observed for 3 days after exposure (Medinsky *et al.*, 1990) or in rats exposed dermally to up to 2530 μmol/kg bw [298 mg/kg bw] (Sabourin *et al.*, 1992b). However, glycine conjugation with the alkoxyacetic acid metabolite has been observed for other glycol ethers (2-methoxyethanol and 2-ethoxyethanol) (Jönsson *et al.*, 1982; Cheever *et al.*, 1984; Moss *et al.*, 1985). Corley *et al.* (1994) did not observe conjugation of 2-butoxyacetic acid with amino acids in samples of blood or urine from rats that were administered single doses of up to 126 mg/kg bw by gavage.

On the basis of these data, it appears that clearance of 2-butoxyacetic acid via conjugation occurs to a greater extent in humans than in rats, although data on this metabolic step in rodents are sparse.

(c) Dealkylation of 2-butoxyethanol to ethylene glycol and butyraldehyde

Only limited data on the occurrence of *O*-dealkylation of 2-butoxyethanol to ethylene glycol and (presumably) butyraldehyde in humans are available. Ethylene glycol, or its metabolite (oxalate), have been detected in the plasma or urine from two individuals who had ingested cleaning products that contained 2-butoxyethanol (250–500 mL of a solution that contained 12% 2-butoxyethanol) (Rambourg-Schepens *et al.*, 1988) and 150 mL of a solution that contained 9.1% 2-butoxyethanol (Nisse *et al.*, 1998). Metabolic acidosis, which is commonly associated with ethylene glycol poisoning, was observed in both cases (Rambourg-Schepens *et al.*, 1988; Nisse *et al.*, 1998). Conversely, neither ethylene glycol nor its metabolites were detected in the serum or urine from two people who had ingested 2-butoxyethanol (200–250 mL of a product that contained 12.7% 2-butoxyethanol (~25–30 g) or 360–480 mL of a product that contained 22% 2-butoxyethanol (~80–105 g)) (Gijsenbergh *et al.*, 1989; Gualtieri *et al.*, 1995), although metabolic acidosis occurred in both cases. Similarly, Corley *et al.* (1997) did not detect ethylene glycol or its metabolic products in the urine of a group of volunteers who were exposed dermally to 50 ppm [242 mg/m^3] 2-butoxyethanol for 2 h.

There is stronger evidence for the occurrence of this metabolic pathway in rats. Medinsky *et al.* (1990) reported that ethylene glycol comprised 14–22% of total urinary radioactive metabolites in rats that were administered up to 2590 ppm [2590 μg/mL] [^{14}C]2-butoxyethanol in the drinking-water for 24 h. It also accounted for 2–11% of total ^{14}C in the urine of rats that were administered doses of 8.6 or 126 mg/kg bw by gavage (Corley *et al.*, 1994), but was not detected in the urine of rats that were administered up to 500 mg/kg bw 2-butoxyethanol by gavage (Ghanayem *et al.*, 1987a). [This discrepancy may have been due to the ^{14}C radiolabel being on the butoxy moiety instead of the ethanol moiety (National Toxicology Program, 2000).] Similarly, Sabourin *et al.* (1992b) identified 4.1–6.5% of urinary metabolites as ethylene glycol in rats that were exposed dermally to up to 2530 μmol/kg bw [298 mg/kg bw] 2-butoxyethanol. Contrary to the increase in the proportion of urinary ethylene glycol observed in rats exposed orally or dermally to increasing levels of 2-butoxyethanol (Medinsky *et al.*, 1990; Sabourin *et al.*, 1992b), the fraction of urinary metabolites identified as ethylene glycol decreased with increasing exposure level in rats exposed to airborne concentrations of 4.3, 49 and

438 ppm [21, 237 and 2119 mg/m³] 2-butoxyethanol for 6 h (i.e. 16, 13.4 and 8%, respectively). The majority of ethylene glycol was excreted after cessation of exposure (Sabourin *et al.*, 1992a).

In an in-vitro study, hepatocytes from both rats and humans (four men and three women) metabolized 2-butoxyethanol to ethylene glycol. However, ethylene glycol represented a greater proportion of total radioactivity in rat cells than in human cells, which indicates a possible greater propensity for this metabolic step in rats than in humans. In both rat and human hepatocytes, the percentage of 2-butoxyethanol that was metabolized to ethylene glycol decreased with increasing dose, which the authors suggested was indicative of saturation of this pathway at relatively low concentrations of 2-butoxyethanol (Green *et al.*,1996).

Haufroid *et al.* (1997) hypothesized that polymorphism for CYP2E1 may influence the extent to which 2-butoxyethanol may be dealkylated to ethylene glycol and butyraldehyde. This was based on the observation that the level of free 2-butoxyacetic acid in the urine of a worker who expressed the heterozygous c2 allele (c1/c2) did not change substantially throughout the workday, unlike the 30 other workers who expressed the homozygous c1 allele (c1/c1) in whom substantial increases in levels of urinary free 2-butoxyacetic acid occurred. The authors suggested that the lack of increase in urinary 2-butoxyacetic acid may be due to greater activity of the c2 allele compared with that of the c1 allele in *O*-dealkylation of 2-butoxyethanol as observed by Hayashi *et al.* (1991). It was noted that urine samples were not analysed for amino acid conjugates of 2-butoxyacetic acid, which could also have influenced the excretion of free 2-butoxyacetic acid. The genetic polymorphism that affects transcriptional regulation of human CYP2E1 could also contribute to interindividual differences in the metabolism of 2-butoxyethanol via the dealkylation pathway.

Although no information was available regarding the formation of butyraldehyde or the subsequent metabolic product, butyric acid, in humans or experimental animals, it is predicted that butyraldehyde is the other metabolite that would result from *O*-dealkylation of 2-butoxyethanol to ethylene glycol.

(d)   Glucuronide and sulfate conjugation of 2-butoxyethanol

Information on the in-vivo formation of glucuronide or sulfate conjugates with 2-butoxyethanol was only available for rats, although the glucuronide conjugate has been tentatively identified in hepatocytes from both rats and humans exposed to 2-butoxyethanol *in vitro* (Green *et al.*, 1996). In rats administered single oral doses of 125 or 500 mg/kg bw radiolabelled 2-butoxyethanol, the glucuronide conjugate represented up to 24% of total urinary metabolites. This conjugate was no longer detectable in the urine 48 h after administration of 125 mg/kg bw, while levels were similar at 8 and 48 h following ingestion of 500 mg/kg bw. The sulfate conjugate was detected in samples of urine taken 8 h after administration of 125 mg/kg bw but was not found in the urine from rats exposed to 500 mg/kg bw. The glucuronide conjugate was the major metabolite in bile and constituted up to 89% of biliary radioactivity 30 min after exposure; however, this proportion declined to 54% after 8 h. The sulfate conjugate was not detected in the bile (Ghanayem *et al.*, 1987a).

The glucuronide conjugate has also been identified as a minor metabolite in the urine of rats exposed to 290–2590 ppm [290–2590 µg/mL] [^{14}C]2-butoxyethanol in the drinking-water for 24 h (8–11% of total radioactive metabolites measured in urine) (Medinsky *et al.*, 1990) and of rats administered 8.6 or 126 mg/kg bw [^{14}C]2-butoxyethanol by gavage (10–15% of total radioactive metabolites) (Corley *et al.*, 1994). The proportion of urinary metabolites identified as 2-butoxyethanol–glucuronide increased with the level of exposure in rats exposed to airborne concentrations of 4.3–438 ppm [21–2119 mg/m^3] 2-butoxy-ethanol for 6 h (i.e. from 10.6 to 62.3%). The glucuronide conjugate is apparently cleared rapidly, since it constituted only 3.6–6.5% of urinary metabolites during the 7–16 h after cessation of exposure (Sabourin *et al.*, 1992a). However, the proportion of urinary meta-bolites identified as the glucuronide conjugate did not increase in rats administered dermal doses of 520–2530 µmol/kg bw, but was similar at all doses (i.e. 13–15%) (Sabourin *et al.*, 1992b).

Inhibition of the principal pathway of metabolism of 2-butoxyethanol (i.e. oxidation to 2-butoxyacetic acid) by injection of pyrazole or cyanamide (inhibitors of ADH and ALDH, respectively) into rats administered a single oral dose of 500 mg/kg bw [^{14}C]-2-butoxyethanol (labelled at C1) resulted in a shift to increased conjugation with glu-curonide and sulfate. The proportions of these conjugates increased from 9–24% (glucu-ronide) and undetectable (sulfate) to 75–85% and 7.5–20%, respectively, of the total radioactivity in the urine. The shift towards the conjugation pathway corresponded with a reduction in 2-butoxyethanol-induced haematotoxicity (Ghanayem *et al.*, 1987b). Following intravenous administration of lower single doses of 2-butoxyethanol to rats (62.5 or 125 mg/kg bw), the glucuronide conjugate was only detected in the blood of ani-mals that had also been administered pyrazole as an inhibitor of ADH (Ghanayem *et al.*, 1990).

Ghanayem *et al.* (1987c) demonstrated that young rats produce a greater proportion of glucuronide conjugates and (as discussed above) proportionally less 2-butoxyacetic acid than older rats, which is consistent with the apparent lower sensitivity of young rats to the haematotoxic effects of 2-butoxyethanol. However, the sulfate conjugate was not detected in the urine of young rats.

4.2   Toxic effects

4.2.1   *Humans*

(*a*)   *Oral exposure*

Several individual cases that involved consumption of a few hundred millilitres of glass cleaners that contained 6.5–35% 2-butoxyethanol have been reported (Gijsenbergh *et al.*, 1989; Rambourg-Schepens *et al.*, 1988; Litovitz *et al.*, 1991; Bauer *et al.*, 1992; Burkhart & Donovan, 1998; Nisse *et al.*, 1998; McKinney *et al.*, 2000; Osterhoudt, 2002;

Gualtieri *et al.*, 2003). The main symptoms were hypotension, poor ventilation, coma, metabolic acidosis (probably due to the formation of butoxyacetic acid), renal impairment, haematuria and effects on the blood (erythropenia, reduced haematocrit and haemoglobin levels, haemoglobinuria and/or hypochromic anaemia) (Table 16). [Treatment by haemodialysis can lead to haemodilution that might account for a lower blood cell count but not for haemoglobinuria.] In a report of 24 cases of ingestion of up to 300 mL of glass-cleaning products that contained 0.5–10% 2-butoxyethanol that were included in a survey of childhood poisonings, all of the children were reported to be asymptomatic. Even at the highest estimated dose of 1850 mg/kg bw (300 mL of a glass cleaner that contained 8% 2-butoxyethanol (~24 g)) that was consumed by a 2-year-old child, no signs of metabolic acidosis or of haematological, renal or neurological adverse effects were manifest (Dean & Krenzelok, 1992).

(b)   Dermal exposure

Percutaneous absorption of 2-butoxyethanol was investigated experimentally in five men, who kept two or four fingers immersed in 2-butoxyethanol for 2 h. None of the subjects exhibited an adverse reaction (Johanson *et al.*, 1988). No evidence of strong adverse dermal effects or skin sensitization was observed in 201 individuals exposed dermally to 0.2 mL 10% 2-butoxyethanol in patches, although repeated applications did produce increasing erythema in several subjects (Greenspan *et al.*, 1995).

(c)   Inhalation exposure

The effects reported by subjects who were exposed to 113 ppm [546 mg/m^3] 2-butoxyethanol for 4 h (two men), 195 ppm [942 mg/m^3] for two 4-h periods separated by a 30-min interval (the same two men and one woman) or 98 ppm [474 mg/m^3] for 8 h (two men and two women) included irritation to the eyes (probably due to direct contact with the vapours), nose and throat, a disturbance of taste, a slight increase in nasal mucous discharge and headache. In this study, the women appeared to be more sensitive to the induction of these effects than the men. In none of these trials was there any evidence of changes from pre-exposure values in erythrocyte fragility, blood pressure, pulse rate or urinary levels of glucose or albumin (Carpenter *et al.*, 1956).

In two studies in which groups of four or seven male volunteers were exposed by inhalation to 20 or 50 ppm [97–242 mg/m^3] 2-butoxyethanol for 2 h, no overt signs of toxicity were observed (Johanson *et al.*, 1986a; Johanson & Boman, 1991). In the earlier investigation, in which the intake of 2-butoxyethanol was estimated to be 2 mg/kg bw for the 2-h exposure at 20 ppm (during which time the men performed light physical exercise), no consistent effects on the lungs (ventilation or breathing rate) or the heart (electrocardiogram readings or heart rate) were observed (Johanson *et al.*, 1986a). In the subsequent study, the investigators distinguished between vapour inhalation (through the mouth alone) and dermal exposure to the vapour (with a mask to prevent inhalation); no toxic effects were evident following either exposure protocol (Johanson & Boman, 1991). In a more recent study, four volunteers exposed to 25 ppm [121 mg/m^3] 2-butoxyethanol for 10 min also did not show overt signs of toxicity shortly after treatment (Kumagai *et al.*, 1999).

Signs of respiratory or ocular irritation, headache, sore throat and a sore nose that would become raw and bleed were reported in small groups of workers exposed to 5 ppm [24 mg/m^3] or less 2-butoxyethanol vapours (Apol, 1986).

The effect of occupational exposure to 2-butoxyethanol on various haematological, renal and hepatic parameters was investigated in 31 male workers at a beverage production plant who were exposed to mean concentrations of 3.64 mg/m^3 2-butoxyethanol (range, 1.77–6.14 mg/m^3; 20 samples) or 2.20 mg/m^3 (range, 0.75–3.35 mg/m^3; 11 samples) for 1–6 years, based on limited exposure data. The workers were also exposed to unspecified concentrations of methyl ethyl ketone. These parameters were also measured in a comparison population of 21 unexposed workers, matched for sex, age and smoking habits. Blood samples were collected at the end of the shift, while urine samples were taken before and after the workshift. No differences were observed in erythrocyte count, reticulocyte count, haemoglobin concentration, mean corpusclar volume, mean corpuscular haemoglobin or erythrocyte osmotic resistance between exposed and unexposed workers. However, haematocrit was significantly lower ($p = 0.03$) in the exposed group, while their mean cell haemoglobin concentration was significantly higher ($p = 0.02$) than that of controls, although the absolute differences in mean values were small (i.e. 43.9 versus 45.5% and 336 versus 329 g/L, respectively) and the ranges of values overlapped. No correlation was found between any of the haematological parameters investigated and levels of butoxyacetic acid in the urine at the end of the workshift or the difference in levels of this acid before and after the workshift (used as parameter of internal exposure), and no differences were observed in the renal parameters investigated (serum creatinine or urinary retinol binding protein). With regard to hepatic parameters, no statistically significant differences in levels of aspartate aminotransferase (20.5 ± 4.9 versus 21.7 ± 6.3 IU/L) or alanine aminotransferase (20.5 ± 13.1 versus 28.6 ± 16.3 UI/L) in the plasma were found between exposed and unexposed workers. However, plasma concentration of alanine aminotransferase and levels of butoxyacetic acid in the urine were statistically significantly correlated ($r = 0.60$; $p = 0.0004$) (Haufroid *et al.*, 1997).

Several hours after the floor in an unventilated office had been stripped using a solvent that contained 2-butoxyethanol and other substances, seven workers were exposed to airborne levels estimated to be 100–300 ppm (483–1449 mg/m^3) (based on symptoms) for 0.5–4 h. Subjects had immediate severe irritation of the eye and upper respiratory tract, nausea and presyncope which subsided within 3 days. [It was not specified in the brief account of these cases whether haematological parameters were examined immediately after exposure.] All but one of these workers reported recurrent upper respiratory irritation and the appearance of cherry angiomas 3 months later. Eight months after exposure, six of the seven workers had an increased blood cell sedimentation rate and mild hypertension, while skin lesions continued to appear and persisted. Follow-up for an additional 5 years in four of these workers revealed gradual disappearance of most of these effects, with the exception of the cherry angiomas that continued to persist and develop (Raymond *et al.*, 1998).

Collinot *et al.* (1996) investigated the potential of 2-butoxyethanol to induce hepatic enzymes in a group of 17 male foundry workers who were exposed to a maximum concentration of 7.5 ppm (36 mg/m³) 2-butoxyethanol. Levels of *D*-glucaric acid (which is the end product of the glucuronic acid pathway and is an indicator of enzyme activity in the liver) in the urine of exposed workers were compared with those in 18 unexposed controls. Urinary excretion of *D*-glucaric acid was significantly greater in exposed subjects than in controls, although significant seasonal variability was also found among exposed workers (increase in *D*-glucaric acid of 165% in winter and 85% in summer when the doors were open and the 2-butoxyethanol concentration was lower). [The Working Group noted that many of these occupational studies involve mixed exposures, the effects of which cannot be ascribed specifically to 2-butoxyethanol.]

4.2.2 *Experimental systems*

(a)   *In-vivo studies with single doses (acute effect)*

Based on LD_{50}s and LC_{50}s that range from 530 to 6700 mg/kg bw and from 450 to 700 ppm [2173–3381 mg/m³], respectively, 2-butoxyethanol produces low to moderate toxicity in experimental animals following acute exposure (Smyth *et al.*, 1941; Werner *et al.*, 1943a; Carpenter *et al.*, 1956; Smyth *et al.*, 1962; Weil & Wright, 1967; Gingell *et al.*, 1998). Haematological effects, as well as effects on the liver, kidney, lung and spleen, some of which may be secondary to haematotoxicity, have been observed in animals exposed acutely to lower doses or concentrations. For example, alterations in haematological parameters that are characteristic of haemolytic anaemia have been observed in rats administered single oral doses as low as 125 mg/kg bw, while haemoglobinuria was noted in older rats following administration of 32 mg/kg bw by gavage (Ghanayem *et al.*, 1987c). Female rats were more sensitive to 2-butoxyethanol-induced haemolysis than male rats following administration of a single dose of 250 mg/kg bw by gavage, as the magnitude of changes in haematological parameters was greater in females than in males; in addition, the onset of haemolysis was faster in females than in males (Ghanayem *et al.*, 2000). Exposure to airborne concentrations of 62 ppm [299 mg/m³] for 4 h resulted in increased osmotic fragility of erythrocytes (Carpenter *et al.*, 1956), whereas dermal exposure to 260 mg/kg bw for 6 h induced haemolysis in rats (Bartnik *et al.*, 1987). Ghanayem *et al.* (1992) and Sivarao and Mehendale (1995) demonstrated that younger blood cells were more resilient to 2-butoxyethanol-induced haemolysis than older cells, as rats that had been bled several days before exposure to a single oral dose were less severely affected than rats that had not been bled.

2-Butoxyethanol is considered to be a mild-to-severe irritant to the skin and eyes of rabbits (range doses, 0.1–0.5 mL neat compound), and severity increased with duration of exposure (range, 1–72 h) (Carpenter & Smyth, 1946; Smyth *et al.*, 1962; Kennah *et al.*,

1989; Jacobs, 1992; Zissu, 1995). There was no evidence of skin sensitization in one investigation in guinea-pigs (Zissu, 1995).

(*b*)   *In-vivo studies with multiple exposures*

(i)   *Short-term exposure*

Oral exposure

In short-term studies in rats exposed by the oral route, the blood was the principal target for the effects of 2-butoxyethanol. Haematological changes that are characteristic of haemolysis (including reductions in red blood cell count, haemoglobin levels and haematocrit values) have been reported by a number of investigators in rats exposed repeatedly to 2-butoxyethanol for 2–65 days (Grant *et al.*, 1985; Krasavage, 1986; National Toxicology Program, 1989; Dieter *et al.*, 1990; Ghanayem *et al.*, 1992; Ezov *et al.*, 2002). In most of the studies in which haematological parameters were measured, these changes were observed at all doses administered by gavage or in the drinking-water (i.e. 100 mg/kg bw per day). However, a no-observed-effect level (NOEL) of 30 mg/kg bw per day was reported in a study in rats exposed for only 3 days (which was designed primarily to investigate developmental toxicity) (National Toxicology Program, 1989). Ghanayem *et al.* (2001) observed an increase in the magnitude of haematological changes that were indicative of severe regenerative anaemia after repeated administration of 250 mg/kg bw 2-butoxyethanol per day by gavage for 1, 2 or 3 days to male and female Fischer 344 rats that were killed 24 or 48 h after the last dose; the onset of effects was faster in females. Thrombosis was observed in the lungs, nasal submucosa, eyes, liver, heart, bones and teeth, together with lesions that were consistent with acute infarction in the vertebrae and femur; again, onset was earlier in female rats than in males, which the authors hypothesized to be precipitated by initial stages of haemolysis induced by 2-butoxyethanol. Similarly, in male and female Fischer F344 rats administered two, three or four daily doses of 250 mg/kg bw 2-butoxyethanol by gavage and examined on days 2, 3, 4 and 29, Ezov *et al.* (2002) reported severe acute regenerative haemolytic anaemia, with faster onset in females, together with thrombosis and infarction in the heart, brain, lungs, eyes and bones mainly in female rats. In a separate report, it was noted that signs of intra-medullary thrombosis in the femur and subsequent new bone growth were observed in rats examined on day 29 (Shabat *et al.*, 2003). Morphological changes were noted in ery-throcytes, the severity of which progressed with increasing exposures and was greater in females than in males. Red blood cells from these exposed rats were found to have increased adherence to an extracellular matrix derived from endothelial cells of the blood vessel wall; it was suggested by the authors that such increased adherence could lead to vascular occlusion and result in the observed thrombosis (Koshkaryev *et al.*, 2003). Nyska *et al.* (1999a) also observed thrombosis of ocular blood vessels with retinal haemorrhage, necrosis and photoreceptor degeneration in female Fischer 344 rats administered 250 mg/kg bw 2-butoxyethanol per day by gavage for 3 consecutive days; thrombosis was also noted in the nasal cavity submucosa, teeth, femur and vertebrae. In a subsequent investigation, Nyska *et al.* (2003) noted a correlation between thrombosis and expression of the vascular cell adhesion molecule, which included severe haemolysis, in the ocular vessels of female Fischer 344 rats administered three or four daily doses of 250 mg/kg bw 2-butoxyethanol. The authors suggested that this molecule functions in the pathogenesis of 2-butoxyethanol-related thrombosis by promoting adhesion of erythrocytes to the endothelium.

In some of the short-term studies in rats, effects on blood were observed to be reversible after cessation of exposure (Grant *et al.*, 1985; Ghanayem *et al.*, 1992). In a preliminary developmental toxicity study in which pregnant rats were exposed daily to 0, 150, 300 or 600 mg/kg bw 2-butoxyethanol on days 9–11 or 11–13 of gestation and then killed on day 20, severe haematological effects were observed in dams 24 h after exposure, although the severity of these effects decreased as time since exposure increased (National Toxicology Program, 1989). In addition, there was evidence that rats developed tolerance to or autoprotection against the haematological effects of 2-butoxyethanol, as the magnitude of the changes was smaller in pre-exposed rats (Ghanayem *et al.*, 1992; Sivarao & Mehendale, 1995). However, an increase in the time between pre-treatment and challenge from 7 to 14 or 21 days resulted in higher mortality, and indicated that the autoprotective effect is gradually lost as the red blood cells age (Sivarao & Mehendale, 1995). Therefore, similar to the results of the acute toxicity studies, these data suggested to the authors that younger blood cells are more resilient to the induction of effects by repeated exposure to 2-butoxyethanol, and that the lethality of 2-butoxyethanol is related to its ability to induce haemolysis.

Other target organs in which 2-butoxyethanol induced effects in short-term oral studies in rats include the spleen, liver and kidneys. Relative weights of the liver and spleen were increased in pregnant rats animals exposed to 100 mg/kg bw per day or more for 3 days (National Toxicology Program, 1989) and in male rats administered 125 mg/kg bw per day for 12 days (Ghanayem *et al.*, 1992), while increased relative kidney weight was observed in pregnant rats exposed to 100 mg/kg bw per day or more for 3 days (National Toxicology Program, 1989). Ezov *et al.* (2002) noted that increases in absolute and relative spleen weights inversely correlated with decreases in red blood cell count in male and female rats administered 250 mg/kg bw 2-butoxyethanol daily for up to 4 days. Microscopic examination revealed congestion of the spleen in rats after 6 weeks of exposure to 222, 443 and 885 mg/kg bw per day, while haemosiderin deposition in the liver and kidneys and haemoglobinuria were noted after exposure to 443 mg/kg bw per day and above (Krasavage, 1986). In contrast, no effects on organ weights were observed in short-term studies in which rats were exposed to up to 506 mg/kg bw per day for up to 21 days (Exon *et al.*, 1991; National Toxicology Program, 1993) or up to 225 mg/kg bw per day for as long as 65 days (Dieter *et al.*, 1990).

Data on the short-term toxicity of orally administered 2-butoxyethanol in mice are more limited. No specific target organs were identified in a limited 2-week range-finding study at doses of up to 627 and 1364 mg/kg bw per day (in males and females, respectively) in the drinking-water, although the relative thymus weight of the males was decreased at 370 mg/kg bw per day and above (National Toxicology Program, 1993). Dehydration was reported in some animals that were exposed to the highest doses (370 and 627 mg/kg bw per day in males and 673 and 1364 mg/kg bw per day in females), although decreased drinking-water consumption was only observed in one of the groups that was reported to have symptoms of dehydration. A reduction in red blood cell count was observed in mice administered 500 or 1000 mg/kg bw per day on 5 days per week for 5 weeks, but haemoglobin levels were not affected (Nagano et al., 1979, 1984).

In an investigation of the potential mode of action of the induction of forestomach tumours in mice, Poet et al. (2003) administered 2-butoxyethanol by gavage to male and female B6C3F₁ mice at doses of 0, 400, 800 or 1200 mg/kg bw per day for 2 days, which were reduced to 0, 200, 400 or 600 mg/kg bw per day for an additional 2 days. Epithelial hyperplasia and inflammation of the forestomach were observed at all doses, and severity increased with dose. Similar effects were also observed in mice administered 400 mg/kg bw per day by intraperitoneal or subcutaneous injection for 4 days. Green et al. (2002) observed hyperkeratosis of the forestomach in female B6C3F₁ mice administered 500 mg/kg bw per day 2-butoxyethanol for 10 days, but not in the forestomach of mice exposed to 150 mg/kg bw per day or less or in the glandular stomach in any dose group.

Inhalation exposure

In short-term inhalation studies in rats, the blood, liver and kidneys were the main targets of 2-butoxyethanol toxicity, although examination was limited to gross pathology (Dodd et al., 1983) or to the microscopic appearance of a limited range of tissues (Carpenter et al., 1956). Increased erythrocyte fragility was reported in an early study in rats after 30 exposures (7 h per day on 5 days per week for 6 weeks) to 54 ppm [261 mg/m³] 2-butoxyethanol and above (Carpenter et al., 1956). In Fischer 344 rats exposed to 0, 20, 86 or 245 ppm [0, 97, 415 or 1183 mg/m³] for 9 days (6 h per day), haematological effects observed at the two higher concentrations included significantly decreased red blood cell count and haemoglobin concentration and increased reticulocyte count and mean corpuscular volume; with the exception of mean corpuscular volume, these changes were reversible during a 14-day recovery period. Increases in relative liver weight were observed at 85 ppm and above, and reversible changes in relative liver weight were also noted at 245 ppm and above. No effects were noted at 20 ppm (Dodd et al., 1983). In another earlier investigation, Werner et al. (1943b) observed decreases in red blood cell count and haemoglobin, accompanied by increases in reticulocyte count, in Wistar rats exposed to 135 or 320 ppm [653 or 1549 mg/m³] 2-butoxyethanol for 5 weeks (7 h per day on 5 days per week).

In a study that was primarily designed to investigate developmental toxicity, pregnant Fischer 344 rats were exposed to 0, 25, 50, 100 or 200 ppm [0, 121, 242, 483 or 966 mg/m³] 2-butoxyethanol for 10 days. The animals were killed on day 21 of gestation and haematological analyses were carried out on the dams. Similar to the effects reported by Dodd et al. (1983), significant decreases in red blood cell count and mean corpuscular haemoglobin concentration and increases in mean corpuscular volume and mean corpuscular haemoglobin were observed in dams exposed to 100 ppm and 200 ppm; significant decreases in haemoglobin and haematocrit and increased relative spleen and relative kidney weights were noted after exposure to 200 ppm. No effects were observed after exposure to 50 and 25 ppm (Tyl et al., 1984).

In the only available short-term inhalation study in mice, a reversible increase in erythrocyte fragility was observed in animals exposed to 100 ppm [483 mg/m^3] for 30 exposures; transient haemoglobinuria was evident after exposure to 200 and 400 ppm [966 and 1932 mg/m^3] (Carpenter et al., 1956).

Exposure of pregnant New Zealand white rabbits to up to 200 ppm [966 mg/m^3] 2-butoxyethanol for 13 days did not result in clear alterations in haematological parameters; however, there was a suggestion of haematuria/haemoglobinuria after exposure to high concentrations (100 and 200 ppm). In addition, mortality and the occurrence of spontaneous abortions were increased by 200 ppm, but not by 100 ppm or less (Tyl et al., 1984).

Limited data are also available on the short-term toxicity of 2-butoxyethanol in other experimental species. No haematological effects were noted in guinea-pigs exposed to up to 494 ppm [2386 mg/m^3] 2-butoxyethanol, although effects were noted in the lungs (congestion) and kidney (tubule swelling and increased relative weight) (Carpenter et al., 1956). However, effects on blood parameters (including increased leukocyte count, decreased erythrocyte count and haemoglobin and increased erythrocyte osmotic fragility) were noted in a small number of dogs exposed to 385 ppm [1860 mg/m^3] and in monkeys exposed to 200 or 100 ppm [966 or 483 mg/m^3] (Carpenter et al., 1956). Werner et al. (1943c) also observed slight, but statistically significant effects on haematological parameters (decreased haematocrit and haemoglobin) in dogs exposed to 415 ppm [2005 mg/m^3] for up to 12 weeks (7 h per day on 5 days per week).

Dermal exposure

Only limited data are available on the short-term dermal toxicity of 2-butoxyethanol. Based on a limited secondary account of an unpublished study (Tyler, 1984), haematological effects (reductions in red blood cell count and haemoglobin concentration) and local skin damage (erythema, oedema and necrosis) were reported in rabbits that received nine applications of an aqueous solution, with a lowest-observable-effect level (LOEL) of 180 mg/kg bw per day (applied as a 50% aqueous dilution) and a NOEL of 90 mg/kg bw per day (applied as a 25% aqueous dilution).

(ii)   *Subchronic exposure*

Based on the limited database available, haematological effects and effects on the liver and kidneys appear to be the critical effects associated with subchronic exposure via ingestion or inhalation in animals.

Oral exposure

In a study conducted by the National Toxicology Program (1993), male and female Fischer 344/N rats were administered 0, 750, 1500, 3000, 4500 or 6000 ppm 2-butoxyethanol in the drinking-water (estimated equivalent doses, 0, 69, 129, 281, 367 or 452 mg/kg bw per day in males and 0, 82, 151, 304, 363 or 470 mg/kg bw per day in females based on drinking-water consumption) for 13 weeks. Haematological effects indicative of anaemia were observed in both males and females exposed to 750–6000 ppm (equivalent to 69–452 mg/kg bw per day in males and 82–470 mg/kg bw per day in females). Females were more sensitive to the haematological effects than males, as alterations in blood parameters (including red blood cell count, haemoglobin concentration, mean cell volume, mean cell haemoglobin and haematocrit) were reported at all doses as early as 1 week after initiation of exposure and were still present at 13 weeks. In males, signs of mild anaemia were only observed at doses of 1500 ppm (129 mg/kg bw per day) and above. The authors suggested from the spectrum of haematological effects that the anaemia was regenerative (as indicated by increased numbers of reticulocytes) and that haemolysis was brought about by cell swelling (increased mean cell volume). Effects were also observed in the liver, including increased relative weights (82 and 367 mg/kg bw per day in females and males, respectively) and histopathological changes (hepatocellular degeneration with 304 and 281 mg/kg bw per day in females and males, respectively, cytoplasmic alterations in all exposed groups and pigmentation with 151 and 452 mg/kg bw per day in females and males, respectively). Although the authors noted that cytoplasmic alterations may be related to the induction of enzymes that are associated with glucuronide and sulfate conjugation of 2-butoxyethanol, an increase in relative liver weight (commonly associated with enzyme induction) was observed at all exposure levels in females, while such increases were only noted in males at higher doses. Hepatic pigmentation was considered to be secondary to haematotoxicity (with similar sex-related differences in sensitivity), while degenerative changes were considered to be compound-related and may represent a primary toxicity of 2-butoxyethanol. The lowest concentration administered (i.e. 750 ppm, or 82 and 69 mg/kg bw per day in females and males for haematological and hepatic effects, respectively) was found to be the LOEL.

In male and female B6C3F$_1$ mice administered 0, 750, 1500, 3000, 4500 or 6000 ppm 2-butoxyethanol in the drinking-water for 13 weeks (estimated equivalent doses, 0, 118, 223, 553, 676 or 694 mg/kg bw per day in males and 0, 185, 370, 676, 861 or 1306 mg/kg bw per day in females based on drinking-water consumption), the only effects observed in mice exposed to up to 6000 ppm (equivalent to 694 and 1306 mg/kg bw per day in males and females, respectively) were slight reductions in body-weight gain (6000 ppm in both sexes) and increased relative kidney weight in females at all exposure levels (i.e. 750 ppm or 185 mg/kg bw per day and above). However, the effects on kidney weight were considered to be secondary to reduced body-weight gain, as no histopathological changes were noted at the highest dose (National Toxicology Program, 1993). [However, the Working Group noted that relative kidney weights were increased at doses lower than those associated with significant reductions in body-weight gain.] In contrast, however, Heindel *et al.* (1990) reported increased mortality in female Swiss CD-1 mice administered drinking-water that contained 1 or 2% 2-butoxyethanol (equivalent doses, 1300 and 2100 mg/kg bw per day) for 15 weeks. Similarly exposed males lost weight during the study. No such effects were observed at doses of 700 mg/kg bw per day. No lesions of the kidney were observed in females exposed to 1300 mg/kg bw per day [the only dose at which examinations appear to have been conducted]. At this dose, relative kidney weights were increased in both sexes and relative liver weight was increased in the females. [It is unclear whether organ weights were examined at other doses.] The NOEL, based on changes in body-weight gain and organ weights, was considered to be 700 mg/kg bw per day; however, it is not indicated whether organ weights were examined at this dose. Haematological parameters were not investigated in either of these two studies.

In a study designed to investigate potential modes of induction of the liver neoplasms observed in a previously reported chronic bioassay in mice (National Toxicology Program, 2000), Siesky *et al.* (2002) administered 2-butoxyethanol by gavage to male B6C3F$_1$ mice and male Fischer 344 rats at doses of 0, 225, 450 and 900 mg/kg bw per day (mice) and 0, 225 and 450 mg/kg bw per day (rats) for up to 90 days; animals were killed after 7, 14, 28 and 90 days of exposure. Dose-related decreases in haematocrit and increases in relative spleen weight were observed in both species, accompanied by an increase in iron deposition in Kupffer cells. Oxidative DNA and lipid damage, as measured by 8-hydroxydeoxyguanosine and malondialdehyde, respectively, and increased DNA synthesis in hepatocytes and endothelial cells were observed in mice after 7 and 90 days of exposure to 2-butoxyethanol, but not in rats at any time point. Park *et al.* (2002a) observed similar indications of oxidative stress in B6C3F$_1$ mice exposed to 450 or 900 mg/kg bw 2-butoxyethanol per day by gavage for 7 days, together with decreased levels of the antioxidant, vitamin E. In an accompanying in-vitro study, these authors induced oxidative stress in isolated mouse hepatocytes exposed to haemolysed red blood cells, but not in hepatocytes exposed to 2-butoxyethanol or 2-butoxyacetic acid, which, they suggested, was indicative that the oxidative stress in the liver in mice was secondary to the accumulation of iron that resulted from 2-butoxyethanol-induced haemolysis. Based on the results of these studies, Park *et al.* (2002a) hypothesized that the liver tumours in mice arise due to stress associated with iron deposition in the liver, although, as noted below, the incidence of hepatic haemosiderin pigmentation did not correlate with the presence of tumours (National Toxicology Program, 2000) (see Section 4.5).

Inhalation exposure

In Fischer 344/N rats exposed to 0, 31, 62.5, 125, 250 or 500 ppm [0, 150, 302, 604, 1208 or 2415 mg/m^3] 2-butoxyethanol by inhalation for 14 weeks (6 h per day on 5 days per week), changes in haematological parameters that were characteristic of macrocytic, normochromic, responsive anaemia (i.e. increased mean cell volume, lack of change in mean cell haemoglobin values and increased reticulocyte count) were observed (National

Toxicology Program, 2000). Females were more sensitive than males; alterations in haematological parameters were observed at the lowest concentration tested (i.e. LOEL, 31 ppm [150 mg/m^3]) in females, while the LOEL in males for these effects was 125 ppm [604 mg/m^3]; the NOEL in males was found to be 62.5 ppm [302 mg/m^3]. The severity of these effects increased with concentration in both sexes. In addition, females that died or were killed before the end of the study had an increased incidence of thrombosis in the blood vessels of several tissues as well as bone infarction. Signs of earlier infarction were also observed in the vertebrae of females exposed to 500 ppm and killed at the end of the study period, although there was no evidence of thrombosis in these animals. These effects were not observed in male rats. It was hypothesized by the authors that the thrombosis resulted from severe acute haemolysis, which caused a release of protocoagulants from erythrocytes, or from anoxic damage to endothelial cells; either of these effects could compromise blood flow (see also Nyska *et al.*, 1999b). Long *et al.* (2000) also reported thrombosis and infarction of the dental pulp of female rats that were exposed to 500 ppm [2415 mg/m^3] for 13 weeks and killed early (day 4 of the treatment) due to their moribund condition, but not in rats that were killed at termination of the study; they suggested that this was indicative of reversibility of the lesions. Other effects consistent with regenerative haemolytic anaemia observed in both male and female rats included excessive haemato-poietic cell proliferation in the spleen, haemosiderin pigmentation in hepatic Kupffer cells and renal cortical tubules and bone marrow hyperplasia. Inflammation and/or hyperplasia of the forestomach also occurred in male and female rats exposed to the higher concentrations (250 and 500 ppm [1208 and 2415 mg/m^3]), while increases in relative kidney and liver weights were noted in females exposed to 62.5 ppm [302 mg/m^3] and above and in males exposed to 250 ppm and above (National Toxicology Program, 2000).

Haematological effects that consisted of slight decreases in red blood cell count and haemoglobin levels and an increase in mean corpuscular haemoglobin were also observed in female Fischer 344 rats exposed to 77 ppm [372 mg/m^3] (6 h per day on 5 days per week) for 6 weeks (Dodd *et al.*, 1983); after 13 weeks of exposure, values for these parameters were generally similar to those of controls [contrary to the observations in this strain of rats by the National Toxicology Program (2000)]. Males appeared to be much less sensitive, as the only effect on blood was a very slight decrease in red blood cell count after 13 weeks of exposure to 77 ppm. No indication of haematotoxicity was observed at doses of 25 and 5 ppm [121 and 24 mg/m^3]. No histopathological changes or alterations in clinical chemistry were noted in exposed rats (Dodd *et al.*, 1983).

Alterations in haematological parameters that were indicative of haemolytic anaemia (haemoglobin, haematocrit and erythrocyte counts) were also the most sensitive end-points observed in B6C3F$_1$ mice exposed to 0, 31, 62.5, 125, 250 or 500 ppm [0, 150, 302, 604, 1208 or 2415 mg/m^3] (6 h per day on 5 days per week) for 14 weeks (National Toxicology Program, 2000). However, the anaemia in mice was considered to be normocytic, normochromic and responsive (compared with the macrocytic anaemia noted in rats), because 2-butoxyethanol did not induce any changes in mean cell volume. In addition, based on the magnitude of the changes, the anaemia was less severe in mice than in rats, although females were again more sensitive than males (LOELs in females and males, 31 ppm [150 mg/m^3] and 125 ppm [604 mg/m^3], respectively). As in rats, effects in the spleen that were consistent with regenerative anaemia (haemosiderin pigmentation at doses of 125 ppm and above in males and 250 ppm and above in females and increased haematopoiesis at doses of 250 ppm and above in males and at 500 ppm in females) were also observed. The incidence of hyperplasia of the forestomach was increased in female mice exposed to 125 ppm or more, while the incidence of forestomach inflammation was increased in females exposed to 250 ppm and above. In males, only non-statistically significant increases in the incidence of forestomach hyperplasia were observed after exposure to the highest concentration. The incidence of haemosiderin pigmentation of hepatic Kupffer cells was increased in male mice at doses of 500 ppm and in female mice at doses of 250 ppm or above; haemosiderin pigmentation was also observed in the renal tubules of both males and females exposed to the highest concentration. Increased mortality was noted in both males and females exposed to 500 ppm.

In an early 90-day study of male C3H mice (Carpenter *et al.*, 1956) that were exposed to 0, 100, 200 or 400 ppm [0, 483, 966 or 1932 mg/m^3] 2-butoxyethanol (7 h per day on 5 days per week) for up to 90 days, transient haemoglobinuria and reversible increased liver weights were observed at the two higher concentrations, although no lesions were observed on microscopic examination of the liver, kidney and lung. The osmotic fragility of the red blood cells from all exposed animals was increased immediately after each exposure, but no increase in severity was apparent throughout the duration of the study. However, the erythrocytes returned to normal during the 17-h rest between exposures. Thus, the LOEL was found to be 100 ppm [483 mg/m^3].

No overt signs of toxicity and no effects on the weight or microscopic appearance of unspecified organs or on haematology (including osmotic fragility) were observed in New Zealand white rabbits that received daily dermal applications (covered) of up to 150 mg/kg bw per day 2-butoxyethanol for 6 h per day on 5 days per week for 13 weeks (Tyler, 1984; ECETOC, 1994, 1995).

(iii) *Chronic inhalation exposure*

A 2-year inhalation bioassay was conducted in groups of 50 male and 50 female Fischer 344/N rats that were exposed to 0, 31.2, 62.5 or 125 ppm [0, 151, 302 or 604 mg/m^3] 2-butoxyethanol (6 h per day on 5 days per week) for 104 weeks. An additional nine or 27 male and female rats per group were evaluated at 3, 6 and 12 months. Similar to the critical end-points observed in shorter-term studies, chronic exposure to 31.2 ppm [151 mg/m^3] 2-butoxyethanol (the lowest concentration tested) or more resulted in haemolytic anaemia (characterized as macrocytic, normochromic anaemia based on decreases in haematocrit, haemoglobin concentrations and erythrocyte counts, increases in mean cell volume and mean cell haemoglobin and the lack of an effect on mean cell haemoglobin concentration) in both male and female rats, which persisted throughout the 12 months that haematological parameters were monitored. The severity of these effects increased with level of exposure and did not improve over time. The anaemia was considered to be responsive, based on the observation of increased reticulocyte and nucleated erythrocyte counts and a decrease in the myeloid:erythroid ratios. Consistent with results observed in earlier studies, toxicokinetic data indicated slower clearance of the active metabolite, 2-butoxyacetic acid, and greater activity of the relevant isoenzyme in females. In general, the severity of haematological effects was greater in females than in males, and alterations in multiple parameters were observed at the lowest concentration tested (i.e. 31.2 ppm [151 mg/m^3], which was considered to be the LOEL), while only mean cell volume was affected in males at this concentration (National Toxicology Program, 2000).

Neoplastic lesions were observed in the adrenal gland of female rats, as described in Section 3. A non-statistically significant increase in the incidence of hyperplasia of the adrenal medulla was also observed in females exposed to 125 ppm [302 mg/m^3]. No such increases were observed in males. Other exposure-related histopathological changes observed in rats exposed to 62.5 ppm and above included increased incidences of minimal hyaline degeneration of the olfactory epithelium in males and females (incidences: 13/48, 21/49, 23/49 and 40/50 males and 13/50, 18/48, 28/50 and 40/49 females exposed to 0, 31.2, 62.5 and 125 ppm, respectively) (which was considered by the authors to be an adaptive/protective effect rather than an adverse effect), increased incidences of pigmentation of Kupffer cells in the liver of males and females (incidences: 23/50, 30/50, 34/50 and 42/50 males and 15/50, 19/50, 36/50 and 47/50 females exposed to 0, 31.2, 62.5 and 125 ppm, respectively) and an increase in splenic fibrosis in males (incidences: 11/50, 14/50, 19/50 and 20/50 exposed to 0, 31.2, 62.5 and 125 ppm, respectively) (National Toxicology Program, 2000).

In a concurrent bioassay (National Toxicology Program, 2000), groups of 50 male and 50 female B6C3F$_1$ mice were exposed by inhalation to 0, 62.5, 125 or 250 ppm [0, 302, 604 or 1208 mg/m^3] 2-butoxyethanol for 6 h per day on 5 days per week for 104 weeks. An additional 30 male and 30 female mice were evaluated at 3, 6 and 12 months. Consistent with the results reported for shorter-term studies, B6C3F$_1$ mice were less sensitive to the haematological effects of 2-butoxyethanol than rats. Anaemia, which was characterized by decreases in haematocrit, haemoglobin concentrations and erythrocyte count, occurred at 3, 6 and 12 months in male and female mice exposed to the two higher concentrations (125 and 250 ppm [604 and 1208 mg/m^3]) and there was some evidence of anaemia in females exposed to 62.5 ppm [302 mg/m^3], but only at one time-point (6 months). In general, based on the lack of consistent changes in mean cell volume (except in females exposed to 250 ppm for 12 months) and mean cell haemoglobin concentrations, the effects observed in mice were consistent with normocytic, normochromic anaemia. Although it was considered to be responsive, based on the increased reticulocyte counts, this response improved over time. In addition, contrary to the observations in rats, there were no decreases in myeloid:erythroid ratios; in fact, increases were observed in some exposed groups. Thrombocytosis was present in both male and female mice at all concentrations, based on the increase in platelet counts; time of appearance was inversely related to concentration. As in rats, female mice were more sensitive than males, and significant alterations in haematological parameters generally occurred earlier and at lower exposure levels in female mice.

The observed neoplastic lesions, including those of the forestomach, liver and circulatory system, are described in Section 3. The incidence of hyperplasia of the epithelium of the forestomach was significantly increased in a concentration-related manner in all exposed groups (1/50, 7/50, 16/50 and 21/50 males and 6/50, 27/50, 42/50 and 44/50 females exposed to 0, 62.5, 125 and 250 ppm, respectively), which was accompanied by a concentration-related trend in the incidence of ulcers of the forestomach in female mice (1/50, 7/50, 13/50 and 22/50). The authors hypothesized that the observed forestomach tumours represented a continuation of the injury/degeneration process, although the potential relationship between these lesions was not investigated. [The authors noted that the mechanism by which the forestomach is exposed is not clear; the role of preening or mucocilliary clearance of the respiratory tract in the exposure is unknown, although similar lesions and accumulation of 2-butoxyethanol in the forestomach of mice were also observed following oral or intraperitoneal administration (Poet *et al.*, 2003).] Minimally severe haemosiderin pigmentation of Kupffer cells was also noted in the liver of exposed mice, which did not appear to be directly correlated to the incidence of neoplastic lesions in this organ, since such pigmentation was not present in all males in which liver tumours were observed but was noted in female mice that did not have an increased incidence of neoplastic lesions at this site. Therefore, although the pathogenesis of neoplastic lesions of the liver could not be determined, the authors suggested that it was unlikely to be related to the accumulation of haemosiderin pigment and was possibly related to oxidative stress. The LOEL for non-neoplastic effects (haematotoxicity and forestomach lesions) was 62.5 ppm [302 mg/m^3] in both sexes of mice.

(iv)   *Other data*

Based on the limited data available, 2-butoxyethanol appears to have some immunomodulating potential, to which mice are more sensitive than rats. Significant effects on indicators of immune function were observed in BALB/c mice administered repeated oral doses of 50 mg/kg bw per day or more for 10 days (Morris *et al.*, 1996), while only slight or no changes in immune function parameters were noted in Fischer 344 and Sprague-Dawley rats administered higher doses (i.e. up to 400 mg/kg bw per day by gavage for 2 days and up to 6000 pm in the drinking-water (equivalent to up to 444 mg/kg bw per day) for 21 days, respectively) (Exon *et al.*, 1991; Smialowicz *et al.*, 1992). Repeated dermal application of 500 mg/kg bw per day for 4 days or longer resulted in a reduced immune response of T cells, but not of B cells, in BALB/c mice (Singh *et al.*, 2001); no similar studies in rats were identified. Topical administration of 4 mg 2-butoxyethanol resulted in a time-dependent decrease in contact hypersensitivity response to oxazolone in female BALB/c mice, whereas higher dermal doses or oral administration of up to 400 mg/kg bw per day for 10 days did not modulate this response (Singh *et al.*, 2002). Reduced weights or histopathological changes were observed in the thymus or spleen of both mice and rats exposed subchronically or chronically to 2-butoxyethanol; however, it was considered that these effects were probably secondary to haemolysis and decreased body weight (National Toxicology Program, 1993, 2000).

No investigations of the neurological effects of 2-butoxyethanol have been identified, although various signs of effects on the central nervous system, including loss of coordination, sluggishness, narcosis, muscular flaccidity and ataxia, have been reported after exposure to high doses or concentrations in numerous short-term studies (Carpenter et al., 1956; Dodd et al., 1983; Hardin et al., 1984; Krasavage, 1986).

(c)   In-vitro investigations of haemolytic effects

Differences in species sensitivity to haemolysis induced by 2-butoxyethanol and its metabolites have been investigated in several studies in vitro. Consistent with the results of in-vivo studies, 2-butoxyacetic acid was more potent than either the parent compound or the acetaldehyde metabolite (Bartnik et al., 1987; Ghanayem, 1989; Sivarao & Mehendale, 1995). Although slight species differences were observed in erythrocytes exposed to 2-butoxyethanol (humans were less sensitive than rats, mice, dogs and guinea-pigs) (Carpenter et al., 1956; Bartnik et al., 1987), variability between species was much more pronounced when cells were exposed to 2-butoxyacetic acid (erythrocytes from humans were less sensitive than those of rats). In a comparison across multiple mammalian species (three to five animals per species), Ghanayem and Sullivan (1993) observed that red blood cells from rats, mice, hamsters, rabbits and baboons were more sensitive to the effects of 2-butoxyacetic acid than those of pigs, dogs, cats, guinea-pigs and humans.

Bartnik et al. (1987) reported that 1.25 mM [165 µg/mL] 2-butoxyacetic acid (the lowest concentration administered) resulted in 25% haemolysis in male Wistar rat erythrocytes after 180 min, while, in contrast, 15 mM [1980 µg/mL] 2-butoxyacetic acid did not produce measurable haemolysis in erythrocytes from healthy humans over the same time. [This study was conducted on washed erythrocytes rather than whole blood, which indicates that the species difference in sensitivity in vitro was probably due to an inherent difference in the erythrocytes, rather than in the extent of plasma protein binding of 2-butoxyacetic acid.] Ghanayem (1989) exposed pooled whole blood from male Fischer 344 rats and healthy human volunteers (three men and women) to 2-butoxyacetic acid for 0.25–4 h and measured haematocrit and free plasma haemoglobin levels as indicators of swelling of the erythrocytes and haemolysis, respectively. Based on observations after 4 h of incubation, 8.0 mM [1056 µg/mL] 2-butoxyacetic acid had less effect in humans than 0.5 mM [66 µg/mL] 2-butoxyacetic acid had in rats. [However, it is not clear from the data presented whether the slight changes in human erythrocytes were produced in relation to the initial control value or were compared with data for a 4-h incubation in the absence of 2-butoxyacetic acid.] Similarly, Udden and Patton (1994) observed no effects in human erythrocytes exposed to 2 mM [264 µg/mL] 2-butoxyacetic acid (the maximum concentration tested) for 4 h, although this concentration induced rapid haemolysis in rat erythrocytes. Exposure of rat erythrocytes to 0.2 mM [26.4 µg/mL] 2-butoxyacetic acid did not result in haemolysis, although reduced cell deformability and increased mean cell volume were noted. In a subsequent investigation, similar sub-haemolytic changes were observed, including loss of deformability and an increase in mean cell volume and cell sodium levels, in human erythrocytes (from up to 14 individuals) that were incubated with 7.5 or 10.0 mM [990 or 1320 µg/mL] 2-butoxyacetic acid and in rat erythrocytes exposed to lower concentrations of 2-butoxyacetic acid (i.e. 0.05, 0.075 or 1.0 mM [6.6, 9.9 or 132 µg/mL]). A slight, but statistically significant increase in haemolysis was observed in red blood cells obtained from 40 hospitalized adults that were exposed *in vitro* to 10 mM 2-butoxyacetic acid; significant increases in haemolysis were not noted in exposed cells from 11 healthy adults or 46 hospitalized children (Udden, 2002).

Following incubation for 4 h with 2 mM [264 µg/mL] 2-butoxyacetic acid, Udden (1994) reported a lack of haemolysis in human red blood cells from groups of different human subjects, including nine healthy young adults (31–56 years old), nine older subjects (64–79 years old), seven patients who had sickle-cell disease and three patients who had spherocytosis. However, these groups differed with regard to the extent of spontaneous haemolysis that occurred after incubation of their red blood cells for 4 h in the absence of 2-butoxyacetic acid.

Unlike the sex-related differences in sensitivity to 2-butoxyethanol-induced haematological effects that have been observed in rats exposed *in vivo*, in-vitro exposure of rat erythrocytes to the metabolite 2-butoxyacetic acid revealed no differences in sensitivity between males and females, as measured by packed cell volume (Ghanayem *et al.*, 2000), which provides further support to the supposition that differences *in vivo* are related to differences in metabolism and toxicokinetics of 2-butoxyethanol rather than to differences in toxicodynamics.

(d) Mode of action that induces haematological effects

Extensive data from comparative toxicity studies with the parent compound and its metabolites, as well as from studies in which oxidation of 2-butoxyethanol to 2-butoxy-acetic acid is inhibited, indicate that 2-butoxyacetic acid is the metabolite that is principally responsible for the haematological effects observed in experimental animals exposed to 2-butoxyethanol (Ghanayam *et al.*, 1987b; Morel *et al.*, 1996). The changes in haematological parameters induced by 2-butoxyacetic acid are characteristic of haemolytic anaemia, although the mode(s) of action by which 2-butoxyacetic acid induces these effects has (have) not been established conclusively. Before the occurrence of haemolysis in red blood cells from rats, erythrocyte swelling, morphological changes (including a change from typical discocytic to spherocytic appearance and stomatocytosis) and decreased deformability have been observed (Udden, 1996). Udden (2000) observed similar morphological changes in rat erythrocytes following in-vivo exposure to 125 mg/kg bw 2-butoxyethanol and in-vitro exposure to 1.0 mM [132 µg/mL] 2-butoxy-acetic acid which are suggestive of a progression from stomatocytosis, or cupping, to spherocytosis and, finally, to lysis. These morphological changes were not observed in human erythrocytes incubated with up to 2.0 mM [264 µg/mL] 2-butoxyacetic acid. The severity of morphological changes in erythrocytes, including stomatocytosis, macro-cytosis, moderate rouleaux formation, spherocytosis, schistocytosis and ghost cell formation, increased progressively in male and female Fischer 344 rats administered 250 mg/kg bw 2-butoxyethanol per day by gavage for 1, 2 or 3 days (Ghanayem *et al.*, 2001). Based on available information from his own research and the investigations of others, Ghanayem (1996) hypothesized that the swelling of erythrocytes was due to increased cell membrane permeability to cations and water and noted that such changes in cellular membranes have been observed in the blood of humans who have hereditary sphero-cytosis, as have stomatocytes, which are associated with altered intracellular levels of sodium and potassium that lead to increased cell water, increased mean cell volume, decreased deformability and increased osmotic fragility. 2-Butoxyacetic acid-induced swelling of rat erythrocytes exposed *in vitro* continued after removal of 2-butoxyacetic acid and was not reversible, although the rate of swelling decreased (Ghanayem *et al.*, 1989). These authors also investigated the partitioning of 2-butoxyacetic acid between erythrocytes and plasma and determined that the concentration in cells increased over time while that in the plasma remained relatively constant (Ghanayem *et al.*, 1989). In a previous study, Ghanayem and Matthews (1990) showed that administration of calcium channel blockers to rats before exposure to 2-butoxyethanol decreased the erythrocyte swelling and improved the associated haemolytic anaemia; it was speculated that homeo-stasis of intracellular calcium or other cations (whose passage through cellular mem-branes may be affected by such blockers) may be involved in 2-butoxyethanol-induced toxicity (Ghanayem, 1996). Conjugation of 2-butoxyethanol with long-chain fatty acids in the liver has been observed in rats (Kaphalia *et al.*, 1996), although it is not known whether such conjugation would occur when lipids were present in erythrocyte mem-branes. In addition, Dartsch *et al.* (1999) reported that the intermediate metabolite, butoxyacetaldehyde, caused depolymerization of intracellular stress fibres that contain actin in mammalian renal epithelial cells, which resulted in morphological alterations in cell shape and volume that were consistent with the hypothesis that cell swelling points to the induction of a necrotic process.

4.3   Reproductive and developmental effects

4.3.1   *Humans*

No data on the potential reproductive or developmental effects of 2-butoxyethanol in humans were available to the Working Group.

4.3.2   *Experimental systems*

(*a*)   *Reproductive toxicity*

Very limited information on the potential reproductive toxicity of 2-butoxyethanol is available. In the only investigation of the potential effect of 2-butoxyethanol on reproduc-tive ability identified (i.e. the multigeneration study by Heindel *et al.* (1990)), adminis-tration of 700–2100 mg/kg bw per day 2-butoxyethanol in the drinking-water to breeding pairs of CD-1 mice throughout mating, pregnancy and lactation did not induce any discernible effects on male reproductive organs or sperm or on the estrous cycle of females. However, fertility was impaired, based on statistically significant reductions in the numbers of litters per pair and live pups per litter after exposure to 1300 and 2100 mg/kg bw per day; these doses were also associated with decreased body-weight gain and drinking-water consumption in the parent mice. Based on the results of a cross-over mating trial, in which exposed males were mated with control females and exposed females were mated with control males, these effects were found to be primarily due to an effect on the treated females. Because of the lack of sufficient pups in the groups treated with 1300 and 2100 mg/kg bw per day, fertility was only examined in the group that was administered 700 mg/kg bw per day. No effects on reproductive ability, as measured by mating and fertility indices, litter size, proportion of live pups or live pup weights, were noted in mice exposed to 2-butoxyethanol *in utero*, from weaning to sexual maturity or until delivery of a litter.

Acute exposure to 800 ppm [3864 mg/m^3] of a saturated vapour of 2-butoxyethanol for 3 h did not result in altered testicular weight in Alpk/Ap rats (Doe, 1984). Similarly, no histopathological effects on the testes, epididymidis or seminal vesicles were observed in Alpk/Ap rats administered a single oral dose of up to 868 mg/kg bw butoxyacetic acid by gavage (Foster *et al.*, 1987).

No effects on testes weight or histopathology were reported in short-term studies in which Fischer 344 (or Fischer 344/N), Sprague-Dawley and Crl:COBS CD (SD)BR rats were administered doses of up to 1000, 506 and 885 mg/kg bw 2-butoxyethanol per day, respectively, and JCL-ICR mice were administered up to 2000 mg/kg bw per day (Nagano *et al.*, 1979, 1984; Grant *et al.*, 1985; Krasavage, 1986; Exon *et al.*, 1991; National Toxicology Program, 1993).

Sperm morphology and vaginal cytology were assessed in Fischer 344/N rats and B6C3F$_1$ mice that received 2-butoxyethanol in the drinking-water for 13 weeks. In mice, no evidence was found of an adverse effect on the estrous cycle of females administered up to 1306 mg/kg bw per day, while a slight reduction in sperm motility was observed in males that received 694 mg/kg bw per day and absolute left testis weights were slightly reduced at all dose levels (i.e. 553 mg/kg bw per day and above). In the corresponding study in rats, uterine atrophy or decreased sperm concentration were evident, with LOELs of 304 and 281 mg/kg bw per day in females and males, respectively (National Toxicology Program, 1993).

Testicular degeneration and necrosis of the epididymis was noted in a subchronic study in B6C3F$_1$ mice that were exposed by inhalation to 500 ppm [2415 mg/m^3] 2-butoxyethanol, a concentration that was associated with decreased survival and lesions in several organs (National Toxicology Program, 2000). No such effects were noted in the concurrent study in Fischer 344/N rats exposed to up to 500 ppm 2-butoxyethanol.

No effects on male or female reproductive organs were reported in a 2-year bioassay in which Fischer 344/N rats and B6C3F$_1$ mice were exposed to up to 125 and 250 ppm [604 and 1208 mg/m^3] 2-butoxyethanol, respectively (National Toxicology Program, 2000).

(b)   Developmental toxicity

In studies in rats and mice, oral administration of 2-butoxyethanol during pregnancy induced fetotoxic and/or embryotoxic effects, but generally only at or above maternally toxic doses. When Fischer 344 rats were administered 0, 30, 100 or 200 mg/kg bw 2-butoxyethanol per day by gavage on days 9–11 of pregnancy (National Toxicology Program, 1989), increased fetal deaths occurred after exposure to 200 mg/kg bw per day. Maternal toxicity (including haemolysis) was evident at doses of 100 mg/kg bw per day or more. The frequency of malformations was not increased at any dose level. Haematological effects (reduced platelet count) were also noted in fetuses of dams that were exposed to 300 mg/kg bw per day on days 11–13 of gestation, although inconsistent changes in mean corpuscular volume were observed at lower doses. The LOELs for developmental and maternal toxicity were considered to be 200 and 100 mg/kg bw per day, respectively; no effects were noted after exposure to 30 mg/kg bw per day.

Pregnant CD-1 mice were administered 0, 350, 650, 1000, 1500 or 2000 mg/kg bw 2-butoxyethanol per day by gavage on days 8–14 of gestation (Wier et al., 1987). An increase in the number of resorbed embryos was observed after oral administration of 1000 mg/kg bw per day or more. Clinical signs of toxicity were observed in dams (staining of cage papers, lethargy, abnormal breathing, failure to right or mortality) treated with 650 mg/kg bw per day and above. The LOEL for maternal toxicity and the no-observed-adverse-effect level (NOAEL) for developmental toxicity were considered to be 650 mg/kg bw per day. In pups of dams administered 650 or 1000 mg/kg bw per day, no effects on survival or growth as of postnatal day 22 were observed. Administration by gavage of 1180 mg/kg bw per day (only dose tested) to CD-1 mice during days 7–14 of pregnancy resulted in maternal deaths (20%) and reductions in the number of viable litters, but did not affect pup weight or postnatal survival (Schuler et al.,1984; Hardin et al., 1987).

Heindel et al. (1990) observed a slight fetotoxic effect at a dose that was not overtly toxic to the parent animals; in a multigeneration study, a small, but statistically significant reduction in live pup weight (by 4.3%) was observed in the F_1 generation after administration of 0.5% 2-butoxyethanol in the drinking-water (equivalent to 700 mg/kg bw per day) to male and female CD-1 mice throughout mating, pregnancy and lactation. Greater reductions in live pup weight were noted at higher doses (1 and 2% in the drinking-water; equivalent to 1300 or 2100 mg/kg bw per day) at which overt maternal toxicity (decreased body weight and fluid consumption, increased kidney weight and/or increased mortality) was observed. This effect was attributed to maternal exposure, since it was only observed in pairings in which exposed females were mated with control males. However, although a 4.4% reduction in live pup weight was noted in the F_2 generation, this decrease was not statistically significant (which indicated that the effect did not worsen in successive generations), and 700 mg/kg bw per day was considered by the investigators to be close to the NOAEL for developmental toxicity.

Developmental toxicity in the form of increased numbers of non-viable implants and resorptions and decreased percentage of live fetuses per litter was observed in Fischer 344 rats exposed to 200 ppm [966 mg/m³] 2-butoxyethanol on days 6–15 of pregnancy. Reduced skeletal ossification was evident at doses of 100 ppm [483 mg/m³] or more (concentrations that were also maternally toxic based on weight loss and haematological effects). Therefore, the LOEL for maternal and developmental toxicity was considered to be 100 ppm, since no effects were observed at doses of 25 or 50 ppm [121 or 242 mg/m³] (Tyl et al., 1984). However, no significant developmental effects occurred in Sprague-Dawley rats exposed to 150 or 200 ppm [726 or 966 mg/m³] 2-butoxyethanol on days 7–15 of pregnancy, although haematuria occurred in dams on the first day of exposure at 200 ppm (Nelson et al., 1984). In rabbits exposed to 2-butoxyethanol on days 6–18 of pregnancy, the LOEL for both maternal and developmental toxicity was 200 ppm [966 mg/m³], based on increased mortality, abortions and weight loss and a slight reduction in the number of viable implants per litter; no significant toxicity was noted in dams or fetuses at doses of 100 ppm [483 mg/m³] or less (Tyl et al., 1984).

In a study of Sprague-Dawley rats that received repeated dermal applications (not specified if the site of application was covered) of neat 2-butoxyethanol on days 7–16 of pregnancy, no overt signs of maternal toxicity and no evidence of developmental toxicity were observed at doses of 0.48 mL per day (~3.6 mmol per day; ~1920 mg/kg bw per day). However, the higher dose of 1.4 mL per day (~10.8 mmole per day; ~5600 mg/kg bw per day) was lethal to the dams (Hardin et al., 1984).

4.4   Genetic and related effects

The genetic toxicology of 2-butoxyethanol and its major metabolites, 2-butoxyacetaldehyde and 2-butoxyacetic acid, has been reviewed (Elliott & Ashby, 1997).

4.4.1   *Humans*

The potential genotoxicity of 2-butoxyethanol and other glycol ethers was studied in a group of 19 workers (15 men and four women) who were occupationally exposed to glycol ethers in a varnish production plant. External and internal exposures were assessed by personal air monitoring on Monday and Tuesday after an exposure-free weekend. In the varnish production area, the concentrations of 2-butoxyethanol, 2-ethoxyethanol and 2-ethoxyethyl acetate in air averaged 0.5, 2.9 and 0.5 ppm, respectively, on Monday and 0.6, 2.1 and 0.1 ppm, respectively, on Tuesday. At the same workplaces, the mean concentrations of 2-butoxyacetic acid and 2-ethoxyacetic acid in the urine of workers were 0.2 and 53.2 mg/L on Monday before the workshift and 16.4 and 53.8 mg/L on Tuesday after the workshift, respectively. On Tuesday after the shift, venous blood samples were collected from the workers, and lymphocyte cultures were prepared and analysed for the frequency of sister chromatid exchange and micronuclei. Fifteen persons who were not occupationally exposed to glycol ethers and who largely matched the exposed group in terms of age and smoking habits served as controls. A comparison of all exposed and unexposed workers as well as of the small subgroups of exposed and unexposed smokers and nonsmokers did not show any increase in the mean frequencies of sister chromatid exchange or micronuclei in the exposed workers (Söhnlein *et al.*, 1993).

No data on the genetic and related effects of 2-butoxyacetaldehyde or 2-butoxyacetic acid in humans were available to the Working Group.

4.4.2   *Experimental systems* (see Table 17 for details and references)

2-Butoxyethanol

   (*a*)   *In-vitro studies*

2-Butoxyethanol has been examined in several bacterial mutagenicity assays both in the absence and in the presence of an exogenous metabolic activation system. In one of these studies (Zeiger *et al.* 1992), postmitochondrial supernatant from both rats and hamsters was used. No induction of gene mutations by 2-butoxyethanol was observed in *Escherichia coli* strain WP2*uvrA* or in *Salmonella typhimurium* strains TA100, TA102, TA1535, TA1537, TA98 or TA97. In a single study, mutagenic activity of 2-butoxyethanol in strain TA97a, which is closely related to strain TA97, was reported. This finding could not be confirmed, however, in a thorough independent study that was specifically designed to investigate this observation. Thus, there is no convincing evidence that 2-butoxyethanol can cause gene mutation in bacteria.

2-Butoxyethanol was also ineffective in inducing mutations in a bacteriophage assay.

In rat and mouse hepatocytes, 2-butoxyethanol did not cause a significant increase in the level of 8-hydroxydeoxyguanosine in DNA, a biomarker of oxidative stress.

In an assay for the induction of mutations in mammalian cells *in vitro*, 2-butoxyethanol did not increase the frequency of *Gpt* mutations in Chinese hamster ovary (CHO-AS52) cells, a subline that has been genetically engineered to allow the detection of both base substitutions and deletions that may result from clastogenic events. In another study, 2-butoxyethanol was reported to induce an increase in mutant frequency in Chinese hamster V79 cells over the concentration range of 20–75 mmol/L [2360–8850 µg/mL]. However, no data and no information on cytotoxicity were presented, and the description was inadequate for evaluation (Elias *et al.*, 1996).

Studies on the capacity of 2-butoxyethanol to induce sister chromatid exchange have yielded inconsistent results. Whereas negative results were reported in Chinese hamster ovary cells, positive findings were obtained in Chinese hamster lung V79 cells and human lymphocytes. A cell cycle delay was observed in 2-butoxyethanol-treated V79 cells (Elias *et al.*, 1996). [As no details on cell cycle kinetics of treated and untreated cells were given for the V79 cells and no data on toxicity or cell cycle were presented for human lymphocytes, the Working Group noted that whether the positive effects reported for these sister chromatid exchange assays are artefacts or not cannot be fully evaluated.]

Table 17. Genetic and related effects of 2-butoxyethanol and its metabolites

Test system	Result[a]		Dose[b] (LED/HID)	Reference
	Without exogenous metabolic system	With exogenous metabolic system		
2-Butoxyethanol				
Escherichia coli WP2*uvrA*, reverse mutation	–	–	10 000 µg/plate	Gollapudi *et al.* (1996)
Salmonella typhimurium TA100, TA1535, TA1537, TA98,TA97, reverse mutation	–	–	10 000 µg/plate	Zeiger *et al.* (1992)
Salmonella typhimurium TA100, TA102, TA98, reverse mutation	–	–	13 600 µg/plate	Hoflack *et al.* (1995)
Salmonella typhimurium TA100, TA97a, reverse mutation	–	–	10 000 µg/plate	Gollapudi *et al.* (1996)
Salmonella typhimurium TA97a, reverse mutation	+	NT	2200	Hoflack *et al.* (1995)
Salmonella typhimurium TA97a, reverse mutation	NT	+	9000 µg/plate	Hoflack *et al.* (1995)
Bacteriophage *T4D*, mutation	–	NT	111.1	Kvelland (1988)
Oxidative DNA damage, 8-OHdG, B6C3F₁ mouse and Fischer 344 rat hepatocytes *in vitro*	–	NT	2954	Park *et al.* (2002a)
Gene mutation, Chinese hamster ovary (CHO-AS52) cells, *Gpt* locus *in vitro*	–	NT	898	Chiewchanwit & Au (1995)
Gene mutation, Chinese hamster V79 cells, *Hprt* locus *in vitro*	(+)	NT	2363[c]	Elias *et al.* (1996)
Sister chromatid exchange, Chinese hamster ovary (CHO) cells *in vitro*	–	NT	3500	National Toxicology Program (1993)
Sister chromatid exchange, Chinese hamster ovary (CHO) cells *in vitro*	NT	–	5 000	National Toxicology Program (1993)
Sister chromatid exchange, Chinese hamster V79 cells *in vitro*	(+)	NT	2363[c]	Elias *et al.* (1996)
Micronucleus formation, Chinese hamster V79 cells *in vitro*	(+)	NT	1005	Elias *et al.* (1996)
Chromosomal aberrations, Chinese hamster ovary (CHO) cells *in vitro*	–	–	5000	National Toxicology Program (1993)
Chromosomal aberrations, Chinese hamster V79 cells *in vitro*	–	NT	NG	Elias *et al.* (1996)
Aneuploidy, Chinese hamster V79 cells *in vitro*	+	NT	993	Elias *et al.* (1996)
Cell transformation, Syrian hamster embryo cells	–	NT	NG	Elias *et al.* (1996)
Cell transformation, Syrian hamster embryo cells	(+)	NT	1000	Kerckaert *et al.* (1996)
Cell transformation, Syrian hamster embryo cells	–	NT	2363	Park *et al.* (2002b)

Table 17 (contd)

Test system	Result[a]		Dose[b] (LED/HID)	Reference
	Without exogenous metabolic system	With exogenous metabolic system		
Sister chromatid exchange, human peripheral lymphocytes *in vitro*	+		500 ppm [500]	Villalobos-Pietrini *et al.* (1989)
Chromosomal aberrations, human peripheral lymphocytes *in vitro*	–		3000 ppm [3000]	Villalobos-Pietrini *et al.* (1989)
Chromosomal aberrations, human peripheral lymphocytes *in vitro*	–	NT	NG	Elias *et al.* (1996)
Oxidative DNA damage, 8-OHdG, mouse liver *in vivo*	+		900 po, 7 d	Park *et al.* (2002a)
Oxidative DNA damage, 8-OHdG, mouse liver *in vivo*	+		450 po × 5/wk, 7–90 d	Siesky *et al.* (2002)
Oxidative DNA damage, 8-OHdG, rat liver *in vivo*	–		450 po × 5/wk, 7–90 d	Siesky *et al.* (2002)
DNA adduct formation (^{32}P-postlabelling), Sprague-Dawley rats, brain, kidney, liver, spleen, testes *in vivo*	–		120 po × 1	Keith *et al.* (1996)
Micronucleus formation, male and female CD-1 mice, polychromatic erythrocytes in bone marrow *in vivo*	–		800 ip × 1	Elias *et al.* (1996)
Micronucleus formation, male B6C3F$_1$ mice, polychromatic erythrocytes in bone marrow *in vivo*	–		550 ip × 3	National Toxicology Program (2000)
Micronucleus formation, male Fischer 344/N rats, polychromatic erythrocytes in bone marrow *in vivo*	–		450 ip × 3	National Toxicology Program (2000)
Inhibition of intercellular communication, Chinese hamster V79 cells *in vitro*	+	NT	1005	Elias *et al.* (1996)
2-Butoxyacetaldehyde				
Salmonella typhimurium TA100, TA102, TA98, TA97a, reverse mutation	–	–	5000 µg/plate	Hoflack *et al.* (1995)
Gene mutation, Chinese hamster ovary (CHO-AS52) cells, *Gpt* locus *in vitro*	–	NT	0.2 % (v/v) 2000	Chiewchanwit & Au (1995)
Gene mutation, Chinese hamster V79 cells, *Hprt* locus *in vitro*	+	NT	232	Elias *et al.* (1996)
Sister chromatid exchange, Chinese hamster V79 cells *in vitro*	+	NT	23.2	Elias *et al.* (1996)

Table 17 (contd)

Test system	Result[a]		Dose[b] (LED/HID)	Reference
	Without exogenous metabolic system	With exogenous metabolic system		
Micronucleus formation, Chinese hamster V79 cells *in vitro*	+	NT	4.7	Elias *et al.* (1996)
Chromosomal aberrations, Chinese hamster V79 cells *in vitro*	+	NT	9.5[c]	Elias *et al.* (1996)
Aneuploidy, Chinese hamster V79 cells *in vitro*	+	NT	10.6	Elias *et al.* (1996)
Cell transformation, Syrian hamster embryo cells *in vitro*	–	NT	NG	Elias *et al.* (1996)
Inhibition of intercellular communication, Chinese hamster V79 cells *in vitro*	–	NT	10	Elias *et al.* (1996)
Chromosomal aberrations, human peripheral lymphocytes *in vitro*	+	NT	9.5[c]	Elias *et al.* (1996)
2-Butoxyacetic acid				
Salmonella typhimurium TA100, TA102, TA98, TA97a, reverse mutation	–	–	1 000 µg/plate	Hoflack *et al.* (1995)
Sister chromatid exchange, Chinese hamster V79 cells *in vitro*	–	NT	105[c]	Elias *et al.* (1996)
Micronucleus formation, Chinese hamster V79 cells *in vitro*	(+)	NT	660	Elias *et al.* (1996)
Chromosomal aberrations, Chinese hamster V79 cells *in vitro*	–	NT	NG	Elias *et al.* (1996)
Aneuploidy, Chinese hamster V79 cells *in vitro*	?	NT	50	Elias *et al.* (1996)
Cell transformation, Syrian hamster embryo cells	–	NT	NG	Elias *et al.* (1996)
Chromosomal aberrations, human peripheral lymphocytes *in vitro*	–	NT	NG	Elias *et al.* (1996)
Micronucleus formation, male and female CD-1 mice, polychromatic erythrocytes in bone marrow *in vivo*	–		200 ip × 1	Elias *et al.* (1996)
Inhibition of intercellular communication, Chinese hamster V79 cells *in vitro*	–	NT	12 408	Elias *et al.* (1996)

8-OHdG, 8-hydroxydeoxyguanosine

[a] +, positive; –, negative; (+), weak positive; ?, inconclusive; NG, not given; NT, not tested

[b] LED, lowest effective dose; HID, highest ineffective dose; in-vitro tests, µg/mL; in-vivo tests, mg/kg bw; po, oral administration; ip, intraperitoneal injection; d, day; wk, week

[c] Estimated from the graph in the article

Consistently negative results were obtained in three independent studies that assessed the ability of 2-butoxyethanol to induce structural chromosomal aberrations in Chinese hamster ovary (CHO) cells and V79 lung cells and human lymphocytes.

In an in-vitro study that examined several genetic or related end-points in Chinese hamster V79 cells, a weak induction of micronuclei, an increased percentage of hyperdiploid cells (aneuploidy) and inhibition of gap-junctional metabolic cooperation between *Hprt*$^+$ and *Hprt*$^-$ cells were observed following treatment of the cells with 2-butoxyethanol. These assays are known to be especially sensitive to interference by the cytotoxic effects of test agents. [The Working Group felt that, in view of the lack of information provided on the toxicity of the treatments, the description of the results was too limited for an evaluation.]

Tests for the ability of 2-butoxyethanol to induce morphological transformation of Syrian hamster embryo cells yielded inconclusive results. Negative results were obtained in two studies in which the cells were incubated with the test compound for 7 days. Positive results were reported in an assay that used an exposure period of 24 h. [The Working Group noted that an inconsistent concentration–effect relationship was evident in this experiment.]

(b)   In-vivo studies

In mice exposed to 2-butoxyethanol by repeated oral administration of 450 and 900 mg/kg bw for 7 days, significantly elevated levels of 8-hydroxydeoxyguanosine were observed in hepatic DNA. This effect was attributed by the authors to oxidative stress induced via the induction of haemolysis and a resulting increase in iron deposition in the liver (Park *et al.*, 2002a). No increase in 8-hydroxydeoxyguanosine was found in liver DNA of similarly exposed rats. This difference is consistent with the species differences in the development of hepatic tumours (see Section 3). No evidence for the genotoxic activity of 2-butoxyethanol was obtained in other in-vivo studies. Oral administration of 120 mg/kg bw to rats did not cause the formation of hydrophilic or hydrophobic DNA adducts detectable by ^{32}P-postlabelling in the brain, liver, kidney spleen or testes. 2-Butoxyethanol did not increase the frequency of micronucleated polychromatic erythrocytes in the bone marrow of mice and rats following repeated intraperitoneal applications or of mice following a single intraperitoneal application. The ratio of polychromatic and normochromatic erythrocytes, a potential indicator of treatment-related cytotoxic effects on the bone marrow, was only determined in the study that used a single application and was found to be unaltered.

(i)   Alterations of proto-oncogenes in tumours

In order to determine whether the induction of mutations in proto-oncogenes by 2-butoxyethanol may have been involved in the formation of forestomach neoplasms induced by this compound in male and female B6C3F$_1$ mice (see Section 3), the spectra of H-*ras* proto-oncogene mutations in forestomach tumours of animals exposed to 2-butoxyethanol and of control animals were compared. Fourteen tumours from exposed mice and 11 from control mice were analysed. Codon 61 mutations in the H-*ras* gene were detected in 57% of the tumours of the exposed animals and in 45% of those of the control animals. The mutation profiles within the forestromach neoplasms of the 2-butoxy-ethanol-exposed animals did not differ significantly from those in the spontaneous neo-plasms. The high frequency of activated H-*ras* gene that was detected in spontaneous neo-plasms suggested that this gene is important for the formation of forestomach tumours in B6C3F$_1$ mice. The findings indicate that 2-butoxyethanol does not increase the mutation frequency of the H-*ras* proto-oncogene and suggest that the compound may enhance tumour formation by promoting clonal growth of spontaneously initiated forestomach cells that primarily contain an activated H-*ras* gene (National Toxicology Program, 2000).

In a related study, the effect of 2-butoxyethanol on the level of DNA methylation was investigated in mice and rats. The continuous treatment of transgenic FVB/N mice (Oncomice Neo 01^{TM}) which carry the viral Harvey *ras* (v-Ha-*ras*) oncogene with ~120 mg/kg bw 2-butoxyethanol per day via subcutaneously implanted minipumps for 2 weeks did not result in an alteration of the methylation status of the Ha-*ras* transgene in testes, spleen, brain, kidney or liver within 5 and 120 days after the start of administration. The authors concluded that it appears unlikely that 2-butoxyethanol causes demethylation of DNA, which would increase the expression of v-Ha-*ras*, or increased methylation of DNA, which would induce mutations through the formation of thymine from 5-methyl-cytosine. A ^{32}P-postlabelling study of the level of 5-methylcytosine from whole genome analyses of male and female v-Ha-*ras* transgenic mice treated with 2-butoxyethanol (mini-pump for up to 120 days) and of male Sprague-Dawley rats (120 mg/kg bw by gavage for 1 day) did not reveal any effect of the compounds on total DNA methylation in mice (brain, bone marrow, spleen and testes) or rats (brain, kidney, liver, spleen and testes) (Keith *et al.*, 1996).

(ii) *Interference with DNA repair*

High concentrations (≥ 8.5 mM) of 2-butoxyethanol have been shown to potentiate the induction of chromosomal aberrations in Chinese hamster V79 cells by methyl methane-sulfonate (Elias *et al.*, 1996). As 2-butoxyethanol alone did not display any clastogenic effect (Elias *et al.*, 1996), it was hypothesized that the compound might inhibit the repair of DNA that was previously damaged by the alkylating agent. In accordance with this hypothesis, Hoflack *et al.* (1997) observed that subsequent exposure to 2-butoxyethanol (5 mM) of Syrian hamster embryo cells that had been treated with methyl methanesulfo-nate (0.2 mM), which rapidly increases the cellular concentration of poly(ADP-ribose), inhibited poly(ADP-ribose) synthesis. No effect of 2-butoxyethanol on poly(ADP-ribose) concentration was observed in cells not pretreated with methyl methanesulfonate. The decrease was not caused by a depletion of NAD$^+$, the substrate of the polymerization reac-tion, by 2-butoxyethanol, and the underlying mechanism remained unclear. As poly(ADP-ribosyl)ation is involved in base-excision repair of DNA damage, this observation supports the notion that high concentrations of 2-butoxyethanol may interfere with the repair of certain types of DNA lesions and the maintenance of chromosomal stability.

2-Butoxyethanol metabolites

(a)   2-Butoxyacetaldehyde

2-Butoxyacetaldehyde did not induce gene mutations in several strains of *S. typhimurium* in the absence or presence of an exogenous metabolic activation system. It was not mutagenic in the Chinese hamster ovary cell subline CHO-AS52, in which the shorter analogue of 2-butoxyacetaldehyde, methoxyacetaldehyde, had been shown to induce mutations (Ma *et al.*, 1993). However, one study reported genotoxic effects at comparatively low concentrations of 2-butoxyacetaldehyde in various assays in Chinese hamster V79 cells without exogenous metabolic activation (an assay for gene mutations at the *Hprt* locus, an assay for the induction of sister chromatid exchange and an assay for the induction chromosomal aberrations, micronucleus formation and aneuploidy). Tests for the inhibition of metabolic cooperation of Chinese hamster V79 cells and for the transformation of Syrian hamster embryo cells yielded negative results. The results of this study may be taken as an indication of a weak genotoxic activity of 2-butoxyacetaldehyde that appears to be predominantly expressed at the chromosomal level. [The Working Group felt that the presentation of the results did not allow a critical examination of the data.]

(b)   2-Butoxyacetic acid

2-Butoxyacetic acid is an aliphatic acid and would not be expected to exhibit any genotoxic activity. The compound did not induce mutations in several strains of *S. typhimurium* in the absence or presence of an exogenous metabolic activation system. In a series of in-vitro assays performed without an exogenous metabolic activation system, it did not increase the frequency of sister chromatid exchange or of structural chromosomal aberrations and did not inhibit gap-junctional metabolic cooperation in Chinese hamster V79 cells. In contrast, weakly positive results were found in a micronucleus assay with V79 cells and, in the same cell line, a weak effect of 2-butoxyacetic acid on the percentage of aneuploid cells was reported. 2-Butoxyacetic acid did not increase the frequency of chromosomal aberrations in human lymphocytes *in vitro*. [The Working Group felt that the limited data presented did not allow any conclusion on the extent to which cytotoxic effects of the treatment or pH changes induced by the acid in culture medium may have contributed to the results reported.]

In the only available in-vivo assay of 2-butoxyacetic acid, the compound did not affect the frequency of micronucleated polychromatic erythrocytes in the bone marrow of mice following a single intraperitoneal injection. In this study, 2-butoxyacetic acid was toxic to the bone marrow, as statistically significant decreases in the ratio of polychromatic and normochromatic erythrocytes were observed at the two highest doses (100 and 200 mg/kg bw).

4.5   Mechanistic considerations

The available data on 2-butoxyethanol largely support the concept that the compound, the structure of which does not carry any alerts for probable genotoxic activity (Ashby &

Tennant, 1991; Tennant & Ashby, 1991; Elliott & Ashby, 1997), exhibits no appreciable genotoxic effects. Although many studies were carried out in the absence of metabolic activation, consistent data show that 2-butoxyethanol does not induce gene mutations in bacteria or structural chromosomal aberrations in mammalian cells *in vitro*, and there is evidence that the compound does not cause oxidative stress that results in genotoxicity in hepatocytes *in vitro*. Weakly positive results have been reported for high concentrations of 2-butoxyethanol in some in-vitro studies of cultured mammalian cells, but the way in which the data were presented and the lack of essential information on experimental details cause uncertainties that prevent their full evaluation. It cannot be excluded, however, that some of the positive findings actually represent true genotoxic effects caused by the metabolite, 2-butoxyacetaldehyde, which may be formed in small amounts *in vitro* depending on the concentration of 2-butoxyethanol, the type of cells and the exogenous metabolic activation system used. Although speculative, this is consistent with a number of potentially positive results that were reported for 2-butoxyacetaldehyde in some assays that mainly used cytogenetic end-points. The genotoxic activity of this aldehyde appears to be lower, however, than that of other glycol ether-derived aldehydes with shorter alkyl groups, since methoxyacetaldehyde is mutagenic in Chinese hamster CHO-AS52 cells and clastogenic in standard Chinese hamster ovary cells, whereas 2-butoxyacetaldehyde is not (Ma *et al.*, 1993; Chiewchanwit & Au, 1995). The metabolic end-product of the oxidation of 2-butoxyethanol and 2-butoxyacetaldehyde, 2-butoxyacetic acid, appears to be non-genotoxic.

Several in-vivo assays with 2-butoxyethanol have shown the absence of detectable genotoxic activity in bone marrow. Studies on the effects of 2-butoxyethanol on mouse liver have indicated, however, that it causes oxidative stress associated with the formation of oxidative base damage in hepatic DNA, as demonstrated by increased levels of 8-hydroxydeoxyguanosine and other biomarkers of oxidative stress (Park *et al.*, 2002a). This hepatic oxidative stress has not been attributed to the action of 2-butoxyethanol *per se*, but to the metabolic formation of 2-butoxyacetic acid via the induction of haemolysis in the liver (see below).

The haematological effects of 2-butoxyethanol have been studied extensively.

The damage to red blood cells that is induced by 2-butoxyethanol appears to proceed through a process known as colloid osmotic haemolysis in which damage to the cell membrane leads to swelling of the red blood cell. In essence, the damage leads to a 'leaky' red cell or to other effects that produce a 'hole' in the red cell membrane that is smaller than the effective radius of the haemoglobin molecule. The extent of such damage governs the different processes that involve removal of damaged red blood cells from the circulation. Red blood cells that have minor damage and are slowly enlarging are removed totally in the spleen which has a particularly efficient mechanism to overcome stress and destroys subtly damaged red blood cells. More extensive damage can be recognized by the liver, which has a much larger capacity for removal of damaged red blood cells, but a higher threshold for recognition of damage. When the capacity of both spleen and liver are overwhelmed by a rapidly progressive swelling of the red blood cell, intravascular haemolysis occurs. Accordingly, in an individual with a spleen, low-level red cell damage does not lead to the build-up of haemosiderin within the liver. It should be noted that some individuals are asplenic at birth or have their spleen removed due to trauma or to treatment for haematological or neoplastic disorders. In such individuals, senescent red blood cells are routinely removed in the liver, as would damaged red blood cells.

Chronic inhalation exposure to 2-butoxyethanol has been shown to result in the formation of hepatic haemangiosarcomas and hepatocellular carcinomas in male mice, but not in female mice or rats of either sex (National Toxicology Program, 2000; see Section 3). The induction of liver neoplasia has been suggested to be the result of oxidative damage secondary to the haemolytic deposition of iron in the liver (Park *et al.*, 2002a; Sielsky *et al.*, 2002; Klaunig & Kamendulis, 2005). It is postulated that the formation of liver tumours is mediated by the production of the haematotoxic metabolite of 2-butoxyethanol, 2-butoxyacetic acid, which causes haemolysis of red blood cells and the release of iron and its deposition in Kupffer cells in both rats and mice. These iron-containing deposits are assumed to catalyse, through Fenton and/or Haber-Weiss reactions, the formation of reactive oxygen species and/or to activate Kupffer cells to produce oxidative species in male mice as well as certain cytokines. The production of reactive oxygen species has been linked to the formation of oxidative DNA damage, i.e. 8-hydroxydeoxyguanosine, observed in hepatocytes (Park *et al.*, 2002a; Siesky *et al.*, 2002) and to the stimulation of DNA synthesis in both endothelial cells and hepatocytes (Siesky *et al.*, 2002) through a postulated modification of gene expression in the livers of male mice. It has been shown that induction of endothelial cell proliferation by the treatment of mice with 2-butoxyethanol occurs at doses that produced haemangiosarcomas in mice (Siesky *et al.*, 2002). The lack of tumour formation in rats has been attributed in part to a higher level of antioxidants, specifically vitamin E (2.5-fold greater), in rat liver than in mouse liver (Siesky *et al.*, 2002). The more effective protection of rats against the consequences of oxidative stress is indicated by the lack of an increase in the formation of oxidative damage and the absence of enhanced proliferation of endothelial cells or hepatocytes, although haemolysis occurred (Siesky *et al.*, 2002). In-vitro results have demonstrated that iron sulfate as well as iron released from haemolysed erythrocytes, but not 2-butoxyethanol, cause oxidative stress in primary cultured mouse hepatocytes and in Syrian hamster embryo cells, together with morphological transformation (Park *et al.*, 2002a,b), which adds support to the hypothesis that iron-induced oxidative stress may play an essential role in the induction of hepatic tumours by 2-butoxyethanol in male mice. Additional strong support for this hypothesis stems from the results of a search for a possible association between chemically induced haemosiderosis and haemangiosarcomas in the liver of mice in selected studies conducted by the National Toxicology Program (Nyska *et al.*, 2004). In addition to 2-butoxyethanol, two other compounds, i.e. *para*-nitroaniline and *para*-chloroaniline, were associated with haemosiderin pigmentation of Kupffer cells in both males and females and with the development of haemangiosarcoma in male mice only. The overall association between liver haemangiosarcoma and pigmentation in Kupffer cells was highly significant ($p < 0.001$). The cause of haemosiderosis in all cases was the haemolytic effect of the compounds (Nyska *et al.*, 2004).

In considering all of the available evidence, a scenario appears conceivable whereby the exposure of male mice to high concentrations of 2-butoxyethanol results in haemolysis and iron-mediated oxidative stress in the liver, which is accompanied by the induction of mutagenic oxidative DNA lesions, such as 8-hydroxydeoxyguanosine, the repair of which by base-excision repair may be impeded by an interference of 2-butoxyethanol with poly-(ADP-ribosyl)ation. The simultaneously induced cell proliferation would increase the probability that DNA damage becomes a fixed mutation and that mutated clones expand and eventually give rise to tumours. However, other mechanisms have not been considered.

None of the known causes of hepatic haemangiosarcoma has been associated with haemolytic anaemia in humans. Similarly, no hepatic angiosarcoma has been reported in groups who have chronic haemolytic processes, such as the autoimmune haemolytic anaemia that is seen in patients who have lupus erythematosus, or individuals who have inherited red cell membrane defects, such as hereditary spherocytosis, for which splenectomy in childhood is the usual treatment. However, it should be noted that hepatic angiosarcomas are relatively rare and may not have been recognized. [The Working Group found no published studies on haemangiosarcomas associated with haemolysis or lupus.] Nevertheless, increased levels of iron in the body have been associated with other forms of cancer in the liver (Nyska *et al.*, 2004).

Compared with that of mice and rats, the blood of humans is much more resistant to induction of haemolysis *in vitro* by 2-butoxyacetic acid. Moreover, the level of vitamin E in human liver is approximately 100-fold higher than that in mouse liver (Rocchi *et al.*, 1997). Thus, it appears that the mechanism of oxidative stress is unlikely to occur in humans and that the hepatic tumours observed in male mice exposed to 2-butoxyethanol are a species- and sex-specific phenomenon that may not be relevant to humans.

Chronic inhalation exposure to 2-butoxyethanol has also been shown to be associated with the formation of forestomach tumours in female mice and, to a lesser extent, in male mice, whereas no forestomach tumours occurred in exposed rats. It has been proposed that tumour induction is the consequence of a sustained exposure of this organ to high concentrations of 2-butoxyethanol and its toxic metabolites, primarily 2-butoxyacetic acid, which results in tissue damage, reparative regeneration and hyperplasia (Green *et al.*, 2002; Poet *et al.*, 2003). Several factors are thought to contribute to a high local burden in the forestomach. These include direct exposure of the tissue, even in inhalation experiments, via the oral route as a consequence of grooming contaminated fur or licking the walls of the exposure chamber, salivary excretion and mucociliary transport of material deposited in the airways followed by ingestion (Green *et al.*, 2002). In addition, other factors result in a prolonged exposure of the forestomach as compared with other organs. These include the physiological function of the forestomach as a storage organ for ingested material and the slow elimination of 2-butoxyethanol from forestomach tissue compared with other tissues or blood, irrespective of the route of application. The reason for the much lower susceptibility of rats to the development of forestomach lesions has not been elucidated fully. However, it has been shown in mice that ADH, which catalyses the first step in the oxidation of 2-butoxyethanol to 2-butoxyacetic acid, has a higher affinity and a higher maximal activity with 2-butoxyethanol as substrate than rat ADH, and that it is expressed at much higher specific activity in areas of the mouse forestomach than in that of rats. These differences have been purported to result in higher local concentrations of toxic metabolites of 2-butoxyethanol in the forestomach of mice compared with that of rats (Green *et al.*, 2002).

It cannot be excluded that the continuous presence of the metabolite 2-butoxyacetaldehyde, which possibly exhibits weak clastogenic activity, can give rise to tumour formation in the regenerating forestomach tissue.

Anatomical and physiological differences between mice and humans limit, but do not entirely rule out, the relevance of mouse forestomach tumours to humans.

5. Summary of Data Reported and Evaluation

5.1 Exposure data

2-Butoxyethanol is a glycol ether that is widely used as a solvent in surface coatings (paints and varnishes), paint thinners, printing inks and glass- and surface-cleaning products (including those used in the printing and silk-screening industries), and as a chemical intermediate. It is also used in a variety of personal care and other consumer products. Occupational exposure occurs through dermal absorption or via inhalation during its manufacture and use as a chemical intermediate, and during the formulation and use of its products. Highest mean exposures have been measured for silk screeners. Exposure of the general population can occur through dermal contact or inhalation during the use of consumer products, particularly cleaning agents.

5.2 Human carcinogenicity data

A case–control study of acute myeloid leukaemia and myelodysplasia found no elevation of risk with exposure to a group of glycol ethers, including 2-butoxyethanol. However, the information provided by this study on 2-butoxyethanol specifically was limited.

5.3 Animal carcinogenicity data

2-Butoxyethanol was tested for carcinogenicity by inhalation exposure in male and female mice and rats. Clear increases in tumour incidence were observed in a single species. Exposure to 2-butoxyethanol induced a dose-related increase in the incidence of haemangiosarcomas of the liver in male mice and a dose-related increase in the incidences of combined forestomach squamous-cell papillomas or carcinomas (mainly papillomas) in female mice. In female rats, a positive trend was observed in the occurrence of combined benign or malignant pheochromocytomas (mainly benign) of the adrenal medulla, but this equivocal result could not be attributed with confidence to exposure to 2-butoxyethanol. There was no increase in the incidence of tumours in male rats.

5.4   Other relevant data

Toxicokinetics and metabolism

2-Butoxyethanol is rapidly absorbed following ingestion, inhalation and dermal exposure in humans and experimental animals. Uptake and metabolism in rats are linear up to 400 ppm. The elimination half-life of 2-butoxyethanol from the blood is much longer in humans than in rats or mice. The principal pathway of metabolism in humans and experimental animals involves oxidation to butoxyacetaldehyde and butoxyacetic acid (the putatively active metabolite for 2-butoxyethanol-induced haematological effects) via alcohol and aldehyde dehydrogenases, respectively. Based on limited data and the results of a physiologically based parmacokinetic model, humans appear to metabolize 2-butoxyethanol to butoxyacetic acid to a lesser extent than rats, which results in greater concentrations of butoxyacetic acid in the blood of rats than in that of humans. The elimination half-life of butoxyacetic acid in the urine is about 6 h in humans, and at least 15–55% of the inhaled dose of 2-butoxyethanol is excreted as free butoxyacetic acid. Although mice metabolize 2-butoxyethanol to butoxyacetic acid at a greater rate than rats, the metabolite is cleared much more slowly in rats, which is consistent with the greater sensitivity of rats to its effects in the blood. Similarly, slower clearance in female rats probably accounts for their greater sensitivity compared with male rats. Detoxification via conjugation of butoxyacetic acid with glutamine and excretion in the urine has been demonstrated in humans, but not to date in rats. The extent of glutamine conjugation varies within and between individuals, with a mean of around 70%. 2-Butoxyethanol may also be *O*-dealkylated to ethylene glycol, based on limited information in humans and more extensive evidence in rodents (conjugation of 2-butoxyethanol with glucuronide or sulfate has been observed in rats, but only tentatively in human hepatocytes *in vitro*).

Toxic effects

Several case reports that involved the consumption of up to several hundred millilitres of glass-cleaning liquid that contained various amounts of 2-butoxyethanol described a variety of effects (hypotension, coma, metabolic acidosis, renal impairment, haematuria, haemoglobinuria, hypochromic anaemia) in adults. In a survey of childhood poisonings, no symptoms were reported in children who had ingested comparable amounts of glass-cleaning liquids.

Incidental cutaneous exposures were not reported to produce adverse skin reactions or skin sensitization. Repeated dermal exposure produced increasing erythema. Exposure to 2-butoxyethanol vapour is irritating to the eyes, nose and throat.

In studies of occupational exposure to airborne 2-butoxyethanol (mean concentrations of 2–4 mg/m^3), effects on blood parameters (lower haematocrit values), but no changes in renal or hepatic function and no correlation with concentrations of 2-butoxyacetic acid in the urine of exposed workers were observed. In one study, airborne levels of 100–300 ppm [483–1450 mg/m^3] 2-butoxyethanol caused acute and severe irritation of the eyes and respiratory tract and the appearance of cherry angiomas (benign cutaneous vascular lesions) after 3 months, which persisted and continued to develop.

Effects on the blood appear to be the most sensitive parameter in experimental animals following acute, short-term, subchronic or chronic exposure via oral, inhalation and dermal routes, based on an extensive database. Alterations in haematological parameters that are consistent with haemolytic anaemia have repeatedly been observed in multiple species, including mice and rats. There is substantial evidence from in-vivo and in-vitro investigations that rats are more sensitive to 2-butoxyethanol-induced haemolysis than other experimental species, and alterations in relevant parameters were observed following long-term exposure to concentrations as low as 31.2 ppm [151 mg/m^3]. Female rats are more sensitive to the haematological effects associated with exposure to 2-butoxyethanol than male rats, which is consistent with sex-related differences in the clearance of the putatively active metabolite, butoxyacetic acid, and greater activity of the enzymes involved in its formation. On the basis of several in-vitro investigations in erythrocytes of humans and rats, humans appear to be much less sensitive. Although the physical–chemical pathway for haemolysis by 2-butoxyethanol has not been fully elucidated, it has been reported that haemolysis involves cell swelling, morphological changes and decreased deformability.

Haemolysis has been proposed to be linked mechanistically to the induction of liver neoplasia in male mice by 2-butoxyethanol. Damage to red blood cells results in the deposition of haemosiderin in Kupffer cells of both mice and rats which in turn apparently mediates the induction of hepatic oxidative stress that has been observed in both species *in vivo*. In mice, but not in rats, oxidative stress results in the formation of the oxidative, mutagenic DNA lesion, 8-hydroxydeoxyguanosine, as well as an increase in the proliferation of endothelial cells; both of these effects are assumed to contribute to the development of liver tumours. The apparent protection of rats against these consequences of oxidative stress, which is not observed in mice, has been attributed to a higher level of protective antioxidants in rat liver than in mouse liver. In view of the much lower sensitivity to haemolysis of human erythrocytes than those of mice and rats, and the fact that the concentration of the antioxidant, vitamin E, is approximately 100-fold higher in human liver than in mouse liver, the induction of liver tumours in humans is unlikely to occur through this pathway. Other potential mechanisms have not been investigated.

Toxic effects have been observed in the forestomach of mice and rats following both oral and inhalation exposure to 2-butoxyethanol; mice were more sensitive than rats. In a chronic inhalation study in mice, toxicity was observed at all concentrations investigated, i.e. at 62.5 ppm [302.5 mg/m^3] and higher. The effects on the forestomach were increased in incidence and severity with increasing exposure concentration, and included irritation, inflammation, hyperplasia and ulceration. Increases in tumour incidences were observed in mice at the higher concentrations. The formation of forestomach tumours in mice is associated with high local exposure of the forestomach to 2-butoxyethanol, even during inhalation exposure, and to high metabolic activity in certain areas of the forestomach, which results in high local concentrations of the toxic metabolite, 2-butoxyacetic acid.

Reproductive and developmental effects

In developmental toxicity studies in rats and mice that involved oral and inhalation exposure to 2-butoxyethanol, embryotoxic or fetotoxic effects were observed at doses or concentrations similar to or greater than those which induced toxicity (including haemato-logical effects) in the dams. Alterations in haematological parameters were also observed in fetuses of exposed dams. Effects on reproductive ability and reproductive organs were also only observed at doses or concentrations of 2-butoxyethanol much greater than those associated with haematological effects.

Genetic and related effects

The available data on 2-butoxyethanol support the concept that the compound itself exhibits no appreciable genotoxicity. The oxidative metabolite, 2-butoxyacetaldehyde, appears to have a weak capacity to cause genotoxic effects *in vitro*, largely at the chromo-somal level. The product of further oxidation, 2-butoxyacetic acid, does not appear to be genotoxic.

5.5   Evaluation

There is *inadequate evidence* in humans for the carcinogenicity of 2-butoxyethanol.
There is *limited evidence* in experimental animals for the carcinogenicity of 2-butoxy-ethanol.

Overall evaluation

2-Butoxyethanol is *not classifiable as to its carcinogenicity to humans (Group 3).*

6.   References

Aasmoe, L. & Aarbakke, J. (1999) Sex-dependent induction of alcohol dehydrogenase activity in rats. *Biochem. Pharmacol.*, **57**, 1067–1072

Aasmoe, L., Winberg, J.-O. & Aarbakke, J. (1998) The role of liver alcohol dehydrogenase iso-enzymes in the oxidation of glycolethers in male and female rats. *Toxicol. appl. Pharmacol.*, **150**, 86–90

ACGIH® Worldwide (2004) *Documentation of the TLVs® and BEIs® with Other Worldwide Occu-pational Exposure Values — CD-ROM — 2004*, Cincinnati, OH

Angerer, J., Lichterbeck, E., Begerow, J., Jekel, S. & Lehnert, G. (1990) Occupational chronic exposure to organic solvents. XIII. Glycolether exposure during the production of varnishes. *Int. Arch. occup. environ. Health*, **62**, 123–126

Apol, A.G. (1981) *Labels West, Inc., Redmond, WA* (Health Hazard Evaluation Report No. HETA 81-105-831), Cincinnati, OH, National Institute for Occupational Safety and Health, Hazard Evaluations and Technical Assistance Branch

Apol, A.G. (1986) *Lamiglas, Woodland, WA* (Health Hazard Evaluation Report No. HETA-86-037-1749), Cincinnati, OH, National Institute for Occupational Safety and Health, Hazard Evaluations and Technical Assistance Branch

Apol, A.G. & Johnson, W.M. (1979) *Associated Grocers, Inc., Seattle, WA* (Health Hazard Evaluation Report No. HETA 78-120-608), Cincinnati, OH, National Institute for occupational Safety and Health, Hazard Evaluations and Technical Assistance Branch

Apol, A.G. & Cone, J. (1983) *Bay Area Hospital, Coos Bay, OR* (Health Hazard Evaluation Report No. HETA 82-053-1263), Cincinnati, OH, National Institute for Occupational Safety and Health, Hazard Evaluations and Technical Assistance Branch

Arbejdstilsynet [Danish Working Environment Authority] (2001) *Re. EU Regulation 793/93. Information from the Danish Product Register*, Copenhagen, Letter dated 04/11/01

Arbejdstilsynet [Danish Working Environment Authority] (2002) *WEA-Guide C.01 — Limit Values for Substances and Materials*, Copenhagen

Ashby, J. & Tennant, R.W. (1991) Definitive relationships among chemical structure, carcinogenicity and mutagenicity for 301 chemicals tested by the US NTP. *Mutat. Res.*, **257**, 229–306

ATSDR (Agency for Toxic Substances and Disease Registry) (1998) *Toxicological Profile for 2-Butoxyethanol and 2-Butoxyethanol Acetate*, Atlanta, GA

Auffarth, J., Hohmann, R. & Tischer, M. (1998) [Exposure to Hazardous Substances in the Screen Printing Industry] (Schriftenreihe der Bundesanstalt für Arbeitsschutz und Arbeitsmedizin GA 53), Dortmund/Berlin (in German)

Baker, E., Smith, T. & Quinn, M. (1985) *Screen Printing Shops Boston, MA and Denton, Maryland Areas* (Health Hazard Evaluation Report HETA 82-212-1553), Cincinati, OH, National Institute for Occupational Safety and Health, Hazard Evaluations and Technical Assistance Branch

Bartnik, F.G., Reddy, A.K., Klecak, G., Zimmermann, V., Hostynek, J.J. & Kunstler, K. (1987) Percutaneous absorption, metabolism, and hemolytic activity of *n*-butoxyethanol. *Fundam. appl. Toxicol.*, **8**, 59–70

Bauer, P., Weber, M., Mur, J.M., Protois, J.C., Bollaert, P.E., Condi, A., Larcan, A. & Lambert, H. (1992) Transient non-cardiogenic pulmonary edema following massive ingestion of ethylene glycol butyl ether. *Intensive Care Med.*, **18**, 250–251

Begerow, J., Heinrich-Ramm, R. & Angerer, J. (1988) Determination of butoxyacetic acid in urine by capillary gas chromatography. *Fresenius Z. anal. Chem.*, **331**, 818–820

Beihoffer, J. & Ferguson, C. (1994) Determination of selected carboxylic acids and alcohols in groundwater by GC–MS. *J. chromatogr. Sci.*, **32**, 102–106

Boatman, R.J. & Knaak, J.B. (2001) Ethers of ethylene glycol and derivatives. In: Bingham, E., Cohrssen, B. & Powell, C.H., eds., *Patty's Toxicology*, 5th Ed., Vol. 7, New York, John Wiley & Sons, pp. 73–84, 136–157, 243–270

Boiano, J.M. (1983) *Downing Displays Inc.* (Health Hazard Evaluation Report HETA No. 82-330-1252), Cincinnati, OH, National Institute for Occupational Safety and Health, Hazard Evaluations and Technical Assistance Branch

Bormett, G.A., Bartels, M.J. & Markham, D.A. (1995) Determination of 2-butoxyethanol and butoxyacetic acid in rat and human blood by gas chromatography–mass spectrometry. *J. Chromatogr.*, **B665**, 315–325

Brown, K.W. & Donnelly, K.C. (1988) An estimation of the risk associated with the organic constituents of hazardous and municipal waste landfill leachates. *Hazard. Waste hazard. Mater.*, **5**, 1–30

Brown, K.K., Cheever, K.L., Butler, M.A., Shaw, P.B. & McLaurin, J.L. (2003) Synthesis, characterization, and use of 2-[(^{2}H$_9$)butoxy]acetic acid and 2-(3-methylbutoxy)acetic acid as an internal standard and an instrument performance surrogate, respectively, for the gas chromatographic–mass spectrometric determination of 2-butoxyacetic acid, a human metabolite of 2-butoxyethanol. *J. Chromatogr.*, **B792**, 153–166

Burkhart K.K. & Donovan J.W. (1998) Hemodialysis following butoxyethanol ingestion. *Clin. Toxicol.*, **36**, 723–725

Cao, X.-L. (1999) *Emissions of Glycol Ethers from Consumer Products — A Final Report for 1998/1999 CEPA Project*, Ottawa, Health Canada

Carpenter, C.P. & Smyth, H.F., Jr (1946) Chemical burns of the rabbit cornea. *Am. J. Ophthalmol.*, **29**, 1363–1372

Carpenter, C.P., Pozzani, U.C., Weil, C.S., Nair, J.H., III, Keck, G.A. & Smyth, H.F., Jr (1956) The toxicity of butyl cellosolve solvent. *Arch. ind. Health*, **14**, 114–131

Cheever, K.L., Plotnick, H.B., Richards, D.E. & Weigel, W.W. (1984) Metabolism and excretion of 2-ethoxyethanol in the adult male rat. *Environ. Health. Perspect.*, **57**, 241–248

Chemical Information Services (2004) *Directory of World Chemical Producers*, Dallas, TX [www.chemicalinfo.com]

Chiewchanwit, T. & Au, W.W. (1995) Mutagenicity and cytotoxicity of 2-butoxyethanol and its metabolite, 2-butoxyacetaldehyde, in Chinese hamster ovary (CHO-AS52) cells. *Mutat. Res.*, **334**, 341–346

Chinn, H., Anderson, E. & Yoneyama, M. (2000) *CEH Marketing Research Report: Glycol Ethers*, Palo Alto, CA, SRI International

Ciccioli, P., Brancaleoni, E., Cecinato, A., Sparapani, R. & Frattoni, M. (1993) Identification and determination of biogenic and anthropogenic volatile organic compounds in forest areas of northern and southern Europe and a remote site of the Himalaya region by high-resolution gas chromatography–mass spectrometry. *J. Chromatogr.*, **643**, 55–69

Ciccioli, P., Cecinato, A., Brancaleoni, E., Frattoni, M., Bruner, F. & Maione, M. (1996) Occurrence of oxygenated volatile organic compounds (VOC) in Antarctica. *Int. J. environ. anal. Chem.*, **62**, 245–253

Clapp, D.E., Zaebst, D.D. & Herrick, R.F. (1984) Measuring exposures to glycol ethers. *Environ. Health Perspect.*, **57**, 91–95

Collinot, J.P., Collinot, J.C., Deschamps, F., Decolin, D., Siest, G. & Galteau, M.M. (1996) Evaluation of urinary D-glucaric acid excretion in workers exposed to butyl glycol. *J. Toxicol. environ. Health*, **48**, 349–358

Corley, R.A., Bormett, G.A. & Ghanayem, B.I. (1994) Physiologically based pharmacokinetics of 2-butoxyethanol and its major metabolite, 2-butoxyacetic acid, in rats and humans. *Toxicol. appl. Pharmacol.*, **129**, 61–79

Corley, R.A., Markham, D.A., Banks, C., Delorme, P., Masterman, A. & Houle, J.M. (1997) Physiologically based pharmacokinetics and the dermal absorption of 2-butoxyethanol vapor by humans. *Fundam. appl. Toxicol.*, **39**, 120–130

CSHPF (Conseil Supérieur d'Hygiène Publique de France) (2002) [Glycol Ethers in Consumer Products and Health] (Progress Report to the Directeur Général de la Santé), Paris, Section des Milieux de Vie (in French)

Daisey, J.M., Hodgson, A.T., Fisk, W.J., Mendell, M.J. & Ten Brinke, J. (1994) Volatile organic compounds in twelve California office buildings: Classes, concentrations and sources. *Atmos. Environ.*, **28**, 3557–3562

Danielson (1992) Toxicity potential of compounds found in parenteral solutions with rubber stoppers. *J. parenteral Sci. Technol.*, **46**, 43–47

Dartsch, P.C., Hildenbrand, S., Gfrörer, W., Kimmel, R. & Schmahl, F.W. (1999) Cytotoxic effects of 2-butoxyethanol in vitro are related to butoxyacetaldehyde, an intermediate oxidation product. *Environ. Toxicol. Pharmacol.*, **7**, 135–142

Dean, B.S. & Krenzelok, E.P. (1992) Clinical evaluation of pediatric ethylene glycol monobutyl ether poisonings. *Clin. Toxicol.*, **30**, 557–563

Deisinger, P.J. & Boatman, R.J. (2004) *In vivo* metabolism and kinetics of ethylene glycol monobutyl ether and its metabolites, 2-butoxyacetaldehyde and 2-butoxyacetic acid, as measured in blood, liver and forestomach of mice. *Xenobiotica*, **34**, 675–685

Delest, A. & Desjeux, F. (1995) [Evaluation of exposure to glycol ethers in 54 building painters.] *Rev. Méd. Trav.*, **22**, 113–117 (in French)

Denkhaus, W., von Steldern, D., Botzenhardt, U. & Konietzko, H. (1986) Lymphocyte subpopulations in solvent-exposed workers. *Int. Arch. occup. environ. Health*, **57**, 109–115

Deutsche Forschungsgemeinschaft (1991) Ethylene glycol derivatives 2-methoxyethanol, 2-ethoxyethanol, 2-butoxyethanol, 2-methoxyethyl acetate, 2-ethoxyethyl acetate. In: Kettrup, A., ed., *Analyses of Hazardous Substances in Air*, Vol. 1, Weinheim, VCH Verlag GmbH

Deutsche Forschungsgemeinschaft (2003) *List of MAK and BAT Values 2003 — Commission for the Investigation of Health Hazards of Chemical Compounds in the Work Area* (Report No. 39), Weinheim, Wiley-VCH Verlag GmbH, pp. 61, 194–195

Dieter, M.P., Jameson, C.W., Maronpot, R.R., Langenbach, R. & Braun, A.G. (1990) The chemotherapeutic potential of glycol alkyl ethers: Structure–activity studies of nine compounds in a Fischer-rat leukemia transplant model. *Cancer Chemother. Pharmacol.*, **26**, 173–180

Dill, J.A., Lee, K.M., Bates, D.J., Anderson, D.J., Johnson, R.E., Chou, B.J., Burka, L.T. & Roycroft, J.H. (1998) Toxicokinetics of inhaled 2-butoxyethanol and its major metabolite, 2-butoxyacetic acid, in F344 rats and B6C3F1 mice. *Toxicol. appl. Pharmacol.*, **153**, 227–242

Dodd, D.E., Snellings, W.M., Maronpot, R.R. & Ballantyne, B. (1983) Ethylene glycol monobutyl ether: Acute, 9-day, and 90-day vapor inhalation studies in Fischer 344 rats. *Toxicol. appl. Pharmacol.*, **68**, 405–414

Doe, J.E. (1984) Further studies on the toxicology of the glycol ethers with emphasis on rapid screening and hazard assessment. *Environ. Health Perspect.*, **57**, 199–206

Dow Chemical Co. (2001) *Sales Specification Sheet: Butyl Cellosolve Solvent*, Midland, MI

Dugard, P.H., Walker, M., Mawdsley, S.J. & Scott, R.C. (1984) Absorption of some glycol ethers through human skin *in vitro*. *Environ. Health Perspect.*, **57**, 193–197

Eastman Chemical Co. (2000a) *Sales Specification: Eastman EB (Ethylene Glycol Monobutyl Ether) Solvent, Stabilized 2* (Specification No. 12211), Longview, TX

Eastman Chemical Co. (2000b) *Sales Specification: Eastman EB Solvent (Ethylene Glycol Mono-butyl Ether)* (Specification No. 650), Longview, TX

Eastman Chemical Co. (2003) *Material Safety Data Sheet: EB Solvent – Stabilized 2*, Kingsport, TN

ECETOC (European Chemical Industry, Ecology and Toxicology Centre) (1985) *The Toxicology of Glycol Ethers and its Relevance to Man: An Up-dating of ECETOC Technical Report No. 4* (Technical Report No. 17), Brussels

ECETOC (European Chemical Industry, Ecology and Toxicology Centre) (1994) *2-Butoxyethanol Criteria Document, including a Supplement for 2-Butoxyethyl Acetate* (Special Report No. 7), Brussels

ECETOC (European Centre for Ecotoxicology and Toxicology of Chemicals) (1995) *The Toxicology of Glycol Ethers and its Relevance to Man* (Technical Report 64), Brussels

Eckel, W., Foster, G. & Ross, B. (1996) Glycol ethers as ground water contaminants. *Occup. Hyg.*, **2**, 97–104

Elias, Z., Danière, M.C., Marande, A.M., Poirot, O., Terzetti, F. & Schneider, O. (1996) Genotoxic and/or epigenetic effects of some glycol ethers: Results of different short-term tests. *Occup. Hyg.*, **2**, 187–212

Elliott, B.M. & Ashby, J. (1997) Review of the genotoxicity of 2-butoxyethanol. *Mutat. Res.*, **387**, 89–96

Environment Canada (1997) *Results of the CEPA Section 16 Notice Respecting the Second Priority Substances List and Di(2-ethylhexyl)phthalate*, Hull, Quebec, Use Patterns Section, Commercial Chemicals Evaluation Branch

Environment Canada/Health Canada (2002) *Priority Substances List Assessment Report: 2-Butoxyethanol*, Quebec/Montreal

European Union (1999) *Council Directive 1999/13/EC of 11 March 1999 on the Limitation of Emissions of Volatile Organic Compounds due to the Use of Organic Solvents in Certain Activities and Installations* (CONSLEG: 1999LOO13), Luxembourg, Office for Official Publications of the European Communities

European Union (2004) *European Union Risk Assessment Report — 2-Butoxyethanol* (Draft Report), Luxembourg, Office for Official Publications of the European Communities

Exon, J.H., Mather, G.G., Bussiere, J.L., Olson, D.P. & Talcott, P.A. (1991) Effects of subchronic exposure of rats to 2-methoxyethanol or 2-butoxyethanol: Thymic atrophy and immunotoxicity. *Fundam. appl. Toxicol.*, **16**, 830–840

Ezov, N., Levin-Harrus, T., Mittelman, M., Redlich, M., Shabat, S., Ward, S.M., Peddada, S., Nyska, M., Yedgar, S. & Nyska, A. (2002) A chemically induced rat model of hemolysis with disseminated thrombosis. *Cardiovasc. Toxicol.*, **2**, 181–193

Foo, S.C., Lwin, S., Chia, S.E. & Jeyaratnam, J. (1994) Chronic neurobehavioural effects in paint formulators exposed to solvents and noise. *Ann. Acad. Med. Singapore*, **23**, 650–654

Foster, P.M.D., Lloyd, S.C. & Blackburn, D.M. (1987) Comparison of the in vivo and in vitro testicular effects produced by methoxy-, ethoxy- and *N*-butoxy acetic acids in the rat. *Toxicology*, **43**, 17–30

Ghanayem, B.I. (1989) Metabolic and cellular basis of 2-butoxyethanol-induced hemolytic anemia in rats and assessment of human risk *in vitro*. *Biochem. Pharmacol.*, **38**, 1679–1684

Ghanayem, B.I. (1996) An overview of the hematotoxicity of ethylene glycol ethers. *Occup. Hyg.*, **2**, 253–268

Ghanayem, B.I. & Matthews, H.B. (1990) Attenuation of 2-butoxyethanol-induced hemolytic anemia by calcium channel blockers (Abstract No. 70). *Pharmacologist*, **32**, 182

Ghanayem, B.I. & Sullivan, C.A. (1993) Assessment of the heamolytic activity of 2-butoxyethanol and its major metabolite, butoxyacetic acid, in various mammals including humans. *Hum. exp. Toxicol.*, **12**, 305–311

Ghanayem, B.I., Burka, L.T., Sanders, J.M. & Matthews, H.B. (1987a) Metabolism and disposition of ethylene glycol monobutyl ether (2-butoxyethanol) in rats. *Drug Metab. Dispos.*, **15**, 478–484

Ghanayem B.I., Burka, L.T. & Matthews, H.B. (1987b) Metabolic basis of ethylene glycol monobutyl ether (2-butoxyethanol) toxicity: Role of alcohol and aldehyde dehydrogenases. *J. Pharmacol. exp. Ther.*, **242**, 222–231

Ghanayem, B.I., Blair, P.C., Thompson, M.B., Maronpot, R.R. & Matthews, H.B. (1987c) Effect of age on the toxicity and metabolism of ethylene glycol monobutyl ether (2-butoxyethanol) in rats. *Toxicol. appl. Pharmacol.*, **91**, 222–234

Ghanayem, B.I., Burka, L.T. & Matthews, H.B. (1989) Structure–activity relationships for the in vitro hematotoxicity of *N*-alkoxyacetic acids, the toxic metabolites of glycol ethers. *Chem.-biol. Interactions*, **70**, 339–352

Ghanayem, B.I., Sanders, J.M., Clark, A.-M., Bailer, J. & Matthews, H.B. (1990) Effects of dose, age, inhibition of metabolism and elimination on the toxicokinetics of 2-butoxyethanol and its metabolites. *J. Pharmacol. exp. Ther.*, **253**, 136–143

Ghanayem, B.I., Sanchez, I.M. & Matthews, H.B. (1992) Development of tolerance to 2-butoxy-ethanol-induced hemolytic anemia and studies to elucidate the underlying mechanisms. *Toxicol. appl. Pharmacol.*, **112**, 198–206

Ghanayem, B.I., Ward, S.M., Chanas, B. & Nyska, A. (2000) Comparison of the acute hemato-toxicity of 2-butoxyethanol in male and female F344 rats. *Hum. exp. Toxicol.*, **19**, 185–192

Ghanayem, B.I., Long, P.H., Ward, S.M., Chanas, B., Nyska, M. & Nyska, A. (2001) Hemolytic anemia, thrombosis, and infarction in male and female F344 rats following gavage exposure to 2-butoxyethanol. *Exp. Toxicol. Pathol.*, **53**, 97–105

Gijsenbergh, F.P., Jenco, M., Veulemans, H., Groeseneken, D., Verberckmoes, R. & Delooz, H.H. (1989) Acute butylglycol intoxication: A case report. *Hum. Toxicol.*, **8**, 243–245

Gingell, R., Boatman, R.J. & Lewis, S. (1998) Acute toxicity of ethylene glycol mono-*n*-butyl ether in the guinea pig. *Food chem. Toxicol.*, **36**, 825–829

Gollapudi, B.B., Barber, E.D., Lawlor, T.E. & Lewis, S.A. (1996) Re-examination of the muta-genicity of ethylene glycol monobutyl ether to Salmonella tester strain TA97a. *Mutat. Res.*, **370**, 61–64

Gourdeau, J., Cocheo, V., Jacob, V., Kaluzni, P., Kirchner, S., Laurent, A.M., Locoge, N., Person, A. & Vasselin, F. (2002) [Volatile Organic Compounds. Protocol of the Pilot Study] (Document de travail, 28/03/2002), Paris, Observatoire de la Qualité de l'Air Intérieur (in French)

Grant, D., Sulsh, S., Jones, H.B., Gangolli, S.D. & Butler, W.H. (1985) Acute toxicity and recovery in the hemopoietic system of rats after treatment with ethylene glycol monomethyl and mono-butyl ethers. *Toxicol. appl. Pharmacol.*, **77**, 187–200

Green, C.E., Gordon, G.R., Cohen, P.M., Nolen, H.W., Peters, J.H. & Tyson, C.A. (1996) *In vitro* metabolism of glycol ethers by human and rat hepatocytes. *Occup. Hyg.*, **2**, 67–75

Green, T., Toghill, A., Lee, R., Moore, R. & Foster, J. (2002) The development of forestomach tumours in the mouse following exposure to 2-butoxyethanol by inhalation: Studies on the mode of action and relevance to humans. *Toxicology*, **180**, 257–273

Greenspan, A.H., Reardon, R.C., Gingell, R. & Rosica, K.A. (1995) Human repeated insult patch test of 2-butoxyethanol. *Contact Derm.*, **33**, 59–60

Groeseneken, D., Veulemans, H., Masschelein, R. & Van Vlem, E. (1989) An improved method for the determination in urine of alkoxyacetic acids. *Int. Arch. occup. environ. Health*, **61**, 249–254

Gualtieri, J., Harris, C., Roy, R., Corley, R. & Manderfield, C. (1995) Multiple 2-butoxyethanol intoxications in the same patient: Clinical findings, pharmacokinetics, and therapy (Abstract No. 170). *J. Toxicol. clin. Toxicol.*, **33**, 550–551

Gualtieri, J.F., DeBoer, L., Harris, C.R. & Corley, R. (2003) Repeated ingestion of 2-butoxy-ethanol: Case report and literature review. *J. Toxicol. clin. Toxicol.*, **41**, 57–62

Hansch, C., Leo, A. & Hoekman, D. (1995) *Exploring QSAR: Hydrophobic, Electronic, and Steric Constants*, Washington DC, American Chemical Society, p. 25

Hansen, M.K., Larsen, M. & Cohr, K.-H. (1987) Waterborne paints. A review of their chemistry and toxicology and the results of determinations made during their use. *Scand. J. Work Environ. Health*, **13**, 473–485

Hardin, B.D., Goad, P.T. & Burg, J.R. (1984) Developmental toxicity of four glycol ethers applied cutaneously to rats. *Environ. Health Perspect.*, **57**, 69–74

Hardin, B.D., Schuler, R.L., Burg, J.R., Booth, G.M., Hazelden, K.P., MacKenzie, K.M., Piccirillo, V.J. & Smith, K.N. (1987) Evaluation of 60 chemicals in a preliminary developmental toxicity test. *Teratog. Carcinog. Mutag.*, **7**, 29–48

Haufroid, V., Thirion, F., Mertens. P., Buchet, J.-P. & Lison, D. (1997) Biological monitoring of workers exposed to low levels of 2-butoxyethanol. *Int. Arch. occup. environ. Health*, **70**, 232–236

Hayashi, S.-J., Watanabe, J. & Kawajiri, K. (1991) Genetic polymorphisms in the 5′-flanking region change transcriptional regulation of the human cytochrome P450IIE1 gene. *J. Biochem.*, **110**, 559–565

Health & Safety Executive (2002) *Occupational Exposure Limits 2002* (EH40/2002), Norwich, Her Majesty' Stationery Office, pp. 13, 29

Heindel, J.J., Gulati, D.K., Russell, V.S., Reel, J.R., Lawton, A.D. & Lamb, J.C., IV (1990) Assess-ment of ethylene glycol monobutyl and monophenyl ether reproductive toxicity using a conti-nuous breeding protocol in Swiss CD-1 mice. *Fundam. appl. Toxicol.*, **15**, 683–696

Hoflack, J.C., Durand, M.J., Poirier, G.G., Maul, A. & Vasseur, P. (1997) Alteration in methyl-methanesulfonate-induced poly(ADP-ribosyl)ation by 2-butoxyethanol in Syrian hamster embryo cells. *Carcinogenesis*, **18**, 2333–2338

Hoflack, J.C., Lambolez, L., Elias, Z. & Vasseur, P. (1995) Mutagenicity of ethylene glycol ethers and of their metabolites in *Salmonella typhimurium* his⁻. *Mutat. Res.*, **341**, 281–287

Hours, M., Dananche, B., Caillat-Vallet, E., Fevotte, J., Philippe, J., Boiron, O. & Fabry, J. (1996) Glycol ethers and myeoloid acute leukemia: A multicenter case control study. *Occup. Hyg.*, **2**, 405–410

INRS (Institut national de Recherche et de Sécurité) (2002) [Glycol ethers: Method 022] In: [Métropol Database (Measurement of Pollutants)], Paris (in French)

INRS (Institut national de Recherche et de Sécurité) (2003) *Extractions from the SEPIA Database for Products containing EGBE* (Internal Document), Paris

INRS (Institut national de Recherche et de Sécurité) (2005) [Threshold Limit Values for Occupa-tional Exposure to Chemicals in France] (Cahiers de Notes documentaires No. 2098), Paris, Hygiène et Sécurité du Travail (in French)

Jacobs, G.A. (1992) Eye irritation tests on two ethylene glycol ethers. *J. Am. Coll. Toxicol.*, **11**, 738

Jakasa, I., Mohammadi, N., Krüse, J. & Kezic, S. (2004) Percutaneous absorption of neat and aqueous solutions of 2-butoxyethanol in volunteers. *Int. Arch. occup. environ. Health*, **77**, 79–84

Jargot, D., Dieudonné, M., Hecht, C., Masson, A., Moulut, O. & Oury, B. (1999) [Water-based Paints for the Automobile Industry] (Cahier de Notes Documentaires No. 177), Paris, Hygiène et Sécurité du Travail (in French)

Johanson, G. (1986) Physiologically based pharmacokinetic modeling of inhaled 2-butoxyethanol in man. *Toxicol. Lett.*, **34**, 23–31

Johanson, G. (1988) Aspects of biological monitoring of exposure to glycol ethers. *Toxicol. Lett.*, **43**, 5–21

Johanson, G. (1989) Analysis of ethylene glycol ether metabolites in urine by extractive alkylation and electron-capture gas chromatography. *Arch. Toxicol.*, **63**, 107–111

Johanson, G. (1994) Inhalation toxicokinetics of butoxyethanol and its metabolite butoxyacetic acid in the male Sprague-Dawley rat. *Arch. Toxicol.*, **68**, 588–594

Johanson, G. & Boman, A. (1991) Percutaneous absorption of 2-butoxyethanol vapour in human subjects. *Br. J. ind. Med.*, **48**, 788–792

Johanson, G. & Dynésius, B. (1988) Liquid/air partition coefficients of six commonly used glycol ethers. *Br. J. ind. Med.*, **45**, 561–564

Johanson, G. & Fernström, P. (1986) Percutaneous uptake rate of 2-butoxyethanol in the guinea pig. *Scand. J. Work Environ. Health*, **12**, 499–503

Johanson, G. & Fernström, P. (1988) Influence of water on the percutaneous absorption of 2-butoxyethanol in guinea pigs. *Scand. J. Work Environ. Health*, **14**, 95–100

Johanson, G. & Näslund P.H. (1988) Spreadsheet programming — A new approach in physiologically based modeling of solvent toxicokinetics. *Toxicol. Lett.*, **41**, 115–127

Johanson, G. & Johnsson, S. (1991) Gas chromatographic determination of butoxyacetic acid in human blood after exposure to 2-butoxyethanol. *Arch. Toxicol.*, **65**, 433–435

Johanson, G., Kronborg, H., Näslund, P.H. & Nordqvist, M.B. (1986a) Toxicokinetics of inhaled 2-butoxyethanol (ethylene glycol monobutyl ether) in man. *Scand. J. Work Environ. Health*, **12**, 594–602

Johanson, G., Wallén, M. & Nordqvist, M.B. (1986b) Elimination kinetics of 2-butoxyethanol in the perfused rat liver — Dose dependence and effect of ethanol. *Toxicol. appl. Pharmacol.*, **83**, 315–320

Johanson, G., Boman, A. & Dynésius, B. (1988) Percutaneous absorption of 2-butoxyethanol in man. *Scand. J. Work Environ. Health*, **14**, 101–109

Jones, K. & Cocker, J. (2003) A human exposure study to investigate biological monitoring methods for 2-butoxyethanol. *Biomarkers*, **8**, 360–370

Jones, K., Cocker, J., Dodd, L.J. & Fraser, I. (2003) Factors affecting the dermal absorption of solvent vapours: A human volunteer study. *Ann. occup. Hyg.*, **47**, 145–150

Jönsson, A.-K., Pedersen, J. & Steen, G. (1982) Ethoxyacetic acid and *N*-ethoxyacetylglycine: Metabolites of ethoxyethanol (ethylcellosolve) in rats. *Acta pharmacol. toxicol.*, **50**, 358–362

Jungclaus, G.A., Games, L.M. & Hites, R.A. (1976) Identification of trace organic compounds in tire manufacturing plant wastewaters. *Anal. Chem.*, **48**, 1894–1896

Kaiser, E.A. & McManus, K.P. (1990) *Graphic Creations, Inc., Warren RI* (Health Hazard Evaluation Report HETA No. 88-346-2030), Cincinnati, OH, National Institute for Occupational Safety and Health, Hazard Evaluations and Technical Assistance Branch

Kaphalia, B.S., Ghanayem, B.I. & Ansari, G.A.S. (1996) Nonoxidative metabolism of 2-butoxy-ethanol via fatty acid conjugation in Fischer 344 rats. *J. Toxicol. environ. Health*, **49**, 463–479

Keith, G., Coulais, C., Edorh, A., Bottin, M.C. & Rihn, B. (1996) Ethylene glycol monobutyl ether has neither epigenetic nor genotoxic effects in acute treated rats and in subchronic treated v-HA-*ras* transgenic mice. *Occup. Hyg.*, **2**, 237–249

Kelly, J.E. (1993) *Ohio University, Athens, OH* (Health Hazard Evaluation Report No. HETA-92-314-2308), Cincinnati, OH, National Institute for Occupational Safety and Health, Hazard Evaluations and Technical Assistance Branch

KEMI (2002) *Information from the Swedish Product Register on 4th Priority List Substances (ESR 793/93)*, Stockholm, Letter dated 04/19/02

Kennah, H.E., II, Hignet, S., Laux, P.E., Dorko, J.D. & Barrow, C.S. (1989) An objective procedure for quantitating eye irritation based upon changes of corneal thickness. *Fundam. appl. Toxicol.*, **12**, 258–268

Kerckaert, G.A., Brauninger, R., LeBoeuf, R.A. & Isfort, R.J. (1996) Use of the Syrian hamster embryo cell transformation assay for carcinogenicity prediction of chemicals currently being tested by the National Toxicology Program in rodent bioassays. *Environ. Health Perspect.*, **104** (Suppl. 5), 1075–1084

Kirchner, S. (2002) [Glycol Ethers and Domestic Environments], Paris, Centre scientifique et technique du Bâtiment (in French)

Klaunig, J.E. & Kamendulis, L.M. (2005) Mode of action of butoxyethanol-induced mouse liver hemangiosarcomas and hepatocellular carcinomas. *Toxicol. Lett.*, **156**, 107–115

Koshkaryev, A., Barshtein, G., Nyska, A., Ezov, N., Levin-Harrus, T., Shabat, S., Nyska, M., Redlich, M., Tsipis, F. & Yedgar, S. (2003) 2-Butoxyethanol enhances the adherence of red blood cells. *Arch. Toxicol.*, **77**, 465–469

Krasavage, W.J. (1986) Subchronic oral toxicity of ethylene glycol monobutyl ether in male rats. *Fundam. appl. Toxicol.*, **6**, 349–355

Kumagai, S., Oda, H., Matsunaga, I., Kosaka, H. & Akasaka, S. (1999) Uptake of 10 polar organic solvents during short-term respiration. *Toxicol. Sci.*, **48**, 255–263

Kvelland, I. (1988) The mutagenic effect of five oil dispersants and of ethyleneglycolmonobutyl-ether in bacteriophage *T4D*. *Hereditas*, **109**, 149–150

Laitenen, J. (1998) Correspondence between occupational exposure limit and biological action level values for alkoxyethanols and their acetates. *Int. Arch. occup. environ. Health*, **71**, 117–124

Lee, S.A. (1988) *Louisiana-Pacific Corp., Missoula, MT* (Health Hazard Evaluation Report No. HETA-87-309-1906), Cincinnati, OH, National Institute for Occupational Safety and Health, Hazard Evaluations and Technical Assistance Branch

Lee, K.M., Dill, J.A., Chou, B.J. & Roycroft, J.H. (1998) Physiologically based pharmacokinetic model for chronic inhalation of 2-butoxyethanol. *Toxicol. appl. Pharmacol.*, **153**, 211–226

Lewis, F.A. & Thoburn, T.W. (1981) *Graphic Color Plate, Inc. Stamford, CT* (Health Hazard Evaluation Report HETA No. 79-020-839), Cincinnati, OH, National Institute for Occupational Safety and Health, Hazard Evaluations and Technical Assistance Branch

Lide, D.R. (2004) *CRC Handbook of Chemistry and Physics*, 84th Ed., Boca Raton, FL, CRC Press, pp. 3-82, 6-84

Litovitz, T.L., Bailey, K.M., Schmitz, B.F., Holm, K.C. & Klein-Schwartz, W. (1991) 1990 Annual Report of the American Association of Poison Control Centers National Data Collection System. *Am. J. emerg. Med.*, **9**, 461–509

Long, P.H., Maronpot, R.R., Ghanayem, B.I., Roycroft, J.H. & Nyska, A. (2000) Dental pulp infarction in female rats following inhalation exposure to 2-butoxyethanol. *Toxicol. Pathol.*, **28**, 246–252

Lucas, S.V. (1984) *GC/MS (Gas Chromatography/Mass Spectrophotometry) Analysis of Organics in Drinking Water Concentrates and Advanced Waste Treatment Concentrates*, Vol. 2, *Computer-printed Tabulations of Compound Identification Results for Large-volume Concentrations* (NC Report No. EPA-600/1-84-0208.397), Columbus, OH, Battelle Laboratories for US Environmental Protection Agency, Office of Research Development, Health Effects Research Laboratories

Ma, H., An, J., Hsie, A.W. & Au, W.W. (1993) Mutagenicity and cytotoxicity of 2-methoxyethanol and its metabolites in Chinese hamster cells (the CHO/HPRT and AS52/GPT assays). *Mutat. Res.*, **298**, 219–225

McKinney, P.E., Palmer, R.B., Blackwell, W. & Benson, B.E. (2000) Butoxyethanol ingestion with prolonged hyperchloremic metabolic acidosis treated with ethanol therapy. *Clin. Toxicol.*, **38**, 787–793

Medinsky, M.A., Singh, G., Bechtold, W.E., Bond, J.A., Sabourin, P.J., Birnbaum, L.S. & Henderson, R.F. (1990) Disposition of three glycol ethers administered in drinking water to male F344/N rats. *Toxicol. appl. Pharmacol.*, **102**, 443–455

Michael, L.C., Pellizzari, E.D. & Wiseman, R.W. (1988) Development and evaluation of a procedure for determining volatile organics in water. *Environ. Sci. Technol.*, **22**, 565–570

Michael, L.C., Pellizzari, E.D. & Norwood, D.L. (1991) Application of the master analytical scheme to the determination of volatile organics in wastewater influents and effluents. *Environ. Sci. Technol.*, **25**, 150–155

Morel, G., Lambert, A.M., Rieger, B. & Subra, I. (1996) Interactive effect of combined exposure to glycol ethers and alcohols on toxicodynamic and toxicokinetic parameters. *Arch. Toxicol.*, **70**, 519–525

Morris, B.J., Shipp, B.K., Bartow, T.A. & Blaylock, B.L. (1996) Oral exposure to 2-butoxyethanol alters immune reponse in BALB/c mice (Abstract No. 1756). *Toxicologist*, **30**, 342

Moss, E.J., Thomas, L.V., Cook, M.W., Walters, D.G., Foster, P.M.D., Creasy, D.M. & Gray, T.J.B. (1985) The role of metabolism in 2-methoxyethanol-induced testicular toxicity. *Toxicol. appl. Pharmacol.*, **79**, 480–489

Nagano, K., Nakayama, E., Koyano, M., Oobayashi, H., Adachi, H. & Yamada, T. (1979) [Testicular atrophy of mice induced by ethylene glycol mono alkyl ethers.] *Jpn. J. ind. Health*, **21**, 29–35 (in Japanese)

Nagano, K., Nakayama, E., Oobayashi, H., Nishizawa, T., Okuda, H. & Yamazaki, K. (1984) Experimental studies on toxicity of ethylene glycol alkyl ethers in Japan. *Environ. Health Perspect.*, **57**, 75–84

National Institute for Occupational Safety and Health (1989) *National Occupational Exposure Survey*, Cincinnati, OH, US Department of Health and Human Services, Centers for Disease Control

National Institute for Occupational Safety and Health (1990) *Criteria for a Recommended Standard: Occupational Exposure to Ethylene Glycol Monobutyl Ether and Ethylene Glycol Monobutyl Ether Acetate* (NTIS No. PB901-173369), Cincinnati, OH

National Institute for Occupational Safety and Health (2003) *NIOSH Manual of Analytical Methods*, 4th Ed., 3rd Suppl., Cincinnati, OH, Method 1403

National Toxicology Program (1989) *Teratologic Evaluation of Ethylene Glycol Monobutyl Ether (CAS No. 111-76-2) Administered to Fischer-344 Rats on Either Gestational Days 9 Through 11 or Days 11 Through 13* (PB 89-165849), Research Triangle Park, NC

National Toxicology Program (1993) *Toxicity Studies of Ethylene Glycol Ethers 2-Methoxyethanol, 2-Ethoxyethanol, 2-Butoxyethanol (CAS Nos. 109-86-4, 110-80-5, 111-76-2) Administered in Drinking Water to F344/N Rats and B6C3F₁ Mice* (NTP Toxicity Report Series No. 26; NIH Publ. No. 93-3349), Research Triangle Park, NC

National Toxicology Program (2000) *Toxicology and Carcinogenesis Studies of 2-Butoxyethanol (CAS No. 111-76-2) in F344/N Rats and B6C3F₁ Mice (Inhalation Studies)* (NTP TR 484; NIH Publication No. 00-3974), Research Triangle Park, NC

Nelson, B.K., Setzer, J.V., Brightwell, W.S., Mathinos, P.R., Kuczuk, M.H., Weaver, T.E. & Goad, P.T. (1984) Comparative inhalation teratogenicity of four glycol ether solvents and an amino derivative in rats. *Environ. Health Perspect.*, **57**, 261–271

Newman, M. & Klein, M. (1990) *Schmidt Cabinet Company, New Salisbury, IN* (Health Hazard Evaluation Report No. HETA-88-068-2077), Cincinnati, OH, National Institute for Occupational Safety and Health, Hazard Evaluations and Technical Assistance Branch

Nguyen, D-K., Bruchet, A. & Arpino, P. (1994) High resolution capillary GC–MS analysis of low molecular weight organic compounds in municipal wastewater. *J. high Resolut. Chromatogr.*, **17**, 153–159

NICNAS (National Industrial Chemicals Notification and Assessment Scheme) (1996) *Priority Existing Chemical No. 6 — 2-Butoxyethanol in Cleaning Products*, Canberra, Australian Government Publishing Service

Nisse, P., Coquelle-Couplet, V., Forceville, X. & Mathieu-Nolf, M. (1998) Renal failure after suicidal ingestion of window cleaner. A case report (Abstract). *Vet. hum. Toxicol.*, **40**, 173

Norbäck, D., Wieslander, G., Edling, C. & Johanson, G. (1996) House painters' exposure to glycols and glycol ethers from water based paints. *Occup. Hyg.*, **2**, 111–117

Nyska, A., Maronpot, R.R. & Ghanayem, B.I. (1999a) Ocular thrombosis and retinal degeneration induced in female F344 rats by 2-butoxyethanol. *Hum. exp. Toxicol.*, **18**, 577–582

Nyska, A., Maranpot, R.R., Long, P.H., Roycroft, J.H., Hailey, J.R., Travlos, G.S. & Ghanayem, B.I. (1999b) Disseminated thrombosis and bone infarction in female rats following inhalation exposure to 2-butoxyethanol. *Toxicol. Pathol.*, **27**, 287–294

Nyska, A., Moomaw, C.R., Ezov, N., Shabat, S., Levin-Harrus, T., Nyska, M., Redlich, M., Mittelman, M., Yedgar, S. & Foley, J.F. (2003) Ocular expression of vascular cell adhesion molecule (VCAM-1) in 2-butoxyethanol-induced hemolysis and thrombosis in female rats. *Exp. Toxicol. Pathol.*, **55**, 231–236

Nyska, A., Haseman, J.K., Kohen, R. & Maronpot, R.R. (2004) Association of liver hemangiosarcoma and secondary iron overload in B6C3F1 mice — The National Toxicology Program experience. *Toxicol. Pathol.*, **32**, 222–228

Occupational Safety & Health Administration (1990) *2-Butoxyethanol (Butyl Cellosolve), 2-Butoxyethyl Acetate (Butyl Cellosolve Acetate), Method 83*, Salt Lake City, UT, Organic Methods Evaluation Branch, OSHA Analytical Laboratory

OECD (Organization for Economic Co-operation and Development) (1997) *SIDS Initial Assessment Report for 6th SIAM, 2-Butoxyethanol (CAS No. 111-76-2)*, Paris, UNEP Publications

Osterhoudt, K.C. (2002) Fomepizole therapy for pediatric butoxyethanol intoxication. *J. Toxicol. clin. Toxicol.*, **40**, 929–930

Oxygenated Solvents Producers Association (2004) *The Glycol Ethers* [http://www.ethers-deglycol.org/english/index.html]

Park, J., Kamendulis, L.M. & Klaunig, J.E. (2002a) Effects of 2-butoxyethanol on hepatic oxidative damage. *Toxicol. Lett.*, **126**, 19–29

Park, J., Kamendulis, L.M. & Klaunig, J.E. (2002b) Mechanisms of 2-butoxyethanol carcinogenicity: Studies on Syrian hamster embryo (SHE) cell transformation. *Toxicol. Sci.*, **68**, 43–50

Poet, T.S., Soelberg, J.J., Weitz, K.K., Mast, T.J., Miller, R.A., Thrall, B.D. & Corley, R.A. (2003) Mode of action and pharmacokinetic studies of 2-butoxyethanol in the mouse with an emphasis on forestomach dosimetry. *Toxicol. Sci.*, **71**, 176–189

Rambourg-Schepens, M.O., Buffet, M., Bertault, R., Jaussaud, M., Journe, B., Fay, R. & Lamiable, D. (1988) Severe ethylene glycol butyl ether poisoning. Kinetics and metabolic pattern. *Hum. Toxicol.*, **7**, 187–189

Raymond, L.W., Williford, L.S. & Burke, W.A. (1998) Eruptive cherry angiomas and irritant symptoms after one acute exposure to the glycol ether solvent 2-butoxyethanol. *J. occup. environ. Med.*, **40**, 1059–1064

Rettenmeier, A.W., Hennigs, R. & Wodarz, R. (1993) Determination of butoxyacetic acid and *N*-butoxyacetylglutamine in urine of lacquerers exposed to 2-butoxyethanol. *Int. Arch. occup. environ. Health*, **65**, S151–S153

Rhyder (1992) *Work Cover Authority NSW, Evaluation of Ethylene Glycol Monobutyl Ether Exposure Levels for GCS School Cleaners in the Coffs Harbour Area, 8–9 August 1992* (cited in NICNAS, 1996)

Rocchi, E., Seium, Y., Camellini, L., Casalgrandi, G., Borghi, A., D'Alimonte, P. & Cioni, G. (1997) Hepatic tocopherol content in primary hepatocellular carcinoma and liver metastases. *Hepatology*, **26**, 67–72

Sabourin, P.J., Medinsky, M.A., Birnbaum, L.S., Griffith, W.C. & Henderson, R.F. (1992a) Effect of exposure concentration of the disposition of inhaled butoxyethanol by F344 rats. *Toxicol. appl. Pharmacol.*, **114**, 232–238

Sabourin, P.J., Medinsky, M.A., Thurmond, F., Birnbaum, L.S. & Henderson, R.F. (1992b) Effect of dose on the disposition of methoxyethanol, ethoxyethanol, and butoxyethanol administered dermally to male F344/N rats. *Fundam. appl. Toxicol.*, **19**, 124–132

Sakai, T., Araki, T. & Masuyama, Y. (1993) Determination of urinary alkoxyacetic acids by a rapid and simple method for biological monitoring of workers exposed to glycol ethers and their acetates. *Int. Arch. occup. environ. Health*, **64**, 495–498

Sakai, T., Araki, T., Morita, Y. & Masuyama, Y. (1994) Gaschromatographic determination of butoxyacetic acid after hydrolysis of conjugated metabolites in urine from workers exposed to 2-butoxyethanol. *Int. Arch. occup. environ. Health*, **66**, 249–254

Salisbury, S., Bennett, D. & Aw, T.-C. (1987) *Tropicana Products, Bradenton, FL* (Health Hazard Evaluation Report HETA No. 83-458-1800), Cincinnati, OH, National Institute for Occupational Safety and Health, Hazard Evaluations and Technical Assistance Branch

Schuler, R.L., Hardin, B.D., Niemeier, R.W., Booth, G., Hazelden, K., Piccirillo, V. & Smith, K. (1984) Results of testing fifteen glycol ethers in a short-term *in vivo* reproductive toxicity assay. *Environ. Health Perspect.*, **57**, 141–146

Shabat, S., Nyska, A., Long, P.H., Goelman, G., Abramovitch, R., Ezov, N., Levin-Harrus, T., Peddada, S., Redlich, M., Yedgar, S. & Nyska, M. (2004) Osteonecrosis in a chemically induced rat model of human hemolytic disorders associated with thrombosis — A new model for avascular necrosis of bone. *Calcif. Tissue int.*, **74**, 220–228

Shah, J.J. & Singh, H.B. (1988) Distribution of volatile organic chemicals in outdoor and indoor air. A national VOCs data base. *Environ. Sci. Technol.*, **22**, 1381–1388

Shell Chemicals (2002) *Data Sheet: Butyl OXITOL*, London

Shell Chemicals (2004) *Data Sheet: Butyl OXITOL (North America)*, Houston, TX

Shields, H.C., Fleischer, D.M. & Weschler, C.J. (1996) Comparisons among VOCs measured in three types of US commercial buildings with different occupant densities. *Indoor Air*, **6**, 2–17

Shih, T.-S., Chou, J.-S., Chen, C.-Y. & Smith, T.J. (1999) Improved method to measure urinary alkoxyacetic acids. *Occup. environ. Med.*, **56**, 460–467

Shyr, L.J., Sabourin, P.J., Medinsky, M.A., Birnbaum, L.S. & Henderson, R.F. (1993) Physiologically based modeling of 2-butoxyethanol disposition in rats following different routes of exposure. *Environ. Res.*, **63**, 202–218

Siesky, A.M., Kamendulis, L.M. & Klaunig, J.E. (2002) Hepatic effects of 2-butoxyethanol in rodents. *Toxicol. Sci.*, **70**, 252–260

Singh, P., Zhao, S. & Blaylock, B.L. (2001) Topical exposure to 2-butoxyethanol alters immune responses in female BALB/c mice. *Int. J. Toxicol.*, **20**, 383–390

Singh, P., Morris, B., Zhao, S. & Blaylock, B.L. (2002) Suppression of the contact hypersensitivity response following topical exposure to 2-butoxyethanol in female BALB/c mice. *Int. J. Toxicol.*, **21**, 107–115

Sivarao, D.V. & Mehendale, H.M. (1995) 2-Butoxyethanol autoprotection is due to resiliance of newly formed erythrocytes to hemolysis. *Arch. Toxicol.*, **69**, 526–532

Smialowicz, R.J., Williams, W.C., Riddle, M.M., Andrews, D.L., Luebke, R.W. & Copeland, C.B. (1992) Comparative immunosuppression of various glycol ethers orally administered to Fischer 344 rats. *Fundam. appl. Toxicol.*, **18**, 621–627

Smyth, H.F., Jr, Seaton, J. & Fischer, L. (1941) The single dose toxicity of some glycols and derivatives. *J. ind. Hyg. Toxicol.*, **23**, 259–268

Smyth, H.F., Jr, Carpenter, C.P., Weil, C.S., Pozzani, U.C. & Striegel, J.A. (1962) Range-finding toxicity data: List VI. *Am. ind. Hyg. Assoc. J.*, **23**, 95–107

Söhnlein, B., Letzel, S., Welte, D., Rüdiger, H.W. & Angerer, J. (1993) Occupational chronic exposure to organic solvents. XIV. Examinations concerning the evaluation of a limit value for 2-ethoxyethanol and 2-ethoxyethyl acetate and the genotoxic effects of these glycol ethers. *Int. Arch. occup. environ. Health*, **64**, 479–484

Stonebreaker, R.D. & Smith, A.J., Jr (1980) Containment and treatment of a mixed chemical discharge from the 'Valley of the Drums' near Louisville, Kentucky Contr. Haz 1-10 (cited in ATSDR, 1998)

Suva (2003) *Grenzwerte am Arbeitsplatz 2003*, Luzern, Swiss Accident Insurance [Swiss OELs]

Tennant, R.W. & Ashby, J. (1991). Classification according to chemical structure, mutagenicity to Salmonella and level of carcinogenicity of a further 39 chemicals tested for carcinogenicity by the US National Toxicology Program. *Mutat. Res.*, **257**, 209–227

ToxEcology Environmental Consulting Ltd (2003) *2-Butoxyethanol and 2-Methoxyethanol. Current Use Patterns in Canada, Toxicology Profiles of Alternatives, and the Feasibility of Performing an Exposure Assessment Study*, Vancouver, BC, Health Canada

Tyl, R.W., Millicovsky, G., Dodd, D.E., Pritts, I.M., France, K.A. & Fisher, L.C. (1984) Teratologic evaluation of ethylene glycol monobutyl ether in Fischer 344 rats and New Zealand white rabbits following inhalation exposure. *Environ. Health Perspect.*, **57**, 47–68

Tyler, T.R. (1984) Acute and subchronic toxicity of ethylene glycol monobutyl ether. *Environ. Health Perspect.*, **57**, 185–191

Työsuojelusäädöksiä (2002) *HTP arvot 2002*, Helsinki, Sosiaali-ja terveysministeriön [Finnish OELs]

Udden, M.M. (1994) Hemolysis and deformability of erythrocytes exposed to butoxyacetic acid, a metabolite of 2-butoxyethanol: II. Resistance in red blood cells from humans with potential susceptibility. *J. appl. Toxicol.*, **14**, 97–102

Udden, M.M. (1996) Effects of butoxyacetic acid on human red cells. *Occup. Hyg.*, **2**, 283–290

Udden, M.M. (2000) Rat erythrocyte morphological changes after gavage dosing with 2-butoxy-ethanol: A comparison with the *in vitro* effects of butoxyacetic acid on rat and human erythrocytes. *J. appl. Toxicol.*, **20**, 381–387

Udden, M.M. (2002) *In vitro* sub-hemolytic effects of butoxyacetic acid on human and rat erythrocytes. *Toxicol. Sci.*, **69**, 258–264

Udden, M.M. & Patton, C.S. (1994) Hemolysis and deformability of erythrocytes exposed to butoxy-acetic acid, a metabolite of 2-butoxyethanol: I. Sensitivity in rats and resistance in normal humans. *J. appl. Toxicol.*, **14**, 91–96

Verschueren, K. (2001) *Handbook of Environmental Data on Organic Chemicals*, 4th Ed., Vol. 1, New York, John Wiley & Sons

Veulemans, H., Groeseneken, D., Masschelein, R. & Van Vlem, E. (1987) Survey of ethylene glycol ether exposures in Belgian industries and workshops. *Am. ind. Hyg. Assoc. J.*, **48**, 671–676

Villalobos-Pietrini, R., Gómez-Arroyo, S., Altamirano-Lozano, M., Orozco, P. & Ríos, P. (1989) Cytogenetic effects of some cellosolves. *Rev. int. Contam. ambient.*, **5**, 41–48

Vincent, R. (1999) [Occupational exposure]. In: [Glycol Ethers, What Health Risks?], Paris, Ed. INSERM, pp. 237–256 (in French)

Vincent, R. & Jeandel, B. (1999) [Evolution of exposure levels between 1987 and 1998.] In: [Glycol Ethers, What Health Risks?], Paris, Ed. INSERM, pp. 257–262 (in French)

Vincent, R., Cicolella, A., Subra, I., Rieger, B., Poirot, P. & Pierre, F. (1993) Occupational exposure to 2-butoxyethanol for workers using window cleaning agents. *Appl. occup. environ. Hyg.*, **8**, 580–586

Vincent, R., Rieger, B., Subra, I. & Poirot, P. (1996) Exposure assessment to glycol ethers by atmos-phere and biological monitoring. *Occup. Hyg.*, **2**, 79–90

Weil, C.S. & Wright, G.J. (1967) Intra- and interlaboratory comparative evaluation of single oral test. *Toxicol. appl. Pharmacol.*, **11**, 378–388

Werner, H.W., Mitchell, J.L., Miller, J.W. & von Oettingen, W.F. (1943a) The acute toxicity of vapors of several monoalkyl ethers of ethylene glycol. *J. ind. Hyg. Toxicol.*, **25**, 157–163

Werner, H.W., Nawrocki, C.Z., Mitchell, J.L., Miller, J.W. & von Oettingen, W.F. (1943b) Effects of repeated exposures of rats to vapors of monoalkyl ethylene glycol ethers. *J. ind. Hyg. Toxicol.*, **25**, 374–379

Werner, H.W., Mitchell, J.L., Miller, J.W. & von Oettingen, W.F. (1943c) Effects of repeated expo-sure of dogs to monoalkyl ethylene glycol ether vapors. *J. ind. Hyg. Toxicol.*, **25**, 409–414

Wesolowski, W. & Gromiec, J.P. (1997) Occupational exposure in Polish paint and lacquer industry. *Int. J. occup. Med. environ. Health*, **10**, 79–88

Wier, P.J., Lewis, S.C. & Traul, K.A. (1987) A comparison of developmental toxicity evident at term to postnatal growth and survival using ethylene glycol monoethyl ether, ethylene glycol monobutyl ether, and ethanol. *Teratog. Carcinog. Mutag.*, **7**, 55–64

Wilkinson, S.C. & Williams, F.J. (2002) Effects of experimental conditions on absorption of glycol ethers through human skin in vitro. *Int. Arch. occup. environ. Health*, **75**, 519–527

Winchester, R.V. (1985) Solvent exposure of workers during printing ink manufacture. *Ann. occup. Hyg.*, **29**, 517–519

Winder, C. & Turner, P.J. (1992) Solvent exposure and related work practices amongst apprentice spray painters in automotive body repair workshops. *Ann. occup. Hyg.*, **36**, 385–394

Yasugi, T., Endo, G., Monna, T., Odachi, T., Yamaoka, K., Kawai, T., Horiguchi, S. & Ikeda, M. (1998) Types of organic solvents used in workplaces and work environment conditions with special references to reproducibility of work environment classification. *Ind. Health*, **36**, 223–233

Yasuhara, A., Shiraishi, H., Tsuji, M. & Okuno, T. (1981) Analysis of organic substances in highly polluted river water by mass spectrometry. *Environ. Sci. Technol.*, **15**, 570–573

Yoshikawa, M. & Tani, C. (2003) Sensitive determination of alkoxyethanols by pre-column derivatization with 1-anthroylnitrile and reversed-phase high-performance liquid chromatography. *J. Chromatog.*, **A1005**, 215–221

Zaebst, D.D. (1984) *In-depth Industrial Hygiene Survey Report of Henredon Furniture Industries, Inc., Morgaton, NC* (Health Hazard Evaluation Report HETA), Cincinnati, OH, National Institute for Occupational Safety and Health, Hazard Evaluations and Technical Assistance Branch

Zeiger, E., Anderson, B., Haworth, S., Lawlor, T. & Mortelmans, K. (1992) Salmonella mutagenicity tests: V. Results from the testing of 311 chemicals. *Environ. mol. Mutag.*, **19** (Suppl. 21), 2–141

Zhu, J., Cao, X.-L. & Beauchamp, R. (2001) Determination of 2-butoxyethanol emissions from selected consumer products and its application in assessment of inhalation exposure associated with cleaning tasks. *Environ. int.*, **26**, 589–597

Zissu, D. (1995) Experimental study of cutaneous tolerance to glycol ethers. *Contact Derm.*, **32**, 74–77

1-*tert*-BUTOXYPROPAN-2-OL

1. Exposure Data

1.1 Chemical and physical data

The chemical that is the subject of this monograph, 1-*tert*-butoxypropan-2-ol, is commonly known as propylene glycol mono-*tert*-butyl ether. However, the latter name is non-specific and could also refer to 2-*tert*-butoxypropan-1-ol or to the mixture of the 1- and 2-isomers (also called α- and β-isomers, respectively). Thus, the name 1-*tert*-butoxypropan-2-ol was chosen for this monograph to avoid ambiguity.

1.1.1 *Nomenclature*

From National Library of Medicine (2004)
Chem. Abstr. Serv. Reg. No.: 57018-52-7
Deleted CAS Reg. No.: 136579-67-4
Chem. Abstr. Name: 1-(1,1-Dimethylethoxy)-2-propanol
Synonyms: 1-*tert*-Butoxy-2-propanol; 1-methyl-2-*tert*-butoxyethanol; propylene glycol 1-(*tert*-butyl ether); propylene glycol mono-*tert*-butyl ether, α-isomer

1.1.2 *Structural and molecular formulae and relative molecular mass*

$$H_3C - \overset{\displaystyle CH_3}{\underset{\displaystyle CH_3}{\overset{|}{\underset{|}{C}}}} - O - CH_2 - \overset{\displaystyle OH}{\overset{|}{CH}} - CH_3$$

$C_7H_{16}O_2$ Relative molecular mass: 132.2

1.1.3 *Chemical and physical properties of the pure substance*

From Lyondell Chemical Co. (2004), unless otherwise specified
(*a*) *Description*: Colourless, combustible liquid with a characteristic odour similar to that of eucalyptus

(b) *Boiling-point*: 151 °C (Boatman, 2001)

(c) *Melting-point*: –27 °C (Staples & Davis, 2002)

(d) *Density*: Specific gravity, 0.87 at 25/4 °C (Boatman, 2001)

(e) *Spectroscopy*: Infrared, nuclear magnetic resonance (proton and carbon-13) and mass spectral data have been reported (National Toxicology Program, 2004a).

(f) *Solubility*: Soluble in water (18% at 20 °C); miscible with many organic solvents; solubility in water is increased by the addition of low-molecular-weight alcohols and other water-miscible glycol ethers.

(g) *Volatility*: Vapour pressure, 2.7 mm Hg at 25 °C (93 Pa at 25 °C; Staples & Davis, 2002); flash-point (Tag closed-cup), 45 °C; flammability limits (lower/upper vol. %), 1.8/6.8

(h) *Octanol/water partition coefficient (P)*: log P, 0.87 (Staples & Davis, 2002)

(i) *Conversion factor*: mg/m^3 = 5.4 × ppm[1]

1.1.4 *Technical products and impurities*

Trade names for 1-*tert*-butoxypropan-2-ol include Arcosolv® PTB. It is commercially available in the USA with the following specifications: purity, min. 99.0%; specific gravity (at 25/25 °C), 0.870–0.874; acidity (% wt as acetic acid, max.), 0.03; and water (% wt, max.), 0.25 (Lyondell Chemical Co., 2004). Potential impurities include: 2-*tert*-butoxy-propan-1-ol (β-isomer; < 0.5%), propylene glycol di-*tert*-butyl ether, propylene glycol, *tert*-butanol and isobutylene (Knifton, 1994).

1.1.5 *Analysis*

1-*tert*-Butoxypropan-2-ol has been quantified in commercial technical products using gas chromatography (GC) with mass spectrometry and GC with flame ionization detection (FID). It has also been determined in air using GC/FID (National Toxicology Program, 2004a).

1.2   Production and use

Glycol ethers began to be used in the 1930s and some have been in general use for nearly 50 years. They form a varied family of more than 30 solvents that commonly dissolve in both water and oil. For this reason, they are very useful in numerous industrial (paints, pharmaceutical industry, inks) and consumer (cosmetics, detergents) applications. Traditionally, a distinction is made between two main groups of glycol ethers: the E series and the P series, which derive from the name of the chemical substances that serve as a starting point for their production (ethylene and propylene, respectively). In each series,

---

[1] Calculated from: mg/m^3 = (relative molecular mass/24.45) × ppm, assuming normal temperature (25 °C) and pressure (103.5 kPa)

different derivatives have been developed to provide the properties of solubility, volatility, compatibility and inflammability that are required for different uses. Since the mid-1980s, concerns about the toxic effects of the E-series glycol ethers have stimulated the development of P-series products as potential substitutes. 1-*tert*-Butoxypropan-2-ol is one of several monoalkyl ethers of propylene glycol that is finding increasing use as a replacement for the E-series glycol ethers (Begley, 1986; Chinn *et al*, 2000; Oxygenated Solvents Producers Association, 2004).

1.2.1   *Production*

The ethers of propylene glycol are prepared commercially by reacting propylene oxide with the alcohol of choice in the presence of a catalyst. They may also be prepared by direct alkylation of the selected glycol with an appropriate alkylating agent such as dialkyl sulfate in the presence of an alkali. Commercial synthesis typically yields products that are mixtures of the α- and β-isomers. The α-isomer has the ether linkage on the terminal hydroxyl group of propylene glycol, while the β-isomer has the ether linkage on the secondary hydroxyl group. The α-isomer is thermodynamically favoured and is the predominant ether formed. By controlling the conditions of synthesis, the proportion of α-isomer may be enhanced to constitute more than 99% of the end-product (Boatman, 2001).

1-*tert*-Butoxypropan-2-ol is generally manufactured by reacting isobutylene with excess propylene glycol in the presence of a solid-resin etherification catalyst. The product is then distilled to produce ≥ 99% of the α-isomer, 1-*tert*-butoxypropan-2-ol (Gupta, 1987). The commercial product contains > 99.5% of the α-isomer (1-*tert*-butoxypropan-2-ol) (Staples & Davies, 2002).

Available information indicates that 1-*tert*-butoxypropan-2-ol was produced by one company in the USA (Chemical Information Services, 2004; Lyondell Chemical Co, 2004). Estimated production of 1-*tert*-butoxypropan-2-ol in the USA between 1989 and 1999 is shown in Table 1 (Chinn *et al*., 2000).

Table 1. Production of 1-*tert*-butoxypropan-2-ol from 1989 to 1999 in the USA (tonnes)

1989	1991	1993	1995	1997	1999
230	1100	1400	1800	1800	2300

From Chinn *et al.* (2000)

1.2.2   *Use*

Butyl ethers have limited solubility in water but are miscible with most organic solvents, which favours their use as coupling, coalescing and dispersing agents. Butyl glycol ethers have been used as solvents for surface coatings, inks, lacquers, paints, resins, dyes, agricultural chemicals and other oils and greases.

1-*tert*-Butoxypropan-2-ol is a better coupling agent and has higher electrolyte solubility than 2-butoxyethanol. It is used commercially as a solvent in water-reducible coatings and in a variety of commercial cleaner formulations including all-purpose, glass- and hard surface-cleaning products. It is also used in inks, adhesives and agricultural, electronic, cosmetic and textile products (Boatman, 2001; Lyondell Chemical Co., 2004).

1.3   Occurrence

1.3.1   *Natural occurrence*

1-*tert*-Butoxypropan-2-ol is not known to occur as a natural product.

1.3.2   *Occupational exposure*

There is a potential for occupational exposure to 1-*tert*-butoxypropan-2-ol mainly via inhalation and dermal absorption during its production and use in a variety of products. Because 1-*tert*-butoxypropan-2-ol is readily absorbed through the skin and has a relatively low vapour pressure, the dermal route may be predominant or may contribute significantly to overall exposure. No data on exposure were available to the Working Group; however, exposure during the manufacturing process is thought to be low since it is largely enclosed (Boatman, 2001).

1.3.3   *Consumer exposure*

1-*tert*-Butoxypropan-2-ol is used in a variety of products and consumer exposure may potentially occur during the handling or use of products that contain this chemical (Boatman, 2001). However, no data were available on levels of consumer exposure.

1.3.4   *Environmental occurrence*

No information was available to the Working Group on environmental exposure to 1-*tert*-butoxypropan-2-ol.

1.4   Regulations and guidelines

No occupational exposure limits (Boatman, 2001) or other occupational or environmental regulations or guidelines have been established for 1-*tert*-butoxypropan-2-ol.

2.   Studies of Cancer in Humans

No data were available to the Working Group.

3.   Studies of Cancer in Experimental Animals

3.1   Inhalation

3.1.1   *Mouse*

Groups of 50 male and 50 female B6C3 F_1 mice, approximately 6 weeks of age, were exposed to 0, 75, 300 or 1200 ppm [0, 405, 1620 or 6480 mg/m^3] 1-*tert*-butoxypropan-2-ol (> 99% pure) vapour by whole-body exposure for 6 h per day on 5 days per week for 104 weeks. Complete necropsies were performed on all mice, when all organs and tissues were examined for macroscopic lesions, and all major tissues were examined microscopically. Exposure to 1-*tert*-butoxypropan-2-ol had no effect on survival of the mice. Survival rates in males were 35/50 (control), 40/50 (low-dose), 40/50 (mid-dose) and 37/50 (high-dose), and those in females were 39/50 (control), 36/50 (low-dose), 42/50 (mid-dose) and 39/50 (high-dose). Increases in the incidences of neoplastic and non-neoplastic lesions were observed in the livers of both male and female mice (Table 2). The incidences of hepato-cellular adenoma and adenoma or carcinoma (combined) occurred with positive trends in males and females ($p \le 0.05$, Poly-3 test); the incidence of hepatoblastoma occurred with a positive trend in males ($p \le 0.05$, Poly-3 test); and the incidences in the high-dose groups were significantly increased ($p \le 0.001$, Poly-3 test). In males, the incidence of combined hepatocellular adenoma and carcinoma in the high-dose group exceeded that seen in histo-rical controls (range, 50–68%). The incidence of hepatoblastomas in historical inhalation controls was 0/250 males and 0/248 females fed NTP-2000 diet. The overall incidence of hepatoblastomas in historical controls following exposure by all routes in all laboratories was 16/1159 (1.38%) males and 0/1152 females fed NTP-2000 diet. In high-dose females, the incidence of combined hepatocellular adenomas and carcinomas also exceeded that seen in historical controls (range, 22–37%). The incidences of hepatocellular foci were generally increased with exposure. The incidence of multinucleated hepatocytes in males exposed to 1200 ppm was significantly greater than that of controls. Multinucleated hepatocytes were randomly distributed; enlarged hepatocytes contained three or more nuclei. The severity of this change was generally mild and based on the number of multinucleated hepatocytes (Doi *et al.*, 2004; National Toxicology Program, 2004a).

Table 2. Incidences[a] of liver lesions in B6C3F$_1$ mice in the 2-year inhalation study of 1-*tert*-butoxypropan-2-ol

Type of tumour or lesion	Controls	75 ppm	300 ppm	1200 ppm
Males				
No. examined	50	49	50	50
Hepatocellular adenoma	18[b]	23	26	36*
Hepatocellular carcinoma	9	8	13	11
Hepatocellular adenoma or carcinoma	25[b]	26	33	41*
Hepatoblastoma	0[b]	0	1	5*
Eosinophilic focus	9	14	11	29*
Hepatocyte, multinucleated	27 (1.0)[c]	23 (1.0)	24 (1.0)	46* (1.8)
Females				
No. examined	49	50	50	49
Hepatocellular adenoma	14[b]	8	10	37*
Hepatocellular carcinoma	4	8	7	10
Hepatocellular adenoma or carcinoma	18[b]	14	16	41*
Hepatoblastoma	0	0	0	2
Eosinophilic focus	11	10	9	27*

From Doi *et al.* (2004); National Toxicology Program (2004a)
* Significantly different ($p \le 0.05$) from concurrent controls by the Poly-3 test
[a] Number of animals with lesion
[b] Overall exposure-related trend ($p \le 0.05$) by the Poly-3 test
[c] Average severity grade of lesions in affected animals is depicted in parentheses: 1, minimal; 2, mild; 3, moderate; 4, marked.

3.1.2   *Rat*

Groups of 50 male and 50 female Fisher 344/N rats, approximately 6 weeks of age, were exposed to 0, 75, 300 or 1200 ppm [0, 405, 1620 or 6480 mg/m^3] 1-*tert*-butoxy-propan-2-ol (> 99% pure) vapour by whole-body exposure for 6 h per day on 5 days per week for 104 weeks. Complete necropsies were performed on all rats, when all organs and tissues were examined for macroscopic lesions, and all major tissues were examined microscopically. Kidneys of male rats were step-sectioned to obtain three to four additional sections. Survival rates in males were 27/50 (control), 29/50 (low-dose), 16/50 (mid-dose) and 22/50 (high-dose); those in females were 33/50 (control), 34/50 (low-dose), 28/50 (mid-dose) and 36/50 (high-dose). No increase in the incidence of tumours was observed in females. Marginal increases in the incidences of kidney and liver tumours were observed in exposed males. The incidence of renal tubule adenomas in exposed males was marginally increased. One renal tubule carcinoma also occurred in the high-dose group. The combined incidences of these tumours were 1/50 (control), 2/50 (low-dose), 5/49 (mid-dose) and 5/50 (high-dose) (not statistically significant by pair-wise comparison and trend test). Historically, no more than one kidney neoplasm has been observed in male control rats fed NTP-2000 diet in National Toxicology Program inhalation studies, and the incidences observed in the current study were greater than the National Toxicology Program historical control range (0–2%). The incidence of hepatocellular adenoma occurred with a positive trend ($p = 0.022$, Poly-3 test) in male rats, and the incidence in the high-dose group exceeded the historical range in controls fed NTP-2000 diet (0–6%) in the National Toxicology Program database. The incidence of liver adenoma in males was 3/50 (control), 0/50 (low-dose), 2/49 (mid-dose) and 6/50 (high-dose) (not statistically significant by pairwise comparison). No hepatocellular carcinomas were observed (Doi *et al.*, 2004; National Toxicology Program, 2004a).

4. Other Data Relevant to an Evaluation of Carcinogenicity and its Mechanisms

4.1 Absorption, distribution, metabolism and excretion

4.1.1 *Humans*

No data were available to the Working Group.

4.1.2 *Experimental systems*

Two studies of the kinetics and metabolism of 1-*tert*-butoxypropan-2-ol were available. The first was part of the National Toxicology Program (1994) study and involved single oral, intravenous or dermal administrations of [^{14}C]1-*tert*-butoxypropan-2-ol to rats and dermal administration of [^{14}C]1-*tert*-butoxypropan-2-ol to mice. The second study was conducted in conjunction with the recent National Toxicology Program chronic bioassay (National Toxicology Program, 2004a) and involved intravenous and inhalation exposure of rats and mice to 1-*tert*-butoxypropan-2-ol (Dill *et al.*, 2004).

(*a*) *Oral administration*

Groups of three male Fischer 344 rats were administered a single oral dose of 3.8, 37.7 and 377.1 mg/kg bw [^{14}C]1-*tert*-butoxypropan-2-ol (which represented 0.1%, 1% and 10% of the LD_{50}) in water at 5 mL/kg and serial samples were collected for 72 h. The cumulative excretion profiles were similar at all dose levels and most of the radioactivity was recovered within 24 h. The predominant route of excretion (48–67% of the administered dose) was via the urine. The major urinary metabolite (23–52%) was the glucuronide conjugate of 1-*tert*-butoxypropan-2-ol (the highest percentage was recovered at the lowest dose); another significant urinary metabolite was the sulfate conjugate (6.7–13%; the highest percentage was recovered after at the highest dose). Unchanged 1-*tert*-butoxypropan-2-ol in urine accounted for less than 2% of the dose. Expiration of [^{14}C]carbon dioxide accounted for 22–26% of the dose, while elimination of exhaled volatile organic compounds was negligible. Faecal elimination accounted for about 4% of the lowest dose but increased to 11% at the highest dose.

Since 26% of the radioactivity was detected as exhaled carbon dioxide, an alternative pathway of metabolism of 1-*tert*-butoxypropan-2-ol, similar to that of other propylene glycol ethers, may occur (Miller *et al.*, 1984). This pathway could involve oxidation (*O*-dealkylation of 1-*tert*-butoxypropan-2-ol) to produce propylene glycol, which could be metabolized further to lactic acid and pyruvic acid, which may undergo tricarboxylic acid cycle conversion to carbon dioxide (Dill *et al.*, 2004), as proposed in Figure 1. However, there are currently no empirical data to support the existence of this pathway for 1-*tert*-butoxypropan-2-ol.

Examination of the distribution of 1-*tert*-butoxypropan-2-ol in tissues after a 3.8-mg/kg dose showed that the five highest levels of radioactivity were in muscle ($2.04 \pm 0.18\%$), skin ($1.39 \pm 0.18\%$), fat ($0.57 \pm 0.12\%$), liver ($0.39 \pm 0.04\%$) and blood ($0.28 \pm 0.04\%$).

(b)   Intravenous administration

Pharmacokinetics were studied in Fischer 344 rats following an intravenous bolus dose of 37.8 mg/kg bw [^{14}C]1-*tert*-butoxypropan-2-ol. The mean plasma half-life was 16 min, the mean clearance was 25.1 mL/min/kg and the volume of distribution at steady state was 0.46 L/kg. Six hours after administration, 40% of the dose was recovered as the glucuronide conjugate in bile, although some of this appeared to be reabsorbed via enterohepatic circulation, as faecal elimination accounted for only 11% of the administered dose. The maximum rate of excretion was 30% of the dose per hour, which was reached between 0.5 and 1 h after administration (National Toxicology Program, 1994).

Fisher F344 rats and B6C3F$_1$ mice received a single intravenous injection of 15 or 200 mg/kg bw 1-*tert*-butoxypropan-2-ol. Serial blood samples were collected (three animals per species per sex per dose per time-point) after treatment for up to 12 h (rats) and 3 h (mice) and were analysed for 1-*tert*-butoxypropan-2-ol. Following the 15-mg/kg bw dose, the elimination half-life was 9.6 min in rats and 3.7 min in mice, but increased after the 200 mg/kg dose to 33.8 min and 9.4 min for rats and mice, respectively. The peak concentration of 1-*tert*-butoxypropan-2-ol in blood increased proportionally with dose (23 µg/g at 15 mg/kg and 284 µg/g at 200 mg/kg) and was not significantly different between the sexes in either species. Clearance in rats was slightly faster in males (30 and 11.5 mL/min/kg) than in females (23.2 and 8.8 mL/min/kg) after both doses (15 and 200 mg/kg) and was reduced with the higher dose; in mice, clearance was also reduced with the higher dose and was not significantly different between sexes (Dill *et al.*, 2004).

(c)   Dermal application

In-vivo dermal absorption was determined in rats and mice using a skin-mounted trap that contained charcoal to maximize recovery of the dose. Following topical application of 4.7 mg/cm^2 [^{14}C]1-*tert*-butoxypropan-2-ol (to 8.4 cm^2 for rats and 0.8 cm^2 for mice), approximately 3% of the applied dose was absorbed in rats (approximately 2% of the dose was recovered in urine and 1% of the dose was exhaled as [^{14}C]carbon dioxide). The

Figure 1. Proposed metabolic pathway for 1-*tert*-butoxypropan-2-ol

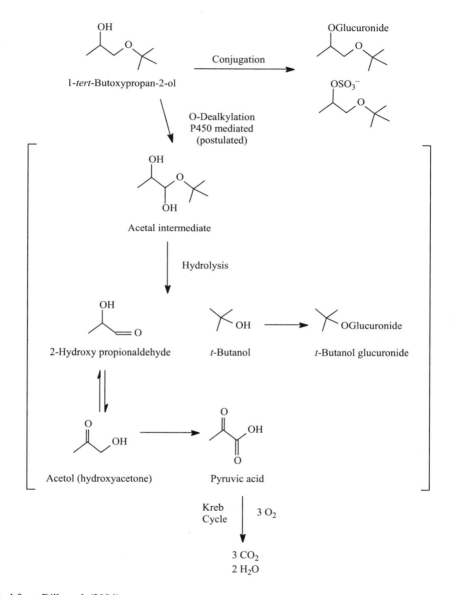

Adapted from Dill *et al.* (2004)

majority of the dose was eliminated within 24 h and about 0.05% of the radioactivity was recovered from the site of application. For mice, a greater proportion of the dose was absorbed (7.8%); urinary radioactivity accounted for 2% and [^{14}C]carbon dioxide for 5% of the dose. The pattern of urinary metabolites was similar to that observed after oral administration (National Toxicology Program, 1994).

(d)   *Inhalation exposure*

Rats and mice received a single 6-h whole-body inhalation exposure to 75, 300 or 1200 ppm [406, 1626 or 6504 mg/m^3] 1-*tert*-butoxypropan-2-ol and serial blood samples were collected for up to 10 h (rats) and 4 h (mice) and analysed for the parent compound. In both species, blood concentrations of 1-*tert*-butoxypropan-2-ol declined rapidly after exposures to 75 or 300 ppm, but decreased more slowly after exposure to 1200 ppm. Although variable, the half-lives, estimated from the exposures to 75 ppm and 300 ppm, were approximately 20 min in rats and 5 min in mice and were not considered to differ within a species as a function of exposure concentration or sex. In rats, the peak blood concentration increased non-linearly with the exposure concentration in both sexes and was slightly but consistently higher (1.2–1.4-fold) in females (3.8, 23 and 368 µg/g at 75, 300 and 1200 ppm, respectively), which suggested saturation of metabolic clearance of 1-*tert*-butoxypropan-2-ol. Following exposure to 1200 ppm, the Michaelis-Menten constant (K_m, ~238 µg/g), maximum elimination rate (V_{max}, ~ 2.6 µg/g/min) and elimination rate constant (K_e, ~0.01 /min) were comparable between sexes. In mice, the peak blood concentration also increased non-linearly with the exposure concentration (around 1.5 µg/g and 16 µg/g for 75 and 300 ppm in both sexes) and, in addition to evidence of saturation of metabolism, there was a difference between the sexes at 1200 ppm (males, 547 µg/g; females, 800 µg/g). The K_m (~98 µg/g), V_{max} (~4.6 µg/g/min) and K_e (~0.04/min) were broadly comparable between sexes. Therefore, compared with rats, mice eliminated 1-*tert*-butoxy-propan-2-ol from blood more rapidly (shorter half-life) and had higher efficiency (lower K_m) and capacity (higher V_{max}) for elimination (Dill *et al.*, 2004).

In the same study (Dill *et al.*, 2004), rats and mice were also exposed by inhalation (whole-body exposure) to 75, 300 or 1200 ppm [406, 1626 or 6504 mg/m^3] 1-*tert*-butoxy-propan-2-ol for 6 h per day on 5 days per week for 14 (rats) or 16 (mice) weeks, as part of the National Toxicology Program 2-year inhalation study (National Toxicology Program, 2004a). At 2, 6, 14 (rats) and 16 (mice) weeks of exposure, a group of animals (three animals per species per sex per exposure concentration per time-point) was bled and samples were analysed for 1-*tert*-butoxypropan-2-ol. In rats, blood concentrations of 1-*tert*-butoxy-propan-2-ol declined rapidly (half-life, approximately 10 min) with similar elimination rates between the groups exposed to 75 ppm and 300 ppm. For the group exposed to 1200 ppm, the initial elimination rate was slower but, after 3–4 h, was similar to that in the groups exposed to lower doses. The peak blood concentration increased in proportion to the dose between 75 ppm and 300 ppm but more than proportionally at 1200 ppm in both sexes. Effects of repeated exposures were insignificant from 2 to 14 weeks. In mice, blood concentrations of 1-*tert*-butoxypropan-2-ol declined rapidly after exposure to 75 and 300 ppm with half-lives of approximately 5 min. Longer half-lives (approximately 14 min) were seen after exposure to 1200 ppm.

Animals in another group (10 animals per species per sex per exposure concentration) were placed in metabolism cages and urine samples were collected (on ice) for 16 h after exposure at 14 weeks (rats) and 16 weeks (mice) in the repeated inhalation study (Dill *et al.*, 2004). Samples were analysed for creatinine, 1-*tert*-butoxypropan-2-ol and its glucuronide and sulfate conjugates. In male and female rats, both the glucuronide and sulfate conjugates were detected in the urine; males excreted more total conjugates than females, which was consistent with a slower rate of clearance of 1-*tert*-butoxypropan-2-ol from the blood in females than in males. However, the conjugation pathway appeared to be saturated at the highest concentration, based on the lower ratio of total urinary conjugates to total exposure. The glucuronide conjugate was the predominant form, with levels 10–40-fold greater than those of the sulfate conjugate. The glucuronide:sulfate ratio decreased with increasing exposure concentration and duration in both sexes. In the earlier study by oral administration (National Toxicology Program, 1994), a relative decline in the glucuronide conjugate with increasing concentration of 1-*tert*-butoxypropan-2-ol was also noted. After exposure to 75 and 300 ppm, female rats excreted relatively more of the glucuronide conjugate than males, although this difference was not apparent after 1200 ppm.

As in rats, both the glucuronide and sulfate conjugates were detected in the urine of mice exposed to 1-*tert*-butoxypropan-2-ol, and the glucuronide was the predominant conjugate in both sexes (31–178-fold in males and 8–25-fold in females). The level of sulfate conjugates increased proportionally with exposure concentration in males exposed to 75 and 300 ppm, and more than proportionally after exposure to 1200 ppm; in females, the increase was proportional to exposure at all concentrations. In general, levels of glucuronide conjugate also increased with exposure concentration, but did not change with duration of exposure. Levels of the two conjugates combined increased more than proportionally with exposure concentration, and male mice excreted more than females. Contrary to the results in rats, male mice excreted relatively more of the glucuronide conjugate compared with the sulfate conjugate than female mice (Dill *et al.*, 2004).

The increase in total conjugated metabolites in the urine over time in both species may be indicative of induction of this metabolic pathway with prolonged exposure (Dill *et al.*, 2004). Since metabolites that arise from the alternative potential pathway which involves oxidation (postulated cytochrome P450-mediated *O*-dealkylation that produces *tert*-butanol or acetol) were not measured, it was not possible to assess the potential for induction of this pathway. Induction of metabolism of 1-*tert*-butoxypropan-2-ol is consistent with the increases in relative liver weight observed in male and female rats and mice exposed for 13 weeks; these changes suggested proliferation of cellular organelles, perhaps those involved in xenobiotic metabolism (National Toxicology Program, 2004a).

(*e*)   *Prediction of metabolic pathways by computer modelling*

In view of the lack of empirical data, the Working Group investigated the probability that the oxidation pathway is important in the metabolism of 1-*tert*-butoxypropan-2-ol in mammals. The expert system computer model META (Multicase, 2002) was used to predict the probable metabolic pathways for this substance and the potential relative contribution of each. Based on the model predictions, the principal pathway involves bio-transformation of 1-*tert*-butoxypropan-2-ol via reductases to 3-(1,1-dimethylethoxy)-1-propene, which is subsequently converted by cytochrome P450 epoxidation of the double bond to the epoxide, *tert*-butyl glycidyl ether.[1] Conjugation with glucuronide is predicted to be the second most probable pathway, with lesser amounts of the sulfate conjugate being formed (consistent with the observations *in vivo*). Based on the model, the oxidation pathway described for other propylene glycol ethers represents only a minor pathway. However, other than conjugation with glucuronide and sulfate, these predicted pathways can only be speculative as they have not been investigated *in vivo*. In addition, elimination of a large proportion of the parent compound as expired carbon dioxide, as observed by Dill *et al.* (2004), was not predicted to be a significant removal process.

4.2   Toxic effects

4.2.1   *Humans*

No data were available to the Working Group.

4.2.2   *Experimental systems*

1-*tert*-Butoxypropan-2-ol has low acute toxicity in rats, with an LD_{50} of 3771 mg/kg bw. Target organs following acute oral exposure to 2239–4467 mg/kg bw were the lungs, stomach, liver and kidneys (Boatman, 2001). In the only acute inhalation study identified, no deaths occurred in Sprague-Dawley rats exposed to 2680 mg/m^3 for 4 h. Mild extra-medullary haematopoiesis was observed in the liver of both males and females. Occluded dermal exposure to 2 g/kg bw 1-*tert*-butoxypropan-2-ol did not cause death, clinical signs or effects on body weight in rabbits exposed for 24 h and observed for a subsequent 14 days, although signs of mild irritation were observed at the site of application in a primary skin irritation assay. However, 1-*tert*-butoxypropan-2-ol was severely irritating to the eyes of rabbits administered 0.1 mL of the neat liquid; slight irritation was observed when the substance was applied as a 20% aqueous solution (Boatman, 2001). [The Working Group

---

[1] The epoxide product, *tert*-butyl glycidyl ether, has been demonstrated to be mutagenic in *Salmonella* (Dabney, 1979; Connor *et al.*, 1980; Canter *et al.*, 1986; National Toxicology Program, 2004b) and to induce unscheduled DNA synthesis in cultured human lymphocytes (Frost & Legator, 1982). However, the root epoxide, glycidol, showed clear evidence of carcinogenicity in rats and mice of both sexes (National Toxicology Program, 1990a) and has been classified as a possible human carcinogen (IARC, 2000). In addition, the linear *n*-butyl glycidyl ether and allyl glycidyl ether were both genotoxic in in-vitro and in-vivo assays (Connor *et al.*, 1980; Frost & Legator, 1982; Whorton *et al.*, 1983; Canter *et al.*, 1986; National Toxicology Program, 1990b, 2004c), while, for the latter substance, the National Toxicology Program (1990b) reported that there was equivocal evidence of carcinogenic activity in male rats and female mice, some evidence in male mice and no evidence in female rats.

noted the lack of detail in this secondary account of studies for which the original data are not publicly available.]

Groups of five male and five female Fischer 344/N rats and five male NBR rats were exposed by inhalation to 0, 75, 150, 300, 600 or 1200 ppm [406, 813, 1626, 3252 or 6504 mg/m^3] 1-*tert*-butoxypropan-2-ol for 6 h per day on 5 days per week for 16 days. NBR rats were used in this study in addition to Fischer 344/N rats because they do not produce hepatic α_{2u}-globulin and, therefore, do not develop nephropathy associated with accumulation of this protein. No effects on body weight gain were observed in any exposed group, although relative liver weights were increased in male and female Fischer 344/N and male NBR rats exposed to the highest concentration and also in male Fischer 344/N rats exposed to 600 ppm; no histopathological changes were noted in the liver at any concentration of 1-*tert*-butoxypropan-2-ol. Relative kidney weights were also increased in male Fischer 344/N rats exposed to 600 ppm and above. Mild hyaline droplet accumulation in the kidneys was observed in all male but not in female Fischer 344/N rats or in NBR rats. In addition, increased cell proliferation was noted in the kidney of male Fischer 344/N rats at 1200 ppm (National Toxicology Program, 2004a).

In a concurrent short-term study, groups of five male and five female B6C3F$_1$ mice were exposed by inhalation to 0, 75, 150, 300, 600 or 1200 ppm [406, 813, 1626, 3252 or 6504 mg/m^3] 1-*tert*-butoxypropan-2-ol for 6 h per day on 5 days per week for 17 days. No clinical signs were noted at any exposure concentration. Although absolute and relative liver weights were significantly greater in females exposed to 300 ppm and above and in males exposed to 600 ppm and above compared with controls, no lesions related to exposure were observed in either sex of exposed mice (National Toxicology Program, 2004a).

In a subchronic study, groups of 10 male and 10 female Fischer 344/N rats were exposed by inhalation to 0, 75, 150, 300, 600 or 1200 ppm [406, 813, 1626, 3252 or 6504 mg/m^3] 1-*tert*-butoxypropan-2-ol for about 6 h per day on 5 days per week for 14 weeks. Additional groups of 10 males and 10 females exposed to the same concentrations were examined at 6 weeks for clinical pathology and renal effects, while renal effects were also examined in five additional male rats at 2 weeks. No effects on survival or body weight were observed in any exposed group. Relative kidney weights were increased in males exposed to all concentrations and in females exposed to 300 ppm or more. Signs of nephropathy, characteristic of that associated with the accumulation of α_{2u}-globulin, included concentration-related increases in the severity or incidence of renal tubular hyaline droplet accumulation, cortical regeneration, medullary granular casts, increased α_{2u}-globulin levels (confirmed by quantitation in kidney homogenates), cell proliferation and alterations in parameters of urinalysis (urine volume, glucose and protein concentrations and activities of aspartate aminotransferase, lactate dehydrogenase and *N*-acetyl-β-D-glucosaminidase) in males exposed to all concentrations of 1-*tert*-butoxypropan-2-ol at 12 and/or 14 weeks. The only changes in urinalysis parameters in female rats were increased activities of lactate dehydrogenase in those exposed to 150 ppm and above and of *N*-acetyl-β-D-glucosaminidase in those exposed to 600 ppm and above. Based on the occurrence of renal effects in female rats, although with less severity than those observed in males, the authors speculated that a mechanism other than that related to α_{2u}-globulin may be involved. Significant increases in relative liver weight were noted in males exposed to 150 ppm and above and in females exposed to 1200 ppm, which the authors hypothesized might be an adaptive response to altered liver function as demonstrated by transient increases in total bile acid concentrations that returned to control levels at termination of the study (14 weeks). Activities of alanine aminotransferase were decreased in females exposed to 150 ppm and above at day 23 but not at 14 weeks; this effect was observed in all exposed groups of males and persisted until the end of the study. No consistent effects on haematological parameters were observed that were considered to be related to exposure to 1-*tert*-butoxypropan-2-ol (National Toxicology Program, 2004a).

Male and female Fischer 344/N rats were exposed by inhalation to 28–709 ppm [152–3843 mg/m^3] 1-*tert*-butoxypropan-2-ol for 6 h per day on 5 days per week for up to 13 weeks. Ten animals per exposure group were killed after 4 weeks of exposure, 13 weeks of exposure or 3 weeks after cessation of exposure. No effects on survival, body weight or haematological or clinical chemistry parameters were observed; similarly, no effects on bone marrow, blood or thymus were noted. Although increased weights of liver, kidneys and spleen were observed [concentrations at which these effects were observed were not specified], no histopathological alterations were found in these organs. The no-observed-adverse-effect level was reported to be 709 ppm (Boatman, 2001). [The Working Group noted the lack of detail in this secondary account of studies for which the original data are not publicly available.]

In the only available subchronic study in mice (National Toxicology Program, 2004a), groups of 10 male and 10 female B6C3F$_1$ mice were exposed by inhalation to 0, 75, 150, 300, 600 or 1200 ppm [406, 813, 1626, 3252 or 6504 mg/m^3] 1-*tert*-butoxypropan-2-ol for 6 h per day on 5 days per week for 14 weeks. Body-weight gain in male mice exposed to 150, 300 and 1200 ppm was significantly lower than that in controls. Liver weight was significantly increased in both sexes at 600 and 1200 ppm; this was accompanied by significant increases in the incidence of minimal-to-mild centrilobular hypertrophy (significant in males exposed to the two higher concentrations and in females only after the highest concentration). Minimal squamous metaplasia was noted in the nasal epithelium of male mice exposed to 1200 ppm 1-*tert*-butoxypropan-2-ol and in one female mouse in each of the groups exposed to 75 and 1200 ppm.

In a 2-year bioassay, groups of 50 male and 50 female Fischer 344/N rats were exposed by inhalation to 0, 75, 300 or 1200 ppm [406, 1626 or 6504 mg/m^3] 1-*tert*-butoxypropan-2-ol for 6 h per day on 5 days per week for 104 weeks. The neoplastic effects observed in this study are reported in Section 3. Survival was decreased in males exposed to 300 ppm, but not to the highest concentration. Body weights were decreased in both sexes exposed to 1200 ppm. A concentration-related increase in the incidence of renal tubule hyperplasia was observed in males, which was significant at the two higher concentrations and was considered by the authors to be part of the continuum of progression to renal neoplasm. The severity of age-related nephropathy increased with increasing concentration of 1-*tert*-butoxypropan-2-ol in both male and female rats. The incidence, but not severity, of mild-to-moderate hyaline droplet accumulation also increased with concentration in males and was significant for the two higher concentrations. It was noted that droplet accumulation was observed most frequently in male rats that died or were killed early during the study period. Other effects on the kidney observed in male rats included a significant increase in mineralization of the renal papilla with all concentrations and a significant increase in hyperplasia of the transitional epithelium of the renal pelvis with 1200 ppm. Similar to their speculations in the 14-week study (see above), the authors suggested that the nephropathy noted in female rats was not related to α_{2u}-globulin. In the liver, a significant increase in the incidence of basophilic foci and clear-cell foci was observed in males and females, respectively, exposed to 1200 ppm. Significant concentration-related increases in the incidence and severity of hyaline degeneration of the olfactory epithelium occurred in both sexes of rats, together with significant increases in the incidence of submucosal gland dilatation in males exposed to 300 ppm and 1200 ppm and goblet-cell hyperplasia in males exposed to 1200 ppm; however, the authors considered these effects to be adaptive or protective responses to an irritant substance. Effects on the eye, including corneal opacity and corneal mineralization, were observed in females exposed to 1200 ppm, although the correlation between the two effects was poor (National Toxicology Program, 2004a).

Groups of 50 male and 50 female B6C3F$_1$ mice were exposed by inhalation to 0, 75, 300 or 1200 ppm [406, 1626 or 6504 mg/m^3] 1-*tert*-butoxypropan-2-ol for approximately 6 h per day on 5 days per week for 104 weeks. A discussion of the observed neoplasms is presented in Section 3. Other than a slight decrease in body weight at the end of the study of females exposed to 1200 ppm, mean body weights were similar in exposed and control mice. In the liver, significant increases in the incidences of eosinophilic foci in both sexes exposed to 1200 ppm, in basophilic foci in males exposed to 300 ppm and in mixed-cell foci in males exposed to 1200 ppm were observed, and also an increase in the incidence of mild multinucleated hepatocytes in male mice exposed to the highest concentration. Male mice also had a significant increase in the incidence of forestomach inflammation after exposure to 300 and 1200 ppm (incidences of 2/48, 3/49, 9/50 and 9/50 at 0, 75, 300 and 1200 ppm, respectively) and of forestomach squamous epithelial hyperplasia with 300 ppm (incidences of 2/48, 5/49, 9/50 and 7/50 at 0, 75, 300 and 1200 ppm, respectively). However, the authors considered that these lesions were not related to exposure to 1-*tert*-butoxypropan-2-ol, as the severity of inflammation and hyperplasia was similar to that observed in controls. Similar to observations in the concurrent bioassay in rats (see above), effects on the cornea were observed in female mice exposed to 1200 ppm, and consisted of pale foci that corresponded partially with mild mineralization and, less frequently, inflammation, erosion and squamous hyperplasia.

4.3   Reproductive and developmental effects

4.3.1   *Humans*

No data were available to the Working Group.

4.3.2   *Experimental systems*

No published studies on the potential effects of exposure to 1-*tert*-butoxypropan-2-ol on reproductive function were identified.

In the 14-week inhalation studies conducted by the National Toxicology Program (2004a), groups of 10 male and 10 female Fischer 344/N rats and groups of 10 male and 10 female B6C3F$_1$ mice were exposed to 0, 300, 600 or 1200 ppm [1626, 3252 or 6504 mg/m^3] 1-*tert*-butoxypropan-2-ol. No effects on testes or epididymal weights or on sperm parameters, including sperm count and motility, were observed in either species. Similarly, no histopathological changes in reproductive organs occurred in either rats or mice. An increase in the length of the estrus cycle (mainly due to lengthened diestrus) was observed in female mice exposed to 1200 ppm, a concentration that was also associated with effects on the liver. No effects on the estrus cycle were observed in rats at any concentration.

Information on the developmental toxicity of 1-*tert*-butoxypropan-2-ol in experimental animals is sparse. Groups of 16 pregnant New Zealand white rabbits were exposed to airborne concentrations of 0, 229, 721 or 984 ppm [1241, 3908 or 5333 mg/m^3] 1-*tert*-butoxypropan-2-ol for 6 h per day on days 7–19 of gestation. No effects on behaviour, weight gain or haematological parameters were noted in the exposed dams, and no morphological effects were observed in fetuses at any concentration (Boatman, 2001). Similarly, no fetal toxicity or developmental effects were observed in groups of 25 pregnant CDF rats exposed to 0, 230, 726 or 990 ppm [1247, 3935 or 5366 mg/m^3] 1-*tert*-butoxypropan-2-ol for 6 h per day on days 6–15 of gestation. However, absolute and relative liver weights were significantly increased in dams exposed to the two higher concentrations and half of the dams exposed to 990 ppm were 'pale in appearance' during most of the exposure period (Boatman, 2001). [The Working Group noted the lack of detail, e.g. on maternal toxicity, in this secondary account of studies for which the original data are not publicly available.]

4.4   Genetic and related effects

4.4.1   *Humans*

No data were available to the Working group.

4.4.2   *Experimental systems* (see Table 3 for references and details)

The genotoxicity of 1-*tert*-butoxypropan-2-ol has been examined in a very limited number of assays, all of which were conducted as part of a study by the National Toxicology Program (2004a). The compound did not induce gene mutations in *Salmonella typhimurium* strains TA100, TA1535 or TA98 either in the absence or presence of an exogenous metabolic activation system (postmitochondrial supernatant) from the livers of Aroclor 1254-treated rats and hamsters. However, in strain TA97, 1-*tert*-butoxypropan-2-ol caused a concentration-related increase in mutant frequency in two repeat experiments in the same laboratory by factors of maximally 2.1 and 2.4, respectively, in the absence of

Table 3. Genetic and related effects of 1-*tert*-butoxypropan-2-ol

Test system	Result[a] Without exogenous metabolic system	Result[a] With exogenous metabolic system	Dose[b] (LED/HID)	Reference
Salmonella typhimurium TA100, TA1535, TA98, reverse mutation	–	–[c]	10 000 µg/plate	National Toxicology Program (2004a)
Salmonella typhimurium TA1537, reverse mutation	–	NT	10 000 µg/plate	National Toxicology Program (2004a)
Salmonella typhimurium TA97, reverse mutation	+	–[c]	10 000 µg/plate	National Toxicology Program (2004a)
Salmonella typhimurium TA97, reverse mutation	+	–[c]	1000 µg/plate	National Toxicology Program (2004a)
Sister chromatid exchange, Chinese hamster ovary (CHO) cells *in vitro*	–	–[d]	1667	National Toxicology Program (2004a)
Sister chromatid exchange, Chinese hamster ovary (CHO) cells *in vitro*	NT[e]	–[d]	5000	National Toxicology Program (2004a)
Chromosomal aberrations, Chinese hamster ovary (CHO) cells *in vitro*	–	–[d]	5000	National Toxicology Program (2004a)
Micronucleus formation, female B6C3F₁ mice, normochromatic erythrocytes in peripheral blood *in vivo*	(+)		1200 ppm, inhal. × 3 mo	National Toxicology Program (2004a)
Micronucleus formation, male B6C3F₁ mice, normochromatic erythrocytes in peripheral blood *in vivo*	–		1200 ppm, inhal. × 3 mo	National Toxicology Program (2004)

[a] +, positive; –, negative; (+), weakly positive; NT, not tested
[b] LED, lowest effective dose; HID, highest ineffective dose; in-vitro studies, µg/mL; inhal., inhalation; mo, month
[c] From the livers of both Aroclor 1254-treated male Sprague-Dawley rats and Syrian hamsters
[d] From the livers of Aroclor 1254-treated male Sprague-Dawley rats
[e] Cytostatic effect without exogenous metabolic activation

an exogenous metabolic activation. No mutagenicity was observed in strain TA97 in the presence of metabolic activation. 1-*tert*-Butoxypropan-2-ol was not mutagenic in another strain that is responsive to frameshift mutations (TA1537) in the absence of an exogenous metabolic activation. This strain is generally regarded as being less sensitive to the action of frameshift mutagens than TA97.

Tests for the induction of sister chromatid exchange and structural chromosomal aberrations in Chinese hamster ovary (CHO) cells yielded negative results both in the absence and in the presence of an exogenous metabolic activation system from the livers of Aroclor 1254-treated rats.

The capacity of 1-*tert*-butoxypropan-2-ol to cause genotoxic effects *in vivo* was assessed by a micronucleus assay in male and female B6C3F$_1$ mice that had been exposed by inhalation to 75–1200 ppm [406–6504 mg/m^3] for 3 months. No increase in the frequency of micronucleated normochromatic erythrocytes was observed in males, and a weak increase was obtained in females. This increase showed a statistically significant trend, and the pairwise comparison of treated animals and the corresponding chamber controls yielded a statistically significant difference at the highest exposure concentration. The treatments did not affect the frequency of polychromatic erythrocytes in males or females, which indicated that the exposures had not been cytotoxic to the bone marrow (National Toxicology Program, 2004a).

4.5   Mechanistic considerations

The available data on the genotoxic potential of 1-*tert*-butoxypropan-2-ol are too limited to draw any sound conclusion regarding the role of potential mutagenic effects of the compound in the etiology of the neoplasms observed in animal studies. There is no plausible explanation for the weak but reproducible mutagenicity in *S. typhimurium* strain TA97, and it it is not clear whether there is a mechanistic link between the induction of mutations in this specific strain and tumour formation. According to the criteria of Ashby and Tennant (1991), the compound carries no structural alerts to genotoxicity, and various other glycol ethers (Zeiger *et al.*, 1985, 1992; National Toxicology Program, 2000) (as well as closely related compounds such as *tert*-butylethyl ether (Zeiger *et al.*, 1992)) were consistently non-mutagenic when tested in various *Salmonella* strains, including TA97. The increase in micronucleus formation in female mice exposed to 1-*tert*-butoxypropan-2-ol might appear to be more relevant to a potential link to tumour formation, but this finding should be viewed with caution, because the effect obtained was very weak, it was not observed in exposed males and, due to the design of the study, the assay was not repeated.

In 2-year studies carried out by the National Toxicology Program (2004a) on Fischer 344/N rats, the kidney was a target organ for the toxicity of 1-*tert*-butoxypropan-2-ol, and the results obtained indicate weak tumorigenicity of the compound in the kidneys of male, but not female rats (Doi *et al.*, 2004; National Toxicology Program, 2004a). The renal lesions observed in male rats were characteristic of α_{2u}-globulin-associated nephropathy, which suggests a possible mechanistic link between renal toxicity and renal tumour response. However, neither the binding of 1-*tert*-butoxypropan-2-ol to α_{2u}-globulin nor the formation of *tert*-butanol, a postulated metabolite of 1-*tert*-butoxy-propan-2-ol (Dill *et al.*, 2004) which has been reported to form a complex with α_{2u}-globulin (Williams & Borghoff, 2001) and to cause α_{2u}-globulin accumulation (Borghoff *et al.*, 2001), were investigated in this study. However, although the binding of 1-*tert*-butoxypropan-2-ol to α_{2u}-globulin has not been investigated, a structurally analogous alcohol compound, a metabolite of trimethylpentane, does bind to this protein and thereby induces nephrotoxicity in male Fischer 344 rats (Lock *et al.*, 1987; Short *et al.*, 1989). In a kidney initiation–promotion model, trimethylpentane has been shown to promote atypical cell foci and renal-cell tumours in male, but not female rats (Short *et al.*, 1989). Data from related investigations suggest that the tumour-promoting potential of trimethylpentane results from reversible binding of its metabolite, 2,4,4-trimethyl-2-pentanol, to α_{2u}-globulin, which leads to decreased renal catabolism of this protein, chronic lysosomal overload, cell death and compensatory cell proliferation (Lock *et al.*, 1987; see also Capen *et al.*, 1999). This alcohol bears a structural resemblance to 1-*tert*-butoxypropan-2-ol (see Fig. 2).

In addition to the renal effects in male rats exposed to 1-*tert*-butoxypropan-2-ol, a significant increase in the severity of age-related nephropathy was also observed in female rats exposed to 1200 ppm and, in the 14-week study, significant increases in absolute and relative kidney weights in females exposed to 300 ppm or higher concentrations; alterations in urinary chemistry parameters were also observed in female rats exposed to concentrations of 150 ppm 1-*tert*-butoxypropan-2-ol or higher. Although these changes were not accompanied by histopathological lesions and were less severe than those in male rats, exposure-related mechanisms of renal injury other than accumulation of α_{2u}-globulin cannot be excluded (Doi *et al.*, 2004). The available data meet some but not all IARC criteria for a compound that induces renal toxicity and tumours via a mechanism associated with α_{2u}-globulin accumulation in male rats (Capen *et al.*, 1999).

No mechanistic information related to the occurrence of increased incidences of liver neoplasms in male rats and both male and female mice exposed to 1-*tert*-butoxypropan-2-ol was available (Doi *et al.*, 2004; National Toxicology Program, 2004a).

Figure 2. Chemical structural resemblance of 1-tert-butoxypropan-2-ol and 2,4,4-trimethyl-2-pentanol

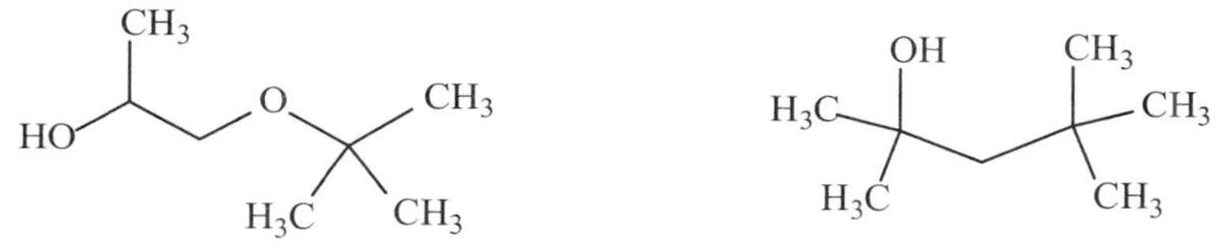

1-*tert*-Butoxypropan-2-ol   2,4,4-Trimethyl-2-pentanol

5.   Summary of Data Reported and Evaluation

5.1   Exposure data

1-*tert*-Butoxypropan-2-ol is a glycol ether that has been increasingly used since the 1980s as a solvent in coatings, glass-cleaning and surface-cleaning products, inks, adhesives and cosmetic products. No data are available on levels of occupational or consumer exposure to 1-*tert*-butoxypropan-2-ol.

5.2   Human carcinogenicity data

No data were available to the Working Group.

5.3   Animal carcinogenicity data

1-*tert*-Butoxypropan-2-ol was tested for carcinogenicity by inhalation in mice and rats. In a single study, a dose-related increase in the combined incidences of liver tumours (hepatocellular adenomas and carcinomas), including hepatoblastomas, was observed in both male and female mice. A significant trend in the increase in malignant tumours was observed in females when hepatocellular carcinomas and hepatoblastomas were combined. In male rats, marginal, non-significant increases in the incidences of renal tubule adenomas (with one carcinoma at the highest dose) and hepatocellular adenomas were observed, but these findings were considered to be equivocal. In female rats, no dose-related increases in tumour incidence were found.

5.4   Other relevant data

No data were available to the Working Group on the kinetics, metabolism, toxic effects, reproductive effects or genetic and related effects of 1-*tert*-butoxypropan-2-ol in humans.

Kinetics and metabolism

1-*tert*-Butoxypropan-2-ol is rapidly absorbed and eliminated in rats and mice. It is eliminated from blood following concentration-dependent non-linear kinetics, with a half-life of approximately 16 and 10 min in rats and mice, respectively. Elimination kinetics were saturable following a single inhalation exposure to 1200 ppm, but saturation was less obvious following repeated exposures. Urinary excretion accounted for 48–67% of an orally administered dose of 1-*tert*-butoxypropan-2-ol; the principal urinary metabolites identified were glucuronide (23–52%) and sulfate (7–13%) conjugates, while expired carbon dioxide accounted for up to 26%. Metabolites resulting from other potential pathways of metabolism have not been investigated experimentally. Biliary excretion of conjugated 1-*tert*-butoxypropan-2-ol may be significant (up to 40% following intravenous administration), although reabsorption may also occur, based on a recovery of only 4–11% of the administered dose in the faeces, which suggests enterohepatic circulation.

Toxic effects

1-*tert*-Butoxypropan-2-ol has low acute toxicity in experimental animals, although it may be irritating to the skin and eyes. Target organs following short-term, subchronic and chronic exposure include the kidneys and liver. Renal effects consistent with α_{2u}-globulin-associated nephropathy, including hyaline droplet accumulation, cell proliferation in the renal cortex and alterations in urinary parameters, were observed in male Fischer 344/N rats following exposure to 1-*tert*-butoxypropan-2-ol, but not in female Fischer 344/N or in male NBR rats, a strain that does not produce α_{2u}-globulin. However, effects on the kidneys were also observed in female Fischer 344/N rats in subchronic and chronic inhalation studies, including increased relative weights, altered urinary parameters and a concentration-related increase in age-related nephropathy, although generally to a lesser degree than that noted in similarly exposed male rats of this strain.

Toxic effects in the liver have also been observed in short-term, subchronic and chronic investigations in both male and female rats and mice, including increased weight and histopathological changes. However, these observations do not elucidate a potential mode of induction of the reported hepatic tumours in mice.

Reproductive and developmental effects

Although there is some evidence for a reproductive effect in female mice exposed to 1-*tert*-butoxypropan-2-ol (altered estrus cycle), this was only observed at concentrations greater than those associated with effects on the liver.

Based on the limited available data, 1-*tert*-butoxypropan-2-ol does not appear to induce developmental toxicity in experimental animals.

Genotoxicity

1-*tert*-Butoxypropan-2-ol, the structure of which does not carry any structural alert to genotoxicity, has been reported to be weakly mutagenic in *Salmonella* strain TA97 and to cause a statistically significant but very weak increase in the frequency of micronuclei in the peripheral blood of female but not male mice. No genotoxicity was observed in assays for the induction of sister chromatid exchange and chromosomal aberrations in the presence or absence of exogenous metabolic activation *in vitro*. In view of the scarcity of the data available, it is not possible to draw any meaningful conclusion regarding the potential genotoxic effects of 1-*tert*-butoxypropan-2-ol in mammalian cells or in mammals *in vivo*.

5.5   Evaluation[1]

There is *inadequate evidence* in humans for the carcinogenicity of 1-*tert*-butoxy-propan-2-ol.

There is *limited evidence* in experimental animals for the carcinogenicity of 1-*tert*-butoxypropan-2-ol.

Overall evaluation

1-*tert*-Butoxypropan-2-ol is *not classifiable as to its carcinogenicity to humans (Group 3)*.

6.   References

Ashby, J. & Tennant, R.W. (1991) Definitive relationships among chemical structure, carcinogenicity and mutagenicity for 301 chemicals tested by the US NTP. *Mutat. Res.*, **257**, 229–306

Begley, R. (1986) Solvent makers eye compliance deadline. *Chem. Mark. Rep.*, **November 3**, 34, 40

Boatman, R.J. (2001) Glycol ethers: Ethers of propylene, butylene glycols, and other glycol derivatives. In: Bingham, E., Cohrssen, B. & Powell, C.H., eds, *Patty's Toxicology*, 5th Ed., Vol. 7, New York, John Wiley & Sons, pp. 271–395

Borghoff, S.J., Prescott, J.S., Janszen, D.B., Wong, B.A. & Everitt, J.I. (2001) α2u-Globulin nephropathy, renal cell proliferation, and dosimetry of inhaled *tert*-butyl alcohol in male and female F-344 rats. *Toxicol. Sci.*, **61**, 176–186

Canter, D.A., Zeiger, E., Haworth, S., Lawlor, T., Mortelmans, K. & Speck, W. (1986) Comparative mutagenicity of aliphatic epoxides in Salmonella. *Mutat. Res.*, **172**, 105–138

Capen, C.C., Dybing, E., Rice, J.M. & Wilbourn, J.D., eds (1999) *Species Differences in Thyroid, Kidney and Urinary Bladder Carcinogenesis* (IARC Scientific Publications No. 147), Lyon, IARC

Chemical Information Services (2004) *Directory of World Chemical Producers*, Dallas, TX [www.chemicalinfo.com]

Chinn, H., Anderson, E. & Yoneyama, M. (2000) *CEH Marketing Research Report: Glycol Ethers*, Palo Alto, CA, SRI International

Connor, T.H., Pullin, T.G., Meyne, J., Frost, A.F. & Legator, M.S. (1980) Evaluation of the mutagenicity of n-BGE and t-BGE in a battery of short-term assays (Abstract No. Ec-12). *Environ. Mutag.*, **2**, 284

[1] After thorough discussion, several members of the Working Group favoured an evaluation of the evidence of carcinogenicity in experimental animals as *sufficient*. This view emphasizes the dose-related induction of hepatoblastomas in male and female mice, because hepatoblastoma is a rare neoplasm with a low spontaneous incidence in mice, especially in females. However, the majority of the Working Group considered the evidence to be *limited* for the reasons discussed in Section 5.3.

Dabney, B.J. (1979) *Mutagenic Evaluation of t-Butyl Glycidyl Ether*, Midland, MI, Dow Chemical Co.

Dill, J.A., Fuciarelli, A.F., Lee, K.M., Mellinger, K.M., Burka, L.T. & Roycroft, J.H. (2004) Toxico-kinetics of propylene glycol mono-*t*-butyl ether following intravenous or inhalation exposure in rats and mice. *Inhal. Toxicol.*, **16**, 1–20

Doi, A.M., Roycroft, J.H., Herbert, R.A., Haseman, J.K., Hailey, J.R., Chou, B.J., Dill, J.A., Grumbein, S.L., Miller, R.A., Renne, R.A. & Bucher, J.R. (2004) Inhalation toxicology and carcinogenesis studies of propylene glycol mono-*t*-butyl ether in rats and mice. *Toxicology*, **199**, 1–22

Frost, A.F. & Legator, M.S. (1982) Unscheduled DNA synthesis induced in human lymphocytes by butyl glycidyl ethers. *Mutat. Res.*, **102**, 193–200

Gupta, V.P. (1987) *Recovery of Propylene Glycol Mono t-Butoxy Ether*. US Patent 4,675,082

IARC (2000) *IARC Monographs on the Evaluation of Carcinogenic Risks to Humans*, Vol. 77, *Some Industrial Chemicals*, Lyon

Knifton, J.F. (1994) *Synthesis of Low Molecular Weight Glycol Ethers from Oxiranes plus Olefins*, US Patent No. 5,349,110

Lock, E.A., Charbonneau, M., Strasser, J., Swenberg, J.A. & Bus, J.S. (1987) 2,2,4-Trimethylpen-tane-induced nephrotoxicity. II. The reversible binding of a TMP metabolite to a renal protein fraction containing α_{2u}-globulin. *Toxicol. appl. Pharmacol.*, **91**, 182–192

Lyondell Chemical Co. (2004) *Technical Data Sheet: ARCOSOLV® PTB (Mono) Propylene Glycol Tertiary Butyl Ether*, Houston, TX

Miller, R.R., Hermann, E.A., Young, J.T., Landry, T.D. & Calhoun, L.L. (1984) Ethylene glycol monomethyl ether and propylene glycol monomethyl ether: Metabolism, disposition, and sub-chronic inhalation toxicity studies. *Environ. Health Perspect.*, **57**, 233–239

Multicase (2002) META Version 1.200. Beechwood, OH

National Library of Medicine (2004) tert-*Butoxypropanol* [http://chem.sis.nlm.gov/chemidplus/chemidlite.jsp] accessed 02/02/2004

National Toxicology Program (1990a) *Toxicology and Carcinogenesis Studies of Glycidol (CAS No. 556-52-5) in F344/N Rats and B6C3F₁ Mice (Gavage Studies)* (NTP TR 374), Research Triangle Park, NC

National Toxicology Program (1990b) *Toxicology and Carcinogenesis Studies of Allyl Glycidyl Ether (CAS No. 106-92-3) in Osborne-Mendel Rats and B6C3F₁ Mice (Inhalation Studies)* (NTP TR 376), Research Triangle Park, NC

National Toxicology Program (1994) *Chemical Disposition in Mammals: The Metabolism and Disposition of Propylene Glycol t-Butyl Ether in the Male Fischer 344 Rat* (Final Report; NIEHS Contract NO1-ES-85320), Research Triangle Park, NC

National Toxicology Program (2000) *NTP Technical Report on the Toxicology and Carcinogenesis Studies of 2-Butoxyethanol (CAS No. 111-76-2) in F344/N Rats and B6C3F₁ Mice (Inhalation Studies)* (Tech. Rep. Ser. No. 484), Research Triangle Park, NC

National Toxicology Program (2004a) *NTP Technical Report on the Toxicology and Carcinogenesis Studies of Propylene Glycol Mono-t-Butyl Ether (CAS No. 57018-52-7) in F344/N Rats and B6C3F₁ Mice and a Toxicology Study of Propylene Glycol Mono-t-Butyl Ether in Male NBR Rats (Inhalation Studies)* (Tech. Rep. Ser. No. 515; NIH Publ. No. 04-4449), Research Triangle Park, NC

National Toxicology Program (2004b) On-line data for *tert*-butyl glycidyl ether [http://ntp-server. nih.gov/htdocs/Results_Status/Resstatb/7665727.html]

National Toxicology Program (2004c) On-line data for N-butyl glycidyl ether [http://ntp-server. nih.gov/htdocs/Results_Status/Resstatb/2426086.html]

Oxygenated Solvents Producers Association (2004) *The Glycol Ethers* [http://www.ethers-de-glycol.org/english/index.html]

Short, B.G., Steinhagen, W.H. & Swenberg, J.A. (1989) Promoting effects of unleaded gasoline and 2,2,4-trimethylpentane on the development of atypical cell foci and renal tubular cell tumors in rats exposed to *N*-ethyl-*N*-hydroxyethylnitrosamine. *Cancer Res.*, **49**, 6369–6378

Staples, C.A. & Davis, J.W. (2002) An examination of the physical properties, fate, ecotoxicity and potential environmental risks for a series of propylene glycol ethers. *Chemosphere*, **49**, 61–73

Whorton, E.B., Jr, Pullin, T.G., Frost, A.F., Onofre, A., Legator, M.S. & Folse, D.S. (1983) Dominant lethal effects of *n*-butyl glycidyl ether in mice. *Mutat. Res.*, **124**, 225–233

Williams, T.M. & Borghoff, S.J. (2001) Characterization of *tert*-butyl alcohol binding to α2u-globulin in F-344 rats. *Toxicol. Sci.*, **62**, 228–235

Zeiger, E., Haworth, S., Mortelmans, K. & Speck, W. (1985) Mutagenicity testing of di(2-ethyl-hexyl)phthalate and related chemicals in *Salmonella*. *Environ. Mutag.*, **7**, 213–232

Zeiger, E., Anderson, B., Haworth, S., Lawlor, T. & Mortelmans, K. (1992) *Salmonella* mutagenicity tests: V. Results from the testing of 311 chemicals. *Environ. mol. Mutag.*, **19** (Suppl. 21), 2–141

SUMMARY OF FINAL EVALUATIONS

Agent	Degree of evidence of carcinogenicity		Overall evaluation of carcinogenicity to humans
	Human	Animal	
Formaldehyde	S	S	1
Glycol ethers			
2-Butoxyethanol	I	L	3
1-*tert*-Butoxypropan-2-ol	I	L	3

S, sufficient evidence of carcinogenicity; L, limited evidence of carcinogenicity; I, inadequate evidence of carcinogenicity; Group 1, carcinogenic to humans; Group 3, cannot be classified as to carcinogenicity to humans. For definitions of criteria for degrees of evidence, see Preamble.

LIST OF ABBREVIATIONS USED IN THIS VOLUME

8-OHdG	8-hydroxydeoxyguanosine
ACGIH	American Conference of Governmental Industrial Chemists
ad-3	adenine-3
ADH	alcohol dehydrogenase
AGT	O^6-alkylguanine–DNA alkyltransferase
AIDS	acquired immunodeficiency syndrome
ALDH	aldehyde dehydrogenase
ATSDR	Agency for Toxic Substances and Disease Registry
AUC	area-under-the-curve
AM	arithmetic mean
AOAC	Association of Official Analytical Chemists
BDO	1,4-butanediol
BL	Burkitt lymphoma
bw	body weight
C	concentration
CAREX	International Information System on Occupational Exposure to Carcinogens
CFD	computational fluid dynamics
CI	confidence interval
C_{max}	maximum blood concentration
COLCHIC	French national occupational exposure data bank
CRCP	cytolethality–regenerative cellular proliferation
CYP	cytochrome P450
d	day
DMBA	7,12-dimethylbenz[a]anthracene
DNA	deoxyribonucleic acid
EBV	Epstein-Barr virus
EXPOLIS	Air Pollution Exposure to Adult Urban Populations in Europe Study
ECETOC	European Chemical Industry, Ecology and Toxicology Centre/ European Centre for Ecotoxicology and Toxicology of Chemicals
FA	Fanconi anaemia
FDH	formaldehyde dehydrogenase
FEV_1	forced expiry volume in 1 sec

FID	flame ionization detection
FTIRS	Fourier transform infrared spectrometry
GAPDH	glyceraldehyde-3-phosphate dehydrogenase
GC	gas chromatography
GM	geometric mean
GSH	glutathione
GST	glutathione *S*-transferase
GSD	geometric standard deviation
HID	highest ineffective dose
HMTA	hexamethylenetetramine
HPLC	high-performance liquid chromatography
I	local irritant
ICD	international code of diseases
IFN	interferon
Ig	immunoglobulin
IL	interleukin
inc.	incident
inhal.	inhalation
INRS	Institut national de Recherche et de Sécurité
instil.	Instillation
K	carcinogenic
K_e	elimination rate constant
K_{eq}	equilibrium constant
K_m	Michaelis-Menten constant
L	substance with ceiling value
LC_{50}	median lethal concentration
LD_{50}	median lethal dose
LDH	lactate dehydrogenase
LOEL	lowest-observable-effect level
LED	lowest effective dose
MAC/MAK	maximum allowable concentration
MDI	4,4′-diphenylmethane diisocyanate
MEL	maximum exposure level
MFR	melamine–formaldehyde resins
MGMT	O^6-methylguanine–DNA transferase
MNNG	*N*-methyl-*N*′-nitro-*N*-nitrosoguanidine
mo	month
MS	mass spectrometry
NA	not applicable
NAD^+	nicotinamide adenine dinucleotide
NCI	National Cancer Institute
ND	not detected

NDEA	*N*-nitrosodiethylamine
NG	not given
NICNAS	National Industrial Chemicals Notification and Assessment Scheme
NIOSH	National Institute for Occupational Safety and Health
NOAEL	no-observed-adverse-effect level
NOEL	no-observed-effect level
NOES	National Occupational Exposure Survey
NR	not reported
NSD	nitrogen selective detection
NSBR	non-specific bronchial hyper-reactivity
NT	not tested
OECD	Organization for Economic Co-operation and Development
OES	occupational exposure limit
OSHA	Occupational Safety and Health Administration
PAR	polyacetal resins
PCMR	proportionate cancer mortality ratio
PCNA	proliferating cell nuclear antigen
PCR	polymerase chain reaction
PE	pentaerythriol
PEL	permissible exposure limit
PFR	phenol–formaldehyde resins
PMR	proportionate mortality rate
po	oral
PTFE	polytetrafluoroethylene
PVC	polyvinyl chloride
REL	recommended exposure limit
RT	reverse transcriptase
SD	standard deviation
SE	standard error
Sen	sensitizer
SEPIA	French product register
Sh	skin sensitizer
SIR	standardized incidence ratio
Sk	skin notation
SMR	standardized mortality ratio
SPICR	standardized proportionate incidence of cancer ratio
SPIR	standardized proportionate incidence ratio
STEL	short-term exposure limit
t	time
TLV	threshold limit value
TMP	trimethylolpropane

TRI	Toxics Release Inventory
TWA	time-weighted average
UFFI	urea–formaldehyde foam insulation
UFR	urea–formaldehyde resins
UV	ultraviolet
V_{max}	maximum elimination rate
wk	wk
wt	weight
XP	xeroderma pigmentosum
y	year

CUMULATIVE CROSS INDEX TO *IARC MONOGRAPHS ON THE EVALUATION OF CARCINOGENIC RISKS TO HUMANS*

The volume, page and year of publication are given. References to corrigenda are given in parentheses.

A

A-α-C	*40*, 245 (1986); *Suppl. 7*, 56 (1987)
Acetaldehyde	*36*, 101 (1985) (*corr. 42*, 263); *Suppl. 7*, 77 (1987); *71*, 319 (1999)
Acetaldehyde formylmethylhydrazone (*see* Gyromitrin)	
Acetamide	*7*, 197 (1974); *Suppl. 7*, 56, 389 (1987); *71*, 1211 (1999)
Acetaminophen (*see* Paracetamol)	
Aciclovir	*76*, 47 (2000)
Acid mists (*see* Sulfuric acid and other strong inorganic acids, occupational exposures to mists and vapours from)	
Acridine orange	*16*, 145 (1978); *Suppl. 7*, 56 (1987)
Acriflavinium chloride	*13*, 31 (1977); *Suppl. 7*, 56 (1987)
Acrolein	*19*, 479 (1979); *36*, 133 (1985); *Suppl. 7*, 78 (1987); *63*, 337 (1995) (*corr. 65*, 549)
Acrylamide	*39*, 41 (1986); *Suppl. 7*, 56 (1987); *60*, 389 (1994)
Acrylic acid	*19*, 47 (1979); *Suppl. 7*, 56 (1987); *71*, 1223 (1999)
Acrylic fibres	*19*, 86 (1979); *Suppl. 7*, 56 (1987)
Acrylonitrile	*19*, 73 (1979); *Suppl. 7*, 79 (1987); *71*, 43 (1999)
Acrylonitrile-butadiene-styrene copolymers	*19*, 91 (1979); *Suppl. 7*, 56 (1987)
Actinolite (*see* Asbestos)	
Actinomycin D (*see also* Actinomycins)	*Suppl. 7*, 80 (1987)
Actinomycins	*10*, 29 (1976) (*corr. 42*, 255)
Adriamycin	*10*, 43 (1976); *Suppl. 7*, 82 (1987)
AF-2	*31*, 47 (1983); *Suppl. 7*, 56 (1987)
Aflatoxins	*1*, 145 (1972) (*corr. 42*, 251); *10*, 51 (1976); *Suppl. 7*, 83 (1987); *56*, 245 (1993); *82*, 171 (2002)
Aflatoxin B₁ (*see* Aflatoxins)	
Aflatoxin B₂ (*see* Aflatoxins)	
Aflatoxin G₁ (*see* Aflatoxins)	
Aflatoxin G₂ (*see* Aflatoxins)	
Aflatoxin M₁ (*see* Aflatoxins)	
Agaritine	*31*, 63 (1983); *Suppl. 7*, 56 (1987)
Alcohol drinking	*44* (1988)
Aldicarb	*53*, 93 (1991)

Aldrin   *5*, 25 (1974); *Suppl. 7*, 88 (1987)
Allyl chloride   *36*, 39 (1985); *Suppl. 7*, 56 (1987);
                                                                          71, 1231 (1999)
Allyl isothiocyanate   *36*, 55 (1985); *Suppl. 7*, 56 (1987);
                                                                          73, 37 (1999)
Allyl isovalerate   *36*, 69 (1985); *Suppl. 7*, 56 (1987);
                                                                          71, 1241 (1999)
Aluminium production   *34*, 37 (1984); *Suppl. 7*, 89 (1987)
Amaranth   *8*, 41 (1975); *Suppl. 7*, 56 (1987)
5-Aminoacenaphthene   *16*, 243 (1978); *Suppl. 7*, 56 (1987)
2-Aminoanthraquinone   *27*, 191 (1982); *Suppl. 7*, 56 (1987)
para-Aminoazobenzene   *8*, 53 (1975); *Suppl. 7*, 56, 390
                                                                          (1987)
ortho-Aminoazotoluene   *8*, 61 (1975) (*corr. 42*, 254);
                                                                          Suppl. 7, 56 (1987)
para-Aminobenzoic acid   *16*, 249 (1978); *Suppl. 7*, 56 (1987)
4-Aminobiphenyl   *1*, 74 (1972) (*corr. 42*, 251);
                                                                          Suppl. 7, 91 (1987)
2-Amino-3,4-dimethylimidazo[4,5-*f*]quinoline (*see* MeIQ)
2-Amino-3,8-dimethylimidazo[4,5-*f*]quinoxaline (*see* MeIQx)
3-Amino-1,4-dimethyl-5*H*-pyrido[4,3-*b*]indole (*see* Trp-P-1)
2-Aminodipyrido[1,2-*a*:3′,2′-*d*]imidazole (*see* Glu-P-2)
1-Amino-2-methylanthraquinone   *27*, 199 (1982); *Suppl. 7*, 57 (1987)
2-Amino-3-methylimidazo[4,5-*f*]quinoline (*see* IQ)
2-Amino-6-methyldipyrido[1,2-*a*:3′,2′-*d*]imidazole (*see* Glu-P-1)
2-Amino-1-methyl-6-phenylimidazo[4,5-*b*]pyridine (*see* PhIP)
2-Amino-3-methyl-9*H*-pyrido[2,3-*b*]indole (*see* MeA-α-C)
3-Amino-1-methyl-5*H*-pyrido[4,3-*b*]indole (*see* Trp-P-2)
2-Amino-5-(5-nitro-2-furyl)-1,3,4-thiadiazole   *7*, 143 (1974); *Suppl. 7*, 57 (1987)
2-Amino-4-nitrophenol   *57*, 167 (1993)
2-Amino-5-nitrophenol   *57*, 177 (1993)
4-Amino-2-nitrophenol   *16*, 43 (1978); *Suppl. 7*, 57 (1987)
2-Amino-5-nitrothiazole   *31*, 71 (1983); *Suppl. 7*, 57 (1987)
2-Amino-9*H*-pyrido[2,3-*b*]indole (*see* A-α-C)
11-Aminoundecanoic acid   *39*, 239 (1986); *Suppl. 7*, 57 (1987)
Amitrole   *7*, 31 (1974); *41*, 293 (1986) (*corr.*
                                                                          52, 513; *Suppl. 7*, 92 (1987);
                                                                          79, 381 (2001)
Ammonium potassium selenide (*see* Selenium and selenium compounds)
Amorphous silica (*see also* Silica)   *42*, 39 (1987); *Suppl. 7*, 341 (1987);
                                                                          68, 41 (1997) (*corr. 81*, 383)
Amosite (*see* Asbestos)
Ampicillin   *50*, 153 (1990)
Amsacrine   *76*, 317 (2000)
Anabolic steroids (*see* Androgenic (anabolic) steroids)
Anaesthetics, volatile   *11*, 285 (1976); *Suppl. 7*, 93 (1987)
Analgesic mixtures containing phenacetin (*see also* Phenacetin)   *Suppl. 7*, 310 (1987)
Androgenic (anabolic) steroids   *Suppl. 7*, 96 (1987)
Angelicin and some synthetic derivatives (*see also* Angelicins)   *40*, 291 (1986)
Angelicin plus ultraviolet radiation (*see also* Angelicin and some   *Suppl. 7*, 57 (1987)
   synthetic derivatives)
Angelicins   *Suppl. 7*, 57 (1987)
Aniline   *4*, 27 (1974) (*corr. 42*, 252);
                                                                          27, 39 (1982); *Suppl. 7*, 99 (1987)

B

Benz[c]acridine	3, 241 (1973); 32, 129 (1983); Suppl. 7, 58 (1987)
Benzal chloride (see also α-Chlorinated toluenes and benzoyl chloride)	29, 65 (1982); Suppl. 7, 148 (1987); 71, 453 (1999)
Benz[a]anthracene	3, 45 (1973); 32, 135 (1983); Suppl. 7, 58 (1987)
Benzene	7, 203 (1974) (corr. 42, 254); 29, 93, 391 (1982); Suppl. 7, 120 (1987)
Benzidine	1, 80 (1972); 29, 149, 391 (1982); Suppl. 7, 123 (1987)
Benzidine-based dyes	Suppl. 7, 125 (1987)
Benzo[b]fluoranthene	3, 69 (1973); 32, 147 (1983); Suppl. 7, 58 (1987)
Benzo[j]fluoranthene	3, 82 (1973); 32, 155 (1983); Suppl. 7, 58 (1987)
Benzo[k]fluoranthene	32, 163 (1983); Suppl. 7, 58 (1987)
Benzo[ghi]fluoranthene	32, 171 (1983); Suppl. 7, 58 (1987)
Benzo[a]fluorene	32, 177 (1983); Suppl. 7, 58 (1987)
Benzo[b]fluorene	32, 183 (1983); Suppl. 7, 58 (1987)
Benzo[c]fluorene	32, 189 (1983); Suppl. 7, 58 (1987)
Benzofuran	63, 431 (1995)
Benzo[ghi]perylene	32, 195 (1983); Suppl. 7, 58 (1987)
Benzo[c]phenanthrene	32, 205 (1983); Suppl. 7, 58 (1987)
Benzo[a]pyrene	3, 91 (1973); 32, 211 (1983) (corr. 68, 477); Suppl. 7, 58 (1987)
Benzo[e]pyrene	3, 137 (1973); 32, 225 (1983); Suppl. 7, 58 (1987)
1,4-Benzoquinone (see para-Quinone)	
1,4-Benzoquinone dioxime	29, 185 (1982); Suppl. 7, 58 (1987); 71, 1251 (1999)
Benzotrichloride (see also α-Chlorinated toluenes and benzoyl chloride)	29, 73 (1982); Suppl. 7, 148 (1987); 71, 453 (1999)
Benzoyl chloride (see also α-Chlorinated toluenes and benzoyl chloride)	29, 83 (1982) (corr. 42, 261); Suppl. 7, 126 (1987); 71, 453 (1999)
Benzoyl peroxide	36, 267 (1985); Suppl. 7, 58 (1987); 71, 345 (1999)
Benzyl acetate	40, 109 (1986); Suppl. 7, 58 (1987); 71, 1255 (1999)
Benzyl chloride (see also α-Chlorinated toluenes and benzoyl chloride)	11, 217 (1976) (corr. 42, 256); 29, 49 (1982); Suppl. 7, 148 (1987); 71, 453 (1999)
Benzyl violet 4B	16, 153 (1978); Suppl. 7, 58 (1987)
Bertrandite (see Beryllium and beryllium compounds)	
Beryllium and beryllium compounds	1, 17 (1972); 23, 143 (1980) (corr. 42, 260); Suppl. 7, 127 (1987); 58, 41 (1993)
Beryllium acetate (see Beryllium and beryllium compounds)	
Beryllium acetate, basic (see Beryllium and beryllium compounds)	
Beryllium-aluminium alloy (see Beryllium and beryllium compounds)	
Beryllium carbonate (see Beryllium and beryllium compounds)	
Beryllium chloride (see Beryllium and beryllium compounds)	
Beryllium-copper alloy (see Beryllium and beryllium compounds)	
Beryllium-copper-cobalt alloy (see Beryllium and beryllium compounds)	

Butylated hydroxytoluene	*40*, 161 (1986); *Suppl. 7*, 59 (1987)
Butyl benzyl phthalate	*29*, 193 (1982) (*corr. 42*, 261);
	Suppl. 7, 59 (1987); *73*, 115 (1999)
β-Butyrolactone	*11*, 225 (1976); *Suppl. 7*, 59
	(1987); *71*, 1317 (1999)
γ-Butyrolactone	*11*, 231 (1976); *Suppl. 7*, 59
	(1987); *71*, 367 (1999)

C

Cabinet-making (*see* Furniture and cabinet-making)	
Cadmium acetate (*see* Cadmium and cadmium compounds)	
Cadmium and cadmium compounds	*2*, 74 (1973); *11*, 39 (1976)
	(*corr. 42*, 255); *Suppl. 7*, 139
	(1987); *58*, 119 (1993)
Cadmium chloride (*see* Cadmium and cadmium compounds)	
Cadmium oxide (*see* Cadmium and cadmium compounds)	
Cadmium sulfate (*see* Cadmium and cadmium compounds)	
Cadmium sulfide (*see* Cadmium and cadmium compounds)	
Caffeic acid	*56*, 115 (1993)
Caffeine	*51*, 291 (1991)
Calcium arsenate (*see* Arsenic in drinking-water)	
Calcium chromate (*see* Chromium and chromium compounds)	
Calcium cyclamate (*see* Cyclamates)	
Calcium saccharin (*see* Saccharin)	
Cantharidin	*10*, 79 (1976); *Suppl. 7*, 59 (1987)
Caprolactam	*19*, 115 (1979) (*corr. 42*, 258);
	39, 247 (1986) (*corr. 42*, 264);
	Suppl. 7, 59, 390 (1987); *71*, 383
	(1999)
Captafol	*53*, 353 (1991)
Captan	*30*, 295 (1983); *Suppl. 7*, 59 (1987)
Carbaryl	*12*, 37 (1976); *Suppl. 7*, 59 (1987)
Carbazole	*32*, 239 (1983); *Suppl. 7*, 59
	(1987); *71*, 1319 (1999)
3-Carbethoxypsoralen	*40*, 317 (1986); *Suppl. 7*, 59 (1987)
Carbon black	*3*, 22 (1973); *33*, 35 (1984);
	Suppl. 7, 142 (1987); *65*, 149
	(1996)
Carbon tetrachloride	*1*, 53 (1972); *20*, 371 (1979);
	Suppl. 7, 143 (1987); *71*, 401
	(1999)
Carmoisine	*8*, 83 (1975); *Suppl. 7*, 59 (1987)
Carpentry and joinery	*25*, 139 (1981); *Suppl. 7*, 378
	(1987)
Carrageenan	*10*, 181 (1976) (*corr. 42*, 255); *31*,
	79 (1983); *Suppl. 7*, 59 (1987)
Cassia occidentalis (*see* Traditional herbal medicines)	
Catechol	*15*, 155 (1977); *Suppl. 7*, 59
	(1987); *71*, 433 (1999)
CCNU (*see* 1-(2-Chloroethyl)-3-cyclohexyl-1-nitrosourea)	
Ceramic fibres (*see* Man-made vitreous fibres)	

Chlorophenols (occupational exposures to)	*41*, 319 (1986)
Chlorophenoxy herbicides	*Suppl. 7*, 156 (1987)
Chlorophenoxy herbicides (occupational exposures to)	*41*, 357 (1986)
4-Chloro-*ortho*-phenylenediamine	*27*, 81 (1982); *Suppl. 7*, 60 (1987)
4-Chloro-*meta*-phenylenediamine	*27*, 82 (1982); *Suppl. 7*, 60 (1987)
Chloroprene	*19*, 131 (1979); *Suppl. 7*, 160 (1987); *71*, 227 (1999)
Chloropropham	*12*, 55 (1976); *Suppl. 7*, 60 (1987)
Chloroquine	*13*, 47 (1977); *Suppl. 7*, 60 (1987)
Chlorothalonil	*30*, 319 (1983); *Suppl. 7*, 60 (1987); *73*, 183 (1999)
para-Chloro-*ortho*-toluidine and its strong acid salts (*see also* Chlordimeform)	*16*, 277 (1978); *30*, 65 (1983); *Suppl. 7*, 60 (1987); *48*, 123 (1990); *77*, 323 (2000)
4-Chloro-*ortho*-toluidine (see *para*-chloro-*ortho*-toluidine)	
5-Chloro-*ortho*-toluidine	*77*, 341 (2000)
Chlorotrianisene (*see also* Nonsteroidal oestrogens)	*21*, 139 (1979); *Suppl. 7*, 280 (1987)
2-Chloro-1,1,1-trifluoroethane	*41*, 253 (1986); *Suppl. 7*, 60 (1987); *71*, 1355 (1999)
Chlorozotocin	*50*, 65 (1990)
Cholesterol	*10*, 99 (1976); *31*, 95 (1983); *Suppl. 7*, 161 (1987)
Chromic acetate (*see* Chromium and chromium compounds)	
Chromic chloride (*see* Chromium and chromium compounds)	
Chromic oxide (*see* Chromium and chromium compounds)	
Chromic phosphate (*see* Chromium and chromium compounds)	
Chromite ore (*see* Chromium and chromium compounds)	
Chromium and chromium compounds (*see also* Implants, surgical)	*2*, 100 (1973); *23*, 205 (1980); *Suppl. 7*, 165 (1987); *49*, 49 (1990) (*corr. 51*, 483)
Chromium carbonyl (*see* Chromium and chromium compounds)	
Chromium potassium sulfate (*see* Chromium and chromium compounds)	
Chromium sulfate (*see* Chromium and chromium compounds)	
Chromium trioxide (*see* Chromium and chromium compounds)	
Chrysazin (*see* Dantron)	
Chrysene	*3*, 159 (1973); *32*, 247 (1983); *Suppl. 7*, 60 (1987)
Chrysoidine	*8*, 91 (1975); *Suppl. 7*, 169 (1987)
Chrysotile (*see* Asbestos)	
CI Acid Orange 3	*57*, 121 (1993)
CI Acid Red 114	*57*, 247 (1993)
CI Basic Red 9 (*see also* Magenta)	*57*, 215 (1993)
Ciclosporin	*50*, 77 (1990)
CI Direct Blue 15	*57*, 235 (1993)
CI Disperse Yellow 3 (see Disperse Yellow 3)	
Cimetidine	*50*, 235 (1990)
Cinnamyl anthranilate	*16*, 287 (1978); *31*, 133 (1983); *Suppl. 7*, 60 (1987); *77*, 177 (2000)
CI Pigment Red 3	*57*, 259 (1993)
CI Pigment Red 53:1 (*see* D&C Red No. 9)	
Cisplatin (*see also* Etoposide)	*26*, 151 (1981); *Suppl. 7*, 170 (1987)
Citrinin	*40*, 67 (1986); *Suppl. 7*, 60 (1987)

Cyclamic acid (*see* Cyclamates)
Cyclochlorotine
Cyclohexanone
Cyclohexylamine (*see* Cyclamates)
Cyclopenta[*cd*]pyrene
Cyclopropane (*see* Anaesthetics, volatile)
Cyclophosphamide

Cyproterone acetate

10, 139 (1976); *Suppl. 7*, 61 (1987)
47, 157 (1989); *71*, 1359 (1999)

32, 269 (1983); *Suppl. 7*, 61 (1987)

9, 135 (1975); *26*, 165 (1981);
Suppl. 7, 182 (1987)
72, 49 (1999)

D

2,4-D (*see also* Chlorophenoxy herbicides; Chlorophenoxy
  herbicides, occupational exposures to)
Dacarbazine

Dantron
D&C Red No. 9

Dapsone
Daunomycin
DDD (*see* DDT)
DDE (*see* DDT)
DDT

Decabromodiphenyl oxide
Deltamethrin
Deoxynivalenol (*see* Toxins derived from *Fusarium graminearum*,
  F. culmorum and *F. crookwellense*)
Diacetylaminoazotoluene
N,N-Diacetylbenzidine
Diallate

2,4-Diaminoanisole and its salts

4,4'-Diaminodiphenyl ether

1,2-Diamino-4-nitrobenzene
1,4-Diamino-2-nitrobenzene

2,6-Diamino-3-(phenylazo)pyridine (*see* Phenazopyridine hydrochloride)
2,4-Diaminotoluene (*see also* Toluene diisocyanates)
2,5-Diaminotoluene (*see also* Toluene diisocyanates)
ortho-Dianisidine (*see* 3,3'-Dimethoxybenzidine)
Diatomaceous earth, uncalcined (*see* Amorphous silica)
Diazepam

Diazomethane
Dibenz[*a,h*]acridine

Dibenz[*a,j*]acridine

15, 111 (1977)

26, 203 (1981); *Suppl. 7*, 184
(1987)
50, 265 (1990) (*corr. 59*, 257)
8, 107 (1975); *Suppl. 7*, 61 (1987);
57, 203 (1993)
24, 59 (1980); *Suppl. 7*, 185 (1987)
10, 145 (1976); *Suppl. 7*, 61 (1987)

5, 83 (1974) (*corr. 42*, 253);
Suppl. 7, 186 (1987); *53*, 179
(1991)
48, 73 (1990); *71*, 1365 (1999)
53, 251 (1991)

8, 113 (1975); *Suppl. 7*, 61 (1987)
16, 293 (1978); *Suppl. 7*, 61 (1987)
12, 69 (1976); *30*, 235 (1983);
Suppl. 7, 61 (1987)
16, 51 (1978); *27*, 103 (1982);
Suppl. 7, 61 (1987); *79*, 619 (2001)
16, 301 (1978); *29*, 203 (1982);
Suppl. 7, 61 (1987)
16, 63 (1978); *Suppl. 7*, 61 (1987)
16, 73 (1978); *Suppl. 7*, 61 (1987);
57, 185 (1993)

16, 83 (1978); *Suppl. 7*, 61 (1987)
16, 97 (1978); *Suppl. 7*, 61 (1987)

13, 57 (1977); *Suppl. 7*, 189
(1987); *66*, 37 (1996)
7, 223 (1974); *Suppl. 7*, 61 (1987)
3, 247 (1973); *32*, 277 (1983);
Suppl. 7, 61 (1987)
3, 254 (1973); *32*, 283 (1983);
Suppl. 7, 61 (1987)

Dichlorvos	*20*, 97 (1979); *Suppl. 7*, 62 (1987); *53*, 267 (1991)
Dicofol	*30*, 87 (1983); *Suppl. 7*, 62 (1987)
Dicyclohexylamine (*see* Cyclamates)	
Didanosine	*76*, 153 (2000)
Dieldrin	*5*, 125 (1974); *Suppl. 7*, 196 (1987)
Dienoestrol (*see also* Nonsteroidal oestrogens)	*21*, 161 (1979); *Suppl. 7*, 278 (1987)
Diepoxybutane (*see also* 1,3-Butadiene)	*11*, 115 (1976) (*corr. 42*, 255); *Suppl. 7*, 62 (1987); *71*, 109 (1999)
Diesel and gasoline engine exhausts	*46*, 41 (1989)
Diesel fuels	*45*, 219 (1989) (*corr. 47*, 505)
Diethanolamine	*77*, 349 (2000)
Diethyl ether (*see* Anaesthetics, volatile)	
Di(2-ethylhexyl) adipate	*29*, 257 (1982); *Suppl. 7*, 62 (1987); *77*, 149 (2000)
Di(2-ethylhexyl) phthalate	*29*, 269 (1982) (*corr. 42*, 261); *Suppl. 7*, 62 (1987); *77*, 41 (2000)
1,2-Diethylhydrazine	*4*, 153 (1974); *Suppl. 7*, 62 (1987); *71*, 1401 (1999)
Diethylstilboestrol	*6*, 55 (1974); *21*, 173 (1979) (*corr. 42*, 259); *Suppl. 7*, 273 (1987)
Diethylstilboestrol dipropionate (*see* Diethylstilboestrol)	
Diethyl sulfate	*4*, 277 (1974); *Suppl. 7*, 198 (1987); *54*, 213 (1992); *71*, 1405 (1999)
N,N'-Diethylthiourea	*79*, 649 (2001)
Diglycidyl resorcinol ether	*11*, 125 (1976); *36*, 181 (1985); *Suppl. 7*, 62 (1987); *71*, 1417 (1999)
Dihydrosafrole	*1*, 170 (1972); *10*, 233 (1976) *Suppl. 7*, 62 (1987)
1,8-Dihydroxyanthraquinone (*see* Dantron)	
Dihydroxybenzenes (*see* Catechol; Hydroquinone; Resorcinol)	
1,3-Dihydroxy-2-hydroxymethylanthraquinone	*82*, 129 (2002)
Dihydroxymethylfuratrizine	*24*, 77 (1980); *Suppl. 7*, 62 (1987)
Diisopropyl sulfate	*54*, 229 (1992); *71*, 1421 (1999)
Dimethisterone (*see also* Progestins; Sequential oral contraceptives)	*6*, 167 (1974); *21*, 377 (1979))
Dimethoxane	*15*, 177 (1977); *Suppl. 7*, 62 (1987)
3,3'-Dimethoxybenzidine	*4*, 41 (1974); *Suppl. 7*, 198 (1987)
3,3'-Dimethoxybenzidine-4,4'-diisocyanate	*39*, 279 (1986); *Suppl. 7*, 62 (1987)
para-Dimethylaminoazobenzene	*8*, 125 (1975); *Suppl. 7*, 62 (1987)
para-Dimethylaminoazobenzenediazo sodium sulfonate	*8*, 147 (1975); *Suppl. 7*, 62 (1987)
trans-2-[(Dimethylamino)methylimino]-5-[2-(5-nitro-2-furyl)-vinyl]-1,3,4-oxadiazole	*7*, 147 (1974) (*corr. 42*, 253); *Suppl. 7*, 62 (1987)
4,4'-Dimethylangelicin plus ultraviolet radiation (*see also* Angelicin and some synthetic derivatives)	*Suppl. 7*, 57 (1987)
4,5'-Dimethylangelicin plus ultraviolet radiation (*see also* Angelicin and some synthetic derivatives)	*Suppl. 7*, 57 (1987)
2,6-Dimethylaniline	*57*, 323 (1993)
N,N-Dimethylaniline	*57*, 337 (1993)
Dimethylarsinic acid (*see* Arsenic and arsenic compounds)	
3,3'-Dimethylbenzidine	*1*, 87 (1972); *Suppl. 7*, 62 (1987)

E

Epstein-Barr virus	*70*, 47 (1997)
d-Equilenin	*72*, 399 (1999)
Equilin	*72*, 399 (1999)
Erionite	*42*, 225 (1987); *Suppl. 7*, 203 (1987)
Estazolam	*66*, 105 (1996)
Ethinyloestradiol	*6*, 77 (1974); *21*, 233 (1979); *Suppl. 7*, 286 (1987); *72*, 49 (1999)
Ethionamide	*13*, 83 (1977); *Suppl. 7*, 63 (1987)
Ethyl acrylate	*19*, 57 (1979); *39*, 81 (1986); *Suppl. 7*, 63 (1987); *71*, 1447 (1999)
Ethylbenzene	*77*, 227 (2000)
Ethylene	*19*, 157 (1979); *Suppl. 7*, 63 (1987); *60*, 45 (1994); *71*, 1447 (1999)
Ethylene dibromide	*15*, 195 (1977); *Suppl. 7*, 204 (1987); *71*, 641 (1999)
Ethylene oxide	*11*, 157 (1976); *36*, 189 (1985) (*corr. 42*, 263); *Suppl. 7*, 205 (1987); *60*, 73 (1994)
Ethylene sulfide	*11*, 257 (1976); *Suppl. 7*, 63 (1987)
Ethylenethiourea	*7*, 45 (1974); *Suppl. 7*, 207 (1987); *79*, 659 (2001)
2-Ethylhexyl acrylate	*60*, 475 (1994)
Ethyl methanesulfonate	*7*, 245 (1974); *Suppl. 7*, 63 (1987)
N-Ethyl-*N*-nitrosourea	*1*, 135 (1972); *17*, 191 (1978); *Suppl. 7*, 63 (1987)
Ethyl selenac (*see also* Selenium and selenium compounds)	*12*, 107 (1976); *Suppl. 7*, 63 (1987)
Ethyl tellurac	*12*, 115 (1976); *Suppl. 7*, 63 (1987)
Ethynodiol diacetate	*6*, 173 (1974); *21*, 387 (1979); *Suppl. 7*, 292 (1987); *72*, 49 (1999)
Etoposide	*76*, 177 (2000)
Eugenol	*36*, 75 (1985); *Suppl. 7*, 63 (1987)
Evans blue	*8*, 151 (1975); *Suppl. 7*, 63 (1987)
Extremely low-frequency electric fields	*80* (2002)
Extremely low-frequency magnetic fields	*80* (2002)

F

Fast Green FCF	*16*, 187 (1978); *Suppl. 7*, 63 (1987)
Fenvalerate	*53*, 309 (1991)
Ferbam	*12*, 121 (1976) (*corr. 42*, 256); *Suppl. 7*, 63 (1987)
Ferric oxide	*1*, 29 (1972); *Suppl. 7*, 216 (1987)
Ferrochromium (*see* Chromium and chromium compounds)	
Fluometuron	*30*, 245 (1983); *Suppl. 7*, 63 (1987)
Fluoranthene	*32*, 355 (1983); *Suppl. 7*, 63 (1987)
Fluorene	*32*, 365 (1983); *Suppl. 7*, 63 (1987)
Fluorescent lighting (exposure to) (*see* Ultraviolet radiation)	
Fluorides (inorganic, used in drinking-water)	*27*, 237 (1982); *Suppl. 7*, 208 (1987)

Gyromitrin	*31*, 163 (1983); *Suppl. 7*, 64, 391 (1987)

H

Haematite	*1*, 29 (1972); *Suppl. 7*, 216 (1987)
Haematite and ferric oxide	*Suppl. 7*, 216 (1987)
Haematite mining, underground, with exposure to radon	*1*, 29 (1972); *Suppl. 7*, 216 (1987)
Hairdressers and barbers (occupational exposure as)	*57*, 43 (1993)
Hair dyes, epidemiology of	*16*, 29 (1978); *27*, 307 (1982);
Halogenated acetonitriles	*52*, 269 (1991); *71*, 1325, 1369, 1375, 1533 (1999)
Halothane (*see* Anaesthetics, volatile)	
HC Blue No. 1	*57*, 129 (1993)
HC Blue No. 2	*57*, 143 (1993)
α-HCH (*see* Hexachlorocyclohexanes)	
β-HCH (*see* Hexachlorocyclohexanes)	
γ-HCH (*see* Hexachlorocyclohexanes)	
HC Red No. 3	*57*, 153 (1993)
HC Yellow No. 4	*57*, 159 (1993)
Heating oils (*see* Fuel oils)	
Helicobacter pylori (infection with)	*61*, 177 (1994)
Hepatitis B virus	*59*, 45 (1994)
Hepatitis C virus	*59*, 165 (1994)
Hepatitis D virus	*59*, 223 (1994)
Heptachlor (*see also* Chlordane/Heptachlor)	*5*, 173 (1974); *20*, 129 (1979)
Hexachlorobenzene	*20*, 155 (1979); *Suppl. 7*, 219 (1987); *79*, 493 (2001)
Hexachlorobutadiene	*20*, 179 (1979); *Suppl. 7*, 64 (1987); *73*, 277 (1999)
Hexachlorocyclohexanes	*5*, 47 (1974); *20*, 195 (1979) (*corr. 42*, 258); *Suppl. 7*, 220 (1987)
Hexachlorocyclohexane, technical-grade (*see* Hexachlorocyclohexanes)	
Hexachloroethane	*20*, 467 (1979); *Suppl. 7*, 64 (1987); *73*, 295 (1999)
Hexachlorophene	*20*, 241 (1979); *Suppl. 7*, 64 (1987)
Hexamethylphosphoramide	*15*, 211 (1977); *Suppl. 7*, 64 (1987); *71*, 1465 (1999)
Hexoestrol (*see also* Nonsteroidal oestrogens)	*Suppl. 7*, 279 (1987)
Hormonal contraceptives, progestogens only	*72*, 339 (1999)
Human herpesvirus 8	*70*, 375 (1997)
Human immunodeficiency viruses	*67*, 31 (1996)
Human papillomaviruses	*64* (1995) (*corr. 66*, 485)
Human T-cell lymphotropic viruses	*67*, 261 (1996)
Hycanthone mesylate	*13*, 91 (1977); *Suppl. 7*, 64 (1987)
Hydralazine	*24*, 85 (1980); *Suppl. 7*, 222 (1987)
Hydrazine	*4*, 127 (1974); *Suppl. 7*, 223 (1987); *71*, 991 (1999)
Hydrochloric acid	*54*, 189 (1992)
Hydrochlorothiazide	*50*, 293 (1990)
Hydrogen peroxide	*36*, 285 (1985); *Suppl. 7*, 64 (1987); *71*, 671 (1999)

Jet fuel   *45*, 203 (1989)
Joinery (*see* Carpentry and joinery)

K

Kaempferol   *31*, 171 (1983); *Suppl. 7*, 65 (1987)
Kaposi's sarcoma herpesvirus   *70*, 375 (1997)
Kepone (*see* Chlordecone)
Kojic acid   *79*, 605 (2001)

L

Lasiocarpine   *10*, 281 (1976); *Suppl. 7*, 65 (1987)
Lauroyl peroxide   *36*, 315 (1985); *Suppl. 7*, 65
                                                            (1987); *71*, 1485 (1999)

Lead acetate (*see* Lead and lead compounds)
Lead and lead compounds (*see also* Foreign bodies)   *1*, 40 (1972) (*corr. 42*, 251); *2*, 52,
                                                            150 (1973); *12*, 131 (1976);
                                                            23, 40, 208, 209, 325 (1980);
                                                            Suppl. 7, 230 (1987); *87* (2006)

Lead arsenate (*see* Arsenic and arsenic compounds)
Lead carbonate (*see* Lead and lead compounds)
Lead chloride (*see* Lead and lead compounds)
Lead chromate (*see* Chromium and chromium compounds)
Lead chromate oxide (*see* Chromium and chromium compounds)
Lead compounds, inorganic and organic   *Suppl. 7*, 230 (1987); *87* (2006)
Lead naphthenate (*see* Lead and lead compounds)
Lead nitrate (*see* Lead and lead compounds)
Lead oxide (*see* Lead and lead compounds)
Lead phosphate (*see* Lead and lead compounds)
Lead subacetate (*see* Lead and lead compounds)
Lead tetroxide (*see* Lead and lead compounds)
Leather goods manufacture   *25*, 279 (1981); *Suppl. 7*, 235
                                                            (1987)
Leather industries   *25*, 199 (1981); *Suppl. 7*, 232
                                                            (1987)
Leather tanning and processing   *25*, 201 (1981); *Suppl. 7*, 236
                                                            (1987)
Ledate (*see also* Lead and lead compounds)   *12*, 131 (1976)
Levonorgestrel   *72*, 49 (1999)
Light Green SF   *16*, 209 (1978); *Suppl. 7*, 65 (1987)
d-Limonene   *56*, 135 (1993); *73*, 307 (1999)
Lindane (*see* Hexachlorocyclohexanes)
Liver flukes (*see Clonorchis sinensis, Opisthorchis felineus* and
        Opisthorchis viverrini)
Lucidin (*see* 1,3-Dihydro-2-hydroxymethylanthraquinone)
Lumber and sawmill industries (including logging)   *25*, 49 (1981); *Suppl. 7*, 383 (1987)
Luteoskyrin   *10*, 163 (1976); *Suppl. 7*, 65 (1987)
Lynoestrenol   *21*, 407 (1979); *Suppl. 7*, 293
                                                            (1987); *72*, 49 (1999)

M

Methoxychlor	*5*, 193 (1974); *20*, 259 (1979); *Suppl. 7*, 66 (1987)
Methoxyflurane (*see* Anaesthetics, volatile)	
5-Methoxypsoralen	*40*, 327 (1986); *Suppl. 7*, 242 (1987)
8-Methoxypsoralen (*see also* 8-Methoxypsoralen plus ultraviolet radiation)	*24*, 101 (1980)
8-Methoxypsoralen plus ultraviolet radiation	*Suppl. 7*, 243 (1987)
Methyl acrylate	*19*, 52 (1979); *39*, 99 (1986); *Suppl. 7*, 66 (1987); *71*, 1489 (1999)
5-Methylangelicin plus ultraviolet radiation (*see also* Angelicin and some synthetic derivatives)	*Suppl. 7*, 57 (1987)
2-Methylaziridine	*9*, 61 (1975); *Suppl. 7*, 66 (1987); *71*, 1497 (1999)
Methylazoxymethanol acetate (*see also* Cycasin)	*1*, 164 (1972); *10*, 131 (1976); *Suppl. 7*, 66 (1987)
Methyl bromide	*41*, 187 (1986) (*corr. 45*, 283); *Suppl. 7*, 245 (1987); *71*, 721 (1999)
Methyl *tert*-butyl ether	*73*, 339 (1999)
Methyl carbamate	*12*, 151 (1976); *Suppl. 7*, 66 (1987)
Methyl-CCNU (*see* 1-(2-Chloroethyl)-3-(4-methylcyclohexyl)-1-nitrosourea)	
Methyl chloride	*41*, 161 (1986); *Suppl. 7*, 246 (1987); *71*, 737 (1999)
1-, 2-, 3-, 4-, 5- and 6-Methylchrysenes	*32*, 379 (1983); *Suppl. 7*, 66 (1987)
N-Methyl-*N*,4-dinitrosoaniline	*1*, 141 (1972); *Suppl. 7*, 66 (1987)
4,4'-Methylene bis(2-chloroaniline)	*4*, 65 (1974) (*corr. 42*, 252); *Suppl. 7*, 246 (1987); *57*, 271 (1993)
4,4'-Methylene bis(*N,N*-dimethyl)benzenamine	*27*, 119 (1982); *Suppl. 7*, 66 (1987)
4,4'-Methylene bis(2-methylaniline)	*4*, 73 (1974); *Suppl. 7*, 248 (1987)
4,4'-Methylenedianiline	*4*, 79 (1974) (*corr. 42*, 252); *39*, 347 (1986); *Suppl. 7*, 66 (1987)
4,4'-Methylenediphenyl diisocyanate	*19*, 314 (1979); *Suppl. 7*, 66 (1987); *71*, 1049 (1999)
2-Methylfluoranthene	*32*, 399 (1983); *Suppl. 7*, 66 (1987)
3-Methylfluoranthene	*32*, 399 (1983); *Suppl. 7*, 66 (1987)
Methylglyoxal	*51*, 443 (1991)
Methyl iodide	*15*, 245 (1977); *41*, 213 (1986); *Suppl. 7*, 66 (1987); *71*, 1503 (1999)
Methylmercury chloride (*see* Mercury and mercury compounds)	
Methylmercury compounds (*see* Mercury and mercury compounds)	
Methyl methacrylate	*19*, 187 (1979); *Suppl. 7*, 66 (1987); *60*, 445 (1994)
Methyl methanesulfonate	*7*, 253 (1974); *Suppl. 7*, 66 (1987); *71*, 1059 (1999)
2-Methyl-1-nitroanthraquinone	*27*, 205 (1982); *Suppl. 7*, 66 (1987)
N-Methyl-*N'*-nitro-*N*-nitrosoguanidine	*4*, 183 (1974); *Suppl. 7*, 248 (1987)
3-Methylnitrosaminopropionaldehyde [*see* 3-(*N*-Nitrosomethylamino)-propionaldehyde]	

N

N-Nitrosopyrrolidine	*17*, 313 (1978); *Suppl. 7*, 68 (1987)
N-Nitrososarcosine	*17*, 327 (1978); *Suppl. 7*, 68 (1987)
Nitrosoureas, chloroethyl (*see* Chloroethyl nitrosoureas)	
5-Nitro-*ortho*-toluidine	*48*, 169 (1990)
2-Nitrotoluene	*65*, 409 (1996)
3-Nitrotoluene	*65*, 409 (1996)
4-Nitrotoluene	*65*, 409 (1996)
Nitrous oxide (*see* Anaesthetics, volatile)	
Nitrovin	*31*, 185 (1983); *Suppl. 7*, 68 (1987)
Nivalenol (*see* Toxins derived from *Fusarium graminearum*, *F. culmorum* and *F. crookwellense*)	
NNA (*see* 4-(*N*-Nitrosomethylamino)-4-(3-pyridyl)-1-butanal)	
NNK (*see* 4-(*N*-Nitrosomethylamino)-1-(3-pyridyl)-1-butanone)	
Nonsteroidal oestrogens	*Suppl. 7*, 273 (1987)
Norethisterone	*6*, 179 (1974); *21*, 461 (1979); *Suppl. 7*, 294 (1987); *72*, 49 (1999)
Norethisterone acetate	*72*, 49 (1999)
Norethynodrel	*6*, 191 (1974); *21*, 461 (1979) (*corr. 42*, 259); *Suppl. 7*, 295 (1987); *72*, 49 (1999)
Norgestrel	*6*, 201 (1974); *21*, 479 (1979); *Suppl. 7*, 295 (1987); *72*, 49 (1999)
Nylon 6	*19*, 120 (1979); *Suppl. 7*, 68 (1987)

O

Ochratoxin A	*10*, 191 (1976); *31*, 191 (1983) (*corr. 42*, 262); *Suppl. 7*, 271 (1987); *56*, 489 (1993)
Oestradiol	*6*, 99 (1974); *21*, 279 (1979); *Suppl. 7*, 284 (1987); *72*, 399 (1999)
Oestradiol-17β (*see* Oestradiol)	
Oestradiol 3-benzoate (*see* Oestradiol)	
Oestradiol dipropionate (*see* Oestradiol)	
Oestradiol mustard	*9*, 217 (1975); *Suppl. 7*, 68 (1987)
Oestradiol valerate (*see* Oestradiol)	
Oestriol	*6*, 117 (1974); *21*, 327 (1979); *Suppl. 7*, 285 (1987); *72*, 399 (1999)
Oestrogen-progestin combinations (*see* Oestrogens, progestins (progestogens) and combinations)	
Oestrogen-progestin replacement therapy (*see* Post-menopausal oestrogen-progestogen therapy)	
Oestrogen replacement therapy (*see* Post-menopausal oestrogen therapy)	
Oestrogens (*see* Oestrogens, progestins and combinations)	
Oestrogens, conjugated (*see* Conjugated oestrogens)	
Oestrogens, nonsteroidal (*see* Nonsteroidal oestrogens)	
Oestrogens, progestins (progestogens) and combinations	*6* (1974); *21* (1979); *Suppl. 7*, 272 (1987); *72*, 49, 339, 399, 531 (1999)

Phenobarbital and its sodium salt	*13*, 157 (1977); *Suppl. 7*, 313 (1987); *79*, 161 (2001)
Phenol	*47*, 263 (1989) (*corr. 50*, 385); *71*, 749 (1999)
Phenolphthalein	*76*, 387 (2000)
Phenoxyacetic acid herbicides (*see* Chlorophenoxy herbicides)	
Phenoxybenzamine hydrochloride	*9*, 223 (1975); *24*, 185 (1980); *Suppl. 7*, 70 (1987)
Phenylbutazone	*13*, 183 (1977); *Suppl. 7*, 316 (1987)
meta-Phenylenediamine	*16*, 111 (1978); *Suppl. 7*, 70 (1987)
para-Phenylenediamine	*16*, 125 (1978); *Suppl. 7*, 70 (1987)
Phenyl glycidyl ether (*see also* Glycidyl ethers)	*71*, 1525 (1999)
N-Phenyl-2-naphthylamine	*16*, 325 (1978) (*corr. 42*, 257); *Suppl. 7*, 318 (1987)
ortho-Phenylphenol	*30*, 329 (1983); *Suppl. 7*, 70 (1987); *73*, 451 (1999)
Phenytoin	*13*, 201 (1977); *Suppl. 7*, 319 (1987); *66*, 175 (1996)
Phillipsite (*see* Zeolites)	
PhIP	*56*, 229 (1993)
Pickled vegetables	*56*, 83 (1993)
Picloram	*53*, 481 (1991)
Piperazine oestrone sulfate (*see* Conjugated oestrogens)	
Piperonyl butoxide	*30*, 183 (1983); *Suppl. 7*, 70 (1987)
Pitches, coal-tar (*see* Coal-tar pitches)	
Polyacrylic acid	*19*, 62 (1979); *Suppl. 7*, 70 (1987)
Polybrominated biphenyls	*18*, 107 (1978); *41*, 261 (1986); *Suppl. 7*, 321 (1987)
Polychlorinated biphenyls	*7*, 261 (1974); *18*, 43 (1978) (*corr. 42*, 258); *Suppl. 7*, 322 (1987)
Polychlorinated camphenes (*see* Toxaphene)	
Polychlorinated dibenzo-*para*-dioxins (other than 2,3,7,8-tetrachlorodibenzodioxin)	*69*, 33 (1997)
Polychlorinated dibenzofurans	*69*, 345 (1997)
Polychlorophenols and their sodium salts	*71*, 769 (1999)
Polychloroprene	*19*, 141 (1979); *Suppl. 7*, 70 (1987)
Polyethylene (*see also* Implants, surgical)	*19*, 164 (1979); *Suppl. 7*, 70 (1987)
Poly(glycolic acid) (*see* Implants, surgical)	
Polymethylene polyphenyl isocyanate (*see also* 4,4′-Methylenediphenyl diisocyanate)	*19*, 314 (1979); *Suppl. 7*, 70 (1987)
Polymethyl methacrylate (*see also* Implants, surgical)	*19*, 195 (1979); *Suppl. 7*, 70 (1987)
Polyoestradiol phosphate (*see* Oestradiol-17β)	
Polypropylene (*see also* Implants, surgical)	*19*, 218 (1979); *Suppl. 7*, 70 (1987)
Polystyrene (*see also* Implants, surgical)	*19*, 245 (1979); *Suppl. 7*, 70 (1987)
Polytetrafluoroethylene (*see also* Implants, surgical)	*19*, 288 (1979); *Suppl. 7*, 70 (1987)
Polyurethane foams (*see also* Implants, surgical)	*19*, 320 (1979); *Suppl. 7*, 70 (1987)
Polyvinyl acetate (*see also* Implants, surgical)	*19*, 346 (1979); *Suppl. 7*, 70 (1987)
Polyvinyl alcohol (*see also* Implants, surgical)	*19*, 351 (1979); *Suppl. 7*, 70 (1987)
Polyvinyl chloride (*see also* Implants, surgical)	*7*, 306 (1974); *19*, 402 (1979); *Suppl. 7*, 70 (1987)
Polyvinyl pyrrolidone	*19*, 463 (1979); *Suppl. 7*, 70 (1987); *71*, 1181 (1999)

Pyrrolizidine alkaloids (*see* Hydroxysenkirkine; Isatidine; Jacobine;
    Lasiocarpine; Monocrotaline; Retrorsine; Riddelliine; Seneciphylline;
    Senkirkine)

Q

Quartz (*see* Crystalline silica)	
Quercetin (*see also* Bracken fern)	*31*, 213 (1983); *Suppl. 7*, 71 (1987); *73*, 497 (1999)
para-Quinone	*15*, 255 (1977); *Suppl. 7*, 71 (1987); *71*, 1245 (1999)
Quintozene	*5*, 211 (1974); *Suppl. 7*, 71 (1987)

R

Radiation (*see* gamma-radiation, neutrons, ultraviolet radiation, X-radiation)	
Radionuclides, internally deposited	*78* (2001)
Radon	*43*, 173 (1988) (*corr. 45*, 283)
Refractory ceramic fibres (*see* Man-made vitreous fibres)	
Reserpine	*10*, 217 (1976); *24*, 211 (1980) (*corr. 42*, 260); *Suppl. 7*, 330 (1987)
Resorcinol	*15*, 155 (1977); *Suppl. 7*, 71 (1987); *71*, 1119 (1990)
Retrorsine	*10*, 303 (1976); *Suppl. 7*, 71 (1987)
Rhodamine B	*16*, 221 (1978); *Suppl. 7*, 71 (1987)
Rhodamine 6G	*16*, 233 (1978); *Suppl. 7*, 71 (1987)
Riddelliine	*10*, 313 (1976); *Suppl. 7*, 71 (1987); *82*, 153 (2002)
Rifampicin	*24*, 243 (1980); *Suppl. 7*, 71 (1987)
Ripazepam	*66*, 157 (1996)
Rock (stone) wool (*see* Man-made vitreous fibres)	
Rubber industry	*28* (1982) (*corr. 42*, 261); *Suppl. 7*, 332 (1987)
Rubia tinctorum (*see also* Madder root, Traditional herbal medicines)	*82*, 129 (2002)
Rugulosin	*40*, 99 (1986); *Suppl. 7*, 71 (1987)

S

Saccharated iron oxide	*2*, 161 (1973); *Suppl. 7*, 71 (1987)
Saccharin and its salts	*22*, 111 (1980) (*corr. 42*, 259); *Suppl. 7*, 334 (1987); *73*, 517 (1999)
Safrole	*1*, 169 (1972); *10*, 231 (1976); *Suppl. 7*, 71 (1987)
Salted fish	*56*, 41 (1993)
Sawmill industry (including logging) (*see* Lumber and sawmill industry (including logging))	
Scarlet Red	*8*, 217 (1975); *Suppl. 7*, 71 (1987)
Schistosoma haematobium (infection with)	*61*, 45 (1994)
Schistosoma japonicum (infection with)	*61*, 45 (1994)

Static electric fields   *80* (2002)
Static magnetic fields   *80* (2002)
Steel founding (*see* Iron and steel founding)
Steel, stainless (*see* Implants, surgical)
Sterigmatocystin   *1*, 175 (1972); *10*, 245 (1976);
                                                               Suppl. 7, 72 (1987)
Steroidal oestrogens   *Suppl. 7,* 280 (1987)
Streptozotocin   *4*, 221 (1974); *17*, 337 (1978);
                                                               Suppl. 7, 72 (1987)
Strobane® (*see* Terpene polychlorinates)
Strong-inorganic-acid mists containing sulfuric acid (*see* Mists and
     vapours from sulfuric acid and other strong inorganic acids)
Strontium chromate (*see* Chromium and chromium compounds)
Styrene   *19*, 231 (1979) (*corr. 42*, 258);
                                                               Suppl. 7, 345 (1987); *60*, 233
                                                               (1994) (*corr. 65*, 549); *82*, 437
                                                               (2002)
Styrene–acrylonitrile copolymers   *19*, 97 (1979); *Suppl. 7*, 72 (1987)
Styrene–butadiene copolymers   *19*, 252 (1979); *Suppl. 7*, 72 (1987)
Styrene-7,8-oxide   *11*, 201 (1976); *19*, 275 (1979);
                                                               36, 245 (1985); *Suppl. 7*, 72
                                                               (1987); *60*, 321 (1994)
Succinic anhydride   *15*, 265 (1977); *Suppl. 7*, 72 (1987)
Sudan I   *8*, 225 (1975); *Suppl. 7*, 72 (1987)
Sudan II   *8*, 233 (1975); *Suppl. 7*, 72 (1987)
Sudan III   *8*, 241 (1975); *Suppl. 7*, 72 (1987)
Sudan Brown RR   *8*, 249 (1975); *Suppl. 7*, 72 (1987)
Sudan Red 7B   *8*, 253 (1975); *Suppl. 7*, 72 (1987)
Sulfadimidine (*see* Sulfamethazine)
Sulfafurazole   *24*, 275 (1980); *Suppl. 7*, 347
                                                               (1987)
Sulfallate   *30*, 283 (1983); *Suppl. 7*, 72 (1987)
Sulfamethazine and its sodium salt   *79*, 341 (2001)
Sulfamethoxazole   *24*, 285 (1980); *Suppl. 7*, 348
                                                               (1987); *79*, 361 (2001)
Sulfites (*see* Sulfur dioxide and some sulfites, bisulfites and metabisulfites)
Sulfur dioxide and some sulfites, bisulfites and metabisulfites   *54*, 131 (1992)
Sulfur mustard (*see* Mustard gas)
Sulfuric acid and other strong inorganic acids, occupational exposures   *54*, 41 (1992)
     to mists and vapours from
Sulfur trioxide   *54*, 121 (1992)
Sulphisoxazole (*see* Sulfafurazole)
Sunset Yellow FCF   *8*, 257 (1975); *Suppl. 7*, 72 (1987)
Symphytine   *31*, 239 (1983); *Suppl. 7*, 72 (1987)

T

2,4,5-T (*see also* Chlorophenoxy herbicides; Chlorophenoxy   *15*, 273 (1977)
     herbicides, occupational exposures to)
Talc   *42*, 185 (1987); *Suppl. 7*, 349
                                                               (1987)
Tamoxifen   *66*, 253 (1996)

2,4-Toluene diisocyanate (*see also* Toluene diisocyanates)	*19*, 303 (1979); *39*, 287 (1986)
2,6-Toluene diisocyanate (*see also* Toluene diisocyanates)	*19*, 303 (1979); *39*, 289 (1986)
Toluene	*47*, 79 (1989); *71*, 829 (1999)
Toluene diisocyanates	*39*, 287 (1986) (*corr. 42*, 264); *Suppl. 7*, 72 (1987); *71*, 865 (1999)
Toluenes, α-chlorinated (*see* α-Chlorinated toluenes and benzoyl chloride)	
ortho-Toluenesulfonamide (*see* Saccharin)	
ortho-Toluidine	*16*, 349 (1978); *27*, 155 (1982) (*corr. 68*, 477); *Suppl. 7*, 362 (1987); *77*, 267 (2000)
Toremifene	*66*, 367 (1996)
Toxaphene	*20*, 327 (1979); *Suppl. 7*, 72 (1987); *79*, 569 (2001)
T-2 Toxin (*see* Toxins derived from *Fusarium sporotrichioides*)	
Toxins derived from *Fusarium graminearum*, *F. culmorum* and *F. crookwellense*	*11*, 169 (1976); *31*, 153, 279 (1983); *Suppl. 7*, 64, 74 (1987); *56*, 397 (1993)
Toxins derived from *Fusarium moniliforme*	*56*, 445 (1993)
Toxins derived from *Fusarium sporotrichioides*	*31*, 265 (1983); *Suppl. 7*, 73 (1987); *56*, 467 (1993)
Traditional herbal medicines	*82*, 41 (2002)
Tremolite (*see* Asbestos)	
Treosulfan	*26*, 341 (1981); *Suppl. 7*, 363 (1987)
Triaziquone (*see* Tris(aziridinyl)-*para*-benzoquinone)	
Trichlorfon	*30*, 207 (1983); *Suppl. 7*, 73 (1987)
Trichlormethine	*9*, 229 (1975); *Suppl. 7*, 73 (1987); *50*, 143 (1990)
Trichloroacetic acid	*63*, 291 (1995) (*corr. 65*, 549); *84* (2004)
Trichloroacetonitrile (*see also* Halogenated acetonitriles)	*71*, 1533 (1999)
1,1,1-Trichloroethane	*20*, 515 (1979); *Suppl. 7*, 73 (1987); *71*, 881 (1999)
1,1,2-Trichloroethane	*20*, 533 (1979); *Suppl. 7*, 73 (1987); *52*, 337 (1991); *71*, 1153 (1999)
Trichloroethylene	*11*, 263 (1976); *20*, 545 (1979); *Suppl. 7*, 364 (1987); *63*, 75 (1995) (*corr. 65*, 549)
2,4,5-Trichlorophenol (*see also* Chlorophenols; Chlorophenols, occupational exposures to; Polychlorophenols and their sodium salts)	*20*, 349 (1979)
2,4,6-Trichlorophenol (*see also* Chlorophenols; Chlorophenols, occupational exposures to; Polychlorophenols and their sodium salts)	*20*, 349 (1979)
(2,4,5-Trichlorophenoxy)acetic acid (*see* 2,4,5-T)	
1,2,3-Trichloropropane	*63*, 223 (1995)
Trichlorotriethylamine-hydrochloride (*see* Trichlormethine)	
T₂-Trichothecene (*see* Toxins derived from *Fusarium sporotrichioides*)	
Tridymite (*see* Crystalline silica)	
Triethanolamine	*77*, 381 (2000)
Triethylene glycol diglycidyl ether	*11*, 209 (1976); *Suppl. 7*, 73 (1987); *71*, 1539 (1999)
Trifluralin	*53*, 515 (1991)
4,4′,6-Trimethylangelicin plus ultraviolet radiation (*see also* Angelicin and some synthetic derivatives)	*Suppl. 7*, 57 (1987)

U

V

Vinyl fluoride								*39*, 147 (1986); *Suppl. 7*, 73
											(1987); *63*, 467 (1995)
Vinylidene chloride							*19*, 439 (1979); *39*, 195 (1986);
											Suppl. 7, 376 (1987); *71*, 1163
											(1999)
Vinylidene chloride-vinyl chloride copolymers				*19*, 448 (1979) (*corr. 42*, 258);
											Suppl. 7, 73 (1987)
Vinylidene fluoride							*39*, 227 (1986); *Suppl. 7*, 73
											(1987); *71*, 1551 (1999)
N-Vinyl-2-pyrrolidone							*19*, 461 (1979); *Suppl. 7*, 73
											(1987); *71*, 1181 (1999)
Vinyl toluene								*60*, 373 (1994)
Vitamin K substances							*76*, 417 (2000)

W

Welding									*49*, 447 (1990) (*corr. 52*, 513)
Wollastonite								*42*, 145 (1987); *Suppl. 7*, 377
											(1987); *68*, 283 (1997)
Wood dust								*62*, 35 (1995)
Wood industries								*25* (1981); *Suppl. 7*, 378 (1987)

X

X-radiation								*75*, 121 (2000)
Xylenes									*47*, 125 (1989); *71*, 1189 (1999)
2,4-Xylidine								*16*, 367 (1978); *Suppl. 7*, 74 (1987)
2,5-Xylidine								*16*, 377 (1978); *Suppl. 7*, 74 (1987)
2,6-Xylidine (*see* 2,6-Dimethylaniline)

Y

Yellow AB								*8*, 279 (1975); *Suppl. 7*, 74 (1987)
Yellow OB								*8*, 287 (1975); *Suppl. 7*, 74 (1987)

Z

Zalcitabine								*76*, 129 (2000)
Zearalenone (*see* Toxins derived from *Fusarium graminearum*,
	F. culmorum and *F. crookwellense*)
Zectran									*12*, 237 (1976); *Suppl. 7*, 74 (1987)
Zeolites other than erionite						*68*, 307 (1997)
Zidovudine								*76*, 73 (2000)
Zinc beryllium silicate (*see* Beryllium and beryllium compounds)
Zinc chromate (*see* Chromium and chromium compounds)
Zinc chromate hydroxide (*see* Chromium and chromium compounds)
Zinc potassium chromate (*see* Chromium and chromium compounds)
Zinc yellow (*see* Chromium and chromium compounds)
Zineb									*12*, 245 (1976); *Suppl. 7*, 74 (1987)
Ziram									*12*, 259 (1976); *Suppl. 7*, 74
											(1987); *53, 423* (1991)

List of IARC Monographs on the Evaluation of Carcinogenic Risks to Humans*

Volume 1
Some Inorganic Substances, Chlorinated Hydrocarbons, Aromatic Amines, *N*-Nitroso Compounds, and Natural Products
1972; 184 pages (out-of-print)

Volume 2
Some Inorganic and Organo-metallic Compounds
1973; 181 pages (out-of-print)

Volume 3
Certain Polycyclic Aromatic Hydrocarbons and Heterocyclic Compounds
1973; 271 pages (out-of-print)

Volume 4
Some Aromatic Amines, Hydra-zine and Related Substances, *N*-Nitroso Compounds and Miscellaneous Alkylating Agents
1974; 286 pages (out-of-print)

Volume 5
Some Organochlorine Pesticides
1974; 241 pages (out-of-print)

Volume 6
Sex Hormones
1974; 243 pages (out-of-print)

Volume 7
Some Anti-Thyroid and Related Substances, Nitrofurans and Industrial Chemicals
1974; 326 pages (out-of-print)

Volume 8
Some Aromatic Azo Compounds
1975; 357 pages (out-of-print)

Volume 9
Some Aziridines, *N*-, *S*- and *O*-Mustards and Selenium
1975; 268 pages (out-of-print)

Volume 10
Some Naturally Occurring Substances
1976; 353 pages (out-of-print)

Volume 11
Cadmium, Nickel, Some Epoxides, Miscellaneous Industrial Chemicals and General Considerations on Volatile Anaesthetics
1976; 306 pages (out-of-print)

Volume 12
Some Carbamates, Thio-carbamates and Carbazides
1976; 282 pages (out-of-print)

Volume 13
Some Miscellaneous Pharmaceutical Substances
1977; 255 pages

Volume 14
Asbestos
1977; 106 pages (out-of-print)

Volume 15
Some Fumigants, the Herbicides 2,4-D and 2,4,5-T, Chlorinated Dibenzodioxins and Miscella-neous Industrial Chemicals
1977; 354 pages (out-of-print)

Volume 16
Some Aromatic Amines and Related Nitro Compounds—Hair Dyes, Colouring Agents and Miscellaneous Industrial Chemicals
1978; 400 pages

Volume 17
Some *N*-Nitroso Compounds
1978; 365 pages

Volume 18
Polychlorinated Biphenyls and Polybrominated Biphenyls
1978; 140 pages (out-of-print)

Volume 19
Some Monomers, Plastics and Synthetic Elastomers, and Acrolein
1979; 513 pages (out-of-print)

Volume 20
Some Halogenated Hydrocarbons
1979; 609 pages (out-of-print)

Volume 21
Sex Hormones (II)
1979; 583 pages

Volume 22
Some Non-Nutritive Sweetening Agents
1980; 208 pages

Volume 23
Some Metals and Metallic Compounds
1980; 438 pages (out-of-print)

Volume 24
Some Pharmaceutical Drugs
1980; 337 pages

Volume 25
Wood, Leather and Some Associated Industries
1981; 412 pages

Volume 26
Some Antineoplastic and Immunosuppressive Agents
1981; 411 pages (out-of-print)

Volume 27
Some Aromatic Amines, Anthraquinones and Nitroso Compounds, and Inorganic Fluorides Used in Drinking-water and Dental Preparations
1982; 341 pages (out-of-print)

Volume 28
The Rubber Industry
1982; 486 pages (out-of-print)

Volume 29
Some Industrial Chemicals and Dyestuffs
1982; 416 pages (out-of-print)

Volume 30
Miscellaneous Pesticides
1983; 424 pages (out-of-print)

---

*High-quality photocopies of all out-of-print volumes may be purchased from University Microfilms International, 300 North Zeeb Road, Ann Arbor, MI 48106-1346, USA (Tel.: +1 313-761-4700, +1 800-521-0600).

Supplement No. 4
Chemicals, Industrial Processes and Industries Associated with Cancer in Humans (*IARC Monographs*, Volumes 1 to 29)
1982; 292 pages (out-of-print)

Supplement No. 5
Cross Index of Synonyms and Trade Names in Volumes 1 to 36 of the *IARC Monographs*
1985; 259 pages (out-of-print)

Supplement No. 6
Genetic and Related Effects: An Updating of Selected *IARC Monographs* from Volumes 1 to 42
1987; 729 pages (out-of-print)

Supplement No. 7
Overall Evaluations of Carcinogenicity: An Updating of *IARC Monographs* Volumes 1–42
1987; 440 pages (out-of-print)

Supplement No. 8
Cross Index of Synonyms and Trade Names in Volumes 1 to 46 of the *IARC Monographs*
1990; 346 pages (out-of-print)

Achevé d'imprimer sur rotative par l'imprimerie Darantiere
à Dijon-Quetigny en décembre 2006

Dépôt légal : décembre 2006 - N° d'impression : 26-1926

Imprimé en France